Comprehensive Management of Arteriovenous Malformations of the Brain and Spine

Comprehensive Management of Arteriovenous Malformations of the Brain and Spine

Edited by

Robert F. Spetzler, MD

JN Harber Chairman of Neurological Surgery and Director, Barrow Neurological Institute, Phoenix, AZ, USA

Douglas S. Kondziolka, MD, MSc, FRCSC, FACS

Professor of Neurosurgery, Vice-Chair Clinical Research (Neurosurgery), Professor of Radiation Oncology, and Director of the Center for Advanced Radiosurgery, NYU Langone Medical Center, New York, NY, USA

Randall T. Higashida, MD

Clinical Professor of Radiology, Neurological Surgery, Neurology, and Anesthesiology, and Chief of the Division of Interventional Neurovascular Radiology, University of California San Francisco Medical Center, San Francisco, CA, USA

M. Yashar S. Kalani, MD, PhD

Assistant Professor of Neurological Surgery, Barrow Neurological Institute, Phoenix, AZ, USA

CAMBRIDGE
UNIVERSITY PRESS

CAMBRIDGE
UNIVERSITY PRESS

University Printing House, Cambridge CB2 8BS, United Kingdom

Cambridge University Press is part of the University of Cambridge.

It furthers the University's mission by disseminating knowledge in the pursuit of education, learning and research at the highest international levels of excellence.

www.cambridge.org
Information on this title: www.cambridge.org/9781107033887

First published 2015

Printed in Spain by Grafos SA, Arte sobre papel

A catalogue record for this publication is available from the British Library

Library of Congress Cataloguing in Publication data
Comprehensive management of arteriovenous malformations of the brain and spine / edited by Robert F.
Spetzler, Douglas Kondziolka, Randall Higashida, Yashar Kalani.
p. ; cm.
Includes bibliographical references and index.
ISBN 978-1-107-03388-7 (hardback)
I. Spetzler, Robert F. (Robert Friedrich), 1944– editor. II. Kondziolka, D. (Douglas), 1961– editor. III. Higashida, Randall T., editor. IV. Kalani, Yashar, editor.
[DNLM: 1. Arteriovenous Malformations – surgery. 2. Central Nervous System Diseases – surgery. 3. Arteriovenous Malformations – diagnosis. 4. Arteriovenous Malformations – physiopathology. 5. Neurosurgical Procedures – methods. WL 301]
RD598.5
617.4′13–dc23

2014014059

ISBN 978-1-107-03388-7 Hardback

To all the patients who have taught me so much.
Robert F. Spetzler

To the many residents and fellows who have worked diligently on AVM science, and to Drs. Pierre Lasjaunias and Raymond Kjellberg who first introduced me to the wonders of this complex disorder.
Douglas S. Kondziolka

To my parents, family, wife, and friends, who gave me constant encouragement throughout my life and career. To my teachers, colleagues, fellows, and students who gave me the chance to teach and also to learn from them.
Randall T. Higashida

To my patients who have inspired me; to my grandmothers, Batool and Fatemeh, who taught me the value of perseverance; to my parents, Afrouz and Mohammad, for their unconditional love and for the sacrifices they made to get me here; to my brother, Maziyar, who has always been my best friend; and, to my fiancée, Kristin, whose love and support helps me march on.
M. Yashar S. Kalani

Contents

Section 4 Medical, endovascular, and radiosurgical treatment of arteriovenous malformations

Videos

Contributors

Francesco Acerbi, MD, PhD
Department of Neurosurgery,
Fondazione IRCCS Istituto Neurologico Carlo Besta,
Milan, Italy

Ayca Akgoz, MD
Departments of Neurosurgery and Radiology,
Brigham and Women's Hospital and Harvard
Medical School,
Boston, MA, USA

Matthew R. Amans, MD, MSc
Department of Radiology and Biomedical Engineering,
Division of Neuroradiology,
Division of Neurointerventional Radiology,
University of California, San Francisco,
San Francisco, CA, USA

Ramsey Ashour, MD
Department of Neurological Surgery,
University of Miami Miller School of
Medicine,
Miami, FL, USA

Mohammed Ali Aziz-Sultan, MD
Department of Neurological Surgery,
University of Miami School of Medicine,
Miami, FL, USA

H. Hunt Batjer, MD
Department of Neurosurgery,
UT Southwestern School of Medicine,
Dallas, TX, USA

Donnie Bell, MD
Division of Interventional Neuroradiology,
Massachusetts General Hospital,
Boston, MA, USA

Bernard R. Bendok, MD, MS
Department of Neurosurgery,
Northwestern University School of Medicine,
Evanston, IL, USA

Giovanni Broggi, MD
Department of Neurosurgery,
Fondazione IRCCS Istituto Neurologico Carlo Besta,
Milan, Italy

Morgan Broggi, MD
Department of Neurosurgery,
Fondazione IRCCS Istituto Neurologico Carlo Besta,
Milan, Italy

Charles A. Bruno Jr., DO
Division of Interventional Neuroradiology,
Department of Radiology,
Columbia University,
College of Physicians and Surgeons,
New York, USA

Steven D. Chang, MD
Department of Neurosurgery,
Stanford University Medical Center,
Stanford, CA, USA

In Sup Choi, MD, FACR
Division of Interventional Neuroradiology,
Lahey Hospital, and Medical Center,
Burlington,
and Tufts University School of Medicine,
Medford, MA, USA

Omar Choudhri, MD
Department of Neurosurgery,
Stanford University Medical Center,
Stanford, CA, USA

Douglas J. Cook, MD
Division of Neurosurgery,
Queen's University,
Kingston, ON, Canada

William P. Dillon, MD
Department of Radiology and Biomedical Imaging,
University of California, San Francisco,
San Francisco, CA, USA

Peter Dirks, MD, PhD, FRCSC
Department of Neurosurgery,
Hospital for Sick Children,
Toronto, Ontario, Canada

Rose Du, MD, PhD
Department of Neurological Surgery,
Brigham and Women's Hospital,
Harvard Medical School,
Boston, MA, USA

Travis M. Dumont, MD
Division of Endovascular Neurosurgery,
Department of Neurosurgery,
School of Medicine and Biomedical Sciences,
University at Buffalo,
State University of New York,
and Department of Neurosurgery,
Gates Vascular Institute,
Kaleida Health,
Buffalo, NY, USA

Tarek Y. El Ahmadieh, MD
Department of Neurosurgery,
Northwestern University School of Medicine,
Evanston, IL, USA

Najib E. El Tecle, MD
Department of Neurosurgery,
Northwestern University School of Medicine,
Evanston, IL, USA

Mohamed Samy Elhammady, MD
Department of Neurological Surgery,
University of Miami School of Medicine,
Miami, FL, USA

Paolo Ferroli, MD
Department of Neurosurgery,
Fondazione IRCCS Istituto Neurologico Carlo Besta,
Milan, Italy

Alana M. Flexman, MD, FRCPC
Department of Anesthesiology, Pharmacology, and Therapeutics,
University of British Columbia
Vancouver, British Columbia, Canada

John C. Flickinger, MD
Department of Radiation Oncology and the Center for Image-Guided Neurosurgery,
University of Pittsburgh School of Medicine,
Pittsburgh, PA, USA

Kai U. Frerichs, MD
Departments of Neurosurgery and Radiology,
Brigham and Women's Hospital and Harvard Medical School,
Boston, MA, USA

Sasikhan Geibprasert, MD
Department of Radiology,
University of Toronto,
Toronto, Ontario, Canada

Adrian W. Gelb, MBChB, FRCPC
Department of Anesthesia and Perioperative Care,
University of California,
San Francisco,
San Francisco, CA, USA

Y. Pierre Gobin, MD
Department of Neurosurgery,
Weill Cornell School of Medicine,
New York, USA

Bradley A. Gross, MD
Department of Neurological Surgery,
Brigham and Women's Hospital,
Harvard Medical School,
Boston, MA, USA

Seunggu J. Han, MD
Department of Neurological Surgery,
University of California, San Francisco,
San Francisco, CA, USA

Tomoki Hashimoto, MD
Department of Anesthesia and Perioperative Care and the Center for Cerebrovascular Research,
University of California, San Francisco,
San Francisco, CA, USA

Juha Hernesniemi, MD, PhD
Department of Neurosurgery,
Helsinki University Central Hospital,
Helsinki, Finland

Roberto C. Heros, MD
Department of Neurological Surgery,
University of Miami School of Medicine,
Miami, FL, USA

Steven W. Hetts, MD
Department of Interventional Neuroradiology,
University of California, San Francisco,
San Francisco, CA, USA

Randall T. Higashida, MD
Departments of Radiology, Neurological Surgery,
Neurology, and Anesthesiology,
University of California, San Francisco
Medical Center,
San Francisco, CA, USA

Joshua A. Hirsch, MD
Division of Interventional Neuroradiology,
Massachusetts General Hospital,
Boston, MA, USA

Nikolai J. Hopf, MD
NeuroChirurgicum, Centre for Endoscopic and Minimally Invasive Neurosurgery,
Stuttgart, Germany

L. Nelson Hopkins MD, FACS
Departments of Neurosurgery and Radiology,
School of Medicine and Biomedical Sciences,
University at Buffalo,
State University of New York,
and Toshiba Stroke and Vascular Research Center and Jacobs Institute,
Buffalo, NY, USA

Maziyar A. Kalani, MD
Department of Neurosurgery,
Stanford University School of Medicine,
Stanford, CA, USA

M. Yashar S. Kalani, MD, PhD
Division of Neurological Surgery,
Barrow Neurological Institute,
St. Joseph's Hospital and Medical Center,
Phoenix, AZ, USA

Hideyuki Kano, MD, PhD
Department of Neurological Surgery and the Center for Image-Guided Neurosurgery,
University of Pittsburgh School of Medicine,
Pittsburgh, PA, USA

Syed Aftab Karim, MD
Department of Neurosurgery,
Stanford University Medical Center,
Stanford, CA, USA

Robert M. Koffie, MD, PhD
Department of Neurological Surgery,
Brigham and Women's Hospital,
Harvard Medical School,
Boston, MA, USA

Douglas S. Kondziolka, MD, MSc, FRCSC, FACS
Departments of Neurosurgery and Radiation Oncology, and Center for Advanced Radiosurgery,
NYU Langone Medical Center,
New York, USA

Timo Krings, MD, PhD, FRCPC
Departments of Radiology and Neurosurgery,
Toronto Western Hospital University of Toronto,
Toronto, Ontario, Canada

Aki Laakso, MD, PhD
Department of Neurosurgery,
Helsinki University Central Hospital,
Helsinki, Finland

Giuseppe Lanzino, MD
Department of Neurological Surgery,
Mayo Clinic,
Rochester, MN, USA

Michael T. Lawton, MD
Department of Neurological Surgery,
Department of Anesthesia and Perioperative Care, and the Center for Cerebrovascular Research,
University of California, San Francisco,
San Francisco, CA, USA

Elad I. Levy, MD, MBA, FACS, FAHA
Departments of Neurosurgery and Radiology,
School of Medicine and Biomedical Sciences,
University at Buffalo,
State University of New York,
and Toshiba Stroke and Vascular Research Center,
Buffalo, NY, USA

L. Dade Lunsford, MD
Department of Neurological Surgery and the Center for Image-Guided Neurosurgery,
University of Pittsburgh School of Medicine,
Pittsburgh, PA, USA

Adel M. Malek, MD, PhD
Cerebrovascular and Endovascular Division,
Department of Neurosurgery,
Tufts Medical Center and Tufts University School of Medicine,
Boston, MA, USA

Michael P. Marks, MD
Departments of Interventional Neuroradiology, Radiology and Neurosurgery,
Stanford University Medical Center,
Stanford, CA, USA

George A. C. Mendes, MD
Division of Neurological Surgery, Barrow Neurological Institute,
St. Joseph's Hospital and Medical Center,
Phoenix, AZ, USA

Philip M. Meyers, MD, FAHA
Departments of Radiology and Neurological Surgery,
Columbia University,
College of Physicians and Surgeons,
Neuroendovascular Service,
New York–Presbyterian Hospital and Columbia Neurological Institute of New York,
New York, USA

Jacques Morcos, MD
Department of Neurological Surgery,
University of Miami Miller School of Medicine,
Miami, FL, USA

Nitin Mukerji, MD, MSc
Department of Neurosurgery,
The James Cook University Hospital,
Middlesborough, UK

Christian Musahl, MD
Department of Neurosurgery,
Dr. Horst Schmidt Klinik,
Wiesbaden, Germany

Ludmila Pawlikowska, PhD
Department of Anesthesia and Perioperative Care and the Center for Cerebrovascular Research,
University of California, San Francisco,
San Francisco, CA, USA

Matthew B. Potts, MD
Department of Neurological Surgery,
University of California, San Francisco,
San Francisco, CA, USA

Ross Puffer, MD
Department of Neurological Surgery,
Mayo Clinic,
Rochester, MN, USA

James D. Rabinov, MD
Division of Interventional Neuroradiology,
Massachusetts General Hospital,
Boston, MA, USA

Jonathan J. Russin, MD
Barrow Neurological Institute,
Phoenix, AZ, USA

Mina G. Safain, MD
Cerebrovascular and Endovascular Division,
Department of Neurosurgery,
Tufts Medical Center and Tufts University School of Medicine,
Boston, MA, USA

Duke Samson, MD
Department of Neurosurgery,
UT Southwestern School of Medicine,
Dallas, TX, USA

Marco Schiariti, MD
Department of Neurosurgery,
Fondazione IRCCS Istituto Neurologico Carlo Besta,
Milan, Italy

R. Michael Scott, MD
Department of Neurosurgery,
Children's Hospital Boston and Harvard Medical School,
Boston, MA, USA

Jason P. Sheehan, MD, PhD
Departments of Neurological Surgery and Radiation Oncology,
University of Virginia,
Charlottesville, VA, USA

Paul Singh, MD, MPH
Department of Neurosurgery,
Weill Cornell School of Medicine,
New York, USA

Edward R. Smith, MD
Department of Neurosurgery,
Children's Hospital Boston and Harvard Medical School,
Boston, MA, USA

Scott G. Soltys, MD
Department of Neurosurgery,
Stanford University Medical Center,
Stanford, CA, USA

Robert F. Spetzler, MD
Division of Neurological Surgery,
Barrow Neurological Institute,
St. Joseph's Hospital and Medical Center,
Phoenix, AZ, USA

Gary K. Steinberg, MD, PhD
Department of Neurosurgery,
Stanford University School of Medicine,
Stanford, CA, USA

Philip E. Stieg, MD, PhD
Department of Neurological Surgery,
Weill Cornell Medical College and New York–Presbyterian Hospital,
New York, USA

Hua Su, PhD
Department of Anesthesia and Perioperative Care and the Center for Cerebrovascular Research,
University of California, San Francisco,
San Francisco, CA, USA

Karel terBrugge, MD, FRCPC
Department of Radiology,
University of Toronto,
Toronto, Ontario, Canada

Kiron Thomas, MD
Division of Interventional Neuroradiology,
Lahey Hospital and Medical Center,
Burlington, MA, USA

Tarik Tihan, MD
Department of Neuropathology,
University of California, San Francisco,
San Francisco, CA, USA

Babu Welch, MD
Department of Neurosurgery,
UT Southwestern School of Medicine,
Dallas, TX, USA

Jonathan White, MD
Department of Neurosurgery,
UT Southwestern School of Medicine,
Dallas, TX, USA

H. Richard Winn, MD
Department of Neurosurgery and Neuroscience,
Mount Sinai Medical School,
New York, NY, USA
and Department of Neurosurgery,
University of Iowa,
Iowa City, IA, USA

Chun-Po Yen, MD
Department of Radiation Oncology,
University of Virginia,
Charlottesville, VA, USA

Jacky T. Yeung, MD
Department of Neurosurgery,
Stanford University Medical Center,
Stanford, CA, USA

Byron Yip, MS
Department of Neurosurgery,
Northwestern University School
of Medicine,
Evanston, IL, USA

Samer G. Zammar, MD
Department of Neurosurgery,
Northwestern University School of Medicine,
Evanston, IL, USA

Foreword

It is truly an honor to have been asked to write a foreword to this truly comprehensive and up-to-date text on arteriovenous malformations (AVMs) of the brain and spine, which has been a favorite topic of mine throughout my career. Clearly, much has been written on this topic and there have been excellent textbooks, frequently on the larger topic of cerebrovascular surgery, which have described in detail one or another aspect of the management of these vascular lesions. However, I know of no other work that "puts it all together" with the most modern available information on this topic.

The first section on development, anatomy, and physiology opens with an excellent chapter by Lawton and his colleagues with beautiful drawings depicting the embryologic development of the vasculature of the nervous system. This section ends with a very good summary of what is known to date about the natural history of AVMs of the brain by Laakso and Hernesniemi. This section also includes an excellent discussion of spinal vascular anatomy by Singh and Gobin. The second section on evaluation and treatment considerations, such as neuromonitoring and neuroanesthesia, concludes with an excellent chapter on the classification of brain and spinal AVMs and fistulae by Du and her colleagues. The next section, on surgical approaches, includes chapters by several of the most experienced cerebrovascular groups, including a beautifully illustrated chapter on the surgery of spinal AVMs and fistulae by the senior editor of this book and his group at the Barrow Neurological Institute. The last section, which includes endovascular and radiosurgical treatments of AVMs, is particularly comprehensive and includes an interesting chapter on the difficult and controversial topic of "palliative" treatment of those lesions that cannot be eliminated with conventional methods. The book concludes with a thoughtful comment by Russin and Spetzler on the ARUBA trial and its impact and possible consequences.

I have truly enjoyed my first cursory look through this excellent textbook. I am looking forward very much to the "banquet" that will be reading leisurely chapter by chapter of the final printed text. Seeing the many beautiful illustrations in almost every chapter in full color will be a special treat. This is a multidisciplinary work that will be equally enjoyed and of great value not only to neurosurgeons but also to neurologists, neuroradiologists, intensivists, and radiation oncologists interested in cerebrovascular disease.

I truly congratulate the editors for gathering a true cast of stars to put together a work of real excellence that will stand as the definite work on the comprehensive management of AVMs of the brain and spine.

Roberto C. Heros, MD
University of Miami

Preface

Arteriovenous malformations and fistulae represent for neurosurgeons rare, but challenging lesions of the brain and spinal vasculature. Historically, many practitioners have been reluctant to tackle these lesions. It was only with advancements in microsurgical techniques that the routine management of patients with these lesions became possible. More recently, advances in the fields of radiation oncology and interventional neuroradiology have resulted in novel adjuncts for treating patients with arteriovenous malformations. With the rapid growth of knowledge about arteriovenous malformations and fistulae, and the development and application of new modalities for their treatment, we felt it essential to produce a comprehensive guide for practitioners at all levels, summarizing the state of the art in the field. Importantly, we wanted to stress the decision-making process associated with patient selection and the thought process used in applying single or multi-modality treatment to these malformations.

Although older texts have reviewed treatment indications and outcomes for brain and spinal vascular malformations, an updated text on the comprehensive management of these lesions is lacking. Here we have gathered a team of international experts in the management of arteriovenous malformations and produced a volume summarizing updated findings on the molecular biology, development, natural history, treatment, and outcomes of patients with these lesions.

This work is intended for practitioners at all levels who work in the fields of neurology, neurosurgery, interventional radiology, radiation oncology, and critical care medicine and who are involved in the care of patients with vascular malformations of the brain and spine. We encourage readers to familiarize themselves with the literature on the natural history of vascular malformations of the brain and spine. In our opinion, no treatment should be attempted or offered until the practitioner understands the risks of morbidity and mortality associated with the natural history of the lesion and how that risk compares with the risks associated with various treatment modalities or with observation alone. Experts in the fields of neurosurgery, interventional radiology, and radiation oncology have written the chapters in this book. Where appropriate, the written chapters are accompanied by videos highlighting the essential techniques used in the treatment of these lesions.

With advances in the fields of genomics and proteomics, we are likely to see a revolution in the way these lesions are identified and treated. Until that time, surgery, interventional techniques, and radiation remain the mainstay of treatment for these lesions.

We thank the expert authors of the chapters for taking time from their busy clinical practices to produce this volume. This work is the result of numerous hours of hard work and dedication to perfection by the editors, illustrators, and animators at the Neuroscience Publications office at Barrow Neurological Institute. A special thanks to Mr. Mark Schornak, Ms. Jaime-Lynn Canales, Ms. Clare Prendergast, Ms. Dawn Mutchler, Ms. Paula Card Higginson, Ms. Marie Clarkson, Mr. Michael Hickman, and Ms. Kristen Larson, without whose efforts this work would not have been possible. The editors wish to extend a note of gratitude to Mr. Nicholas Dunton and Ms. Joanna Chamberlin at Cambridge University Press for their assistance with the work.

Chapter 1

Development of the central nervous system vasculature and the pathogenesis of brain arteriovenous malformations

Steven W. Hetts, Hua Su, Tarik Tihan, Tomoki Hashimoto, Ludmila Pawlikowska, and Michael T. Lawton

Introduction

An arteriovenous malformations (AVM) is a spectacular freak of nature, a tangle of hemodynamic energy and red fury, throbbing and swirling in the sulci and gyri of the brain. There is nothing like it in the realm of brain pathology, at once so beautiful and so fearsome. Where do these lesions come from and how do they form? These questions have been without answers for as long as we have known about AVMs, and in our ignorance, we simply say that they are congenital. But are they really? Maybe they arise from miscues or miscommunications during embryogenesis when arteries and veins are in direct contact without intervening capillaries, and then persist after birth as AVMs rather than remodeling and maturing into normal circulatory architecture during vasculogenesis. Maybe they arise as a result of underlying genetic abnormalities that produce signaling errors and structural defects leading to arteriovenous pathology. Maybe AVMs are not congenital at all but acquired, as are dural arteriovenous fistulae after an injury where they are an abnormal response to that injury. The pathogenesis of brain AVMs remains a mystery, although tantalizing clues are emerging. This chapter will examine the development of the vasculature of the central nervous system (CNS), experimental AVM models, inflammation, and genetics in order to explore some of these ideas about AVM pathogenesis.

Vasculogenesis

Vessels exist to transmit nutrients to and remove waste from tissues. The arteries of the brain and spinal cord develop to supply the CNS during early embryonic stages in response to the metabolic needs of the neural tube. By the end of the third gestational week, the neuroectoderm differentiates into the neural plate, which itself folds longitudinally into a tube. Before the neural tube closes, nutrients and metabolites diffuse freely across the inner (ependymal) surface of the neural tissue from the amniotic fluid [1]. On the 23rd day of development in the human, the cephalic end of the neural tube (the anterior neuropore) closes to form the lamina terminalis (third ventricle anterior wall); the caudal neural tube will become the spinal cord [1]. After anterior neuropore closure, during the prechoroidal stage, the neural tube is surrounded by *meninx primitiva*, a connective tissue derived from the neural crest that supplies nutrition by diffusion across the neural tube's outer (meningeal) surface (Fig. 1.1) [1]. In the choroidal phase, as the cerebral tissues grow and convolute, the meninx invaginates into the neural tube (ventricular lumen) to become the choroid plexus [1]. Consequently, metabolic exchange is possible across both ependymal and meningeal surfaces of the neural tissue. The locations of choroid plexus in relation to the thickening neural cortex dictate the morphology of the early afferent arterial tree to the prosencephalon (forebrain), mesencephalon (midbrain), and rhombencephalon (hindbrain) [1,2].

As the cortical mantle continues to thicken and fold, the parenchymatous stage of cerebral vascularization consists of angiogenesis from the superficial anastomotic vascular network stimulated by the metabolic demands of the primitive brain tissue [1]. The neurovascular unit, a functional partnership of neural tissue and blood vessels, may arise during this period [3,4]. The basic arterial pattern laid down in the early embryonic period (Fig. 1.2) persists but is subsequently partially reorganized as a result of metabolic demands and concomitant hemodynamic changes of the later embryonic and fetal periods.

Development of craniocervical arteries: aortic arch and great vessels

The complex development of the craniocervical arteries can be broken down by embryonic stages and anatomical locations. Early embryonic development of the aortic arch and great vessels consists of formation and partial regression of undifferentiated plexiform paired vascular arches along the surface of the pharyngeal arches connecting the ventral aorta (aortic sac) with paired dorsal aortae (Table 1.1) [5]. The first pair of pharyngeal arches appears about day 22 and the concomitant first aortic vascular arches appear about day 24. The second pharyngeal arches appear by day 24 and, while the first pair of aortic arches regress, the second aortic arches appear by day 26. The third through sixth aortic arches have appeared by day 28 and 29. Blood flow to the brain is supplied mainly by the

Comprehensive Management of Arteriovenous Malformations of the Brain and Spine, ed. Robert F. Spetzler, Douglas S. Kondziolka, Randall T. Higashida, and M. Yashar S. Kalani. Published by Cambridge University Press.

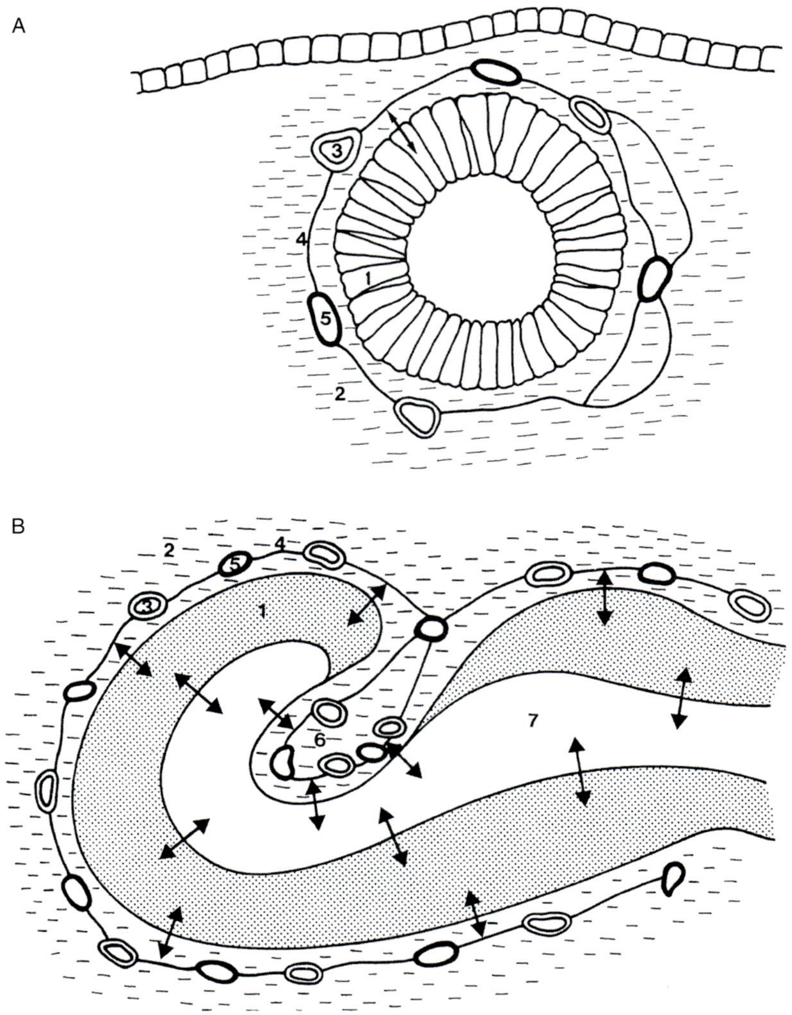

Fig. 1.1. Supply of nutrients to the neural tube. (A) After the neural tube (1) has closed, it is surrounded by the meninx primitiva (2), which contains arterial (3), capillary (4), and venous (5) channels. Metabolites diffuse from the capillary channels into the meninx and from there centripetally into the neural tissue (arrow). (B) As the neural tube thickens, centripetal diffusion cannot meet its metabolic demands. Invagination of the meninx primitiva into the ventricular lumen (choroid plexus; 6), allows exchange of metabolites between the capillaries of the meninx and the ventricular fluid (7), and between the ventricular fluid and the neural tissue via the ependymal surface. Metabolic exchanges across the external surface of the brain and spinal cord also persist as development continues.

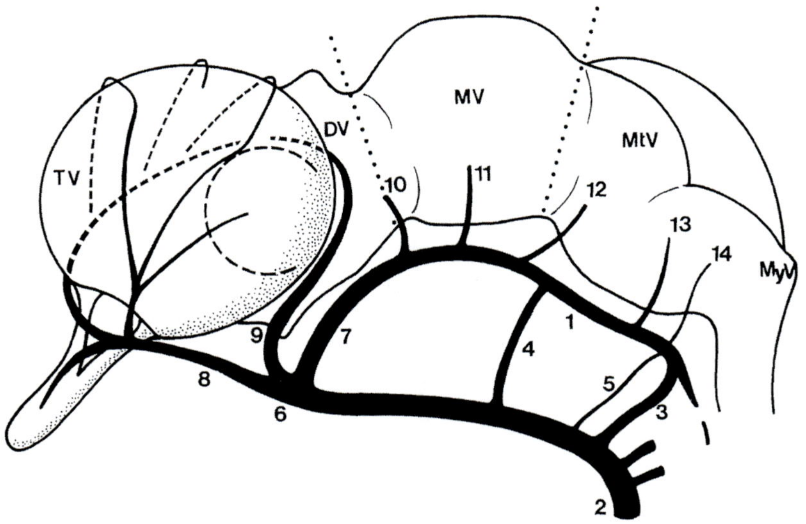

Fig. 1.2. Development of the arterial vascularization of the brain. The longitudinal neural artery (1) of the ventral aspect of the rhombencephalon is supplied by branches of the primitive common carotid artery (2), the proatlantal artery (3) caudally, the trigeminal artery (4) and cranially by the hypoglossal artery (5). The longitudinal system of anastomoses between the cervical intersegmental arteries has not yet evolved into the vertebral arteries. More cranially, the primitive carotid artery ends as a rostral (6, olfactory artery) and a caudal (posterior communicating artery; 7) division. The anterior branch subdivides into the anterior cerebral (8) and future anterior choroidal (9) arteries, and both encircle the neck of the telencephalic vesicle (TV) and anastomose. Their lateral branches form the pericerebral arterial network of the hemispheres, including what is to become the middle cerebral artery. The posterior branch of the primitive carotid artery sends secondary branches toward the diencephalon (DV) (posterior choroidal arteries; 10), the mesencephalon (MV) (collicular arteries; 11), and the metencephalon (MtV) (superior cerebellar artery; 12). It connects with the longitudinal neural artery, thereby causing the trigeminal artery to regress, while the development of the vertebral artery supplies the caudal arterial system in place of the proatlantal artery, which then also regresses. 13, anterior inferior cerebellar artery; 14, posterior inferior cerebellar artery; MyV, myelencephalic vesicle.

Table 1.1. Development of aortic arch, great vessels, and craniocervical arteries

Embryonic precursor	Primitive artery formed	Regression/remodeling	Becomes
Bulbus cordis	Truncus arteriosus	Aorticopulmonary septum forms	Ascending aorta, pulmonary trunk
Aortic sac	Ventral aorta	Persists	Ascending aorta, brachiocephalic trunk
Dorsal aortae (paired)	Carotid arteries (distal)	Right partially regresses (distal to SCA); left persists	Right: part of right SCA, right distal ICA, right ACA (from primitive ICA and olfactory artery), right MCA, right PComA (variable regression), right PCA (often annexed by basilar) Left: descending aorta, left distal ICA, left ACA (from primitive ICA and olfactory artery), left MCA, left PComA (variable regression), left PCA (often annexed by basilar) Fusion of midline plexus between ACAs: anterior communicating artery
Cervical plexi	Cervical intersegmental arteries	C1–C6 (proximal segments regress); C7	C1–C6: vertebral arteries C7: subclavian arteries
Dorsal plexi	Longitudinal neural arteries (paired)	Midline fusion	Basilar artery
Aortic arches			
I	Mandibular arteries	Involute	± distal ECA
II	Hyoid arteries	Mostly involute	Caroticotympanic arteries
	Stapedial arteries	Partially involute	Distal segments persist as middle meningeal artery and internal maxillary artery
III	Carotid arteries (proximal)	Persist	Common carotid arteries, proximal ICAs, ECA
IV	Right and left primitive aortic arches	Asymmetric remodeling	Right becomes proximal right SCA; left becomes definitive aortic arch
V	None		
VI	Ductus arteriosus	Asymmetric remodeling	Bilateral pulmonary arteries; ductus arteriosus

ACA, anterior cerebral artery; ECA external carotid artery; ICA, internal carotid artery; MCA, middle cerebral artery; SCA, subclavian artery; PCA, posterior cerebral artery; PComA, posterior communicating artery.
Source: adapted with permission of Wolters Kluwer Health from Osborn, 1999 [5].

primitive carotid arteries whose proximal aspects (future definitive common carotid arteries [CCAs]) are derived from the ventral aorta and third aortic arches and whose distal aspects (future definitive internal carotid arteries [ICAs]) are derived from the paired dorsal aortae [5].

During the fifth week of embryonic development, the dorsal aortic segments between the third and fourth aortic arches regress (Fig. 1.3), leaving the ICAs supplied by the ventral aorta and third aortic arches. Around the same time, two vascular plexi – the longitudinal neural arteries – form dorsal to the third and fourth arches and supply the developing rhombencephalon. These arteries are supplied from below via cervical intersegmental arteries and also anastomose with the primitive carotid arteries via the primitive trigeminal, otic, hypoglossal, and proatlantal intersegmental arteries (some of which occasionally persist into adulthood as variant caroticobasilar anastomoses). The external carotid arteries also begin to develop in the fifth week, sprouting from the third aortic arches (CCAs) and possibly with contributions from the first and second arches.

During the sixth week, the caudal division of the ICA anastomoses with the longitudinal neural artery to become the posterior communicating artery. Plexiform connections between the cervical intersegmental arteries fuse to form the vertebral arteries while the first six intersegmental arterial connections to the dorsal aortae regress. The subclavian arteries form from the seventh cervical intersegmental arteries.

In the seventh week, further remodeling of the primitive aortic arches occurs. The paired longitudinal neural arteries fuse in the midline to form the definitive basilar artery which itself anastomoses to the vertebral arteries. By the eighth week of development, the definitive adult configuration of the aortic arch and great vessels – including the ICAs and external carotid arteries arising from CCA trunks – has been achieved.

Development of craniocervical arteries: the circle of Willis and its branches

By embryonic week 6, the ICAs have divided into cranial and caudal divisions (Fig. 1.4). The cranial ICA divisions subsequently give rise to the primitive olfactory arteries, the anterior cerebral arteries, the anterior choroidal arteries, and the middle cerebral arteries. The anterior communicating

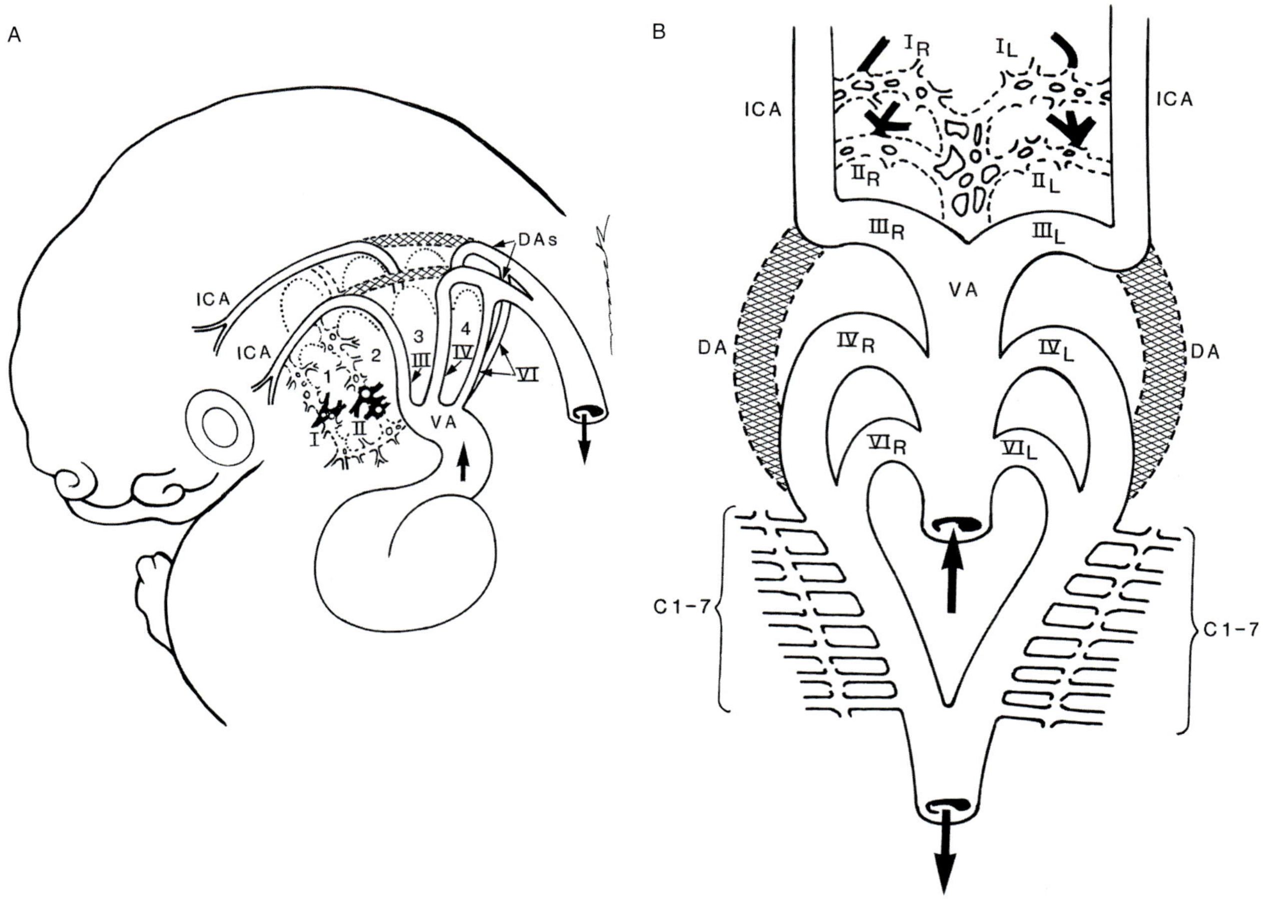

Fig. 1.3. Craniocerebral and aortocervical arterial development at approximately 4 weeks of gestation (6–8 mm crown–rump length). (A) Oblique three-dimensional anatomical sketch depicts the craniocerebral vasculature. The relationship between the embryonic pharyngeal pouches (1–4) and the developing aortic arches (I–VI) is shown. The third, fourth, and sixth arches (solid lines) have appeared. The plexiform first and second arches have regressed (dotted lines) except for some small remnants (solid black areas) that may persist as part of the future distal external carotid arteries. The primitive internal carotid arteries (ICAs) are formed from cephalad continuation of the dorsal aortae (DAs), whereas the common carotid arteries are derived from the ventral aorta (VA) and third arches. The DA segments between the third and fourth arches (cross-hatched areas) are still patent at this stage but will eventually regress completely. (B) This diagrammatic sketch (anteroposterior view) depicts the developing aortic arches (I–VI) and craniocervical vasculature. The plexiform first and second arches (dotted lines) have largely regressed, except for small remnants (solid black areas) that are annexed later by the future external carotid arteries. The third and fourth arches are prominent; the sixth arches are beginning to develop. The DA segments between the third and fourth arches (cross-hatched areas) are still present but will soon regress. Cephalad continuation of the right and left dorsal aortic segments from their junction with the third arches forms the primitive ICAs; their more proximal segments (i.e., the future common carotid arteries) are formed by the ventral aorta (VA) and third arches. The seven cervical intersegmental arteries are also depicted (C1–C7). Their midsegments are beginning to coalesce and will eventually form the definitive vertebral arteries. Direction of blood flow is indicated by large black arrows. (From Osborn 1999 [5], reprinted with permission of Wolters Kluwer Health.)

artery coalesces from a plexiform midline vascular network, connecting the two anterior cerebral arteries. Although initial branches of the middle cerebral arteries form in the embryonic period, the massive growth of the neocortex during fetal development results in a deepening sylvian fissure, an insula buried under opercula, and a highly convoluted mature middle cerebral artery architecture.

The caudal ICA divisions anastomose with the longitudinal neural arteries to become the posterior communicating arteries and proximal segments of the posterior cerebral arteries. After the longitudinal neural arteries fuse to become the basilar artery, the posterior communicating arteries regress to a variable degree, resulting in some individuals deriving supply to the distal posterior cerebral arteries primarily from the anterior (ICA) circulation and some primarily from the posterior (vertebrobasilar) circulation.

Development of cranial veins and sinuses

The cranial veins can be divided into several groups familiar in the mature human brain, including the superficial cortical veins, the deep subependymal veins, the posterior fossa veins, and the dural venous sinuses. They can also be divided based on evolutionary patterns in vertebrates into a dorsal venous system, a lateral–ventral venous system, and a ventricular venous system [6]. Development will be discussed in terms of the dural venous sinuses and the cerebral veins.

Analogous to, although more variable than, the development of the cerebral arteries, the dural venous sinuses arise from fusion of multiple plexi along the surfaces of developing brain. A primary head sinus arises from the primary dorsal hindbrain venous channel [5,7]. Anterior, middle, and posterior dural plexi drain their respective developing cerebral

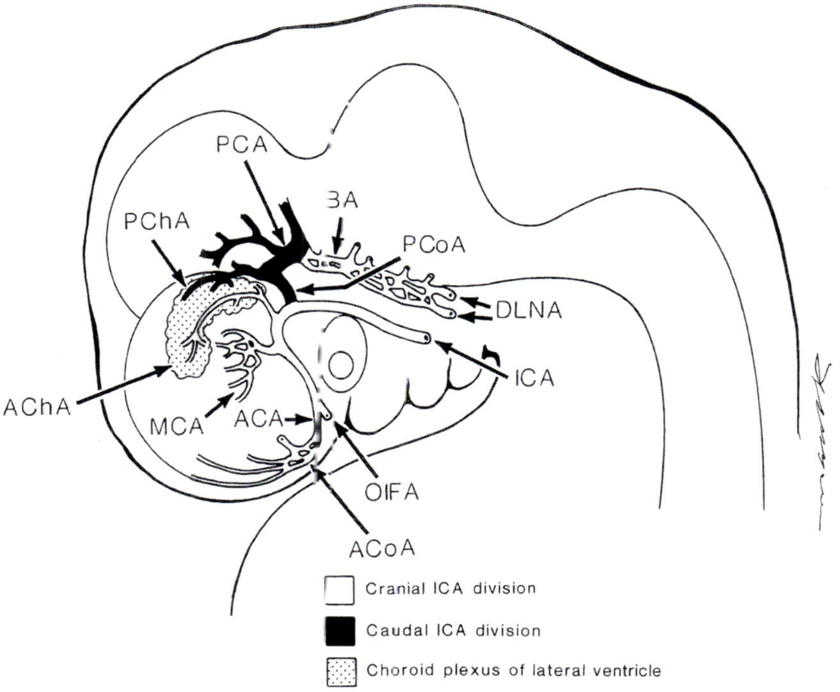

Fig. 1.4. Embryonic intracranial arteries at approximately 5 to 6 weeks of gestation. The primitive internal carotid arteries (ICAs) each have a cranial and a caudal division. The cranial divisions give rise to the primitive olfactory arteries (OlFA) as well as to the anterior cerebral arteries (ACAs), anterior choroidal arteries (AChA), and middle cerebral arteries (MCAs). The anterior communicating artery (ACoA) forms from coalescence of a midline plexiform network. The caudal divisions will become the posterior communicating arteries (PCoAs) and also supply the stems of the posterior cerebral arteries (PCAs). The basilar artery (BA) will be formed from fusion of the paired dorsal longitudinal neural arteries (DLNAs). (From Osborn 1999 [5], reprinted with permission of Wolters Kluwer Health.)

vesicles. By approximately eight weeks of embryonic development, paired primitive marginal sinuses extend from the anterior dural plexus along the sides of the anterior cerebral vesicle; these eventually fuse to form the superior sagittal sinus and the transverse sinuses (Fig. 1.5) [5]. The embryonic tentorial plexus gives rise to the straight sinus.

The median prosencephalic vein of Markowski drains the choroid plexus of the lateral ventricles by eight weeks, emptying into the falcine sinus, a midline dorsal interhemispheric plexus. As the basal ganglia and choroid plexus enlarge, the definitive internal cerebral veins develop and the median prosencephalic vein regresses, leaving its caudal remnant as the definitive vein of Galen connecting the internal cerebral veins to the straight sinus. It is thought that if the median prosencephalic vein persists as an outlet for deep venous drainage, a vein of Galen malformations results, along with concomitant atresia of the straight sinus and persistent falcine sinus. Many types of vascular malformations seen in postnatal life may have their origins in the primitive vascular plexus remodeling that normally occurs during embryogenesis, either as persistence of primitive connections during development or as aberrant activations of developmental genes later in life [5,8].

Pathogenesis and progression of brain arteriovenous malformations

The pathogenesis of brain AVM is not completely understood. Recent studies suggest that the initiation and progression of AVM require interplay among several factors, including (1) homozygous loss of function of causative genes in somatic endothelial cells, (2) angiogenic stimulation (response to injury), (3) participation of bone marrow-derived cells (BMDCs), (4) alteration of monocyte/macrophage function, and (5) hemodynamic changes (Fig. 1.6).

Homozygous causative gene mutations

The genesis of sporadic brain AVM has been observed in a handful of reported patients. An important conceptual advance is that hereditary hemorrhagic telangiectasia (HHT) can serve as a familial form of the more common sporadic brain AVM disorder, similar to the homology between familial and sporadic cavernous malformations [9–12]. The two most prevalent causative genes for HHT are *ALK1* (encoding activin-like kinase) and *ENG* (encoding endoglin). The prevailing view is that HHT is caused by haploinsufficiency of one of its causative genes in somatic endothelial cells. However, inactivation of the remaining wild-type allele appears to have powerful effect, irrespective of the mechanism by which it is inactivated (e.g., loss of heterozygosity or loss of protein during inflammation) [13]. For example, the loss of a single allele of genes such as *Eng* or *Alk1* in animal models reproduces certain aspects of the human disease and is primarily found in older animals [14,15]. In contrast, loss of both alleles of any HHT-causative gene is embryonically lethal in mice [16,17], and conditional (tissue/time-specific) homozygous deletion of *Eng* [13] or *Alk1* [18,19] results in striking vascular malformations resembling the AVMs found in HHT. It has been shown that homozygous knockout of *Eng* in only around 1% of endothelial cells in mice resulted in a more severe cerebrovascular dysplasia after vascular endothelial growth factor (VEGF) stimulation than in $Eng^{+/-}$ mice [20]. Moreover, analysis of human brain and lung AVMs in HHT indicates that haploinsufficiency of *ENG* is not sufficient to cause lesion development [21]. A tenable model explaining this phenotypic heterogeneity is that loss of function in the second allele locally or in

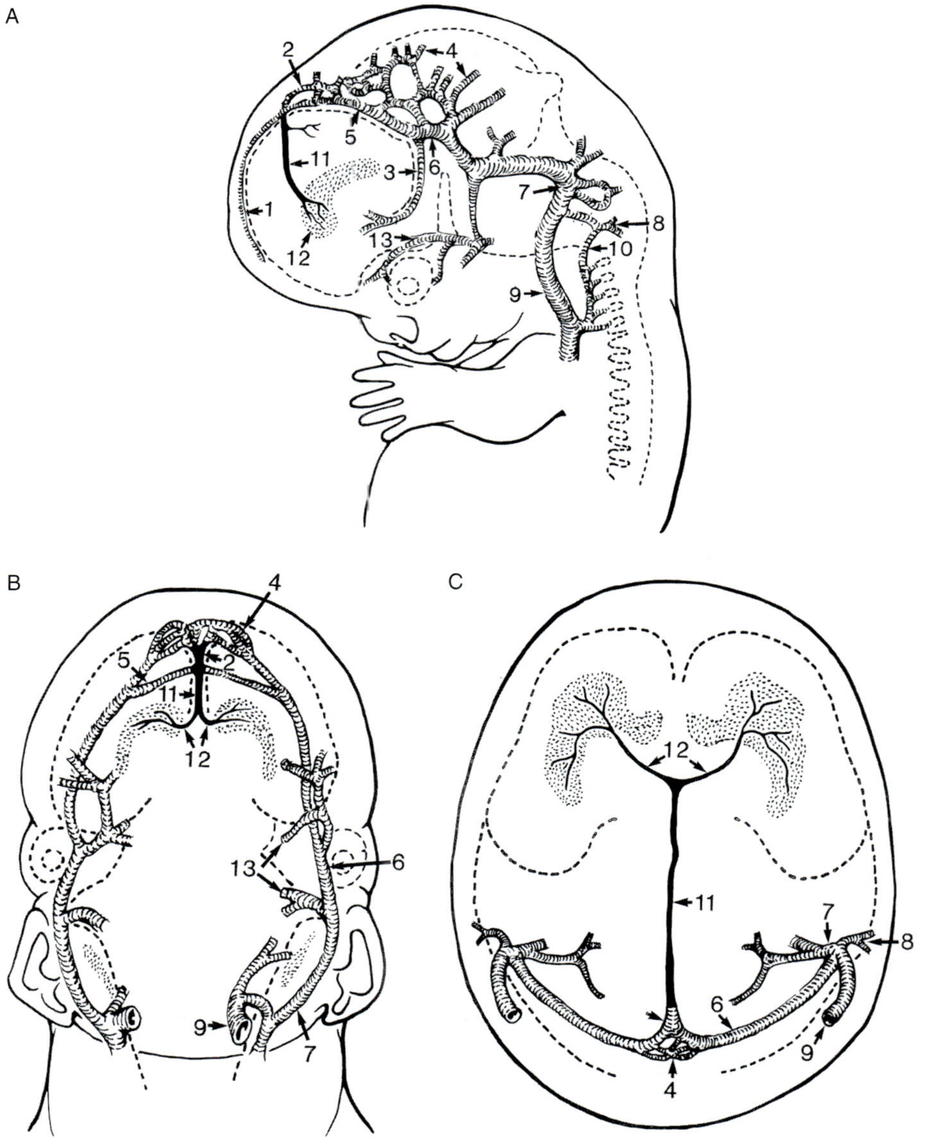

Fig. 1.5. Dural venous sinuses and cerebral veins at approximately 8 weeks of gestation. The choroid plexus is indicated by the dotted areas in the lateral (A), frontal (B), and axial (C) views. A single midline deep cerebral vein (the median prosencephalic vein of Markowski or primitive internal cerebral vein) drains the choroid plexi and is indicated by the solid black lines. (1) superior sagittal sinus; (2) primitive straight (falcine) sinus; (3) tentorial sinus; (4) tentorial plexi; (5) primitive marginal sinus; (6) primitive transverse sinus; (7) sigmoid sinus; (8) condylar, hypoglossal emissary veins; (9) internal jugular vein; (10) vertebral veins; (11) primitive internal cerebral vein (median prosencephalic vein); (12) choroid veins; (13) primitive supraorbital, maxillary veins. (From Osborn 1999 [5], reprinted with permission of Wolters Kluwer Health.)

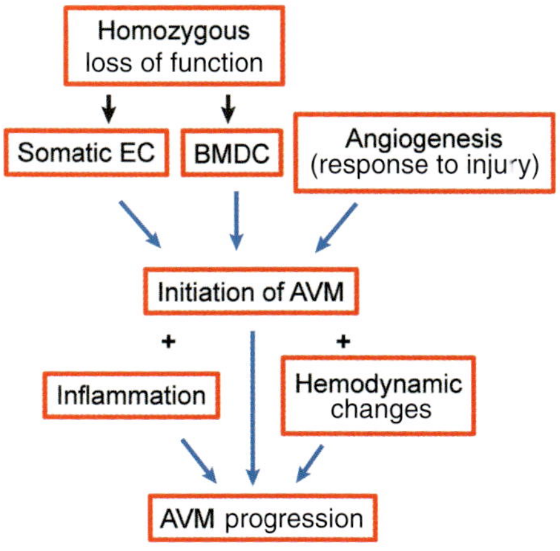

Fig. 1.6. Novel theories of arteriovenous malformations initiation and progression. AVM, arteriovenous malformations; EC, endothelial cell; BMDC, bone marrow-derived cells.

bone marrow-derived endothelial precursor cells contributes to the AVM phenotype. There is compelling proof-of-principle evidence that loss of function of the wild-type allele is relevant to vascular malformations, demonstrated for two related disorders: somatic mucocutaneous venous malformations [22] and cerebral cavernous malformations [23].

Angiogenesis and the "response to injury" hypothesis

The brain AVM lesional phenotype includes an active angiogenic and inflammatory component that is inconsistent with a static congenital anomaly [24]. A "response to injury" hypothesis may explain incomplete penetrance of brain AVM in patients with HHT. It is known that both $Eng^{+/-}$ [25] and $Alk1^{+/-}$ [14] adult mice develop vascular lesions in various organs, but spontaneous lesions in the brain are quite modest and only seen in older mice

[14,26]. However, more pronounced forms of cerebral microvascular dysplasia were induced using focal VEGF stimulation in $Eng^{+/-}$ or $Alk1^{+/-}$ mice [27–29].

Antenatal conditional deletion of *Alk1* causes anteriovenous fistula in neonatal brain and intracranial hemorrhage [19]. Conditional global *Alk1* deletion in adult mice induced AVM and hemorrhage in the lung and gastrointestinal tract, but not in the skin or brain. However, upon wounding, *Alk1*-deleted mice developed vascular dysplasia and direct arteriovenous connections around the skin wound, suggesting an abnormal response to injury. Direct arteriovenous connections have also been detected in the retina of *Eng*-deficient neonatal mice [13]. The combination of local angiogenic stimulation (Matrigel [a gelatinous protein mixture secreted by mouse sarcoma cells] plus VEGF/fibroblast growth factor) and *Eng* deletion led to gross venous enlargement [13]. Walker *et al.* described the brain AVM phenotype in mice with apparent arteriovenous shunting after focal VEGF stimulation in animals subjected to regional conditional *Alk1* deletion (Fig. 1.7) [30].

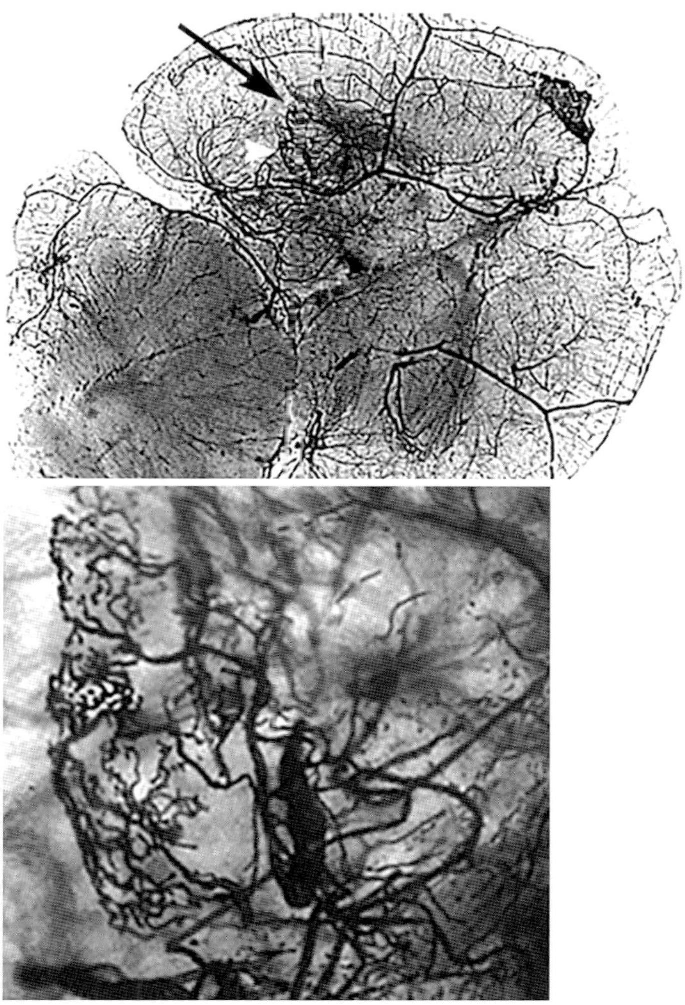

Fig. 1.7. Vessel casting showing arteriovenous malformations (AVM) in the brain angiogenic region. Top. Large tangled vessels resembling an AVM were detected in the brain angiogenic focus of an *Alk1*-deficient mouse (black arrow). Bottom. An enlarged image of angiogenic foci shows tangle dilated vessels. Scale bar, 100 µm.

Taken together, both genetic manipulation and angiogenic stimulation seem to be required for AVM development. The angiogenic stimulus can be a minor injury, exogenous growth factor delivery, or high endogenous angiogenic factors in the brain of young and perinatal individuals.

Bone marrow-derived cells

Several studies support a pivotal role for BMDCs in AVM formation [31]. After VEGF stimulation in the brain, wild-type mice with $Eng^{+/-}$ bone marrow developed a similar degree of dysplasia as somatically heterozygous $Eng^{+/-}$ mice, suggesting that the loss of even one allele of a causative gene in BMDCs is sufficient to cause an abnormal vascular phenotype [31]. Similarly, $Eng^{+/-}$ mice with wild-type bone marrow had fewer dysplastic vessels compared with $Eng^{+/-}$ mice with $Eng^{+/-}$ bone marrow. These data suggest that BMDCs contribute to AVM formation and indicate that the tendency to form AVMs might be rescued by transplantation of normal bone marrow.

So far, the cell type(s) in the bone marrow underlying AVM formation are unknown. There is evidence for two primary – probably complementary – BMDC types that serve as a locus for the phenomena: endothelial cells that incorporate into the angiogenic neovasculature [31,32] and monocytes/macrophages, which may provide critical repair function in response to injury [33–35] and/or provide guidance involving NOTCH signaling during angiogenesis [36,37].

The involvement of bone marrow-derived endothelial cells in focal angiogenesis has been shown in several conditions, such as tumor formation. Bone marrow-derived endothelial cells seed tumor vascular beds and regulate tumor angiogenesis [38,39]. Bone marrow-derived endothelial cells can incorporate into vessels in the brain angiogenic foci in mouse models [31,32,40]. In addition, endothelial precursor cells have been identified in vessels in adult human sporadic brain AVMs [41].

Inflammatory cells

Supporting evidence for myeloid cells playing a critical role in AVM progression includes (1) that most of the BMDCs that home to the brain angiogenic foci are CD68+ or CD45+ [31,40] and (2) that intraperitoneal administration of neutrophil neutralizing antibody reduces VEGF-mediated angiogenesis and matrix metalloproteinase (MMP)-9 activity [42]. Other experiments suggest that both neutrophils and macrophages are also relevant to large vessel remodeling [43].

Further, normal human monocytes rescue the impairment of $Eng^{+/-}$ mice in repairing myocardial injury, whereas monocytes from patients with HHT fail to improve the myocardial repair [33,35]. The monocytes from patients with HHT type 1 migrate to stromal cell-derived factor 1 less effectively than normal monocytes, which is associated with an increase of CD26 expression [33,35]. These data suggest that the function of monocytes in vascular repair or remodeling is defective in patients with HHT, which could result in abnormal vascular remodeling and thus promote AVM progression.

Hemodynamic changes in arteriovenous malformations

Vessels in an AVM are subjected to abnormally high flow rates. High vascular flow rates in *Alk1*$^{+/-}$ mice induced by vasodilators (i.e. nicardipine or hydralazine) after focal VEGF stimulation increased the number of dysplastic vessels in the brain angiogenic foci [28].

Cerebral venous hypertension is a common symptom in brain AVMs [44]. Venous hypertension has been implicated in the formation of dural arteriovenous fistula [45,46] through a mechanism that involves the induction of angiogenesis [46]. In rats, non-ischemic levels of venous hypertension (15–23 mmHg) cause expression of hypoxia-inducible factor 1α and its downstream signal VEGF [47]. Further, hypoxia-inducible factor 1α, VEGF, stromal cell-derived factor 1 expression, neutrophils, macrophages, and MMP-9 activity all increase in the brains of the mice with venous hypertension. Capillary density in the parasagittal cortex also increases in the mouse venous hypertension model. These findings suggest that mild non-ischemic venous hypertension results in a pro-angiogenic state [48]. Consequently, venous hypertension could represent a kind of injury that triggers AVM development in subjects carrying mutant genes.

Inflammation in arteriovenous malformations formation and remodeling

A number of possibilities exist for the role of inflammation in the genesis and modulation of brain AVMs, apart from the fact that inflammatory infiltrates can be introduced into lesions through surgical manipulations, embolization, or secondary infectious processes [49–51]. The latter factors often confuse the interpretation of inflammatory cells such as lymphocytes and macrophages within AVM tissue specimens. In addition, hemorrhagic complications such as AVM rupture are associated with extravasation of hemosiderin and subsequent accumulation of macrophages and other reactive cells as a response to tissue damage. Therefore, the finding of inflammatory cells and cytokines within AVMs should be interpreted with caution.

However, even in the absence of obvious inciting processes, abnormal expression patterns of inflammatory mediators and cytokines, as well as influx of inflammatory cells into AVMs, have been observed by a number of investigators [52–56]. Studies on genetic and cytokine expression in AVMs suggest that inflammation is associated with AVM formation, progression, and rupture [24]. The typical findings in unruptured brain AVMs include perivascular inflammatory infiltrates (Fig. 1.8A) and intraparenchymal macrophages (Fig. 1.8B), occasionally associated with microscopic deposits of hemosiderin.

In humans and in animal models, AVMs have been associated with an increased inflammatory response [57–61]. Inflammatory markers are overexpressed in human AVMs, including myeloperoxidase and interleukin (IL)-6, both of which highly correlate with MMP-9 levels. Levels of MMP-9, in turn, correlate with the expression of lipocalin–MMP-9 complex within AVMs, suggesting that neutrophils may play a role in their pathophysiology. Substantial numbers of neutrophils and macrophages occupy the perivascular spaces and the intervening stroma around even unruptured and non-embolized AVMs. While their presence does not indicate a causal association, inflammatory cells and cytokines may influence the formation and evolution of AVMs.

Remodeling of the vascular network in AVMs is facilitated by a number of proteases, which can enlarge the vascular elements in the nidus. This remodeling is partially mediated through VEGF activity and modulated by pro-angiogenic signals such as MMP. The MMPs maintain and remodel the extracellular matrix [62] and the MMPs, including MMP-9, are major components of neutrophilic tertiary granules and are also synthesized by monocytes and lymphocytes. There are significantly higher levels of MMP-9 in brain AVMs than in control tissue [53,63], but the source of this increase is unclear. Both production and activity of MMP-9 are stimulated during inflammation by the cytokines IL-8, IL-1β, and IL-6. Matrix metalloproteinase-9 degrades key components of the cerebrovascular matrix including laminin, denatured collagen, and tight junction proteins such as zona occuldens 1, leading to blood–brain barrier leakage and hemorrhage [64,65]. The MMP-9 signal colocalizes with myeloperoxidase and correlates with both myeloperoxidase and IL-6 levels, which suggests that the source of the MMP-9 may be the inflammatory cells in the environment [53].

Soluble ENG (extracellular domain) has been shown to contribute to another vascular disease, pre-eclampsia [66]. Soluble ENG is distinct from long- and short-form ENG, which have cytoplasmic tails of 47 and 14 amino acid residues, respectively [67]. Soluble ENG is also increased in brain AVMs [68]. It is not clear how soluble ENG is formed. A related type III transforming growth factor-β (TGFβ) receptor, β-glycan, appears to be shed through a process that is mediated by MMP-1 [69]. Several different MMPs are also found in AVM nidal tissue [53,70,71], suggesting that similar mechanisms may contribute to the formation of soluble ENG or soluble ALK1 [66]. Tumor necrosis factor-α (TNFα) can induce the release of soluble ENG from normal placental villous explants [72]. Therefore, inflammatory proteins and cytokines in AVMs could cause shedding of soluble ENG and promote brain AVM instability. Another interesting observation is the increased levels of immunoglobulins within brain AVMs when compared with control brain [54].

Vascular inflammation is central to the pathogenesis of several vascular diseases, including intracranial aneurysm growth [73] and abdominal aortic aneurysm formation [74,75]. In addition to findings of vascular inflammation, associations between single nucleotide polymorphisms in genes encoding cytokines such as TNFα and increased brain AVM intracerebral hemorrhage risk have been described [76]. In addition, single nucleotide polymorphisms in the gene encoding IL-6 were also associated with a hemorrhagic clinical presentation in patients with brain AVM [52], and the highest risk *IL6* genotype (GG) was associated with the highest production of IL-6 in brain AVM tissue [71].

A

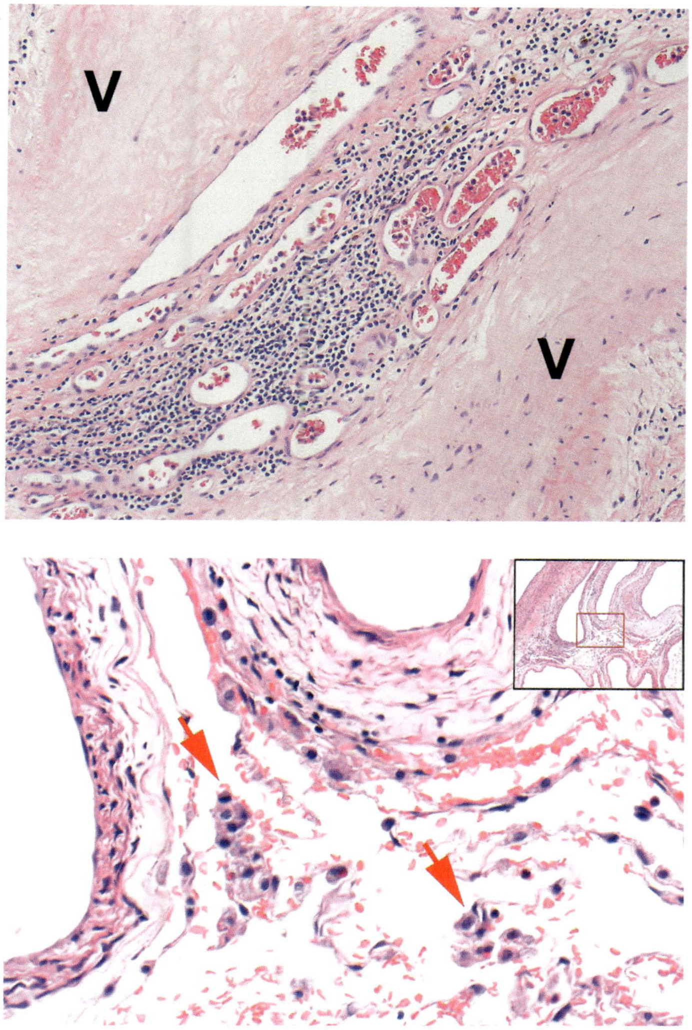

B

Fig. 1.8. Unruptured arteriovenous malformations without clinical or radiological evidence of hemorrhage. (A) Medium power magnification of perivascular lymphoplasmacytic infiltrate. The inflammatory cells are in the perivascular region between two large, abnormal vessels (V) along with numerous smaller capillaries (hematoxylin & eosin, original magnification ×200). (B) High power magnification of perivascular macrophage aggregates. The inset demonstrates the region within the malformations at low power. The red square highlights the magnified area. Collections of macrophages (arrows) as well as scattered individual macrophages can be seen in the perivascular spaces (hematoxylin & eosin, original magnification ×400; inset original magnification ×20).

Hemodynamic stress can trigger vascular inflammation that initiates vascular remodeling and angiogenesis. High shear stress activates endothelial cells and upregulates leukocyte adhesion molecules, including intercellular adhesion molecule 1 and monocyte chemotactic protein 1 [77–80]. Shear stress activates endothelial and smooth muscle cells and promotes their production and release of angiogenic factors and other cytokines critical for vascular remodeling [81,82]. Along with activated endothelial and smooth muscle cells, these inflammatory cells secrete proteinases, including MMPs and elastases [77], that digest the vascular wall and surrounding matrix to facilitate vascular remodeling and the release of angiogenic factors [83,84]. The MMPs and proinflammatory cytokines can interact to carry out both physiological and pathological vascular remodeling.

Clinical and experimental evidence suggests that AVMs undergo significant vascular remodeling and angiogenesis in adult life. The variable nature of AVMs, with respect to their growth, regression, and spontaneous hemorrhage [85], strongly suggests that AVMs are unstable blood vessels that must continuously remodel and repair in response to abnormally high flow conditions. A review of studies examining interval angiography in 106 patients with mean follow-up periods of 8.4 years showed that over half of the AVMs increased in size and one-fifth decreased in size or vanished [86], suggesting active remodeling processes.

Histological studies further support the notion of active vascular remodeling and angiogenesis in AVMs. Endothelial cell proliferation rates measured using the Ki-67 index were higher in adult AVM specimens than the control brain (2.5 vs. 0.5%) [87]. Another study examining 37 AVMs and 5 control specimens found a seven-fold increase in non-nesting endothelial cells in AVMs compared with control brain [86], providing more evidence for active vascular remodeling and angiogenesis in AVMs. Underlying mechanisms for active vascular remodeling and angiogenesis in AVMs are under vigorous investigation [86,88–92].

An abnormal pattern of MMP-9 and tissue inhibitors of metalloproteinases has been found in AVM tissues [63]. There is markedly increased MMP-9 activity in AVMs compared with control brain samples and MMP-9 is found in the endothelial cell/peri-endothelial cell layer of AVMs. Along with endothelial and smooth muscle cells, inflammatory cells seem to be a major contributor to the abnormally high levels of MMP-9 in AVM

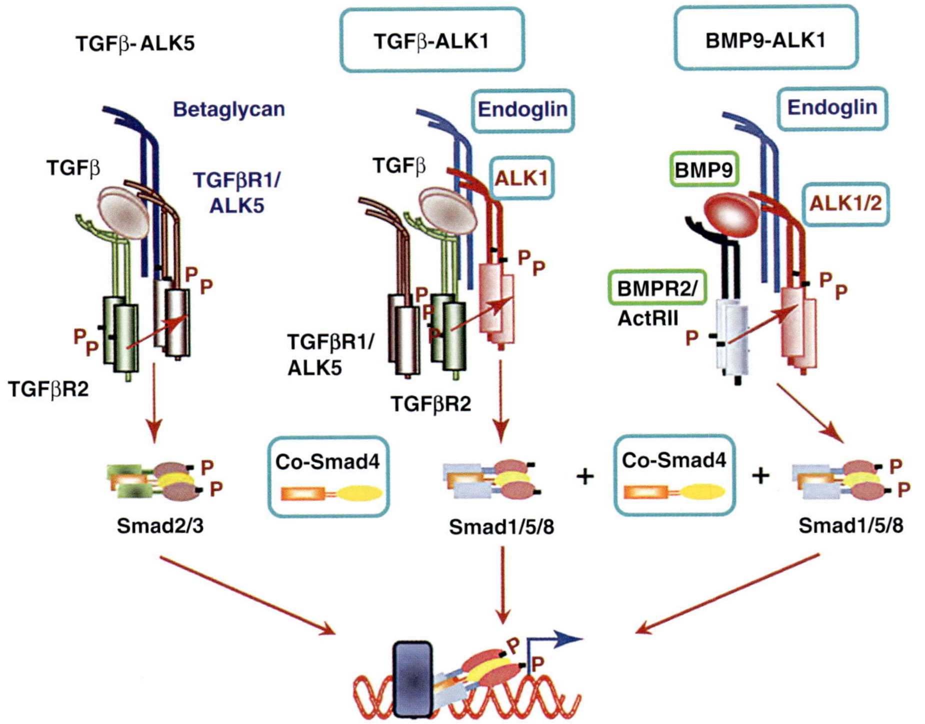

Fig. 1.9. A working model of transforming growth factor-β (TGFβ) and bone morphogenetic protein 9 (BMP9) signaling relevant to arteriovenous malformations (AVM). TGFβ signals through two pathways in endothelial cells, via the activin receptor-like kinases (ALK) 1 and 5. BMP9 signals via ALK1 and the BMP receptor type 2 (BMPR2). Endoglin is a membrane accessory protein required for efficient TGFβ/ALK1 signaling. Genes linked to hereditary hemorrhagic telangiectasia are boxed in teal; other AVM syndrome genes within the pathway are boxed in green. (Adapted from Pardali E, Goumans MJ, ten Dijke P. Signaling by members of the TGF-β family in vascular morphogenesis and disease, *Trends Cell Biol* 2010;20: 556–67, with permission from Elsevier.)

tissue [53]. The increased MMP-9 activity can be expected to cause degradation of the vascular matrix, impairing structural stability of AVM vessels. Interestingly, higher levels of MMP-9 were associated with clinical characteristics that were linked to AVM hemorrhage [63]. There is interest in utilizing MMP inhibitors to stabilize fragile or inflamed blood vessels and prevent their rupture [93–96] and MMP-9 may serve as a pharmacological target to modify clinical behavior of AVMs [70].

Genetics, biomarkers, and implications for arteriovenous malformations management

Genetics of inherited syndromes

Studies of rare Mendelian forms of a disease often generate the first insights into understanding its molecular mechanisms. In the case of brain AVMs, insights into the pathogenesis and pathobiology have come from studies of HHT, a recessively inherited syndrome of mucocutaneous fragility and abnormal artery–vein connections, ranging in size from smaller telangiectases to larger AVMs [97,98]. In HHT, AVMs occur in brain and in visceral organs (lung, liver, gastrointestinal tract). There is significant morbidity and mortality associated with HHT, with the most serious manifestations related to severe bleeding or stroke, most commonly from complications of pulmonary AVM, or from brain AVM rupture. Sporadic AVMs and brain AVMs in HHT are morphologically and functionally similar; however, brain AVM multiplicity is much more likely in HHT than in sporadic AVM [99]. Over 85% of HHT is caused by heterozygous, presumed loss-of-function, mutations in three genes encoding proteins that function in the TGFβ–bone morphogenetic protein (BMP)-9 signaling pathway: *ENG*, *ALK1*, and *SMAD4* (Fig. 1.9) [97,100–105]. Mutations in two other genes encoding proteins in this pathway have been found in patients with HHT-like syndromes that feature lesions similar to AVMs: in *BMPR2* encoding a receptor [106] and in *BMP9*, encoding the ligand [107]. Taken together with mechanistic studies in mouse models, these findings suggest that it is BMP-9 signaling rather than canonical TGFβ signaling that may be deranged in AVM lesions (Fig. 1.9).

Another pathway implicated in brain AVM pathobiology by studies of inherited syndromes is RAS/MAP kinase signaling. Capillary malformations–arteriovenous malformations syndrome, an autosomal dominant disorder featuring both cutaneous capillary malformations ("port-wine stain") and arteriovenous fistulae or AVMs in organs including the brain, is caused by heterozygous inactivating mutations in *RASA1* [108,109]. These mutations have also been found in patients with spinal arteriovenous anomalies [110]. *RASA1* encodes p120-RasGTPase activating protein, a negative inhibitor of the Ras/MAP kinase signaling pathway, which mediates signaling from growth factor receptors and has effects on endothelial cell motility and apoptosis.

Genotype–phenotype correlations

Patients with HHT with different mutated genes show differences in AVM phenotypes. Both pulmonary AVMs [111–114] and brain AVMs [112–114] are more common among patients with *ENG* mutations than *ALK1* mutations; however, differences in brain AVM hemorrhagic presentation are not related to which gene is mutated [115]. Other genetic modifier effects could further alter HHT and AVM clinical manifestations; common polymorphisms in genes located in *TGFB* modifier loci identified in studies of *Tgfβ1* knockout mice have been associated with presence of pulmonary AVM in HHT [116].

Genetics of sporadic brain arteriovenous malformations

Inspired by findings in familial AVM syndromes and in related disorders, candidate gene and, more recently, genome-wide association studies (GWAS) have investigated genetic influences on sporadic AVM etiology. A common non-coding polymorphism in *ALK1*, IVS3-35A>G, was associated with sporadic brain AVM in white patients [117]; this association has been replicated in two independent AVM cohorts [118,119]. Associations with brain AVM have also been reported for common polymorphisms in *ENG* [117], *ITGB8* (encoding integrin-$\alpha_v\beta_8$) [120], *IL1B* [121], *ANGPTL4* (encoding angiopoietin-like protein 4) [122], *GPR124* (encoding G protein-coupled receptor 124) [123], *VEGF* [124], and *MMP3* [125]. The first GWAS, which is taking a hypothesis-free approach and evaluating both single nucleotide polymorphisms [126] and copy number variations [127], is in progress. No associations with brain AVM have yet been replicated [126], and it appears that no other common variants in the known familial AVM syndrome genes have strong genetic associations with sporadic brain AVM [128]. Finally, an association has been reported between brain AVM and genetic variation at the chromosome 9p21 locus [129], which is reproducibly associated with a variety of cardiovascular phenotypes including aortic and intracranial aneurysms [130,131]. This association may be explained by the presence of AVM-associated aneurysms [132].

Somatic mutation hypothesis

In some familial vascular malformations syndromes, patients heterozygous for a germline loss-of-function mutation bear a second-hit somatic inactivating mutation in their wild-type copy of the same gene in lesion cells [133]. This two-hit mechanism has been demonstrated in cerebral cavernous malformations [23] and in multiple cutaneous and mucosal venous malformations [22]. Somatic activating mutations in *GNAQ* have recently been discovered in Sturge–Weber syndrome [134], another vascular malformations syndrome. These precedents, and findings from the mouse models discussed above, suggest that somatic mutations could be involved in HHT and sporadic AVM lesion development. These hypotheses are currently under investigation by high throughput sequencing approaches.

Genetic modifiers of clinical course and biomarkers of disease severity

Whether or not genetic risk factors underlie sporadic AVM etiology, it is well established from other diseases that genetic modifiers can influence disease severity, clinical course, or response to treatment by modulating biological mechanisms such as inflammation, angiogenesis, or response to injury [135–137]. Predictors of brain AVM clinical course and response to therapy would have considerable immediate clinical utility, and the need for biomarkers of hemorrhage risk in both unruptured AVMs and untreatable brain AVMs is particularly urgent. Candidate gene studies of sporadic brain AVM have reported common polymorphisms associated with hemorrhagic presentation of brain AVM (the best currently known risk factor for subsequent hemorrhage) in *IL6* [52] and in *EPHB4* (encoding ephrin B receptor 4) [138] and with hemorrhage in natural course in *IL1B* [121] (also associated with brain AVM risk, see above). Examination of intracerebral hemorrhage presentation of brain AVM using GWAS is underway [139]. The *APOE* (encoding apolipoprotein E) e2 allele [140] and *TNFA* 238G>A [141] have been associated with increased risk of new hemorrhage in the natural course of brain AVM, and also with increased risk of new hemorrhage after treatment [76]. Finally, genetic influences on outcomes after brain AVM surgery are suggested by studies of the brain-derived neurotrophic factor (BDNF) Val66Met variant, which has been implicated in cerebrovascular disease outcomes [142–144]. The Met variant was associated with worse functional outcomes after resection in patients presenting with unruptured AVM [145]. Multiple lines of evidence from genetic studies, imaging studies in AVM tissue and animal models, and imaging studies in patients indicate that inflammation may play a role in sporadic brain AVM pathobiology and clinical behavior, possibly in the context of response-to-injury mechanisms (Table 1.2).

Implications for clinical management

In summary, replication in independent cohorts is still needed to validate the genetic associations reported so far, as well as the preliminary and as yet unpublished results from GWAS of sporadic brain AVM risk and hemorrhagic presentation. Currently only the *ALK1* IVS3-35A>G association has been replicated for white patients. Some of the reported associations are with genomic markers that tag a particular group of genetic variants in the genome (haplotype-tagging variants), while the actual functional variant remains to be identified. However, such markers, if replicated, can still be used as risk predictors even without a known molecular function. A further challenge is that large cohorts are needed to study genetic associations with clinical course and brain AVM subphenotypes. Additional studies are also needed to test the relevance of these associations in other race/ethnic groups. Variant frequencies and biological effects can differ among populations because of epistasis (interaction) with other genetic variants (in sporadic brain AVM, an effect of ancestry was shown for *IL6* 174G>C among Hispanic patients [146]), or with environmental factors. The goal for the future of clinical management of brain AVM is to develop a prediction score for specific clinical course and surgical/therapeutic outcomes that will incorporate genotypes of common polymorphisms alongside epidemiological and morphological risk factors (e.g., type of presentation, AVM size, location, age, sex, ethnicity). The advent of personal genomes will increase future availability of genotype information for screening and risk assessment.

Table 1.2. Common genetic polymorphisms associated with sporadic brain arteriovenous malformations phenotypes

Brain phenotype	Variant	Functional or tagging variant
Brain AVM	*ALK1* IVS3–35A>G	Unknown, potential splicing? [117,119]
	ENG 207A>G	Unknown, synonymous Leu69 [117]
	ITGB8 rs10486391	Tagging/marker [120]
	ANGPTL4 rs11672433	Tagging (synonymous Pro389) [122]
	IL1B 31T>C, 511T>C	Promoter; transcription [121]
	GPR124 rs7015566	Tagging/marker [123]
Brain AVM aneurysm	chr9p21 rs1333040	Tagging/marker [129,132]
Hemorrhagic presentation	*EPHB4* rs314308, rs314313	Tagging/marker [138]
	IL6 174G>C	Promoter; transcription [52]
New hemorrhage in natural course and after treatment	*APOE* e2	Coding (alters protein function) [76,140]
	IL1B 31T>C,–511T>C	Promoter, transcription [121]
Outcome after surgery (unruptured only)	*TNFα* 238G>A	Promoter, transcription [76,141]
	BDNF rs6265 Val66Met	Coding, affects activity-dependent brain-derived neurotrophic factor secretion [145]

AVM, arteriovenous malformations.
See text for more details of genes.

Conclusions

The pathogenesis and pathophysiology of brain AVMs are complex and currently unclear. However, it is quite clear that these are not static lesions that can be dismissed as congenital anomalies. Rather, they are dynamic lesions that may be the result of vasculogenesis gone awry or may develop after birth. Genetic abnormalities appear to be involved with AVM pathogenesis, as are events such as injury that lead to angiogenesis. While AVMs have long been considered to be present at birth, this idea has been challenged by experimental models in animals and clinical case reports showing de novo AVM formation. Hemodynamic forces are constantly degrading AVMs, leading to inflammation and vascular instability. Angiogenesis appears to be involved with ongoing repair of AVMs, and imbalances between degradation and repair can lead to rupture with catastrophic consequences. The body of research presented in this chapter demonstrates that the mystery of AVM formation has yet to be solved. Progress is being made, and that progress will eventually lead not only to answers but also to better models with which to study AVM pathophysiology and novel therapies to stabilize those AVMs deemed too risky for therapeutic intervention.

References

1. Lasjaunias P, Berenstein A, terBrugge KG. *Surgical Neuroangiography:* Vol. 1 *Clinical Vascular Anatomy and Variations*, 2nd edn. Berlin: Springer, 2001.
2. Padget DH. The development of the cranial arteries in the human embryo. *Contrib Embryol* 1948;**212**:207–61.
3. Bautch VL, James JM. Neurovascular development: the beginning of a beautiful friendship. *Cell Adh Migr* 2009;**3**:199–204.
4. Lo EH, Rosenberg GA. The neurovascular unit in health and disease: introduction. *Stroke* 2009;**40**:S2–S3.
5. Osborn AG. *Diagnostic Cerebral Angiography*, 2nd edn. Philadelphia, PA: Lippincott, Williams & Wilkins, 1999.
6. Aurboonyawat T, Suthipongchai S, Pereira V, *et al.* Patterns of cranial venous system from the comparative anatomy in vertebrates. Part I, introduction and the dorsal venous system. *Interv Neuroradiol* 2007;**13**:335–44.
7. Padget DH. The development of the cranial venous system in man: From the viewpoint of comparative anatomy. *Contrib Embryol* 1957;**221**:81–139.
8. Meyers PM, Halbach VV, Barkovich AJ. Anomalies of cerebral vasculature: Diagnostic and endovascular considerations. In Barkovich AJ, ed. *Pediatric Neuroimaging*, 4th edn. Philadelphia, PA: Lippincott, Williams & Wilkins, 2005, pp. 870–911.
9. McDonald DA, Shi C, Shenkar R, *et al.* Fasudil decreases lesion burden in a murine model of cerebral cavernous malformation disease. *Stroke* 2012;**43**:571–4.
10. Cavalcanti DD, Kalani MY, Martirosyan NL, *et al.* Cerebral cavernous malformations: from genes to proteins to disease. *J Neurosurg* 2012;**116**:122–32.

11. McDonald DA, Shenkar R, Shi C, *et al.* A novel mouse model of cerebral cavernous malformations based on the two-hit mutation hypothesis recapitulates the human disease. *Hum Mol Genet* 2011;**20**:211–22.

12. Riant F, Bergametti F, Ayrignac X, *et al.* Recent insights into cerebral cavernous malformations: the molecular genetics of CCM. *FEBS J* 2010;**277**:1070–5.

13. Mahmoud M, Allinson KR, Zhai Z, *et al.* Pathogenesis of arteriovenous malformations in the absence of endoglin. *Circ Res* 2010;**106**:1425–33.

14. Srinivasan S, Hanes MA, Dickens T, *et al.* A mouse model for hereditary hemorrhagic telangiectasia (HHT) type 2. *Hum Mol Genet* 2003;**12**:473–82.

15. Bourdeau A, Faughnan ME, Letarte M. Endoglin-deficient mice, a unique model to study hereditary hemorrhagic telangiectasia. *Trends Cardiovasc Med* 2000;**10**:279–85.

16. Urness LD, Sorensen LK, Li DY. Arteriovenous malformations in mice lacking activin receptor-like kinase-1. *Nat Genet* 2000;**26**:328–31.

17. Sorensen LK, Brooke BS, Li DY, *et al.* Loss of distinct arterial and venous boundaries in mice lacking endoglin, a vascular-specific TGFβ coreceptor. *Dev Biol* 2003;**261**:235–50.

18. Milton I, Ouyang D, Allen CJ, *et al.* Age-dependent lethality in novel transgenic mouse models of central nervous system arteriovenous malformations. *Stroke* 2012;**43**:1432–5.

19. Park SO, Wankhede M, Lee YJ, *et al.* Real-time imaging of de novo arteriovenous malformation in a mouse model of hereditary hemorrhagic telangiectasia. *J Clin Invest* 2009;**119**:3487–96.

20. Choi EJ, Walker EJ, Shen F, *et al.* Minimal homozygous endothelial deletion of *Eng* with VEGF stimulation is sufficient to cause cerebrovascular dysplasia in the adult mouse. *Cerebrovasc Dis* 2012;**33**:540–7.

21. Bourdeau A, Cymerman U, Paquet ME, *et al.* Endoglin expression is reduced in normal vessels but still detectable in arteriovenous malformations of patients with hereditary hemorrhagic telangiectasia type 1. *Am J Pathol* 2000;**156**:911–23.

22. Limaye N, Wouters V, Uebelhoer M, *et al.* Somatic mutations in angiopoietin receptor gene TEK cause solitary and multiple sporadic venous malformations. *Nat Genet* 2009;**41**:118–24.

23. Akers AL, Johnson E, Steinberg GK, *et al.* Biallelic somatic and germline mutations in cerebral cavernous malformations (CCMs): evidence for a two-hit mechanism of CCM pathogenesis. *Hum Mol Genet* 2009;**18**:919–30.

24. Chen Y, Zhu W, Bollen AW, *et al.* Evidence of inflammatory cell involvement in brain arteriovenous malformations. *Neurosurgery* 2008;**62**:1340–9.

25. Torsney E, Charlton R, Diamond AG, *et al.* Mouse model for hereditary hemorrhagic telangiectasia has a generalized vascular abnormality. *Circulation* 2003;**107**:1653–7.

26. Satomi J, Mount RJ, Toporsian M, *et al.* Cerebral vascular abnormalities in a murine model of hereditary hemorrhagic telangiectasia. *Stroke* 2003;**34**:783–9.

27. Xu B, Wu YQ, Huey M, *et al.* Vascular endothelial growth factor induces abnormal microvasculature in the endoglin heterozygous mouse brain. *J Cereb Blood Flow Metab* 2004;**24**:237–44.

28. Hao Q, Su H, Marchuk DA, *et al.* Increased tissue perfusion promotes capillary dysplasia in the ALK1-deficient mouse brain following VEGF stimulation. *Am J Physiol Heart Circ Physiol* 2008;**295**:H2250–6.

29. Hao Q, Zhu Y, Su H, *et al.* VEGF induces more severe cerebrovascular dysplasia in endoglin than in Alk1 mice. *Transl Stroke Res* 2010;**1**:197–201.

30. Walker E, Shen F, Halprin R, *et al.* Regional deletion of *Smad4* plus VEGF stimulation leads to vascular dysplasia in the adult mouse brain. *Stroke* 2010;**41**:e20.

31. Choi EJ, Walker EJ, Degos V, *et al.* Endoglin deficiency in bone marrow is sufficient to cause cerebrovascular dysplasia in the adult mouse after vascular endothelial growth factor stimulation. *Stroke* 2013;**44**:795–8.

32. Hao Q, Su H, Palmer D, *et al.* Bone marrow-derived cells contribute to vascular endothelial growth factor-induced angiogenesis in the adult mouse brain by supplying matrix metalloproteinase-9. *Stroke* 2011;**42**:453–8.

33. van Laake LW, van den Driesche S, Post S, *et al.* Endoglin has a crucial role in blood cell-mediated vascular repair. *Circulation* 2006;**114**:2288–97.

34. Li Y, Hiroi Y, Ngoy S, *et al.* Notch1 in bone marrow-derived cells mediates cardiac repair after myocardial infarction. *Circulation* 2011;**123**:866–76.

35. Post S, Smits AM, van den Broek AJ, *et al.* Impaired recruitment of HHT-1 mononuclear cells to the ischaemic heart is due to an altered CXCR4/CD26 balance. *Cardiovasc Res* 2010;**85**:494–502.

36. Fantin A, Vieira JM, Gestri G, *et al.* Tissue macrophages act as cellular chaperones for vascular anastomosis downstream of VEGF-mediated endothelial tip cell induction. *Blood* 2010;**116**:829–40.

37. Outtz HH, Tattersall IW, Kofler NM, *et al.* Notch1 controls macrophage recruitment and Notch signaling is activated at sites of endothelial cell anastomosis during retinal angiogenesis in mice. *Blood* 2011;**118**:3436–9.

38. Rafii S, Lyden D. Cancer. A few to flip the angiogenic switch. *Science* 2008;**319**:163–4.

39. Gao D, Nolan DJ, Mellick AS, *et al.* Endothelial progenitor cells control the angiogenic switch in mouse lung metastasis. *Science* 2008;**319**:195–8.

40. Hao Q, Liu J, Pappu R, *et al.* Contribution of bone marrow-derived cells associated with brain angiogenesis is primarily through leukocytes and macrophages. *Arterioscler Thromb Vasc Biol* 2008;**28**:2151–7.

41. Gao P, Chen Y, Lawton MT, *et al.* Evidence of endothelial progenitor cells in the human brain and spinal cord arteriovenous malformations. *Neurosurgery* 2010;**67**:1029–35.

42. Hao Q, Chen Y, Zhu Y, *et al.* Neutrophil depletion decreases VEGF-induced focal angiogenesis in the mature mouse brain. *J Cereb Blood Flow Metab* 2007;**27**:1853–60.

43. Hashimoto T, Matsumoto M, Tsang EJ, *et al.* Critical roles of neutrophils and macrophages in flow-induced adaptive outward vascular remodeling. *J Neurosurg Anesthesiol* 2006;**18**:293.

44. Young WL, Kader A, Pile-Spellman J, *et al.* Arteriovenous malformation draining vein physiology and determinants of transnidal pressure gradients. The Columbia University AVM Study Project. *Neurosurgery* 1994;**35**:389–95.

45. Terada T, Higashida RT, Halbach VV, *et al.* Development of acquired arteriovenous fistulas in rats due to venous hypertension. *J Neurosurg* 1994;**80**:884–9.

46. Lawton MT, Jacobowitz R, Spetzler RF. Redefined role of angiogenesis in the pathogenesis of dural arteriovenous malformations. *J Neurosurg* 1997;**87**:267–74.

47. Zhu Y, Lawton MT, Du R, *et al.* Expression of hypoxia-inducible factor-1 and vascular endothelial growth factor in response to venous hypertension. *Neurosurgery* 2006;**59**:687–96.

48. Gao P, Zhu Y, Ling F, *et al.* Nonischemic cerebral venous hypertension promotes a pro-angiogenic stage through HIF-1 downstream genes and leukocyte-derived MMP-9. *J Cereb Blood Flow Metab* 2009;**29**:1482–90.

49. Germano IM, Davis RL, Wilson CB, *et al.* Histopathological follow-up study of 66 cerebral arteriovenous malformations after therapeutic embolization with polyvinyl alcohol. *J Neurosurg* 1992;**76**:607–14.

50. Hernandez-Rodriguez J, Molloy ES, Calabrese LH, *et al.* Arteriovenous malformation of the brain mimicking primary central nervous system vasculitis. *Scand J Rheumatol* 2008;**37**:481–4.

51. Natarajan SK, Born D, Ghodke B, *et al.* Histopathological changes in brain arteriovenous malformations after embolization using Onyx or *N*-butyl cyanoacrylate. *J Neurosurg* 2009;**111**:105–13.

52. Pawlikowska L, Tran MN, Achrol AS, *et al.* Polymorphisms in genes involved in inflammatory and angiogenic pathways and the risk of hemorrhagic presentation of brain arteriovenous malformations. *Stroke* 2004;**35**:2294–300.

53. Chen Y, Fan Y, Poon KY, *et al.* MMP-9 expression is associated with leukocytic but not endothelial markers in brain arteriovenous malformations. *Front Biosci* 2006;**11**:3121–8.

54. Shenkar R, Shi C, Check IJ, *et al.* Concepts and hypotheses: inflammatory hypothesis in the pathogenesis of cerebral cavernous malformations. *Neurosurgery* 2007;**61**:693–702.

55. Aziz MM, Takagi Y, Hashimoto N, *et al.* Activation of nuclear factor kappaB in cerebral arteriovenous malformations. *Neurosurgery* 2010;**67**:1669–79.

56. Sturiale CL, Puca A, Sebastiani P, *et al.* Single nucleotide polymorphisms associated with sporadic brain arteriovenous malformations: where do we stand? *Brain* 2013;**136**:665–81.

57. Chen W, Guo Y, Walker EJ, *et al.* Reduced mural cell coverage and impaired vessel integrity after angiogenic stimulation in the Alk1-deficient brain. *Arterioscler Thromb Vasc Biol* 2013;**33**:305–10.

58. Chen W, Guo Y, Bollen AW, Hua S, Young WL. Reduced PDGFR-beta expression after regional Alk1 deletion and VEGF stimulation in the brain is associated with reduced mural cell coverage. *Stroke* 2012;**43**:A3169.

59. Chen W, Guo Y, Jun K, *et al.* Alk1 deficiency impairs mural cell recruitment during brain angiogenesis. *Stroke* 2013;**44**:ATMP118.

60. Guo Y, Saunders T, Su H, *et al.* Silent intralesional microhemorrhage as a risk factor for brain arteriovenous malformation rupture. *Stroke* 2012;**43**:1240–6.

61. Braverman IM, Keh A, Jacobson BS. Ultrastructure and three-dimensional organization of the telangiectases of hereditary hemorrhagic telangiectasia. *J Invest Dermatol* 1990;**95**:422–7.

62. Nagase H, Meng Q, Malinovskii V, *et al.* Engineering of selective TIMPs. *Ann N Y Acad Sci* 1999;**878**:1–11.

63. Hashimoto T, Wen G, Lawton MT, *et al.* Abnormal expression of matrix metalloproteinases and tissue inhibitors of metalloproteinases in brain arteriovenous malformations. *Stroke* 2003;**34**:925–31.

64. Rosenberg GA. Matrix metalloproteinases in neuroinflammation. *Glia* 2002;**39**:279–91.

65. Visse R, Nagase H. Matrix metalloproteinases and tissue inhibitors of metalloproteinases: structure, function, and biochemistry. *Circ Res* 2003;**92**:827–39.

66. Venkatesha S, Toporsian M, Lam C, *et al.* Soluble endoglin contributes to the pathogenesis of preeclampsia. *Nat Med* 2006;**12**:642–9.

67. Velasco S, varez-Munoz P, Pericacho M, *et al.* L- and S-endoglin differentially modulate TGFbeta1 signaling mediated by ALK1 and ALK5 in L6E9 myoblasts. *J Cell Sci* 2008;**121**:913–19.

68. Chen Y, Hao Q, Kim H, *et al.* Soluble endoglin modulates aberrant cerebral vascular remodeling. *Ann Neurol* 2009;**66**:19–27.

69. Velasco-Loyden G, Arribas J, Lopez-Casillas F. The shedding of betaglycan is regulated by pervanadate and mediated by membrane type matrix metalloprotease-1. *J Biol Chem* 2004;**279**:7721–33.

70. Hashimoto T, Matsumoto MM, Li JF, *et al.* Suppression of MMP-9 by doxycycline in brain arteriovenous malformations. *BMC Neurol* 2005;**5**:1.

71. Chen Y, Pawlikowska L, Yao JS, *et al.* Interleukin-6 involvement in brain arteriovenous malformations. *Ann Neurol* 2006;**59**:72–80.

72. Cudmore M, Ahmad S, Al-Ani B, *et al.* Negative regulation of soluble Flt-1 and soluble endoglin release by heme oxygenase-1. *Circulation* 2007;**115**:1789–97.

73. Chyatte D, Bruno G, Desai S, *et al.* Inflammation and intracranial aneurysms. *Neurosurgery* 1999;**45**:1137–46.

74. Eliason JL, Hannawa KK, Ailawadi G, *et al.* Neutrophil depletion inhibits experimental abdominal aortic aneurysm formation. *Circulation* 2005;**112**:232–40.

75. Thompson S, Kim L, Scott A. Screening for abdominal aortic aneurysm: screening reduces deaths related to aneurysm. *BMJ* 2005;**330**:601–2.

76. Achrol AS, Kim H, Pawlikowska L, *et al.* Association of tumor necrosis factor-alpha-238G>A and apolipoprotein E2 polymorphisms with intracranial hemorrhage after brain arteriovenous malformation treatment. *Neurosurgery* 2007;**61**:731–9.

77. Hoefer IE, van Royen N, Rectenwald JE, *et al.* Arteriogenesis proceeds via ICAM-1/Mac-1-mediated mechanisms. *Circ Res* 2004;**94**:1179–85.

78. Tzima E, del Pozo MA, Shattil SJ, *et al.* Activation of integrins in endothelial cells by fluid shear stress mediates Rho-dependent cytoskeletal alignment. *EMBO J* 2001;**20**:4639–47.

79. Shyy JY, Chien S. Role of integrins in cellular responses to mechanical stress and adhesion. *Curr Opin Cell Biol* 1997;**9**:707–13.

80. Shyy YJ, Hsieh HJ, Usami S, *et al.* Fluid shear stress induces a biphasic response of human monocyte chemotactic protein 1 gene expression in vascular endothelium. *Proc Natl Acad Sci USA* 1994;**91**:4678–82.

81. Chien S, Li S, Shyy YJ. Effects of mechanical forces on signal transduction and gene expression in endothelial cells. *Hypertension* 1998;**31**:162–9.

82. Malek AM, Gibbons GH, Dzau VJ, *et al.* Fluid shear stress differentially modulates expression of genes encoding basic fibroblast growth factor and platelet-derived growth factor B chain in vascular endothelium. *J Clin Invest* 1993;**92**:2013–21.

83. Tronc F, Mallat Z, Lehoux S, *et al.* Role of matrix metalloproteinases in blood flow-induced arterial enlargement: interaction with NO. *Arterioscler Thromb Vasc Biol* 2000;**20**:E120–6.

84. Bergers G, Brekken R, McMahon G, *et al.* Matrix metalloproteinase-9 triggers the angiogenic switch during carcinogenesis. *Nat Cell Biol* 2000;**2**:737–44.

85. Arteriovenous Malformation Study Group. Arteriovenous malformation of the brain in adults. *N Engl J Med* 1999;**340**:1812–18.

86. Hashimoto T, Mesa-Tejada R, Quick CM, *et al.* Evidence of increased endothelial cell turnover in brain arteriovenous malformations. *Neurosurgery* 2001;**49**:124–31.

87. Hatva E, Jaaskelainen J, Hirvonen H, *et al.* Tie endothelial cell-specific receptor tyrosine kinase is upregulated in the vasculature of arteriovenous malformations. *J Neuropathol Exp Neurol* 1996;**55**:1124–33.

88. Kader A, Goodrich JT, Sonstein WJ, *et al.* Recurrent cerebral arteriovenous malformations after negative postoperative angiograms. *J Neurosurg* 1996;**85**:14–18.

89. Sonstein WJ, Kader A, Michelsen WJ, *et al.* Expression of vascular endothelial growth factor in pediatric and adult cerebral arteriovenous malformations: an immunocytochemical study. *J Neurosurg* 1996;**85**:838–45.

90. Hashimoto T, Emala CW, Joshi S, *et al.* Abnormal pattern of Tie-2 and vascular endothelial growth factor receptor expression in human cerebral arteriovenous malformations. *Neurosurgery* 2000;**47**:910–18.

91. Shenkar R, Elliott JP, Diener K, *et al.* Differential gene expression in human cerebrovascular malformations. *Neurosurgery* 2003;**52**:465–77.

92. Uranishi R, Baev NI, Kim JH, *et al.* Vascular smooth muscle cell differentiation in human cerebral vascular malformations. *Neurosurgery* 2001;**49**:671–9.

93. Rosenberg GA. Growth and bleeding in BAVM: another role for MMPs. *Stroke* 2003;**34**:925–31.

94. Curci JA, Mao D, Bohner DG, *et al.* Preoperative treatment with doxycycline reduces aortic wall expression and activation of matrix metalloproteinases in patients with abdominal aortic aneurysms. *J Vasc Surg* 2000;**31**:325–42.

95. Axisa B, Loftus IM, Naylor AR, *et al.* Prospective, randomized, double-blind trial investigating the effect of doxycycline on matrix metalloproteinase expression within atherosclerotic carotid plaques. *Stroke* 2002;**33**:2858–64.

96. Lee CZ, Xu B, Hashimoto T, *et al.* Doxycycline suppresses cerebral matrix metalloproteinase-9 and angiogenesis induced by focal hyperstimulation of vascular endothelial growth factor in a mouse model. *Stroke* 2004;**35**:1715–19.

97. Faughnan ME, Palda VA, Garcia-Tsao G, *et al.* International guidelines for the diagnosis and management of hereditary haemorrhagic telangiectasia. *J Med Genet* 2011;**48**:73–87.

98. Shovlin CL. Hereditary haemorrhagic telangiectasia: pathophysiology, diagnosis and treatment. *Blood Rev* 2010;**24**:203–19.

99. Bharatha A, Faughnan ME, Kim H, *et al.* Brain arteriovenous malformation multiplicity predicts the diagnosis of hereditary hemorrhagic telangiectasia: quantitative assessment. *Stroke* 2012;**43**:72–8.

100. McAllister KA, Grogg KM, Johnson DW, *et al.* Endoglin, a TGF-beta binding protein of endothelial cells, is the gene for hereditary haemorrhagic telangiectasia type 1. *Nat Genet* 1994;**8**:345–51.

101. Shovlin CL, Hughes JM, Tuddenham EG, *et al.* A gene for hereditary haemorrhagic telangiectasia maps to chromosome 9q3. *Nat Genet* 1994;**6**:205–9.

102. Johnson DW, Berg JN, Gallione CJ, *et al.* A second locus for hereditary hemorrhagic telangiectasia maps to chromosome 12. *Genome Res* 1995;**5**:21–8.

103. Vincent P, Plauchu H, Hazan J, *et al.* A third locus for hereditary haemorrhagic telangiectasia maps to chromosome 12q. *Hum Mol Genet* 1995;**4**:945–9.

104. Gallione CJ, Repetto GM, Legius E, *et al.* A combined syndrome of juvenile polyposis and hereditary haemorrhagic telangiectasia associated with mutations in *MADH4 (SMAD4)*. *Lancet* 2004;**363**:852–9.

105. Gallione CJ, Richards JA, Letteboer TG, *et al.* *SMAD4* mutations found in unselected HHT patients. *J Med Genet* 2006;**43**:793–7.

106. Rigelsky CM, Jennings C, Lehtonen R, *et al.* *BMPR2* mutation in a patient with pulmonary arterial hypertension and suspected hereditary hemorrhagic telangiectasia. *Am J Med Genet A* 2008;**146**:2551–6.

107. Wooderchak-Donahue WL, McDonald J, O'Fallon B, *et al.* *BMP9* mutations cause a vascular-anomaly syndrome with phenotypic overlap with hereditary hemorrhagic telangiectasia. *Am J Hum Genet* 2013;**93**:530–7.

108. Eerola I, Boon LM, Mulliken JB, *et al.* Capillary malformation-arteriovenous malformation, a new clinical and genetic disorder caused by *RASA1* mutations. *Am J Hum Genet* 2003;**73**:1240–9.

109. Wooderchak-Donahue W, Stevenson DA, McDonald J, *et al.* RASA1 analysis: clinical and molecular findings in a series of consecutive cases. *Eur J Med Genet* 2012;**55**:91–5.

110. Thiex R, Mulliken JB, Revencu N, *et al.* A novel association between *RASA1* mutations and spinal arteriovenous anomalies. *AJNR Am J Neuroradiol* 2010;**31**:775–9.

111. Lesca G, Olivieri C, Burnichon N, *et al.* Genotype–phenotype correlations in hereditary hemorrhagic telangiectasia: data from the French-Italian HHT network. *Genet Med* 2007;**9**:14–22.
112. Letteboer TG, Mager JJ, Snijder RJ, *et al.* Genotype–phenotype relationship in hereditary haemorrhagic telangiectasia. *J Med Genet* 2006;**43**:371–7.
113. Sabba C, Pasculli G, Lenato GM, *et al.* Hereditary hemorrhagic telangiectasia: clinical features in *ENG* and *ALK1* mutation carriers. *J Thromb Haemost* 2007;**5**:1149–57.
114. Bayrak-Toydemir P, McDonald J, Markewitz B, *et al.* Genotype–phenotype correlation in hereditary hemorrhagic telangiectasia: mutations and manifestations. *Am J Med Genet A* 2006;**140**:463–70.
115. Nishida T, Faughnan ME, Chakinala M. Correlations between genotypes and clinical manifestations in brain AVMs with HHT. *Hematol Rep* 2011;**3**:10–11.
116. Benzinou M, Clermont FF, Letteboer TG, *et al.* Mouse and human strategies identify PTPN14 as a modifier of angiogenesis and hereditary haemorrhagic telangiectasia. *Nat Commun* 2012;**3**:616.
117. Pawlikowska L, Tran MN, Achrol AS, *et al.* Polymorphisms in transforming growth factor-beta-related genes *ALK1* and *ENG* are associated with sporadic brain arteriovenous malformations. *Stroke* 2005;**36**:2278–80.
118. Simon M, Schramm J, Ludwig M, *et al.* Author reply to letter by Young WL et al., "Arteriovenous malformation." *J Neurosurg* 2007;**106**:732–3.
119. Simon M, Franke D, Ludwig M, *et al.* Association of a polymorphism of the *ACVRL1* gene with sporadic arteriovenous malformations of the central nervous system. *J Neurosurg* 2006;**104**:945–9.
120. Su H, Kim H, Pawlikowska L, *et al.* Reduced expression of integrin alphavbeta8 is associated with brain arteriovenous malformation pathogenesis. *Am J Pathol* 2010;**176**:1018–27.
121. Kim H, Hysi PG, Pawlikowska L, *et al.* Common variants in interleukin-1-beta gene are associated with intracranial hemorrhage and susceptibility to brain arteriovenous malformation. *Cerebrovasc Dis* 2009;**27**:176–82.
122. Mikhak B, Weinsheimer S, Pawlikowska L, *et al.* Angiopoietin-like 4 (*ANGPTL4*) gene polymorphisms and risk of brain arteriovenous malformations. *Cerebrovasc Dis* 2011;**31**:338–45.
123. Weinsheimer S, Brettman AD, Pawlikowska L, *et al.* G protein-coupled receptor 124 (*GPR124*) gene polymorphisms and risk of brain arteriovenous malformation. *Transl Stroke Res* 2012;**3**:418–27.
124. Chen H, Gu Y, Wu W, *et al.* Polymorphisms of the vascular endothelial growth factor A gene and susceptibility to sporadic brain arteriovenous malformation in a Chinese population. *J Clin Neurosci* 2011;**18**:549–53.
125. Zhao Y, Li P, Fan W, *et al.* The rs522616 polymorphism in the matrix metalloproteinase-3 (MMP-3) gene is associated with sporadic brain arteriovenous malformation in a Chinese population. *J Clin Neurosci* 2010;**17**:1568–72.
126. Weinsheimer S, Kim H, Pawlikowska L, *et al.* Genome-wide association study of brain arteriovenous malformation patients. *Stroke* 2011; **42**:e135.
127. Bendjilali N, Kim H, Weinsheimer S, *et al.* A genome-wide investigation of copy number variation in patients with sporadic brain arteriovenous malformation. *PLoS One* 2013;**8**:e71434.
128. Weinsheimer S, Bendjilali N, Pawlikowska L, *et al.* Common polymorphisms in familial vascular malformation genes do not show association with sporadic brain arteriovenous malformation. *Stroke* 2012; abstract 3666.
129. Sturiale CL, Gatto I, Puca A, *et al.* Association between the rs1333040 polymorphism on the chromosomal 9p21 locus and sporadic brain arteriovenous malformations. *J Neurol Neurosurg Psychiatry* 2013;**84**:1059–62.
130. Holdt LM, Teupser D. Recent studies of the human chromosome 9p21 locus, which is associated with atherosclerosis in human populations. *Arterioscler Thromb Vasc Biol* 2012;**32**:196–206.
131. Helgadottir A, Thorleifsson G, Magnusson KP, *et al.* The same sequence variant on 9p21 associates with myocardial infarction, abdominal aortic aneurysm and intracranial aneurysm. *Nat Genet* 2008;**40**:217–24.
132. Bendjilali N, Nelson J, Weinsheimer S, *et al.* Genetic variants on 9p21.3 are associated with brain arteriovenous malformations with associated arterial aneurysms. *J Neurol Neurosurg Psychiatry* 2014;in press.
133. Brouillard P, Vikkula M. Genetic causes of vascular malformations. *Hum Mol Genet* 2007;**16**(Spec No. 2):R140–9.
134. Shirley MD, Tang H, Gallione CJ, *et al.* Sturge–Weber syndrome and port-wine stains caused by somatic mutation in GNAQ. *N Engl J Med* 2013;**368**:1971–9.
135. Emond MJ, Louie T, Emerson J, *et al.* Exome sequencing of extreme phenotypes identifies DCTN4 as a modifier of chronic *Pseudomonas aeruginosa* infection in cystic fibrosis. *Nat Genet* 2012;**44**:886–9.
136. Wright FA, Strug LJ, Doshi VK, *et al.* Genome-wide association and linkage identify modifier loci of lung disease severity in cystic fibrosis at 11p13 and 20q13.2. *Nat Genet* 2011;**43**:539–46.
137. Drumm ML, Konstan MW, Schluchter MD, *et al.* Genetic modifiers of lung disease in cystic fibrosis. *N Engl J Med* 2005;**353**:1443–53.
138. Weinsheimer S, Kim H, Pawlikowska L, *et al.* *EPHB4* gene polymorphisms and risk of intracranial hemorrhage in patients with brain arteriovenous malformations. *Circ Cardiovasc Genet* 2009;**2**:476–82.
139. Weinsheimer S, Pawlikowska L, Xu H. Integration of genome-wide SNP and expression profiling data to identify candidate genes for brain arteriovenous malformation hemorrhage. In *American Society of Human Genetics 59th Annual Meeting Honolulu*, 2009.
140. Pawlikowska L, Poon KY, Achrol AS, *et al.* Apolipoprotein E epsilon 2 is associated with new hemorrhage risk in brain arteriovenous malformations. *Neurosurgery* 2006;**58**:838–43.
141. Achrol AS, Pawlikowska L, McCulloch CE, *et al.* Tumor necrosis factor-α: 238G>A promoter polymorphism is associated with increased risk of new hemorrhage in the natural course of patients with brain arteriovenous malformations. *J Neurosurg Anesthesiol* 2005;**17**:217–218.
142. McAllister TW, Tyler AL, Flashman LA, *et al.* Polymorphisms in the brain-derived neurotrophic factor gene influence memory and

processing speed one month after brain injury. *J Neurotrauma* 2012;**29**:1111–18.

143. Qin L, Kim E, Ratan R, *et al.* Genetic variant of BDNF (Val66Met) polymorphism attenuates stroke-induced angiogenic responses by enhancing anti-angiogenic mediator CD36 expression. *J Neurosci* 2011;**31**:775–83.

144. Siironen J, Juvela S, Kanarek K, *et al.* The Met allele of the *BDNF* Val66Met polymorphism predicts poor outcome among survivors of aneurysmal subarachnoid hemorrhage. *Stroke* 2007;**38**:2858–60.

145. Westbroek EM, Pawlikowska L, Lawton MT, *et al.* Brain-derived neurotrophic factor Val66Met polymorphism predicts worse functional outcome after surgery in patients with unruptured brain arteriovenous malformation. *Stroke* 2012;**43**:2255–7.

146. Kim H, Hysi PG, Pawlikowska L, *et al.* Population stratification in a case-control study of brain arteriovenous malformation in Latinos. *Neuroepidemiology* 2008;**31**:224–8.

Chapter 2

Cranial vascular anatomy and implications for treatment of arteriovenous malformations and dural arteriovenous fistulae

James D. Rabinov, Donnie Bell, and Joshua A. Hirsch

Introduction

There are many facets of cranial vascular anatomy and physiology that influence natural history and treatment strategies of brain arteriovenous malformations (AVM) and dural arteriovenous fistula (DAVF). This chapter will describe the anatomy of the native cerebral vasculature and the normal variants and types of collateral circulation that are recruited by these lesions. It will discuss how these anatomical elements are altered to serve the angioarchitecture of AVMs and DAVFs. The goal is to provide a rational basis for treatment considerations that will be discussed in the following chapters.

Cervical and cranial vascular anatomy has a plasticity that adjusts to the vascular needs of the normal tissue range of physiology as well as to a number of pathological conditions. Brain AVM nidus can have a variety of appearances from a compact mass to a diffuse infiltrative pattern with intervening parenchyma. Discrete arteriovenous shunts or aneurysms are architectural elements that bear on the natural history of these lesions. Local arterial anatomy of a brain AVM may include direct arterial vessels or indirect supply. By analogy, DAVFs may also have a focal point of shunt into a single venous channel or a diffuse surface over a dural sinus. Collateral circulation can play a major role in both brain AVMs and DAVFs. While intracranial collateral circulation plays a dominant role for brain AVMs, the extracranial collateral circulation plays a dominant role for DAVFs through the skull base. Finally, venous anatomy and physiology have a major role in the natural history and risks of treatment of these lesions.

Cervical and intracranial arterial anatomy

Anterior circulation anatomy

The internal carotid artery (ICA) can be divided into two segments: the proximal segment derived from the third branchial arch consisting of the carotid bulb, ascending cervical, and foramen lacerum segments, and the distal segment derived from the bilateral paired dorsal aortae, consisting of the cavernous, clinoid, ophthalmic, and communicating segments.

Bouthillier *et al.* described seven segments of the ICA [1]. The C1 segment extends from the common carotid bifurcation to the carotid canal of the petrous bone. There are no branches that arise from this portion.

The petrous segment or C2 portion of the ICA begins as the vessel enters the carotid canal and can be divided into vertical and horizontal components. There are two branches of the C2 portion of the ICA, the vidian and the caroticotympanic arteries. The vidian artery exits the cranium via the foramen lacerum and may have anastomosis with the internal maxillary artery. The caroticotympanic artery arises from the C2 segment near the genu, and passes superiorly through the stapes to supply the middle ear cavity. This artery may anastomose with the external carotid artery via the inferior tympanic branch of the ascending pharyngeal artery.

The C3 segment, or lacerum segment, of the ICA typically has no branches.

The C4 segment traverses the cavernous sinus. There are three branch arteries that may arise from the C4 segment including the meningohypophyseal artery (posterior), inferior lateral trunk (ILT; lateral), and the capsular artery of McConnell (medial). The meningohypophyseal artery arises from the posterior genu of the C4 segment and supplies the pituitary gland, clivus, and tentorium. The ILT arises from the lateral aspect of the horizontal component of the C4 segment and crosses cranial nerve VI as it courses through the cavernous sinus. This artery is significant for two reasons: first, it supplies cranial nerves III, IV, and VI, the Gasserion ganglion, and the cavernous sinus dura; second it forms external carotid artery (ECA) to ICA (ECA–ICA) collaterals via the artery of foramen rotundum with the internal maxillary artery and via posterior branches with the middle meningeal artery and maxillary artery. The least consistent of the C4 segment branches is the capsular artery of McConnell, which is seen in 28% of individuals and supplies the pituitary gland.

The C5 segment, the clinoid ICA, passes through the dural ring adjacent to the anterior clinoid process. The ophthalmic artery may occasionally arise from the C5 segment.

Comprehensive Management of Arteriovenous Malformations of the Brain and Spine, ed. Robert F. Spetzler, Douglas S. Kondziolka, Randall T. Higashida, and M. Yashar S. Kalani. Published by Cambridge University Press. © Cambridge University Press 2015.

The C6 segment, the ophthalmic ICA, is the first intradural segment of the ICA. The major branches of the C6 segment are the ophthalmic and superior hypophyseal arteries. The ophthalmic artery enters the optic canal with the optic nerve. It has three main branch types: ocular, orbital, and extraorbital. The ocular branches include the central retinal and ciliary arteries; the orbital branches include the lacrimal and muscular arteries; and the extraocular branches include the supraorbital, anterior and posterior ethmoidal, dorsal nasal, palpebral, medial frontal, and supratrochlear arteries. Of note, the ocular and extraocular branches may provide ECA–ICA anastomoses; these include the recurrent meningeal branch of the lacrimal artery, which may anastomose with the middle meningeal artery, as well as the extraocular branches that may anastomose with ethmoidal and facial branches of the ECA. One dominant or several separate superior hypophyseal arteries may arise from the posterior medial aspect of the C6 segment and supply the anterior pituitary and pituitary stalk as well as the optic nerve and chiasm.

The C7 segment, the communicating ICA, originates at the origin of the posterior communicating artery and ends where the ICA bifurcates into the anterior and middle cerebral arteries (ACA and MCA, respectively) just below the anterior perforated substance along the medial aspect of the sylvian fissure. The two branches of the C7 segment are the posterior communicating artery and the anterior choroidal artery. The posterior communicating artery courses posteriorly above cranial nerve III and anastomoses with the P1 segment of the posterior cerebral artery (PCA). The anterior choroidal artery, which may be a single vessel or a plexus of small vessels, arises from the posterior medial C7 segment superior to the posterior communicating artery. There are two branches of the anterior choroidal artery, cisternal and intraventricular. The cisternal branch courses posteromedially within the crural cistern around the cerebral peduncle towards the lateral geniculate body of the thalamus, turning sharply medially to enter the temporal horn through the choroidal fissure. The intraventricular branch begins in the temporal horn and courses posteriorly along the choroid plexus before turning anteriosuperiorly around the thalamus and heading towards the foramen of Monro. The anterior choroidal artery supplies vital structures, including the optic tract, posterior limb of the internal capsule, choroid plexus, and medial temporal lobe.

Aberrant ICA is the term designating ICA agenesis with collateral vascular development; ICA hypoplasia and agenesis is rare, occurring in approximately 0.01% and 0.08%, respectively. In aberrant ICA, the ICA and carotid canal are absent. Instead, there is hypertrophy of the inferior tympanic artery, which courses through the floor of the middle ear cavity and enters the skull base through the foramen lacerum where it anastomoses with the caroticotympanic artery [2,3].

The stapedial artery, a proximal branch of the hyoid artery, is a developmentally transient vessel that gives rise to the anlage of the inferior alveolar, infraorbital, middle meningeal, anterior ethmoidal, frontal, supraorbital, and lacrimal arteries. Persistent stapedial artery is a rare variant with a prevalence of approximately 0.02%. In this variant, the middle meningeal artery arises from the persistent stapedial artery, thus having an aberrant course resulting in agenesis of the foramen spinosum. The usual course of the persistent stapedial artery arises from the petrous ICA and passes through the anteromedial hypotympanum in Jacobson's canal, into the anterior facial nerve canal before exiting at the geniculate ganglion into the extradural middle cranial fossa. Of note, aberrant ICAs as described above, are frequently associated with persistent stapedial arteries. The persistent stapedial artery provides ECA–ICA collaterals via its connections to the ophthalmic artery through the supraorbital branches and to the maxillary artery through the infraorbital branches.

The ACA arises as a network from the primitive olfactory artery and courses rostrally around the growing hemispheric vesicle. Its initial growth is driven by the choroid plexus. In its final formation, the A1 segment extends horizontally from the ICA bifurcation coursing medially towards the interhemispheric fissure over the optic chiasm (70%) or sometimes over the optic nerves (30%). The anterior communicating artery junction lies within or just below the interhemispheric fissure. An average of eight perforating branches arise from the A1 segment, including medial lenticulostriate perforators and optic perforators. The medial lenticulostriate perforators course posterosuperiorly through the anterior perforated substance to supply the suprachiasmatic hypothalamus, inferior frontal lobe, and third ventricle while the optic perforators course inferiorly to supply the optic chiasm and optic nerves. In 14% of people, the recurrent artery of Heubner may also arise from the A1 segment and in 78% from the A2. The recurrent artery of Heubner forms a hairpin loop back towards the ACA and supplies the anterior part of the caudate nucleus, the anterior third of the putamen, the tip of the outer segment of the globus pallidus, and the anterior limb of the internal capsule.

The distal ACA originates deep within the interhemispheric fissure ascending anterior to the lamina terminalis into the longitudinal fissure between the cerebral hemispheres; it becomes the pericallosal artery as it curves over the corpus callosum to terminate at the choroid plexus in the roof of the third ventricle. There are, on average, five central perforating branches that pass posteriorly to enter the optic chiasm, lamina terminalis, and anterior forebrain to supply the anterior hypothalamus, the septum pellucidum, the medial portion of the anterior commissure, the pillars of the fornix, and the anterior–inferior part of the striatum.

The most common cortical cerebral branch origins include the orbitofrontal and frontopolar arteries (A2), the anterior and middle internal frontal and callosomarginal arteries (A3), the paracentral artery (A4), and the superior and inferior parietal arteries (A5). The short and long callosal branches that arise from the pericallosal artery supply the corpus callosum and septum pellucidum.

Several variant conditions exist for ACA development. The most common variant of the A1 segment is hypoplasia, which is present in 10% of subjects.

The accessory ACA arises from the anterior communicating artery as a triplicate A2 segment with an incidence of 3.3–15%. Persistence of the median callosal artery beyond 7 weeks of gestation, when it normally involutes, is also possible. The accessory ACA may be associated with cerebral aneurysms.

The azygous ACA variant results in a solitary A2 segment and has an incidence of 0.2–2.0%. Azygous ACAs are associated with cerebral aneurysm formation and may also be seen in holoprosencephaly.

The ACA originating from the internal cerebral artery at the level of the ophthalmic artery is a rare variant, reported approximately 15 times in the literature. Anomalous origin of the ACA may be seen with an ipsilateral hypoplastic A1 segment, suggesting persistence of a prechiasmatic anastomotic loop. This entity is associated with a myriad of additional abnormalities, including aneurysms, carotid agenesis, Moyamoya disease, and incomplete cleidocranial dysostosis.

Infraoptic origin of the ACA is a rarer variant than anomalous origin. It may represent an anastomotic vessel between the primitive maxillary artery and the primitive olfactory artery. This entity can be associated with high incidence of cerebral aneurysms, carotid–basilar anastomosis, agenesis of the contralateral ICA, anomalous origin of the ophthalmic artery from the ECA, fused pericallosal arteries, and Moyamoya disease.

The primitive olfactory artery is an embryological precursor to the formation of the definitive ACA (the ACA arises from the primitive olfactory artery as the medial olfactory artery) that normally regresses at seven weeks of gestation. Persistence of the primitive olfactory artery is rare, with an incidence of 0.14% and no laterality. There are three types of the persistent primitive olfactory artery described in the literature; in type 1, the anomalous artery arises from the ICA, courses within the olfactory tract, and hairpin turns to supply the ACA territory; in type 2, the anomalous artery arises from the ACA, traverses the cribriform plate, and supplies the nasal cavity; and in the recently described type 3 (thought to be a hybrid of types 1 and 2), there are two main branches to the persistent artery, one traversing the cribriform plate to supply the nasal cavity and a second with a hairpin turn supplying the distal ACA territory. The etiology of this variant likely results from abnormal morphogenesis of the primitive olfactory artery. Persistent primitive olfactory arteries are associated with an increased incidence of cerebral aneurysm formation.

The MCA is subdivided into four divisions; M1, the horizontal/sphenoidal segment; M2, the insular segment; M3, the opercular segment; and M4, the cortical branches. The M1 segment extends from the ICA laterally in a horizontal plane towards the sylvian fissure where it turns posterior–superior at the limen insulae to form the genu. This segment consists of two components, the pre- and the postbifurcation segments. Perforator arteries arise from the M1 segment and are divided into medial and lateral lenticulostriate arteries. The medial lenticulostriate arteries enter the anterior perforated substance and course superiorly to directly supply the lentiform nucleus, caudate nucleus, and internal capsule; the lateral lenticulostriate arteries are typically larger and course laterally around the lentiform nucleus and superiorly within the external capsule, where they turn medially to supply the caudate nucleus. Small cortical branches may arise from the M1 segment to supply the temporal lobe (48%). In roughly 80% of individuals, the MCA M1 segment bifurcates; in the remaining individuals, the MCA M1 segment trifurcates (~10%) or demonstrates greater branching complexity (~10%).

The six to eight M2/insular branches extend to the circular sulcus of the insula. The M3/opercular branches extend to the surface of the sylvian fissure, and the M4 branches supply the cerebral cortex. These branches include anterior (orbitofrontal and prefrontal), intermediate (precentral, central, and postcentral), and posterior (posterior parietal, angular, temporo-occipital, posterior temporal, intermediate temporal, and anterior temporal) branches.

Several variant conditions affect MCA development. Hypoplasia/aplasia of MCA M1 is a rare phenomenon and must be differentiated from Moyamoya and degenerative steno-occlusive disease.

An MCA M1 branch that arises from the ICA and courses inferior to the native MCA M1 segment is a duplicated MCA M1 segment. This variant occurs with a frequency of 1–3%.

An additional MCA branch that arises from the ACA A1 segment near the anterior communicating artery is known as an accessory MCA and typically supplies the anterior–inferior frontal lobe. This variant can be seen in roughly 3% of individuals. Care must be taken to avoid confusing this variant with a normal recurrent artery of Heubner. An accessory MCA is differentiated from the recurrent artery of Heubner by the fact that accessory MCAs will supply cortical areas typically supplied by the MCA.

Additional MCA M1 variants include a fenestrated MCA, anomalous origin of the MCA, and single non-bifurcating MCA; these are seen in less than 5% of individuals.

Posterior circulation anatomy

During stage 1 of arterial development, the vertebrobasilar vascular distribution is supplied via the transient carotid–vertebrobasilar connections, including the trigeminal, otic, hypoglossal, and proatlantic arteries, to bilateral paired longitudinal neural arteries. In stage 2, the paired longitudinal neural arteries begin to fuse axially along the midline, forming the primordial basilar artery, yet supply to the posterior circulation is still derived from the carotid–vertebrobasilar connections. In stage 3, the basilar artery is more distinctive and, in addition, the vertebral arteries begin to form from longitudinal fusion of the intersegmental cervical arteries from C1–C7. During stages 4–5, the basilar artery usually joins with the posterior communicating arteries to supply the PCAs [2,4].

The vertebral artery can be divided into four segments: the V1 or extraosseous segment from the subclavian to the entrance of the foramen transversarium; the V2 or foraminal segment typically extending from C6 to C3 vertebra; the V3 extraspinal segment; and V4, the intradural segment. The V1 segment typically arises from the subclavian arteries and courses posterior–superiorly to enter the transverse neuroforamen of the C6 vertebral body. The V2 segment begins at the C6 level and ascends vertically within the neuroforamen from C6 to C1. The V3 segment extends from the C1 neuroforamen to the dura, and the V4 segment extends from the dura to the vertebrobasilar junction at the lower margin of the pons.

The vertebral arteries have several branches along their course providing supply for cervical musculature, dura mater, the spinal cord, the brainstem, as well as the cerebellum. Vertebral artery branches include V2 muscular, spinal, and anterior meningeal branches; V3; and V4 anterior and posterior spinal arteries, posterior inferior cerebellar artery (PICA), and olivary and peduncular perforators, which have variations according to the individual pattern of fusion and regression.

The basilar artery lies anterior to the pons and terminates in the suprasellar cistern at the floor of the third ventricle. It gives rise to the bilateral anterior inferior cerebellar arteries (AICAs), pontine perforators, superior cerebellar arteries, PCAs, as well as paramedial, circumferential, and thalamic perforator arteries. The AICAs are the first branches of the basilar artery, arising on average 9.5 mm from the vertebrobasilar junction. The AICAs course posteriorly along the surface of the pons across cranial nerve IV to the cerebellopontine cistern. The superior cerebellar arteries typically arise within 1–3 mm of the basilar artery bifurcation. The superior cerebellar artery wraps around the brainstem in a groove between the pons and the midbrain and extends through the cerebellomesencephalic fissure to the tentorial edge. It has intimate associations with multiple cranial nerves as it courses below the oculomotor and trochlear nerves and above the trigeminal nerve. The PCAs arise from the basilar apex and course laterally around the brainstem through the ambient and crural cisterns. There are four posterior cerebellar artery segments: P1 precommunicating segment; P2 segment, extending from the posterior communicating artery to the common temporal branch origin; P3 segment, extending from the common temporal branch to the origins of the parieto-occipital and calcarine arteries; and P4, the cortical segment. The PCAs also provide perforators, including the thalamoperforators and the circumflex perforators arising from the P1 segment, as well as the thalamogeniculate, peduncular, circumflex branches, and medial and lateral posterior choroidal arteries.

Numerous variant conditions can affect posterior circulation development. The vertebral arteries typically arise from the subclavian arteries; however in 5% of the population, the vertebral artery arises from the aortic arch directly. There is variability in the vertebral artery dominance patterns but approximately half are left dominant, one-quarter are right dominant, and one-quarter codominant.

Fenestrated and bifid vertebral arteries are rare entities seen in less than 1% of the population. Of note, fenestrated vertebral arteries are associated with other abnormalities, including fused vertebrae and vascular lesions, including aneurysms and vascular malformations. A fenestrated basilar artery is seen in approximately 1% of anatomical dissections. Fenestrated basilar arteries are also associated with basilar artery aneurysms. Rare cases of non-fusion of the basilar artery have been reported in the literature.

The PICA most commonly arises from the V4 segment of the vertebral artery. However, several variants that involve the PICA exist, including vertebral artery PICA termination, AICA–PICA common trunk, extradural PICA origin, and a duplicated PICA; these variants occur in 2% or less of the population. A single branch arising from the basilar artery may bifurcate into AICA and PICA. In up to 20% of the population, an accessory AICA is present. In approximately 10%, there can be duplicate or triplicate superior cerebellar arteries.

Aside from the posterior communicating arteries, there are four other carotid–basilar congenital anastomoses that have been described, including persistent hypoglosssal, proatlantal, trigeminal, and otic arteries. The most common carotid–basilar anastomosis is the persistent trigeminal artery, which has a prevalence of up to 0.6 %. The artery may course posteriorly in a medial or lateral fashion: the medial course is intrasellar, may compress the pituitary gland, and penetrates the dorsum sellae; the lateral course follows along the trigeminal nerve. There are two types of persistent trigeminal arteries, Saltzmann types I and II, determined by the configuration of the ipsilateral PCA. In Saltzmann type I anastomoses, the posterior communicating artery is absent and the persistent trigeminal artery supplies the entire vertebrobasilar system on that side. In Saltzmann type II anastomoses, there is a fetal ipsilateral posterior communicating artery and no PCA P1 segment. Of note, persistent trigeminal arteries are associated with a 25% incidence of intracranial vascular malformations and a 14% incidence of intracranial aneurysms. Persistent trigeminal artery variants that connect directly to cerebellar arteries have also been described but are much less common than persistent trigeminal arteries that connect with the basilar artery. The remaining carotid–basilar anastomoses are rare, with incidences of less than 0.1%.

Cerebral arteriovenous malformations angioarchitecture

Annual rates of hemorrhage for brain AVMs are 2–4%, with rehemorrhage rates of 8–35% depending on the lesion [5–8]. The angioarchitecture of cerebral AVMs provides significant prognosticators, impacting natural history and management strategies. Anatomical factors include AVM location and characterization (compact or diffuse), size, direct versus en passage arterial feeders, aneurysms, discrete shunts, vasculopathies and venous drainage pattern. The revised three-tier Spetzler–Martin scale factors size (<3 cm, 3–6 cm, and >6 cm), location (± eloquent), and venous drainage (superficial or deep); from this the most widely accepted and used recommendations are surgical resection for class A (Spetzler–Martin grade I and II); multimodal therapy, including surgery, radiosurgery, and/or endovascular embolization for class B (Spetzler–Martin grade III); and conservative management for class C (Spetzler–Martin grade IV and V) [5,6,9]

Arterial supply of AVMs has many facets that bear on natural history and treatment risks. The focus of treatment is to close the nidus by embolization, surgery, and/or radiotherapy. Size of a feeding pedicle is important. Direct AVM arterial feeders terminate in the AVM nidus (Fig. 2.1). En passage feeders contribute branches to the AVM nidus while the parent artery continues to course distally and supply normal cerebral

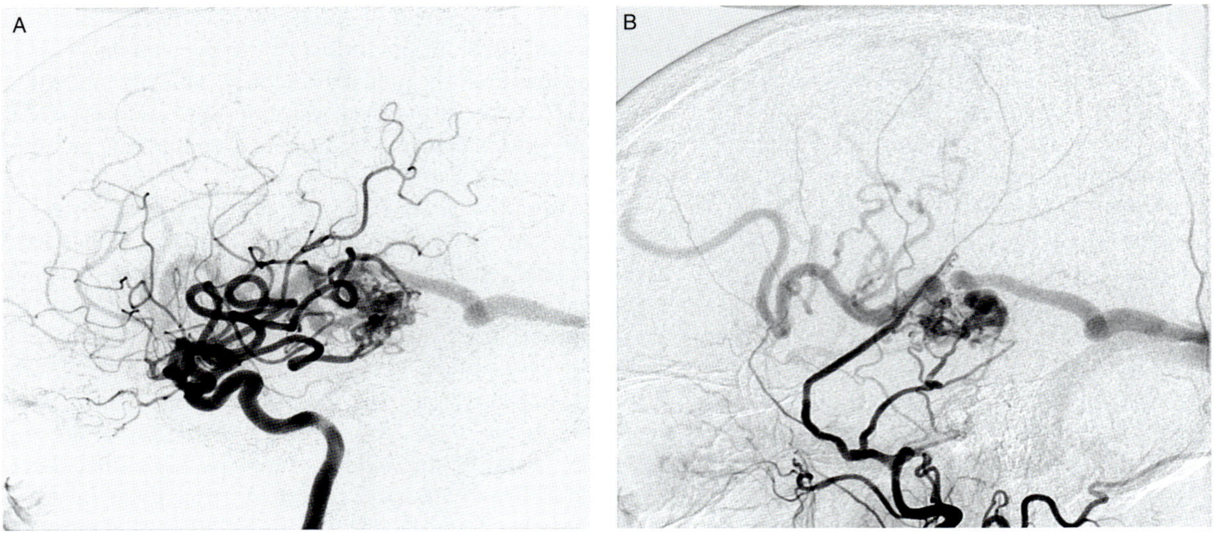

Fig. 2.1. Spetzler–Martin grade I arteriovenous malformations of the right temporal lobe with end vessel supply from the right middle cerebral artery. Different zones are supplied by the right middle meningeal artery, but there is a common set of draining veins indicating the arteriovenous malformations has one compartment.

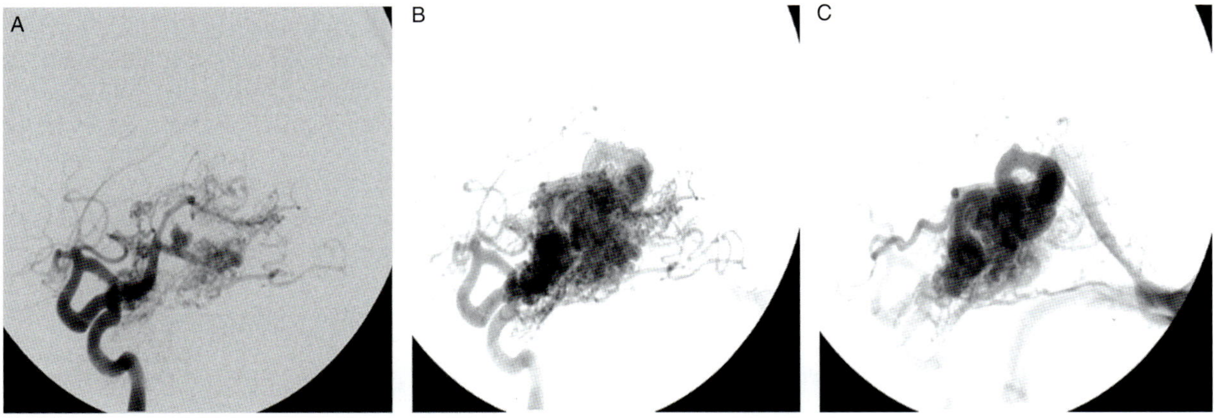

Fig. 2.2. Spetzler–Martin grade IV arteriovenous malformations of the medial temporal lobe of the left cerebral hemisphere. Note the numerous en passage branches arising from the left posterior communicating artery and the posterior cerebral artery.

parenchyma (Fig. 2.2). The AVM arterial feeder type does not seem to impact hemorrhage risk. However, en passage feeders are less amenable to endovascular treatment because of their diminutive nature, right angle orientation from the parent vessel, and the presence of perfusion of normal cerebral parenchyma distally.

The next level of flow augmentation is via collaterals from one intracranial circulation to another. This can be from direct ACA to MCA branches into an AVM or via pial collaterals providing indirect racemose connections. There can be similar connections between deep perforator branches and the ACA, MCA, or PCA (Fig. 2.3). Finally, there can be collateral circulation between ECA and ICA/vertebrobasilar circulations (Fig. 2.1). These can be related to increased flow through native developmental arteries such as the ILT of the ICA or via neovascularity, such as seen when flow is parasitized from the middle meningeal artery into a parenchymal AVM via intervening MCA branches. This applies to DAVFs in the opposite direction, with augmentation of supply from parenchymal arteries into the dural shunt.

There are a few reports in the literature of proliferative angiopathy, which can appear similar to AVMs [10–12]. These lesions show exuberant direct and collateral flow to diffuse regions interspersed with brain parenchyma (Fig. 2.4). There is often focal stenosis of a major arterial branch and prominent external carotid collaterals. Finally, there is variable shunting.

Direct arteriovenous shunts within a nidus are present in 10–20% of parenchymal AVMs. Soderman *et al.* [7] described intranidal fistulae as potential weak spots for hemorrhage. This is consistent with data from Crawford *et al.* [8], who demonstrated that the overall risk of hemorrhage decreased by 24–78% when an intranidal aneurysm or fistula was embolized. Marks *et al.* [10] demonstrated that closure of fistulae within an AVM could be accomplished safely compared with overall risks of AVM treatment.

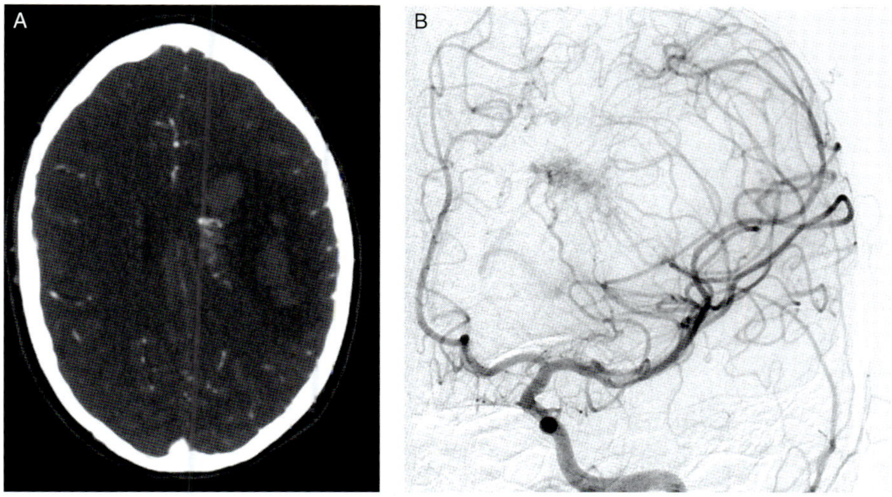

Fig. 2.3. Spetzler–Martin grade III arteriovenous malformations of the left centrum semiovale. Arterial supply is via the left middle cerebral artery lenticulostriate and middle cerebral artery cortical branches. Small aneurysm of a lenticulostriate artery is noted on CT scan (A) and angiogram (B).

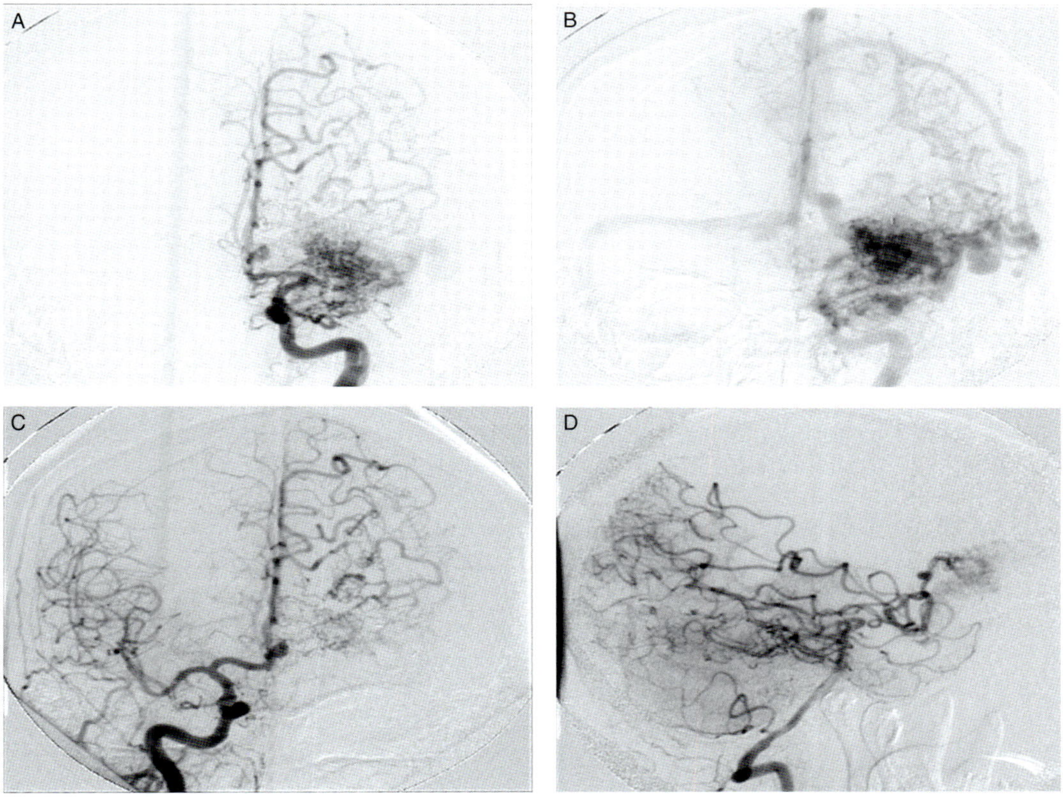

Fig. 2.4. Proliferative angiopathy of the medial left temporal lobe. The angiogram is notable for occlusive pathology of the left M1. Collateral flow is via the right carotid and the anterior communicating artery and from the left posterior communicating artery. There is a flow-related aneurysm of the anterior communicating artery. In this case, there is some degree of arteriovenous shunting.

There are three types of aneurysm associated with AVMs, with a reported incidence of 10–58%, including arterial feeder flow-related aneurysms, peri- or intranidal aneurysms, or aneurysms unrelated to the AVM. In addition to Spetzler–Martin grading criteria, AVM management is predicated on the type of associated aneurysm, as they carry a greater risk profile than AVMs not associated with aneurysms. Intranidal aneurysms pose the greatest risk, with an annual hemorrhage rate of 10% compared with the typical AVM crude annual hemorrhage rate of 2–4%. Most flow-related aneurysms of proximal vessels are not associated with higher AVM hemorrhage rates and typically regress following resolution of arteriovenous shunting and the high flow state. It is not known whether aneurysms on perforator branches, such as lenticulostriate arteries, which supply AVMs have higher rates of hemorrhage. For these reasons, and the belief that treatment of an AVM with an intranidal aneurysm before securing the aneurysm may precipitate rupture through the abrupt changes in hemodynamics, intranidal aneurysms of AVMs are typically secured prior to AVM treatment, while proximal flow-related aneurysms are managed conservatively [13–18].

Venous elements, including deep venous drainage, a single draining vein, and venous stenosis, thrombosis or occlusion, increase the risk of AVM hemorrhage. In a study of the Columbia AVM database including 622 patients, deep venous drainage was associated with a model estimated annual rupture risk of 11.4% in patients presenting with hemorrhage [13]. Miyasaka *et al.* demonstrated a single draining vein and venous outflow obstruction as risk factors for increased hemorrhage [19]. In addition, venous hypertension secondary to venous stenosis or outflow obstruction may lead to cerebral ischemia, prompting release of angiogenic factors leading to the development of arteriovenous fistulae and thereby increasing the complexity of the lesion and possibly its risk for hemorrhage [20]. Closing a nidal fistula does not carry additional risk beyond standard AVM embolization [21]. Compartmentalization of an AVM is important to assess. For an individual region, the arterial input must be closed before occluding the vein.

Dural arteriovenous fistula angioarchitecture

Dural arteriovenous fistulae are the other type of high-flow vascular shunt discussed in this chapter. Formal classification by Cognard *et al.* is based on a detailed description and natural history risks based on venous outflow [22]. Type I is a shunt from ECAs into a venous sinus with flow remaining antegrade. Type II has reversal of flow into the main sinus but not the cortical veins (IIa), into the cortical veins but not the sinus (IIb), or into both (IIab). Type IIb and type IIab carry a 10% risk of intracranial hemorrhage. Type III has direct cortical venous reflux, with a 40% risk of intracranial hemorrhage, and type IV has venous ectasia with a 65% risk. Type V drains into the spinal veins, causing myelopathy in 50% of patients. Arterial supply can arise from ECAs, the extracranial cervical circulation, and the parenchymal vessels (ICA and vertebrobasilar circulations). It is important to control such lesions with embolization of safe pedicles (Fig. 2.5). Compared with brain AVMs, the key to closing these lesions is to close the venous confluence. The routes of arterial embolization demand knowledge of collateral circulation around the skull base between the intracranial and extracranial circulations. Treatment options may include transarterial embolization via low-risk branches or transvenous embolization of the affected venous sinus. The next section describes in detail these developmental collateral pathways.

Extracranial to intracranial collateral vasculature

Anastomoses of ECA–intracranial artery are important anatomical considerations in both DAVFs and cerebral AVMs. Between 14 and 50% of cerebral AVMs may have an extracranial supply. Newton and Cronqvist defined these lesions as mixed pial–dural arteriovenous malformations and noted that extracranial supply was more common in temporal, parietal, or occipital location, superficial lesions, diffuse lesions, high-flow lesions, and large AVMs (>10 mL volume) [23].

The ECA, ICA, and vertebral arteries share anastomoses during embryonic development, as described in Chapter 1. Mature analogues and persistence of transient embryological structures form the anatomical basis for the three vascular territories described as functional vascular anatomy [3]. This concept suggests that adjacent head and neck vascular territories are linked by these anastomoses and, in the setting of vascular occlusion, arteriovenous shunting, or pressurized contrast injection, may provide collateral flow. The general architecture of these anastomoses is ECA (internal maxillary artery and/or ascending pharyngeal artery)-to-intermediary network (orbital, petrocavernous, or upper cervical)-to-intracranial vessel (ICA or vertebral artery). As the two constant components of the anastomoses are the ECA branches and the intracranial vessels, the most practical way of organizing these connections is centered on the variable, the intermediary networks. It is important to note that although the intermediary networks organize the extracranial–intracranial anastomoses into anatomical regions that facilitate an understanding of the collateral pathways, there is considerable internetwork communication [12,23–26].

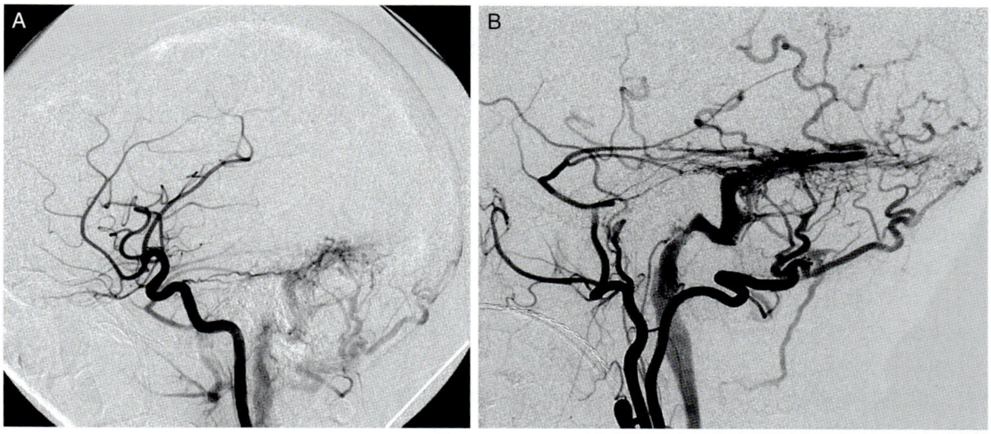

Fig. 2.5. Dural arteriovenous fistula of the left transverse and sigmoid sinuses demonstrates numerous high-risk internal and external carotid arteries supplying the lesion. These branches include the lateral tentorial branch of the internal carotid artery, neuromeningeal trunk, and petrous branch of the left middle meningeal artery. The lesion has a low-risk arterial supply from the left occipital artery and the squamosal branch of the left middle meningeal artery.

Orbital network

The orbital network consists of three components: the internal maxillary artery arising from the ECA, the intermediary ophthalmic artery arising from the ICA, and ICA itself. Utilizing a unidirectional ECA to ICA system, these pathways may be subdivided according to their place of origin from the internal maxillary artery or their place of transit through the orbital network. Given that the location of occlusion in the orbital network has implications on vision through central retinal artery occlusion and stroke from retrograde flow of embolic material into the ICA, in this discussion, the place of transit through the orbital network will be taken as the frame of reference.

The ophthalmic artery branches may be categorized based on the compartment or structures that the arteries supply or the location of the origins of the branches along the artery.

The most frequently encountered orbital network anastomosis is the meningo-ophthalmic artery, which is seen in approximately 16% of patients. This anatomical variant is an analogue of the stapedial artery and arises from the middle meningeal artery, supplying the distal ophthalmic artery including the central retinal and ciliary arteries. Angiographic evidence of this variant is the lack of an ophthalmic artery arising from the ICA and a choroidal blush seen following external carotid artery contrast injection.

The orbital network is extensive, with many additional anastomotic routes of collateral flow. The ophthalmic artery can be divided into three segments: segment 1, originating at the orbital foramen and terminating as the vessel crosses under the optic nerve; segment 2, passing over or under the optic nerve; and segment 3, extending from the bend in the vessel on the medial aspect of the optic nerve to the edge of the orbit. The segmental anatomy of the ophthalmic artery is essential to determining the risk of injury to vision as occlusion beyond the second segment generally does not lead to blockage of the central retinal artery.

Anastomoses arising from segment 2 of the ophthalmic artery include the proximal lacrimal branches that anastomose with the middle meningeal artery, the distal lacrimal branch that anastomoses with the anterior deep temporal and infraorbital arteries, and the posterior ethmoidal branches (which may also arise from segment 3) that anastomose with the sphenopalatine, greater palatine, and middle meningeal arteries. Those branches arising from segment 3 include the anterior ethmoidal branches that anastomose with the septal, sphenopalatine, and middle meningeal arteries, and the supraorbital branch that anastomoses with the superficial temporal artery. Those branches that arise from the terminal portion include the dorsal nasal branch that anastomoses with the facial arteries and infraorbital arteries.

Petrous–cavernous network

In contrast to the orbital network where there was only one intermediary artery between the ECA–ICA anastomoses, in the petrous–cavernous network, there are three intermediary nodes with their respective arteries: the petrous node comprising the caroticotympanic and mandibular arteries, the clival node comprising the meningohypophyseal trunk and lateral clival artery, and cavernous node comprising the ILT of the ICA.

Petrous node

The petrous node ECA–ICA anastomoses are supplied via the ascending pharyngeal and internal maxillary arteries.

The mandibular anastomosis arises from the ascending pharyngeal artery as well as the proximal and distal internal maxillary artery. The ascending pharyngeal artery gives off two main trunks, the pharyngeal and the neuromeningeal. The pharyngeal trunk is further divided into the inferior, middle, and superior branches, with the superior branch giving rise to the most clinically significant ECA–ICA collaterals via the eustachian tube anastomotic circle; this circle connects the ascending pharyngeal artery to the mandibular artery. In addition, the mandibular artery may anastomose with another ascending pharyngeal artery branch, the inferior tympanic artery, as described below. The distal internal maxillary artery, vidian, and pterygovaginal branches also anastomose with the mandibular artery. The vidian artery is distinguished by its horizontal course through the vidian canal. The pterygovaginal artery typically arises adjacent to the vidian artery and has a more inferior course along the roof of the nasopharynx. The pterygovaginal artery connects with the eustachian tube anastomotic circle, thereby connecting to the mandibular artery. Finally, the accessory meningeal artery, a branch of the proximal internal maxillary artery, supplies small vessels to the eustachian tube anastomotic circle, which leads to the mandibular artery.

The caroticotympanic anastomosis arises from the inferior tympanic artery. The inferior tympanic artery may arise from the ascending pharyngeal artery itself or from one of its major branches and it anastomoses with the caroticotympanic artery via the tympanic foramen.

Clival node

The clival node ECA–ICA anastomoses are supplied via the ascending pharyngeal artery, internal maxillary artery, and occipital/posterior auricular arteries.

The ascending pharyngeal artery neuromeningeal trunk gives rise to jugular and hypoglossal arteries, which travel via the jugular and hypoglossal foramina, respectively. After exiting these foramina, both arteries give rise to medial and lateral clival branches, which, in turn, anastomose with the meningohypophyseal trunk and the lateral clival artery. The middle meningeal artery petrosquamosal branch may also form anastomoses with the meningohypophyseal trunk via its marginal artery of the tentorium branch (this branch may also arise from the ophthalmic artery or the ILT of the ICA).

The stylomastoid artery, a branch of either the occipital artery or the posterior auricular artery, may also anastomose with the meningohypophyseal trunk.

The distal internal maxillary artery branch, the artery passing through the foramen rotundum, has a characteristic corkscrew appearance and may rarely anastomose with the lateral clival artery. The carotid canal branch of the ascending pharyngeal artery, which courses through the foramen lacerum, may anastomose with the lateral clival artery (as well as the ILT of the ICA), as described below.

Cavernous node

The cavernous node anastomoses are supplied via the ascending pharyngeal artery carotid canal branch and the internal maxillary artery.

The ascending pharyngeal artery carotid canal branch courses through the foramen lacerum where it may anastomose with the ILT or lateral clival artery, as mentioned above.

The proximal internal maxillary artery supply is through the middle meningeal artery cavernous, orbital, and petrosquamosal branches. The branches arise as the middle meningeal artery exits the foramen spinosum and anastomoses with the superior/tentorial branches of the ILT of the ICA. The orbital branches of the middle meningeal artery anastomose with the anteromedial ILT branches in the superior orbital fissure. In addition, the petrosquamosal branches of the middle meningeal artery may anastomose with the marginal artery of the tentorium branch of the ILT. The accessory meningeal artery courses through the foramen ovale to anastomose with the posteromedial branches of the ILT. In 20% of the population, the accessory meningeal artery may supply the entire ILT territory.

The distal internal maxillary artery supply is via the artery of the foramen rotundum, which can anastomose with the anterolateral branch of the ILT.

Finally, the stylomastoid artery, which may arise from the posterior auricular artery or the occipital artery, may anastomose with the ILT to form an internetwork connection.

Upper cervical network

The upper cervical network is an extracranial–intracranial network connecting the ECA and other extracranial vessels to the vertebral artery. The anastomoses of the upper cervical network are supplied by the occipital artery, posterior auricular artery, the ascending pharyngeal artery, and the ascending and deep cervical arteries of the subclavian artery.

The major anastomoses of the upper cervical network are the posterior anastomotic auricular branches that arise from the horizontal portion of the occipital artery at C1/C2 and connect with the vertebral artery. An additional anastomosis that may arise from the occipital or posterior auricular artery is the stylomastoid artery connection with the posterior meningeal artery branch of the vertebral artery.

The ascending pharyngeal musculospinal and prevertebral branches anastomose with the vertebral artery. The musculospinal artery anastomoses with the C3 branches of the vertebral artery. The prevertebral branch anastomoses with the odontoid arch, which later connects with the C3 branches of the vertebral artery. The prevertebral branch has a characteristic U-shaped appearance medially overlying the C2 dens in lateral views. The prevertebral branches may arise either from the ascending pharyngeal main trunk or the neuromeningeal trunk.

Cervical anastomoses arising from the thyrocervical trunk via the ascending cervical artery and the costocervical trunk via the deep cervical artery are also present. These arteries typically anastomose at the C2–C4 level. Rarely, the vertebral artery may share a common origin with the thyrocervical trunk.

Cranial nerve vascular supply

An important subtype of the extracranial–intracranial functional anatomy that is not classically described this way is the vascularity and anastomoses associated with cranial nerves. In this system, the essential architecture is an extracranial artery, cranial nerves with arterial supply from the functional anatomy intermediary branches (described above), and the intracranial arteries (or vertebral artery). The anatomical locations of the cranial nerves serve as the basis for their groupings into orbital, cavernous sinus, cerebellopontine angle, and lower cranial nerve networks. A general theme emerges from this categorization of the relationship between cranial nerve anatomy, their arterial supply, and extracranial–intracranial anastomoses; the extracranial–intracranial anastomoses functional anatomy overlies the anatomical groupings of cranial nerves such that the anastomotic pathways also identify cranial nerves at risk during embolization. The most important extracranial artery supply to the cranial nerves is typically considered to be cranial nerve V as well as the lower cranial nerves (IX–XII). Another facet of the cranial nerve arterial supply to note is that, in the lower cranial nerves, the cisternal supply is generally from the ipsilateral vertebral artery and the foraminal supply is generally from the neuromeningeal trunk of the ascending pharyngeal artery.

The orbital network is similar to that noted above for extracranial–intracranial anastomoses and will not be covered further here.

The cavernous sinus contains cranial nerves III, IV, V1, V2, and VI. These nerves are supplied via the ascending pharyngeal artery, meningohypophyseal artery, the ILT of the ICA, and the middle meningeal artery branches of the internal maxillary artery.

Cranial nerve III receives its arterial supply from the ILT while cranial nerve IV receives arterial supply from the marginal artery of the tentorium cerebelli branch of the menigohypophyseal trunk and the ILT. These vessels may serve as intermediary arteries in the petrous–cavernous network.

Cranial nerve V1 receives arterial supply from the basilar vestige of the trigeminal artery, lateral artery of the trigeminal ganglion, the cavernous branch of the middle meningeal artery, the carotid branch of the ascending pharyngeal artery, and the ILT. Cranial nerve V2 receives arterial supply from the artery of the foramen rotundum. The petrous–cavernous network includes the ILT while the upper cervical network includes the ascending pharyngeal artery.

Cranial nerve VI receives arterial supply from the jugular branch of the ascending pharyngeal artery, medial branch of the lateral clival artery, meningohypophyseal trunk, and the ILT. The ascending pharyngeal artery, lateral clival artery, meningohypophyseal trunk, and ILT are components of the petrous–cavernous and upper cervical networks.

The cerebellopontine network consists of the cranial nerves V3, VII, and VIII. These nerves are supplied via the ILT, accessory meningeal artery, internal auditory branch of the AICA, petrosal branch of the middle meningeal artery, stylomastoid branch of the posterior auricular or occipital arteries, and the jugular branch of the neuromeningeal trunk of the ascending pharyngeal artery.

Cranial nerve V3 is supplied via the posterior medial branch of the ILT and the accessory meningeal artery. These arteries are components of the petrous–cavernous network.

Cranial nerves VII and VIII are supplied via the internal auditory branch of the AICA, petrosal branch of the middle meningeal artery, stylomastoid branch of the posterior auricular or occipital arteries, and jugular branch of the neuromeningeal trunk of the ascending pharyngeal artery. These arteries are components of the petrous–cavernous and upper cervical networks.

Cranial nerves IX–XII are supplied via the C3 segmental branches of the vertebral arteries and the jugular and hypoglossal branches of the neuromeningeal trunk of the ascending pharyngeal artery. These arteries are a component of the upper cervical network.

Conclusions

Several points should be kept in mind when considering treatment of a brain AVM. First, it is important to determine whether the goal is curative or palliative and then to plan for single or multimodality methodology. Focal lesions such as aneurysms and fistulae can be targeted by embolization. Flow reduction can be done in preparation for surgery or radiosurgery. The focus is to close the nidus fully before closing the venous drainage.

The goal of DAVF treatment is to close the abnormal draining vein. In most cases, high-risk arterial input may be closed via lower-risk arterial input from ECA branches.

It is important to keep in mind during any embolization that, while collaterals may not be visualized by angiography because of flow phenomena, it must be assumed that they may be present.

References

1. Bouthillier A, van Loveren HR, Keller JT. Segments of the internal carotid artery: a new classification. *Neurosurgery* 1996;**38**:425–32.
2. Padget DH. The development of the cranial arteries in the human embryo. *Contrib Embryol* 1948;**212**:207–61.
3. Lasjaunias P. Internal carotid artery anatomy. In Lasjaunias P, Berenstein A, terBrugge KG, eds. *Surgical Neuroangiography*. New York: Springer, 2001, pp. 479–630.
4. Lasjaunias P. Posterior circulation. In Lasjaunias P, Berenstein A, terBrugge KG, eds. *Surgical Neuroangiography*. New York: Springer, 2001, pp. 479–630.
5. Spetzler RF, Ponce FA. A 3-tier classification of cerebral arteriovenous malformations. Clinical article. *J Neurosurg* 2011;**114**:842–9.
6. Pollock BE, Flickinger JC. A proposed radiosurgery-based grading system for arteriovenous malformation. *J Neurosurg* 2002;**96**:79–85.
7. Soderman M, Andersson T, Karlsson B, *et al.* Management of patients with brain arteriovenous malformation. *Eur J Radiol* 2003;**46**:195–205.
8. Crawford PM, West CR, Chadwick DW, *et al.* Arteriovenous malformation of the brain: natural history in unoperated patients. *J Neurol Neurosurg Psychiatry* 1986;**49**:1–10.
9. Hartmann A, Pile-Spellman J, Stapf C, *et al.* Risk of endovascular treatment of brain arteriovenous malformation. *Stroke* 2002;**33**:1816–20.
10. Marks MP, Lane B, Steinberg G, *et al.* Vascular characteristics of intracerebral arteriovenous malformation in patients with clinical steal. *AJNR Am J Neuroradiol* 1991;**12**:489–96.
11. Mawad ME, Hilal SK, Michelsen WJ, *et al.* Occlusive vascular disease associated with cerebral arteriovenous malformation. *Radiology* 1984;**153**:401–8.
12. Lasjaunias PL, Landrieu P, Rodesch G, *et al.* Cerebral proliferative angiopathy. Clinical and angiographic description of an entity different from cerebral AVMs. *Stroke* 2008;**39**:878–85.
13. Stapf C, Mast H, Sciacca RR, *et al.* Predictors of hemorrhage in patients with untreated brain arteriovenous malformation. *Neurology* 2006;**66**:1350–5.
14. Pollock BE, Flickinger JC, Lunsford LD, *et al.* Factors that predict the bleeding risk of cerebral arteriovenous malformation. *Stroke* 1996;**27**:1–6.
15. Lv X, Wu Z, Jiang C, *et al.* Angioarchitectural characteristics of brain arteriovenous malformation with and without hemorrhage. *World Neurosurg* 2011;**76**:95–9.
16. Hernesniemi JA, Dashti R, Juvela S, *et al.* Natural history of brain arteriovenous malformation: a long-term follow-up study of risk of hemorrhage in 238 patients. *Neurosurgery* 2008;**63**:823–9.
17. Almefty K, Spetzler RF. Arteriovenous malformation and associated aneurysms. *World Neurosurg* 2011;**76**:396–7.
18. Liu Y, Zhu S, Jiao L, *et al.* Cerebral arteriovenous malformation associated with aneurysms: a report of 10 cases and literature review. *J Clin Neurosci* 2000;**7**:254–6.
19. Miyasaka Y, Yada K, Ohwada T, *et al.* An analysis of the venous drainage system as a factor in hemorrhage from arteriovenous malformation. *J Neurosurg* 1992;**76**:239–43.
20. Moftakhar P, Hauptman JS, Malkasian D, *et al.* Cerebral arteriovenous malformation, Part 2: physiology. *Neurosurg Focus* 2009;**26**:E11.
21. Yuki I, Kim RH, Duckwiler G, *et al.* Treatment of brain arteriovenous malformations with high-flow arteriovenous fistulas: risk and complications associated with endovascular embolization in multimodality treatment. Clinical article. *J Neurosurg* 2010;**113**:715–22.
22. Cognard C, Gobin YP, Pierot L, *et al.* Cerebral dural arteriovenous fistulas:

clinical and angiographic correlation with a revised classification of venous drainage. *Radiology* 1995;**194**:671–80.

23. Newton TH, Cronqvist S. Involvement of dural arteries in intracranial arteriovenous malformation. *Radiology* 1969;**93**:1071–8.

24. Geibprasert S, Pongpech S, Armstrong D, *et al.* Dangerous extracranial-intracranial anastomoses and supply to the cranial nerves: vessels the neurointerventionalist needs to know. *AJNR Am J Neuroradiol* 2009;**30**:1459–68.

25. Hayreh SS. Arteries of the orbit in the human being. *Br J Surg* 1963;**50**:938–53.

26. Lasjaunias P. Skull base and external carotid arteries. In Lasjaunias P, Berenstein A, terBrugge KG, eds. *Surgical Neuroangiography*. New York: Springer, 2001, pp. 387–478.

Chapter 3 Spinal vascular anatomy and implications for treatment of arteriovenous malformations

Paul Singh and Y. Pierre Gobin

Spinal vascular anatomy

Arterial system

Spinal vascular anatomy incorporates not only the vascular supply to the cord but also that to the adjacent structures which share common networks for blood supply, including the nerve roots, dura, and paraspinal musculature. It is important to understand the complex anatomical detail of the spinal column and its anomalies prior to undergoing extensive diagnostic or therapeutic spinal vascular procedures. Because vessel origins vary with progression from the cervical to the thoracic, lumbar, and sacral levels, this chapter starts by outlining the arteriovenous system macroscopically (Fig. 3.1).

Superficially, the anterior two-thirds of the spinal cord is supplied by the anterior spinal artery (ASA) and the posterior one-third is supplied by the posterior spinal arteries (PSAs). These vessels also anastomose over the peripheral cord to form a pial plexus, the vasocorona (Fig. 3.2) [1].

Deeper in the spinal cord, the ASA feeds into the sulcal arteries, which propagate into the anterior median fissure. These central arteries then centrifugally supply the gray matter. The vasocorona has perforators that centripetally supply the white matter of the peripheral spinal cord (rami perforantes) [2].

Neuroanatomically, when incorporating the extrinsic and intrinsic systems, the ASA supplies the anterior commissure, dorsal nucleus of Clarke, corticospinal tract, spinothalamic tract, and the anterior portions of fasciculi cuneatus and gracilis. The PSAs supply the posterior horns, parts of the corticospinal tracts, and the posterior third of the spinal cord [1].

Segmental arteries

The level of each segmental artery corresponds to the spinal level it supplies rather than its site of origin from the aorta. In the upper thoracic spine, the segmental arteries can exit the aorta up to two levels caudal to the vertebral levels they supply. The midthoracic segmental arteries generally exit just below their corresponding vertebral levels, and the lumbar segmental vessels arise typically at their respective vertebral levels. The

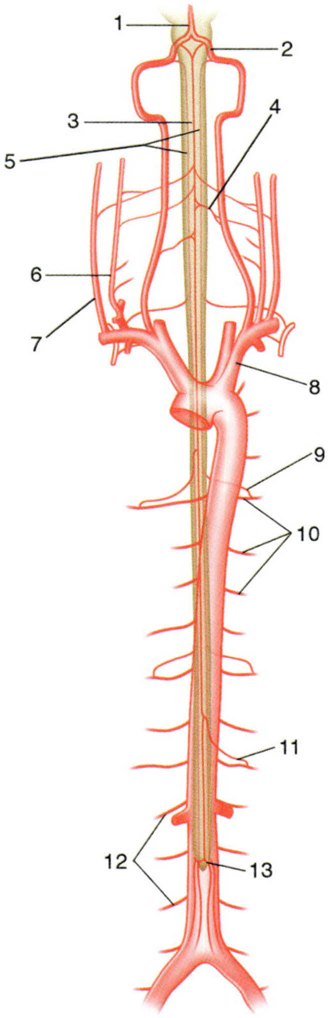

Fig. 3.1. Arteries supplying the spinal cord. (1) Basilar artery; (2) vertebral artery; (3) anterior spinal artery; (4) anterior radiculomedullary artery; (5) posterior spinal arteries; (6) ascending cervical artery; (7) deep cervical artery; (8) subclavian artery; (9) posterior radiculomedullary artery; (10) segmental arteries (intercostal arteries); (11) great anterior radiculomedullary artery (artery of Adamkiewicz); (12) segmental arteries (lumbar arteries); (13) rami cruciantes. (Reprinted from Santillan *et al.* 2012 [1], with permission from BMJ Publishing Group.)

Comprehensive Management of Arteriovenous Malformations of the Brain and Spine, ed. Robert F. Spetzler, Douglas S. Kondziolka, Randall T. Higashida, and M. Yashar S. Kalani. Published by Cambridge University Press.

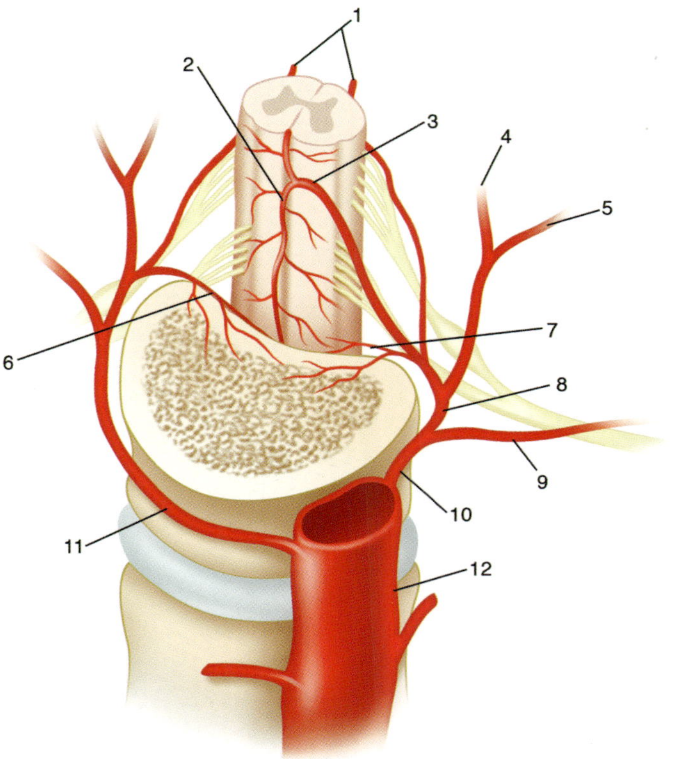

Fig. 3.2. Segmental arteries supplying the spinal cord. (1) Posterior spinal arteries; (2) anterior spinal artery; (3) anterior radiculomedullary artery; (4) medial musculocutaneous branch; (5) lateral musculocutaneous branch; (6 & 7) retrocorporeal arteries; (8) posterior (spinal) branch; (9) anterior branch; (10 & 11) trunk of the segmental (intercostal or lumbar) artery; (12) aorta. (Reprinted from Santillan *et al.* 2012 [1], with permission from BMJ Publishing Group.)

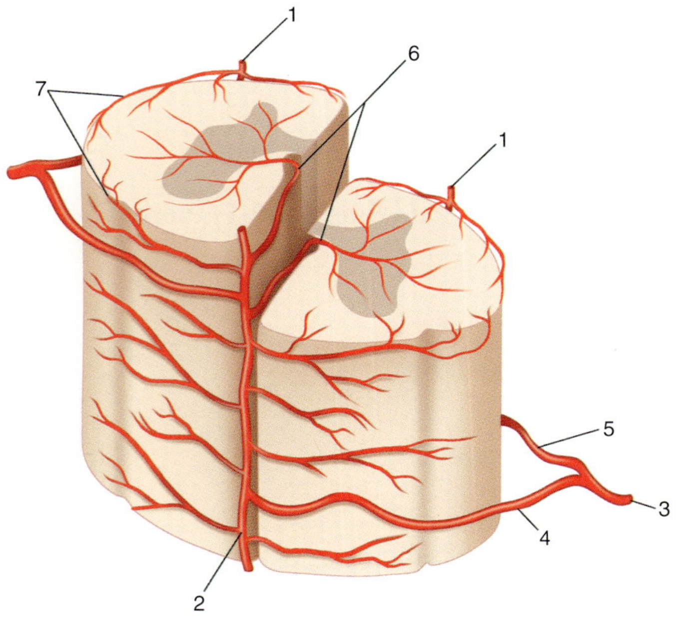

Fig. 3.3. Posterior and anterior spinal cord arteries. (1) Posterior spinal arteries; (2) anterior spinal artery; (3) spinal branch; (4) anterior radiculomedullary artery; (5) posterior radiculomedullary artery; (6) central (sulcal) arteries; (7) vasocorona. (Reprinted from Santillan *et al.* 2012 [1], with permission from BMJ Publishing Group.)

lower lumbar and sacral supply originates from branches of the internal iliac arteries.

Because the aorta is located anterior to the spinal cord, the left segmental arteries generally exit the aorta posteriorly and the right segmental arteries originate medially [3]. Each segmental artery has a ventral, dorsal, and spinal branch. The spinal branch enters the intervertebral foramen and splits into (1) the retrocorporeal (anterior spinal canal) and prelaminar (posterior spinal canal) arteries, and (2) a radicular artery. The radicular artery supplies nerve roots and dura at every level as the radiculoradial or radiculomeningeal arteries. At certain levels, the radicular artery supplies the spinal cord via branches known as the radiculomedullary arteries. The anterior radiculomedullary arteries supply the ASA and the posterior radiculomedullary arteries supply the PSAs (Fig. 3.3) [4].

Anterior spinal artery

At the cervical level, the ASA originates from a medial branch of each intracranial vertebral artery, which join together in the midcervical spine (C2–C4)(Fig. 3.4). This vessel descends over the central sulcus of the anterior cord all the way to the conus medullaris [5]. En route, it acquires multiple feeders. In

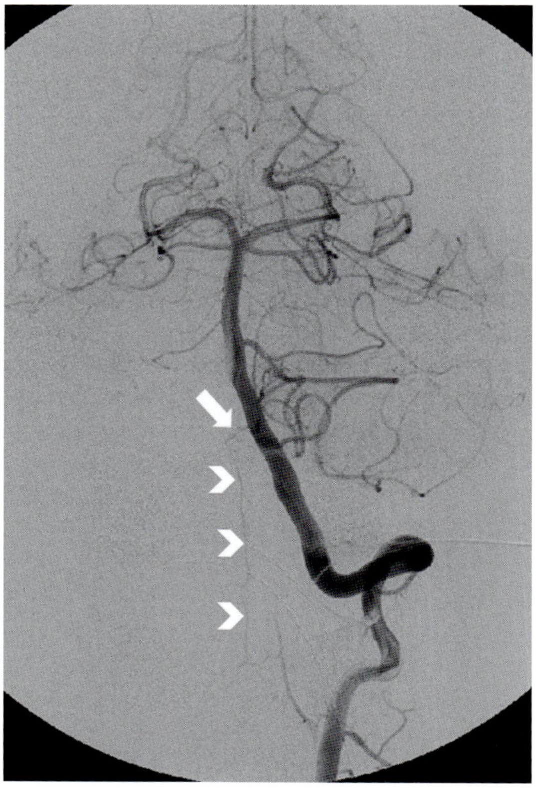

Fig. 3.4. Selective right vertebral artery catheter angiogram (frontal view) demonstrates the artery of cervical enlargement (arrow) supplying the anterior spinal artery (arrowheads). (Reprinted from Santillan *et al.* 2012 [1], with permission from BMJ Publishing Group.)

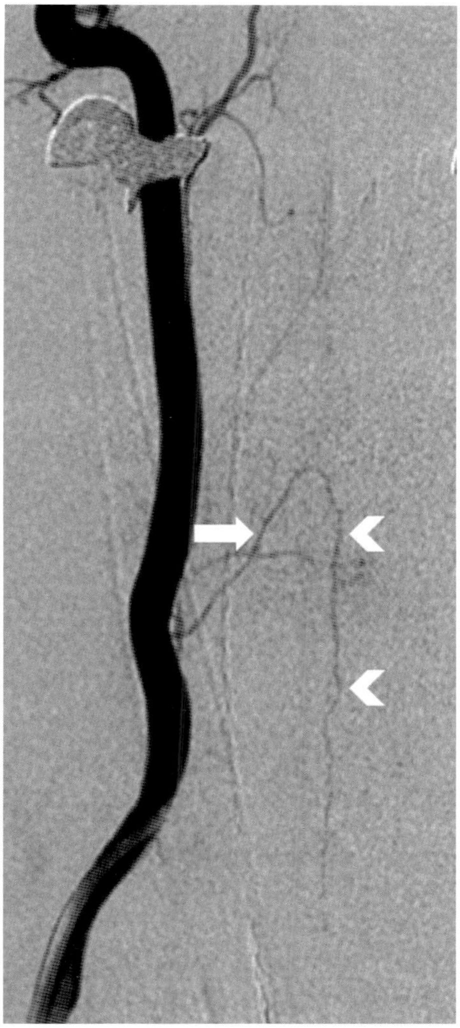

Fig. 3.5. Selective left vertebral artery catheter angiogram (frontal view) shows the anterior spinal artery (arrowheads) originating from the left vertebral artery (arrow) distal to the posterior inferior cerebellar artery origin. (Reprinted from Santillan *et al.* 2012 [1], with permission from BMJ Publishing Group.)

the cervical spine, the most prominent feeder is the artery of cervical enlargement, which is typically a branch of the deep cervical artery from the costocervical trunk at the C4–C8 level (Fig. 3.5) [6].

Additional arterial supply can arise from branches of the vertebral artery (usually around C3), the thyrocervical trunk (C4–C6), and the costocervical trunk (C6–C8) (Fig. 3.1) [2].

In the thoracolumbar spine, multiple anterior radiculomedullary feeders (usually six on average) from segmental branches directly from the aorta give supply to the ASA [2,7]. It is worth delineating the course of these arteries from the aorta to the spinal cord. In the thoracic spine, caudally from the T3 level, there are, on average, 10 pairs of segmental arteries exiting from the aorta. Above T3, a supreme intercostal artery emanates from the aorta and can divide into multiple segmental artery branches in order to supply the upper thoracic spine.

In the lumbar spine, there are normally four pairs of lumbar segmental arteries from L1–L4 (Fig. 3.2) [3]. Although there is much variability in the exact segmental arteries supplying the ASA, the anterior great radiculomedullary artery (artery of Adamkiewicz [AKA]), is a large feeder that originates from a segmental branch from T8 to L2 in the majority of individuals, although it can exit higher or lower than these levels [8]. It is typically found on the left side, taking a "hairpin" turn cranially prior to its downward course (Fig. 3.6) [3].

The lower lumbar segmental arteries, specifically at L4 and L5, can originate below the level of the aorta (i.e., the common iliac arteries and the median sacral artery), which are normally seen at the aortic bifurcation (Fig. 3.7).

Posterior spinal artery

At the level of the foramen magnum, two PSAs originate from branches of the vertebral arteries or posterior inferior cerebellar arteries. As mentioned above, the PSAs supply the posterior one-third of the spinal cord, specifically the posterior columns, dorsal lateral columns, and dorsal gray matter. Each PSA descends along the posterolateral surface of the spinal cord, receiving arterial feeders from 6 to 11 posterior radiculomedullary arteries as they descend caudally [5]. It should be noted that, unlike the ASA, the PSAs are discontinuous in their course (Fig. 3.8).

Venous system

The venous anatomy of the spinal cord is more variable than that of the arterial system. It is convenient to subdivide the anatomy of the venous side into a similar manner to the arterial side: into an intrinsic system and an extrinsic system (Fig. 3.9).

Intrinsic system

Venous drainage is not directly analogous to the arterial anatomy. Drainage is more regional with a central and peripheral venous system. The peripheral, or radial, veins originate in the capillaries at the gray–white junction and are directed centrifugally. The central, or sulcal, veins drain from the medial aspects of both halves of the spinal cord, specifically from the anterior horns, anterior commissure, and the white matter in the anterior funiculus [1].

Extrinsic system

Unlike the intrinsic system, it is convenient to correlate the superficial extrinsic venous system with the arterial system. The anterior median spinal vein is the closest corollary to the ASA and descends ventrally, receiving venous drainage from the sulcal veins and veins of the

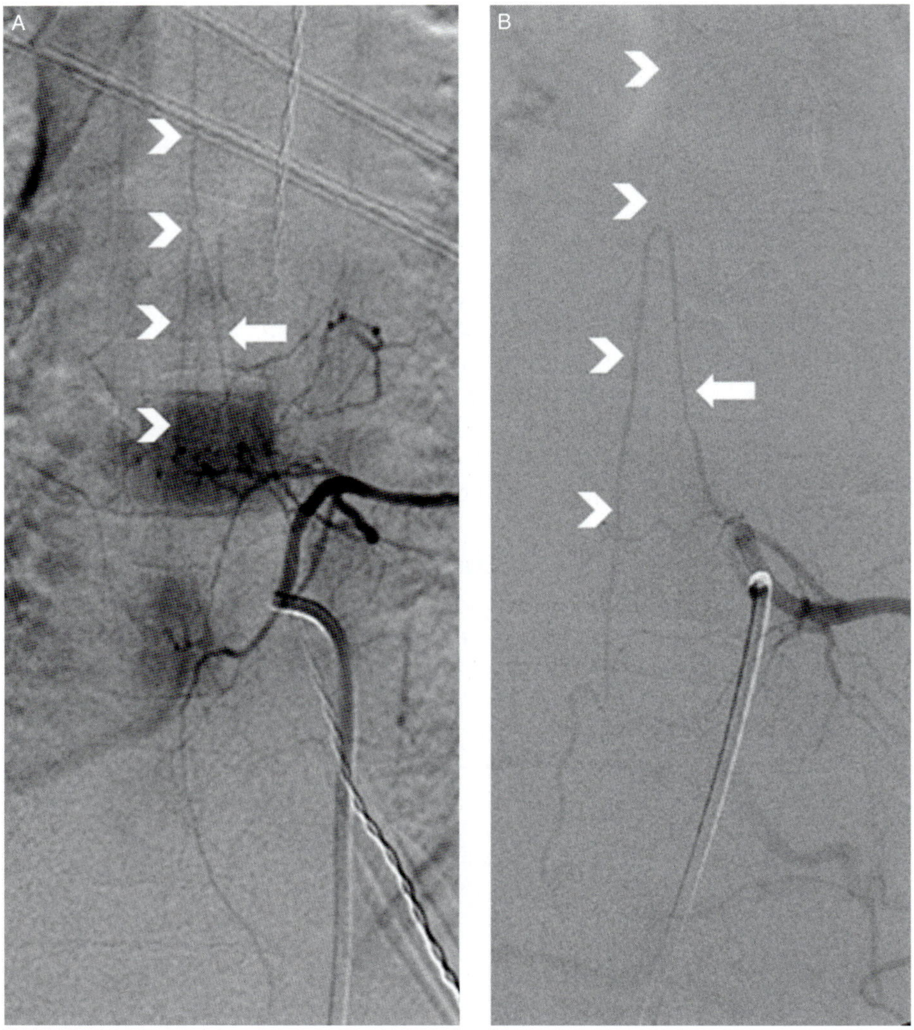

Fig. 3.6. Two lower thoracic selective catheter spinal angiograms (frontal views) depicting the typical "hairpin" turn of the artery of Adamkiewicz (arrow), which supplies the anterior spinal artery (arrowheads). The hemivertebral blush is noted in (A), confirming the midline position of the anterior spinal artery. (Reprinted from Santillan *et al.* 2012 [1], with permission from BMJ Publishing Group.)

ventral fissure. Posteriorly, there is usually a dominant posterior median vein, but smaller posterolateral veins often accompany this vessel [1]. These veins receive drainage from the peripheral veins of the spinal cord. The anterior and posterior median spinal veins subsequently drain into the anterior and posterior radiculomedullary veins, respectively, which then drain into epidural venous plexi. There are, on average, 8–14 anterior radiculomedullary veins [9] and 5–10 posterior radiculomedullary veins [5]. The largest anterior draining vein is the great anterior radiculomedullary vein, which drains the anterior thoracolumbar spine and is the closest corollary to AKA, given its proximity to the AKA. It is usually found from T11 to L3 (Fig. 3.10). It should be noted that venous drainage is normally difficult to visualize, except when injecting the AKA. The venous phase must appear within 10 seconds, otherwise it should be considered an abnormal finding and a spinal dural arteriovenous fistula must be suspected.

On average, three tortuous posterior median spinal veins and the anterior median spinal vein descend towards the epidural venous plexus via the posterior and anterior radiculomedullary veins [1].

On axial views, the epidural venous plexi are best represented diagrammatically with the anterior external vertebral venous plexus and basivertebral vein draining the vertebral body and the anterior internal vertebral venous plexus draining the epidural space. Posterior external and internal venous plexi are also present at each level. The internal venous plexi communicate with the aforementioned radiculomedullary veins and with the external venous plexi via the intervertebral veins in a valveless system (Fig. 3.11).

The intervertebral veins subsequently drain into segmental veins, which empty into the ascending lumbar and azygos systems before entering the superior vena cava (Fig. 3.9) [10,11].

When discussing the normal anatomy of the spinal venous system, it is necessary to discuss physiological mechanisms behind the venous drainage in the lower spinal cord. Many theories exist as to how autoregulation of venous pressure occurs in the spinal cord to prevent venous reflux under the umbrella of

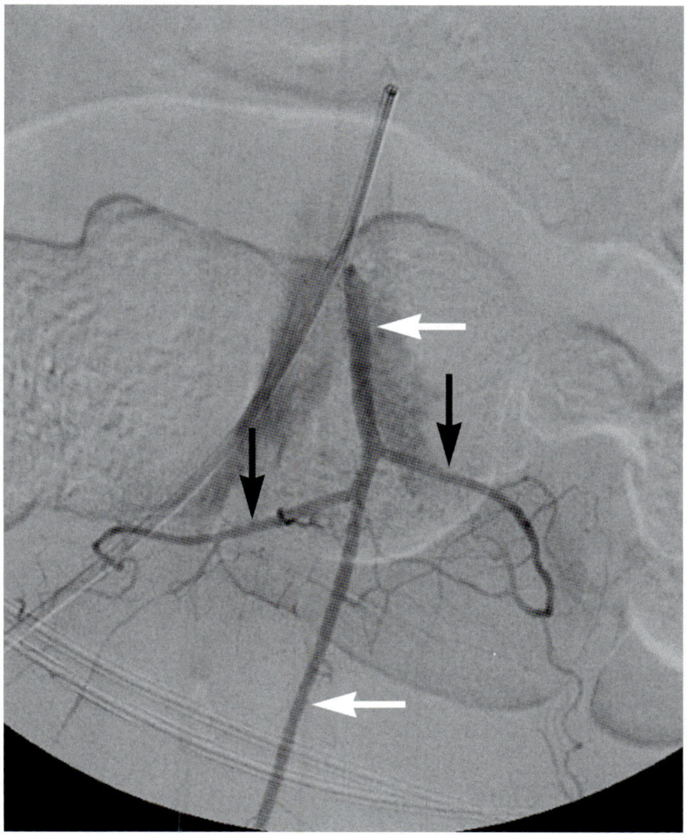

Fig. 3.7. Selective median sacral artery angiogram (frontal view) originating from the aorta (white arrows). Bilateral L5 segmental arteries are seen originating from this vessel (black arrows).

the "anti-reflux mechanism." Early theories ascribed this to the presence of radicular venous valves, but these valves are not found universally in cadaveric studies. Other structures to explain the anti-reflux mechanism have been discovered that will help to control venous pressure, including intravenous intradural folds, narrowing of radicular veins upon their entrance to the dura, increased smooth muscle fibers in these veins to assist in regulating waves in pressure, and a tortuous course to assist in siphoning increases in venous pressure [12,13].

Embryology

Embryologically, bilateral capillary networks on the ventrolateral surface of the cord connect with segmental branches of the aorta. These networks slowly transform into longitudinal systems that eventually form the ASA by the end of the second embryological month [5]. At this stage, there are 31 pairs of segmental arteries feeding the ASA. By the end of the fourth embryological month, variable regression of these vessels leaves four to eight ventral arteries supplying the ASA, with the artery of cervical enlargement and the AKA being the dominant vessels [14]. This variable segmental artery regression also leads to the origination of the vertebral arteries, thyrocervical trunks, and costocervical trunks in the cervical region and the iliac arteries in the lumbar region [15]. Venous networks are forming as these arterial anastomoses develop early in the embryo. It is thought that many vascular malformations can originate at this critical time, three to six weeks after gestation [16]. The premise of

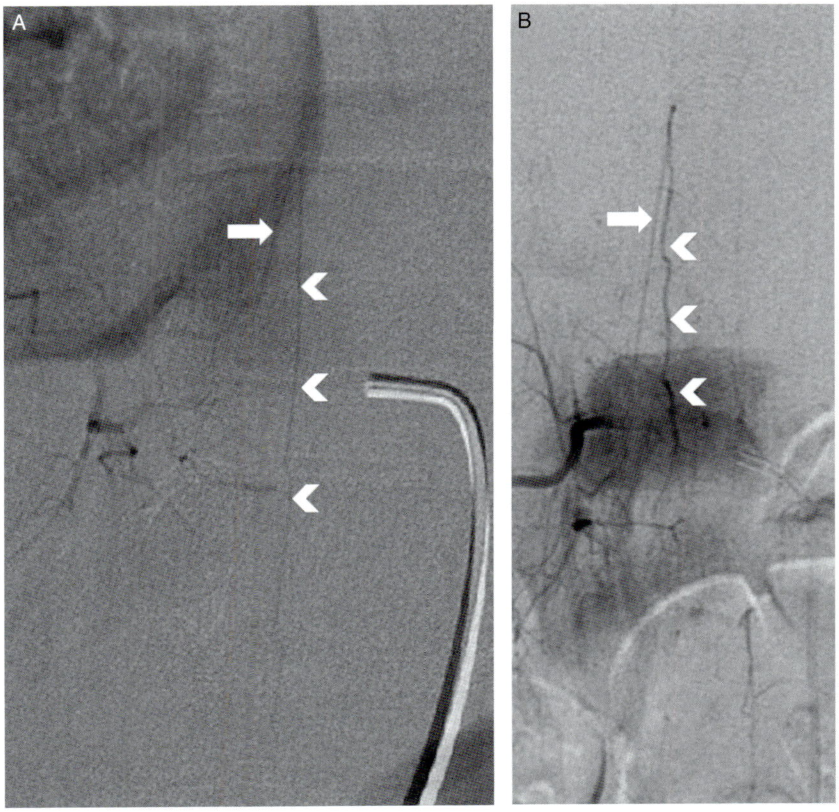

Fig. 3.8. Selective catheter spinal angiograms showing the differences between the anterior (A) and posterior (B) radiculomedullary arteries. (A) The hairpin curve formed when the anterior radiculomedullary artery (arrow) joins the anterior spinal artery (arrowheads) is round. (B) The posterior radiculomedullary artery (arrow) makes a sharper turn when reaching the posterior spinal artery (arrowheads). (Reprinted from Santillan *et al.* 2012 [1], with permission from BMJ Publishing Group.)

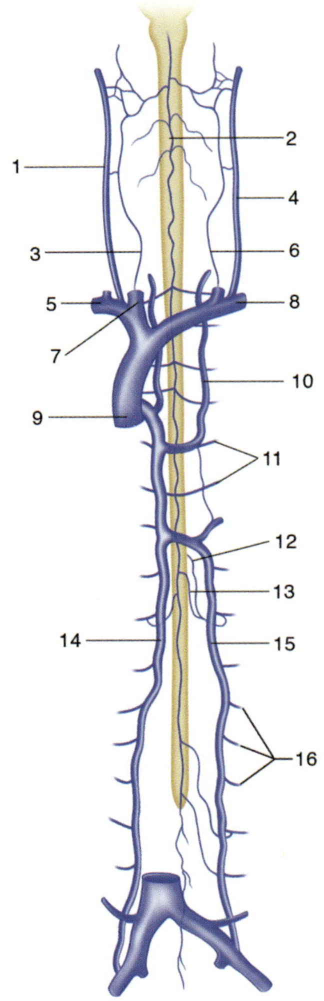

Fig. 3.9. Venous drainage of the spinal cord. (1) Right vertebral vein; (2) anterior median vein; (3) right deep cervical vein; (4) left vertebral vein; (5) subclavian vein (6) left deep cervical vein; (7) internal jugular vein; (8) left subclavian vein; (9) superior vena cava; (10) accessory hemiazygos vein; (11) intercostal veins; (12) posterior radiculomedullary vein; (13) anterior radiculomedullary vein; (14) azygos vein; (15) hemiazygos vein; (16) lumbar veins. (Reprinted from Santillan *et al.* 2012 [1], with permission from BMJ Publishing Group.)

variable arterial regression in altering the vascular supply of the spinal cord at any given level underscores the need for an exhaustive angiogram of all potential feeding vessels for spinal vascular anomalies (Fig. 3.12). There are fewer data on the embryological development of the venous system [5].

Spinal anastomoses

Knowledge of spinal anastomotic networks is essential for an adequate characterization of spinal vascular lesions and subsequent treatment of these abnormalities. Failure to do so may result in inaccurate false-negative spinal angiograms or incompletely treated arteriovenous malformations [17].

Arterial anastomoses

Extradural anastomoses

The extradural anastomoses are divided into intraspinal and extraspinal systems. The extraspinal system, also known as the paravertebral anastomotic network, is a longitudinal network that runs along the lateral aspect of the vertebral bodies and is best defined in the cervical spine where the vertebral artery, ascending cervical artery, and deep cervical arteries can communicate [18]. It is also evident between adjacent segmental arteries. The intraspinal system, or retrocorporeal arterial network, is primarily a transverse network that connects the right and left segmental arteries and is best recognized as a diamond-shaped network located in the dorsal epidural space posterior to the vertebral bodies [15].

Pial anastomoses

The pial arterial network, also known as the vasocorona, is an arterioarterial connection between the anterior and posterior spinal systems that is not visualized on a normal spinal angiogram because of the small caliber of these vessels, although it visible in high-flow lesions such as arteriovenous malformations [15].

Conus anastomoses

Commonly referred to as the "arterial basket" the conus anastomosis is the anastomotic arcade located at the conus medullaris that connects the ASA to two PSAs via the rami cruciantes [15]. Radicular arteries from the cauda equina also go through this network because of the abundant vascular arterial supply [15].

Venous anastomoses

Although not uniform in their anatomy, venous anastomoses can be subdivided into central–peripheral and transmedullary types. The central–peripheral type connects sulcal and radial veins and the transmedullary type is a midline anastomosis of the left and right median veins [18]. The latter is a larger, more important, network that can sometimes be visualized on MRI as well as angiography. It should be noted that the transmedullary system is largest in the cervicothoracic spine [5].

Although a thorough investigation of all potential spinal anastomoses is needed to diagnose a treatable lesion, occasionally angiography must look beyond the spine itself. One additional pathological anastomosis is the type 5 craniocervical dural arteriovenous fistula, which can clinically present as dysfunction of the upper cord or lower brainstem and radiographically with edema in the cervical spine and/or brainstem. The existence of these fistulae underlines the need not only for a spinal angiogram but also for cerebral angiography when searching for treatable lesions [19–23].

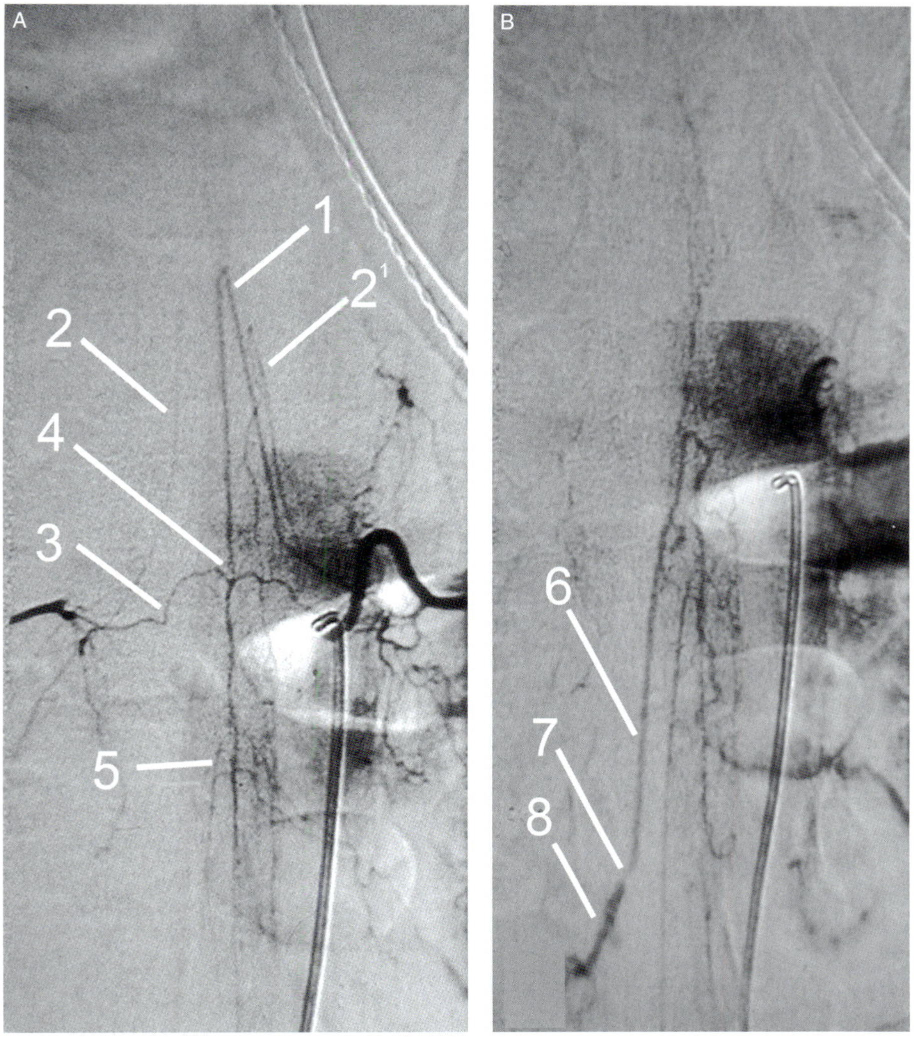

Fig. 3.10. Selective spinal angiography demonstrating the greater anterior radicular vein. Left T11 angiograms with a prolonged injection of contrast to better visualize the angioanatomy at the conus medullaris. (A) Late arterial phase. In this particular patient, all three radiculomedullary arteries of the conus medullaris are seen: (1) the artery of Adamkiewicz; (2 & 2') the right and left posterior radiculomedullary arteries; (3) the right retrocorporeal artery; (4) transmedian anastomosis of the retrocoporeal arteries (note how the right retrocorporeal arteries fill via this anastomosis on this left intercostal artery angiogram); (5) capillary blush of the conus medullaris. (B) Late venous phase (10–12 seconds). (6) The greater anterior radicular vein is well visualized; (7) narrowing at the dural passage that has been identified as a potential anti-reflux mechanism; (8) epidural vein. Note also other veins following the nerve roots of the filum terminale.

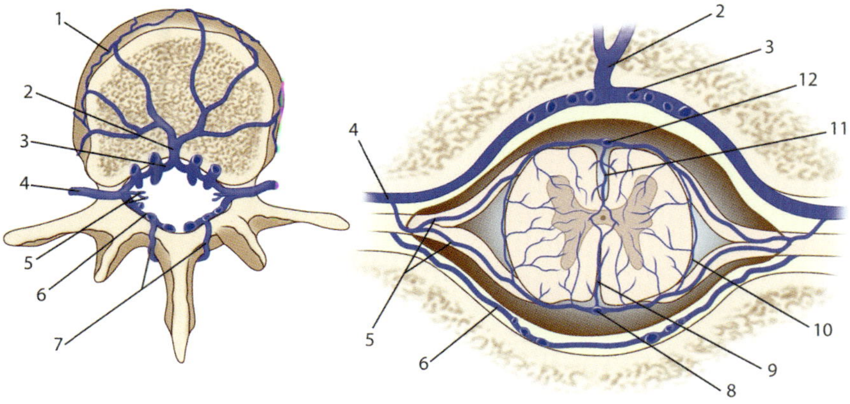

Fig. 3.11. Veins of the spinal cord in axial views. (1) Anterior external vertebral venous plexus; (2) basivertebral vein; (3) anterior internal vertebral venous plexus; (4) intervertebral vein; (5) anterior and posterior radicular veins; (6) posterior internal vertebral venous plexus; (7) posterior external vertebral venous plexus; (8) posterior spinal vein; (9) posterior central vein; (10) pial venous plexus; (11) anterior central vein; (12) anterior spinal vein.

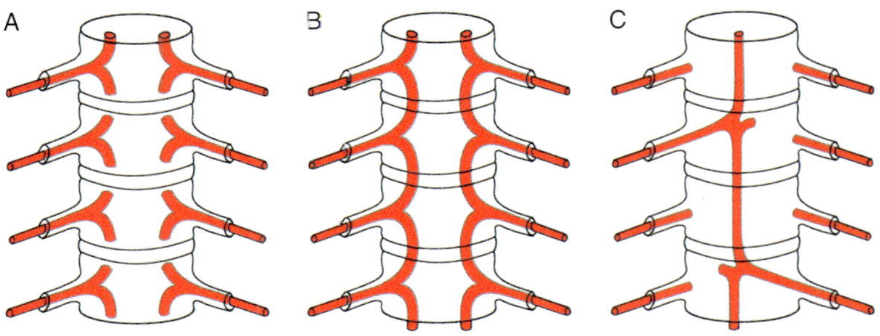

Fig. 3.12. Embryological development of the arterial system. (A) Metameric stage with individual arteries supplying each spinal level. (B) Formation of longitudinal anastomoses. (C) Segmental regression and fusion of arteries with formation of a central artery.

References

1. Santillan A, Nacarino V, Greenberg E, *et al.* Vascular anatomy of the spinal cord. *J Neurointerv Surg* 2012;**4**:67–74.
2. Brockstein B, Johns L, Gewertz BL. Blood supply to the spinal cord: anatomical and physiologic correlations. *Ann Vasc Surg* 1994;**8**:394–9.
3. Shimizu S, Tanaka R, Kan S, *et al.* Origins of the segmental arteries in the aorta: an anatomical study for selective catheterization with spinal arteriography. *AJNR Am J Neuroradiol* 2005;**26**:922–8.
4. Manelfe C, Lazorthes G, Roulleau J. [Arteries of the human spinal dura mater.] *Acta Radiol Diagn (Stockh)* 1972;**13**:829–41.
5. Thron AK. *Vascular Anatomy of the Spinal Cord: Neuroradiological Investigations and Clinical Syndromes.* New York: Springer, 1989.
6. Lazorthes G, Poulhes J, Bastide G, *et al.* [Arterial vascularization of the spine; anatomical research and applications in pathology of the spinal cord and aorta.] *Neurochirurgie* 1958;**4**:3–19.
7. Djindjian R. *L'Angiographie de la Moelle Epiniere*. Paris: Masson, 1970.
8. Hong MK, Hong MK, Pan WR, *et al.* The angiosome territories of the spinal cord: exploring the issue of preoperative spinal angiography. Laboratory investigation. *J Neurosurg Spine* 2008;**8**:352–64.
9. Gillilan LA. Veins of the spinal cord. Anatomical details; suggested clinical applications. *Neurology* 1970;**20**:860–8.
10. Groen RJ, du Toit DF, Phillips FM, *et al.* Anatomical and pathological considerations in percutaneous vertebroplasty and kyphoplasty: a reappraisal of the vertebral venous system. *Spine (Phila Pa 1976)* 2004;**29**: 1465–71.
11. Medscape. Anatomy of the CSVS. *Medscape* 2006 (http://www.medscape.org/viewarticle/522597_2 accessed 16 May 2014).
12. van der Kuip M, Hoogland PV, Groen RJ. Human radicular veins: regulation of venous reflux in the absence of valves. *Anat Rec* 1999;**254**:173–80.
13. Goyal M, Willinsky R, Montanera W, *et al.* Paravertebral arteriovenous malformations with epidural drainage: clinical spectrum, imaging features, and results of treatment. *AJNR Am J Neuroradiol* 1999;**20**:749–55.
14. Lamin SBJ. *Practical Neurology: Vascular Anatomy of the Spinal Cord and Spinal Cord Ischaemia*. Oxford: Blackwell, 2003.
15. Neuroangio.org. *Spinal Arterial Anatomy*, 2013 (http://neuroangio.org/spinal-vascular-anatomy/spinal-arterial-anatomy/ accessed 16 May 2014).
16. Deshaies EM, Eddleman CS, Boulos AS. *Handbook of Neuroendovascular Surgery*. Stuttgart: Thieme, 2011.
17. Patsalides A, Santillan A, Knopman J, *et al.* Endovascular management of spinal dural arteriovenous fistulas. *J Neurointerv Surg* 2011;**3**:80–4.
18. Hurst RW, Rosenwasser RH. *Interventional Neuroradiology*. New York: Informa Healthcare, 2008.
19. Kulwin C, Bohnstedt BN, Scott JA, *et al.* Dural arteriovenous fistulas presenting with brainstem dysfunction: diagnosis and surgical treatment. *Neurosurg Focus* 2012;**32**:E10.
20. Gobin YP. Classification and endovascular treatment of spinal cord arteriovenous malformations and fistulas. *J Stroke Cerebrovasc Dis* 1997;**6**:282–6.
21. Cognard C, Gobin YP, Pierot L, *et al.* Cerebral dural arteriovenous fistulas: clinical and angiographic correlation with a revised classification of venous drainage. *Radiology* 1995;**194**:671–80.
22. Gobin YP, Rogopoulos A, Aymard A, *et al.* Endovascular treatment of intracranial dural arteriovenous fistulas with spinal perimedullary venous drainage. *J Neurosurg* 1992;**77**:718–23.
23. Brunereau L, Gobin YP, Meder JF, *et al.* Intracranial dural arteriovenous fistulas with spinal venous drainage: relation between clinical presentation and angiographic findings. *AJNR Am J Neuroradiol* 1996;**17**:1549–54.

Chapter 4

Physiology and hemodynamics of arteriovenous malformations

H. Richard Winn and Philip E. Stieg

Introduction

This chapter will review the physiology and hemodynamics of arteriovenous malformations (AVMs). These malformations are characterized by a direct connection between the arterial and venous systems. This low resistance connection has physiological and pathological consequences on the surrounding and, in some cases, distant nervous tissue. These effects are best understood by knowledge of the relevant anatomy of the cerebral circulation and the factors involved in regulation of cerebral blood flow (CBF).

There are many studies of CBF and metabolism in patients with AVMs, but the data and the conclusions derived from these studies are not uniform and this chapter will attempt to clarify some of these disparate observations. Some of the confusion may stem from the fact that these clinical observations are based on a mature or relative steady-state lesion where the present status has been created by dynamic and reactive physiological and pathological forces.

We recognize that uncertainty exists about the CBF and brain metabolism in patients with AVMs but suggest that the preponderance of data supports the existence of the following three factors: shunt, steal, and elevated venous pressure.

- A shunt exists between the high-pressure arterial system and the low-pressure venous system. This shunt is an anatomical pathological entity with low cerebrovascular resistance. In normal human brain, direct arterial–venous connection is absent [1].
- A steal exists or, in the past did exist, as a consequence of the shunt and its low resistance. Arterial blood, destined for surrounding "normal" brain, is diverted from higher-resistant vessels perfusing surrounding normal brain tissue into the low-resistant shunt. This steal has metabolic and CBF effects on the surrounding tissue.
- Venous hypertension occurs because of the increased blood flow through the shunt; the "afterload" or blood volume of the venous system is increased and, depending on the capacitance of the venous system (i.e., adequacy of drainage), venous pressure is increased in the surrounding brain and possibly elsewhere throughout the brain. The increase in venous blood volume and venous hypertension has metabolic and CBF effects on the peri-AVM tissue, and in some instances, on brain distant from the AVM.

These three factors are critical to understanding the mechanisms regulating CBF and metabolism in the brains of patients harboring AVMs.

Anatomy

A comprehensive review of the blood supply of the CNS is presented in Chapter 2 whereas the discussion below is focused on the relevant anatomy as it pertains to AVMs.

The cerebral circulation can be divided into macro (arteries and veins) and micro (arterioles, capillaries, and venules) components. In considering the vascular anatomy as it pertains to AVMs, changes in normal vascular anatomy and the development of collateral circulation will be considered.

Macrocirculation

Arteries

The arterial component of the macrocirculation comprises large conductance vessels whose walls contain vascular smooth muscle [2]. Both intraluminal blood pressure (generally ≥90% of aorta mean pressure) and flow are high (Fig. 4.1) [3]. Little gas or nutrient exchange occurs at this level of the circulation. The branching architecture influences the flow pattern with acute angle branches (<30 degrees) receiving more flow than arteries whose branching is less acute (60–90 degrees). In AVMs, the angle of branches may also change as dominant feeding arteries enlarge, thicken, and become tortuous.

The presence of an AVM and the shunt has an impact on arterial and venous macrocirculatory vessels. In general, the feeding and draining vessels enlarge and undergo anatomical changes in their walls. The mechanisms responsible for these changes are not comprehensively understood, but the initiating event is clearly related to increased arterial flow, which is defined by the general principles of fluid dynamics:

$$F = P/R$$

Comprehensive Management of Arteriovenous Malformations of the Brain and Spine, ed. Robert F. Spetzler, Douglas S. Kondziolka, Randall T. Higashida, and M. Yashar S. Kalani. Published by Cambridge University Press.

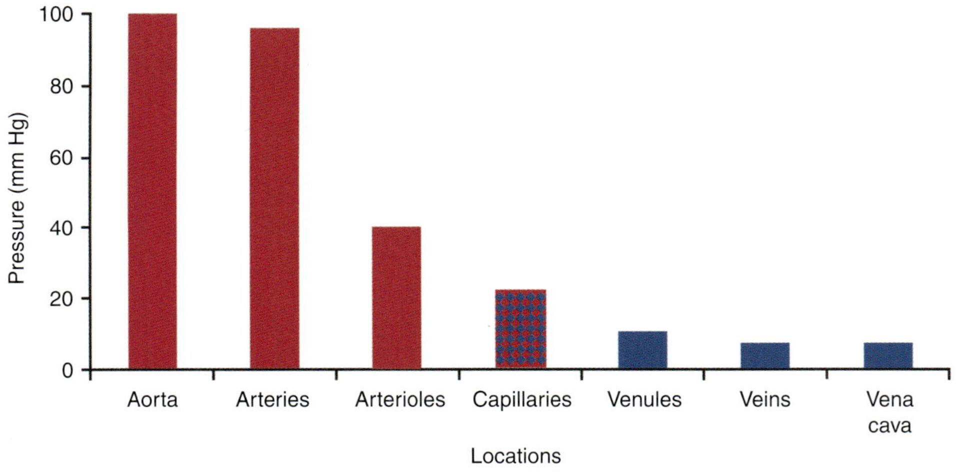

Fig. 4.1. Average intraluminal pressure at various locations within the circulation under physiological conditions. Note the greatest drop in blood pressure occurs between the arteries and the arterioles. The arteriolar component of the circulation is critical for flow regulation.

where *F* is flow (CBF), *P* is pressure, and *R* is resistance. In turn, resistance is inversely related to the fourth power of the diameter [4]. Consequently, small increases in the diameter of the arterioles result in significant decreases in resistance and, assuming that there is sufficient perfusion pressure, flow will increase dramatically.

The ability of arteries to sense alteration of flow is an inherent property of the arterial wall [5]. This can be demonstrated in the laboratory with isolated perfused and pressurized brain arterioles, where acute increase in flow results in vasodilatation even in the absence of any parenchyma [6]. This flow response appears to involve nitric oxide [6].

The above observations illustrate the arterial response to acute change in flow and may or may not be applicable to the chronic state. Any discussion of the changes in the vascular anatomy of human AVMs must take into consideration that, in general, most AVMs are not recognized at birth and are only discovered in a more mature state. This is true even now with the availability of MRI, which allows a non-invasive window into the brain. Therefore, discussions about the change in vascular anatomy (and brain metabolism) are, to a large part speculative, based on extrapolations of limited clinical observations in patients with AVMs. Data obtained from perinidal "mature" AVMs may not reflect the dynamic response to a "distress" signal in the perinidal tissue, a resultant response (arterial enlargement), and the re-establishment of new "normal" steady state [7].

Some insights in regard to the steal phenomenon and perinidal conditions might be gained by evaluating animal models of AVM [8–11]. Most models are in rodents and are created by anastomosing a component of the carotid artery to the venous system and then studying the distant responses in brain and vascular tissue. Unfortunately, these surgically created fistulae, while ingenious, are not intracranial and may, therefore, not mimic the human condition. In addition, as has been recently recognized, rodent models have distinct limitations for simulating human diseases [12].

An alternative to animal models is to evaluate the changes occurring in humans after the surgical creation of an arteriovenous fistulae in the forearm for hemodialysis [13], where zero time is known (surgery) and subsequent changes in the peri-AVM tissue can then be documented. In this situation, steal does occasionally occur in the distal hand. However, the comparison with human brain AVM is not parallel because the metabolism of tissue around this arteriovenous fistula (muscle and bone) is distinctly different from that of the brain. Moreover, there are recognized systemic abnormalities associated with kidney failure that make comparisons problematic [13].

With these caveats in mind, enlargement of the feeding arteries appears to be related to increase in flow and the ability of the vascular endothelium to sense change in flow and wall stress [14,15]. Shear stress (tau) is defined as a measure of the force of friction from a fluid acting on a body in the path of that fluid [7]. Endothelial cells are capable of discerning flow and change in flow rates [14]. Like the similar cellular mechanisms in the inner ear, transformation of mechanical energy to a biological signal occurs in the endothelium. The biological signaling results in vascular smooth muscle growth and enlargement of the vessel diameter [14]. With prolonged time and stress, arteries undergo hypertrophy and changes that are characteristic of aging vessels: wall thickening, vascular smooth muscle hypertrophy, and, eventually, atherosclerosis [7,16]. These changes, either individually or in combination, alter the hemodynamic characteristics of the feeding arteries by varying wall stiffness, pulsatility, and shear stress. Flow-related arterial aneurysms can develop [17]. On the venous side of the macrocirculation, similar changes can be observed [18]. Comparable changes have been well documented in patients after traumatically or surgically induced arteriovenous fistulae [13].

Arteriovenous malformations: development of collateral arterial circulation

In the setting of an AVM, macrocirculatory arterial collateral flow can originate from two sources: the branches of the circle of Willis and/or branches of the external carotid arteries. Two different mechanisms can account for the recruitment of collateral blood flow: the low resistance of the shunt and brain tissue hypoperfusion.

The low resistance of the shunt. The low vascular resistance caused by the absence of a capillary network leads to increased flow in the upstream large arteries. Depending on the degree of the shunt, increased flow may extend even to the cervical arteries. As noted above, the ability of arteries and arterioles to sense alteration of flow is an inherent property of the arterial wall. At the macro level of the cerebral circulation, flow is diverted toward the low resistance shunt and feeding arteries enlarge. The plasticity and reversibility of these events and processes are well illustrated by observations in 50 patients with AVMs treated by radiosurgery [19]. The diameters of branches of the circle of Willis were not static. Following AVM treatment and closure, feeding arteries regressed whereas other arteries became better perfused.

Brain tissue hypoperfusion. A different mechanism appears to be responsible for the recruitment of flow from the external carotid. Here the initiating mechanisms are related indirectly to the shunt but directly to the lowered perfusion of normal tissue surrounding the AVM. The lowered perfusion comes about because of the diversion of arterial flow away from the surrounding tissue towards the AVM because of lower resistance in the shunt and increased venous pressure. As a result of the diversion of arterial flow, the surrounding tissue is marginally perfused, simulating ischemic and/or hypoxic conditions. As in other ischemic or hypoxic conditions, the resultant chronic metabolic stress would be expected to elaborate substances such as adenosine, endothelial growth factor, and hypoxia-inducible factor 1, which induce blood vessel formation, growth, and eventually collateral flow from the external carotid circulation into the brain [20,21]. Venous hypertension, in the absence of ischemia, has also been shown experimentally to cause the elaboration of these factors [22]. In addition, in brain tissue from patients with AVMs, there appears to be an abnormal balance in the angiopoietin–tie2 system [23].

Veins of the macrocirculation

The venous system is characterized by low resistance, low intraluminal pressure, and a syncytial-like interconnection, which allows for large capacitance and redistribution of draining blood.

In humans and other animals, two different types of venous system exist and have been characterized by their degree of compliance: large and small. The large compliant venous beds, such as the splanchnic and cutaneous circulations, have significant ability for storage of venous blood. In contrast, the cerebral circulation has a low storage capacity and the veins serve primarily as conduits. The lack of capacitance is related to the rigidity of the skull and the restriction on the expansion of intracranial volume, as dictated by the Monro–Kellie doctrine [24,25]:

$$K = V_P + V_{CSF} + V_B$$

where K is a constant, V_P is the volume of the parenchyma, V_{CSF} is the volume of the cerebrospinal fluid, and V_B is the volume of blood. In the setting of an AVM and increased venous volume, this relative lack of capacitance becomes a factor in altering the circulation to normal brain tissue and may, in the long term, decrease the parenchymal volume.

In patients with AVM, the geographic extent of the venous drainage is increased compared with the venous drainage in the absence of an AVM.

The pathognomonic sign of the presence of an AVM is an "early" filling vein seen on catheter angiography. The arteriovenous circulation time (as compared with transit time) is defined as the duration between maximal contrast filling in the carotid siphon to the maximal contrast filling of the parietal veins and has been measured to be 4.13 ± 0.74 seconds [26]. Transit time is sometimes used interchangeably with circulation time or more commonly applied to a specific component (i.e., peak concentration) of the circulation (i.e., shunt, peri-AVM tissue).

The normal sequence of venous contrast filling after carotid arteriography is as follows. The superficial draining veins emptying into the sagittal sinus fill from anterior to posterior with the deep venous draining filling later; the veins of Labbé and Trolard in normal conditions may fill out of sequence. With AVMs, as noted above, there will be early filling of veins draining the shunt, but the surrounding venous drainage may be delayed or poorly visualized on arteriography. As a consequence, the circulation time may be an unreliable measurement. Some investigators have found that transit times in the peri-AVM tissues are delayed and predictive of hemorrhage [27].

During laboratory observations of the pial circulation through a rigid clear cranial window, cerebral veins, unlike arteries and arterioles, do not enlarge their diameter [2] during an increase in CBF caused by multiple physiological stimuli (e.g., hypoxia, hypercarbia, neuronal activation). However, chronic increase in venous flow and pressure, as occurs in AVM, usually leads to progressive enlargement of individual veins and the extent of the collection system.

As noted with the arterial macrocirculation, pathological changes in the venous wall can occur as a consequence of the increased venous volume and flow. These changes would include wall thickening, vascular smooth muscle hypertrophy, and calcification. Taken in sum, these and other pathological changes can lead to venous tortuosity, aneurysm formation, and relative or absolute constriction. The last can extenuate the degree of venous hypertension and has been correlated with increased risk of AVM hemorrhage (as has the presence of venous aneurysms) [18].

In studies during surgical exposure [28–30] in humans with AVMs, the open cranial state may inadvertently lead to misleading results. An open cranial system violates the characteristic restrictions of the Monro–Kellie doctrine [24,25] (see above) since the intracranial volume has been expanded by the craniotomy. Moreover, as has been clearly demonstrated in animals with exposure of the cortex to the atmosphere [31], loss of carbon dioxide from the exposed surface of the brain results in rapid (<10 minutes) alteration in cerebrospinal fluid and interstitial fluid pH (alkalinization). This change in pH causes significant (~20%) vasoconstriction, thereby altering the baseline CBF and vessel diameter measurements [31]. With an open window preparation, hypercarbic vasodilatation and response to norepinephrine are exaggerated [31]. Other investigators have also noted a pH sensitive to catecholamines

[32]. Therefore, data analyzing intraoperative vascular reactions obtained during craniotomy (i.e., open window) for AVM resection may not represent normal physiological responses and should be interpreted with caution[28,33].

Microcirculation

The microcirculation consists of arterioles, capillaries, and venules. The regulation of CBF and exchange of materials and nutrients occurs predominantly at the microcirculatory level. This component of the circulation is absent in the AVM circulation but present in the surrounding brain. An understanding of the physiology and anatomy of the microcirculation is important since the microcirculation of the brain surrounding an AVM has been shown to be impaired.

Arterioles

The first component of the microcirculation is the largest arterioles (arteries <300–400 μm), which are located on the pial surface. Smaller branches (60–20 μm) arising from the pial arterioles then plunge down through the Virchow–Robin space to achieve an intraparenchymal location. These "terminal" arterioles are 8–20 μm in diameter and consist of two layers: an outer vascular smooth muscle and an inner endothelium.

The greatest fall in blood pressure is observed when comparing the pressure in the arteries and the arterioles (Fig. 4.1). Thus the arteriolar circulation accounts for a significant amount of the vascular resistance. The pressure drop "shields" the fragile capillaries from exposure to high intraluminal blood pressure. The critical role of the arteriolar circulation in brain is illustrated by the study of Kontos *et al.* [34], who observed through a closed, clear cranial window different-sized pial arteries and arterioles as blood pressure dropped from 130 to 40 mmHg. The smallest (~40 μm) arterioles dilated the most (~60%) and continued to increase in diameter as blood pressure fell below 50 mmHg. In contrast, arteries (>300 μm) dilated the least (~10%) and remained stable as blood pressure fell from 90 to 70 mmHg.

The rheology of the microcirculation will be influenced by hematocrit, erythrocyte flexibility, platelet aggregation, and plasma viscosity [35]. In vessels smaller than 200–300 μm in diameter, red blood cells move into the central rapid moving part of the flow stream, while white blood cells and other constituents of the plasma move more slowly next to the vessel wall [36]. At asymmetrical branch points, the cells are distributed in an uneven fashion, the greater proportion going to the branches deviating the least from the original direction and to those with higher flow. Tributaries close to a right angle may receive only plasma, platelets, and a few white cells. As a result, the hematocrit in the microvasculature is lower than in the average large blood vessel [36]. White blood cells, by comparison, are represented in a higher proportion in the microcirculation [36].

Under normal conditions, acute microvascular vasodilatation (e.g., in response to neuronal activation) requires coordinated response in the upstream arterial tree in order to provide sufficient flow to the dilated arterioles. In the absence of upstream vasodilatation, there would be insufficient flow to the microcirculation, leading to diversion ("steal") of blood from the surrounding tissue. The mechanisms responsible for coordinating the upstream responses are unclear. Potentially, changes in upstream shear could cause larger arteries to dilate, but vasodilatation and flow in pial arteries has been shown to occur before a measureable change in shear stress [37]. Under physiological conditions, the conducted signal for vasodilatation may travel in the arterial wall, as occurs in the non-cerebral circulation [38]. Alternatively, the pathway of this conducted signal may involve astrocytes and their extensions into the glia-limitans [39]. However, astrocytic signaling is an unlikely mechanism in the large arteries, which are not in direct contact with the brain. Here, vascular wall signaling appears to be the most likely mechanism coordinating upstream vasodilatation. In the setting of an AVM, no studies have evaluated these upstream coordinating mechanisms. Conceivably, enlargement of arteries upstream to the shunt may be partially related to vessel wall- or astrocyte-mediated mechanisms. In the peri-AVM tissue, failure of these coordinating mechanisms may contribute to steal.

While the arterial macro- and microcirculation responses to a variety of challenges (i.e., changes in carbon dioxide) are similar and differ only in degree, clear distinctions occur, particularly in their response to injury. For example, following experimental head injury in cats with a cranial window, both arterioles and larger arteries failed to dilate with topical application of acetylcholine [40]. However, the arterioles regained their vasomotor response within minutes whereas the large arterial response remained impaired for 8–12 hours [40]. The macrocirculatory and microcirculatory responses in patients with AVMs before and after treatment remain to be determined. Perhaps, as with trauma, clear distinctions exist.

Capillaries

Each terminal arteriole gives rise to 8–32 capillaries. Capillaries are composed of a unique endothelium (largely responsible for the blood–brain barrier) and a basement membrane. In peri-AVM tissue, enlarged and congested capillaries has been documented [41].

Venules

The smallest (20–30 μm) components of the venous system are the non-muscular venules, which together with the capillaries form the "exchange" component of the circulation. These vessels (capillaries and non-muscular venules) have the thinnest walls and the largest surface area in the circulation. Moreover, the velocity of the blood flow is the lowest in the circulation, thereby allowing more time for exchange of materials.

Exchange of materials between the intravascular compartment and the extravascular compartment involves movement of water and solutes across the endothelium. Amongst other mechanisms, diffusion and ultrafiltration (or osmosis) are critical. Diffusion depends on random motion of individual molecules and ions, but it can be influenced by blood flow, particularly where permeability is high. In the CNS, another factor affecting diffusion is the tight junctions of the capillaries.

In general, diffusion depends on differences in concentration in blood and tissue (interstitial fluid). The latter will be affected by local metabolic production and consumption. Diffusion can also be flow limited, especially in regard to oxygen and carbon dioxide. In the brain surrounding an AVM where flow is reduced, relative hypoxia and hypercarbia may ensue.

Ultrafiltration is the movements of fluids and solutes together through a membrane unidirectionally and is driven by the difference between hydrostatic and osmotic pressure. As with diffusion, ultrafiltration can be influenced by the blood–brain barrier. Ultrafiltration is the principal mechanism for controlling interstitial fluid volumes. Since ultrafiltration follows Starling's hypothesis (ultrafiltration is determined by the balance between hydrostatic and osmotic forces) and is susceptible to intravascular pressure, theoretically increased venous pressure should lead to brain edema. Most AVM studies in humans, despite documentation of elevated venous pressure, fail to document increase in brain edema. This absence of edema may be related to adaptive changes in the next order of the circulation, the muscular venules. These muscular venules are known to control exchange vessel pressures and venular volumes and thereby play a role in blood flow and exchange function. The absence of brain edema in the setting of increased venous pressure in most patients with AVMs again emphasizes that analysis of the "mature" AVM may not be the ideal setting to uncover the dynamic forces affecting surrounding brain.

Physiology of cerebral blood flow

To understand the pathophysiology of CBF in patients with AVMs, it is important to understand the physiology of CBF regulation. There are three main hypotheses to explain CBF regulation [2]: the neural hypothesis, metabolic hypothesis, and myogenic hypothesis.

The neural hypothesis states that nerves have a direct influence on vascular tone [2]. Nerve fibers associated with cerebral vessels have been identified mainly within the macrocirculation [42], although innervation of the microcirculation has also been suggested [42].

There are two proposed origins of these nerves: intrinsic and extrinsic to the brain [2]. The former involves brainstem and cerebellar and cortical mechanisms. The extrinsic system arises extracerebrally and consists of sympathetic and parasympathetic autonomic fibers (particularly those arising from the trigeminal system), which are found to terminate in the vicinity of large and small conductance vessels with innervation sparse in the pial arterioles (<50 mm) and absent in penetrating arterioles [43]. Studies employing stimulation or ablation of these nerves and their ganglia have demonstrated a limited effect on the CBF under physiological conditions [44–46].

However, neural mechanisms may influence CBF under pathological conditions. Bill and Linder first showed that sympathetic stimulation was capable of preventing hyperemic flow, passive increases in CBF, and the breakthrough of autoregulation observed with sudden elevation in blood pressure into the hypertensive range [47]. Sympathectomized animals have a higher frequency of intracerebral hemorrhage and it was hypothesized that sympathetically induced vasoconstriction protected the brain from intracerebral bleeding during hypertension [48]. The importance of the trigeminal influence on CBF under a number of pathological conditions has been demonstrated, together with the release of vasoactive neuropeptides from perivascular sensory nerves via axon reflex-like mechanisms [49].

There has been very limited evaluation of the integrity of the sympathetic and parasympathetic innervation of cerebral arteries in patients with AVMs [50]. Impairment of innervation could play a role in perfusion breakthrough following AVM resection. It is possible that remodeling of large feeding arteries interferes with the normal sympathetic and parasympathetic mechanisms. Some experimental models have demonstrated alteration in the blood–brain barrier after closure of the experimental shunt, but these models do not address the integrity of the neural innervations of the large arteries feeding the AVM [8,10,11].

The metabolic hypothesis states, in most basic form, that the metabolic status of neural tissue regulates CBF through a process by which the parenchyma (neurons and/or glia) communicates with the vascular compartment. This hypothesis is presently the most widely accepted and has the most supportive data. Moreover, it appears to be the dominant process in regulation of CBF [2]. Thus, when CBF is insufficient to maintain metabolism, the parenchyma expresses an error signal, which results in vasodilatation. Insufficiency could result from either lack of supply (e.g., of oxygen or metabolites) or from increased demand (neuronal activity). When supply equals or exceeds demand, the signal is attenuated and CBF decreases.

Metabolic regulation of CBF is best illustrated during hypoxia (lack of supply) or neuronal activation (increased demand). In hypoxia, CBF is rapidly (~5–10 seconds) increased two- to three-fold when the partial pressure of oxygen approaches 50 mmHg [51]. With neuronal activation caused by sciatic nerve stimulation, pial arteriolar vasodilatation is observed within 1.7 seconds of somatosensory activation [52].

While the existence of metabolic regulation of CBF is well established, uncertainty exists about the cells (i.e., neurons or astrocytes) responsible for the error signal, the mechanism(s) involved in transmission of the error signal from the parenchyma to the vascular compartment, and the identity of the chemical factor(s) acting as a signal between the parenchyma and the vascular compartment. A variety of metabolites, individually or in combination, have been implicated as serving as the chemical link between metabolism and CBF [2]. In patients with AVMs, there are a limited number of studies of these agents linking blood flow to metabolism [53,54].

The myogenic hypothesis envisions that vascular tone is preset and reflects a balance between the intraluminal and abluminal pressure. Bayliss in 1902 reported direct contraction and relaxation of canine hind limb arteries in response to an increase or decrease of intravascular pressure, respectively, a reaction attributed to intrinsic properties of vascular smooth muscle [55].

Multiple mechanisms have been proposed to explain the myogenic response. One suggestion is that the myogenic response

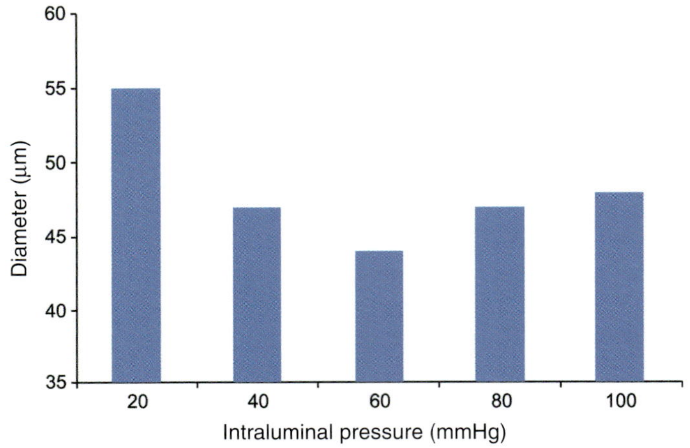

Fig. 4.2. In vitro penetrating cerebral arterioles and the steady-state changes in diameter of intracerebral arterioles with changes in intraluminal pressure. Note that with increasing pressure, the arterioles (average diameter 45 μm) constrict. All diameters differed significantly ($p < 0.05$) from the diameter at 20 mmHg intraluminal pressure. (Data taken from Ngai and Winn, 1995 [6].)

involves vascular smooth muscle metabolism of arachidonic acid via a P4504A-dependent pathway to 20-hydroxyeicosatetraenoic acid [14,56]. With a decrease in intraluminal pressure and possibly flow, the endothelium presumably acts as a mechanoreceptor, transducing variations in transmural pressure and shear stress into altered vascular tone. As will be discussed below, the parenchyma may also participate in the vascular response.

The existence of a myogenic mechanism in the cerebral microcirculation can be demonstrated in isolated intracerebral arterioles (Fig. 4.2) [6]. Intraluminal hypotension results in vasodilatation whereas intraluminal hypertension results in vasoconstriction. This compensatory mechanism is most likely involved in maintaining relatively stable CBF with alteration in perfusion pressure (P_P):

$$P_P = P_A - P_V \text{ or } P_A - P_{ICP}$$

where P_A is equal to mean arterial pressure (diastolic + 1/3 systolic), P_V is venous pressure, and P_{ICP} is intracranial pressure. In most circumstances, brain perfusion pressure is equal to $P_A - P_{ICP}$. When $P_{ICP} > P_V$, P_{ICP} must be used to determine perfusion pressure. If interstitial tissue pressure is elevated (e.g., brain edema), venous outflow may be impaired and then perfusion pressure will be determined by $P_A - P_T$, where P_T represents tissue pressure. A local increase in P_T may not be reflected in measurement of P_{ICP}, a situation that may occur in patients with AVM.

In vivo, as blood pressure (or perfusion pressure) changes, CBF over a wide range remains relatively (but not absolutely) constant [2]. This phenomenon is known as autoregulation. At either extremes of the autoregulatory range, compensatory changes in arterial tone fail and CBF varies directly with blood pressure. In humans without a history of hypertension, the lower and upper limit of autoregulation is usually stated to be 60–70 mmHg and 130–140 mmHg, respectively, whereas in patients with chronic hypertension, the curve is shifted to the right. It has been suggested that in peri-AVM tissue not only is the autoregulatory curve preserved but it is also shifted to the left [50,57].

In the peri-AVM tissue, perfusion pressure may be decreased by increased venous pressure. As a consequence, increased pressure is transmitted across the capillary network into the precapillary arterioles. Based on the myogenic hypothesis, and as demonstrated in the isolated arteriolar preparation (Fig. 4.2), arterioles should react to the increase in intraluminal pressure by contracting [6].

However, in vivo animal studies have demonstrated precisely the opposite: increased venous pressure results in pial arteriolar dilatation, as shown in both cats [58] and monkeys [24].

Subsequently, Wei and Kontos [59] elevated venous pressure and, using a closed cranial window, observed pial arterioles in the presence of cerebrospinal fluid containing oxygen-enriched fluorocarbons. In the presence of high oxygen (but not with normal oxygen levels), the vasodilatation induced by elevated venous pressure was converted to vasoconstriction. This observation with oxygen-enriched fluorocarbons indicates that venous hypertension results in cortical hypoxia and/or ischemia of a degree sufficient to cause the release of a metabolic factor from the parenchyma to counteract the myogenic response induced by the venous hypertension. In summary, the metabolic influence predominates over the myogenic mechanism. Other studies support the influence of metabolic factors in autoregulation [60].

Many studies of vascular control in peri-AVM tissue in patients have focused on investigating vasomotor reserve (or autoregulation) while ignoring the over-riding influence of metabolic influence.

Clinical studies of physiology and hemodynamic regulation in brain tissue surrounding arteriovenous malformations

This section reviews the relevant physiological and hemodynamic factors affecting patients with AVM.

There are multiple studies of patients with AVMs analyzing a variety of parameters such as CBF, cerebral blood volume, oxygen saturation (SaO_2), transit time, vascular reserve, and brain metabolism using multiple methods (angiography, CT angiography, transcranial Doppler, positron emission tomography [PET], MRI). These studies evaluate the pre-, intra-, and/or postoperative period. Some investigators focused on the shunt while others have analyzed peri-AVM or distant brain tissue. Early studies reached varying conclusions because of the limitations and diversity of investigative methods. With time, instrumentation has improved and methodological limitations were recognized. Nevertheless, even now, most reports involve a limited number of patients, which restricts their statistical power, randomized evaluations are lacking, and blinded analysis rare [61]. Lastly, almost all human AVM studies are, by their nature, selective since most patients come to attention because of symptoms such as seizures, headaches, neurological impairment, or hemorrhage. Bias is thus the norm and definitive conclusions about hemodynamic factors must be considered with caution.

Normal pressure breakthrough

To a considerable extent, analysis of AVM physiology has been stimulated by the desire to identify hemodynamic factors that could explain postsurgical events such as normal pressure perfusion breakthrough (NPPB), which was first proposed by Spetzler and colleagues in 1978 [11]. This hypothesizes that the AVM shunt causes peri-AVM tissue to be hypoperfused. As a consequence of the decreased perfusion pressure and as dictated by the Bayliss effect, the peri-AVM arterioles dilate. An additional impact of the shunt would be to increase venous volume and pressure; this, in turn, would also decrease perfusion of the microcirculation of the peri-AVM tissue. Spetzler *et al.* [11] hypothesized that the dilated arterioles are suddenly exposed to an increased arterial pressure with surgical obliteration of the shunt. Because of their prolonged exposure to low pressure, the dilated arterioles would be unable to contract ("vasomotor paralysis") and this would expose the remaining microcirculation (capillaries and venules) to unregulated high pressure and flow. Postoperative brain edema and hemorrhage could, therefore, ensue in a small number of patients.

This hypothesis remains controversial, related in part to the infrequency of NPPB and the consequent lack of a robust patient base for statistical analysis. Furthermore, postoperative swelling and bleeding following AVM resection has other causes and so the patient pool for NPPB may be mixed, further complicating the ability to establish strong statistical correlations, much less causal relationships. In addition, hemodynamic and physiological parameters before and after surgical resection or endovascular embolization may not be uniform [62–64] even in patients with clear-cut NPPB [65]. An inconsistent temporal component of the hemodynamic and physiological changes may not be recognized, leading to clouding of the data [66]. Lastly, many of the techniques used to measure CBF and other physiological parameters (e.g., PET, single-photon emission computed tomography, SaO_2) do not have sufficient precision to clarify events occurring in the microcirculation.

Despite the limitations of studies noted above, there is considerable support for aspects of this hypothesis [11] based on both patient and laboratory studies. Data indicate that peri-AVM tissue is (or at one time was) hypoperfused [7]. However, other aspects of the hypothesis do not appear to be strongly supported. For example, arterioles do not appear to be maximally dilated [67] and they are capable of constricting and dilating; they are not in a state of vasomotor paralysis [30,50,54,67–70]. Moreover, there is limited clarity or consistency in describing patient conditions, preoperative findings, or treatment factors that are unequivocally associated with or predictive of NPPB. However, some investigators found that NPPB was related to pre/postoperative global CBF [67], size of the AVM (large AVMs having increased risk), or areas of severe hypoxia [28]. What is clear is that the hypothesis has fulfilled one of the main purposes, in general, of hypothesis creation: to stimulate interest and hypothesis-testing studies.

Most studies designed to evaluate the underlying mechanisms of NPPB consider the arterial circulatory system as being one entity rather than divided into macro- and microcomponents. Indeed, under normal physiological conditions, pial arterial diameter and CBF (reflecting the microcirculation) are linked [71]. However, under pathological conditions, such as following the removal of an AVM, flow in the micro- and macrocirculation may vary. For example, following experimental head injury [40], there is vasomotor paralysis in both the micro- and macrocirculation. However, the arterioles are able to vasodilate within minutes whereas the larger arteries remain unresponsive for 8–12 hours. Most recent analyses of vascular function after AVM resection have focused on processes under the control of the microcirculation (i.e., CBF, SaO_2, cerebral metabolic rate of oxygen), with less information available about the macrocirculation. Information about the macrocirculation largely stems from an earlier era and is based on data derived from arteriography, which does reveal the existence of large persistent dilated arteries in patients with NPPB [72]. Potentially, if the macro- and microcirculations could be compared individually in the setting of NPPB, the hypothesis of vasomotor failure in the macrocirculation might be confirmed.

Physiology and hemodynamic factors found in patients

As discussed above, a limitation of all the clinical studies is the fact that AVMs are rarely discovered early in patients and so are in a "mature" state. Therefore, the conditions and responses in the peri-AVM and distant brain tissues represent a response to the vascular and metabolic challenge of the underlying lesion (the shunt). Assuming that the peri-AVM tissue is or was hypoperfused, the peri-AVM tissue will respond to this challenge by attempting to establish a normal physiological state (e.g., CBF, SaO_2, oxygen extraction) [28]. To the extent that normalization occurs, investigations designed to evaluate CBF, SaO_2, and metabolism may find minimal or no differences compared with normal values [28,50,73,74] and, therefore, conclude that hemodynamic and physiological status and responses of the peri-AVM and distant tissues are "normal" [41,73,74]. This may be correct, but it may not recognize the dynamic changes that have produced the "normal" conditions.

Recognizing the caveats outlined above, a review of the literature relating to the physiological and hemodynamic data indicate that a number of factors are significant in peri-AVM tissues and these are summarized below.

Arterial macrocirculation

The degree and extent of arterial dilatation may increase with time [11]. In most studies, blood flow through the shunt correlates to the size of the AVM [74]. In regard to risk of hemorrhage a number of factors appear to be significant.

Size of AVM. There is substantial support for the correlation between small size of the nidus and increased risk of hemorrhage [75–78], although Norris *et al.* failed to confirm this association, which may reflect the size of the studied population and the methodology used [61]. In addition, 12 of

27 patients (44%) with large AVMs (>5 cm) presented with a bleed [79].

Feeding arterial pressure. There are good data supporting an inverse correlation between high feeding artery pressures and AVM size [75–77,80]: higher pressures are found with small AVMs [76–78,81]. Moreover, feeding artery pressure correlates with increased risk of hemorrhaging. Some investigators found that the relationship between feeding arterial pressure and risk of hemorrhage was independent of size and location or the AVM. Young *et al.* [67] noted an absence of correlation between feeding arterial pressure and NPPB.

Flow rate. Slow flow (i.e., transit time) on angiography in peri-AVM tissue was correlated with increased risk of hemorrhage [61]. In contrast, transit time through the nidus had no relationship with clinical presentation [61].

Location. Some studies have found a correlation between the location of the AVM and the likelihood of bleeding: deep location (basal ganglion, intra- or periventricular, and posterior fossa) having a higher risk (Fig. 4.3) [75,81–87]. Perhaps, the deep locations are less likely to come to medical attention except with hemorrhage, since others investigations have not substantiated the relationship between location and hemorrhage risk [72].

A long parenchymal or perforating artery. Some studies have found a correlation between artery length and increased risk of hemorrhage [75,81].

Venous macrocirculation

Venous blood volumes in the peri-AVM regions are increased. Similar to the arterial macrocirculation, the extent and degree of venous dilatation can increase with time. Deep venous pressure is not affected by presence of deep venous drainage, AVM size, AVM location, prior embolization, or clinical presentation (i.e., hemorrhage or none) [33]. A number of factors have been associated with risk of hemorrhage.

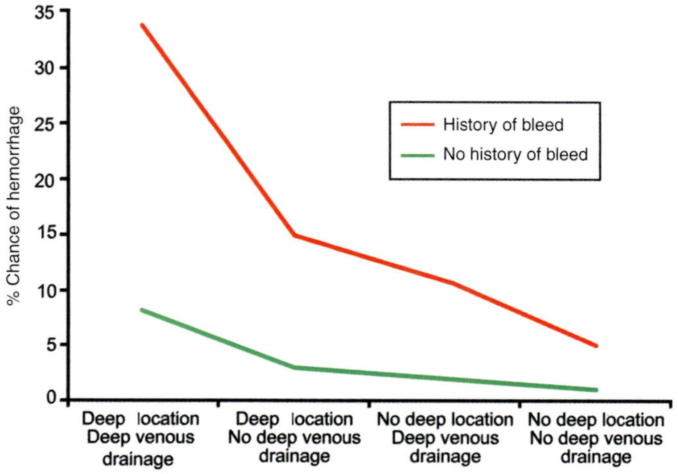

Fig. 4.3 Annual percentage chance of hemorrhage. Correlation between hemorrhage and arteriovenous malformations location, venous drainage, and history based on data from 622 untreated patients. (Data taken from Stapf *et al.*, 2006 [17].)

Deep venous drainage. This is correlated (Fig. 4.3) with increased risk of hemorrhage and may be an independent predictor of propensity to hemorrhage [17,72,75,81,86]; even large AVMs with deep venous drainage had a high propensity to bleed [17].

Draining vein. Other investigators have noted that AVMs with a solitary draining vein, whether deep or superficial, have a higher propensity to bleed [76,87,88], but some studies do not support an association [89].

Venous structure. Aneurysms, stenosis, occlusion, and/or vessel wall irregularity have been suggested as being correlated with risk of hemorrhage [18,90]. However, the lack of association has also been noted [72,81].

Venous pressure. The degree of venous hypertension will depend on the size of the shunt, the capacitance of the venous drainage in general, and the vagaries specific to individual venous systems [33]. These multifactorial conditions, seen in both small and large AVMs, have weakened the ability of investigators to establish strong correlation between venous flow and pressure and propensity to bleed [75]. Young *et al.* [33] found no relationship between draining venous pressure and patient presentation, deep (vs. superficial) drainage, size of the AVM, location, or prior embolization. Feeding arterial pressure correlated with venous pressure [33]. Ruptured AVMs had higher venous pressure compared with those that had a benign course and there was an inverse relationship between the number of draining veins and intravascular (both arterial and venous) pressure [76]; however, this relationship has not been supported by all studies [75].

Trans-AVM pressure differential. The fall in pressure across an AVM (feeding arterial pressure minus draining venous pressure) has been found to be inversely correlated with the size of the AVM (large AVMs have smaller transnidal differences between feeding arterial and draining venous pressure).

Steal

Although disparate observations exist, peri-AVM hypoperfusion appears to be a factor in the peri-AVM tissue.

Flow in the peri-AVM tissue. This is decreased (i.e., steal exists) [50,63,91–93]. Early studies based on contrast angiography revealed a paucity or delayed filling of perinidal arteries and tissue. The existence of steal has been demonstrated in many [92,94,95], but not all [74,89,96], studies. Some of the disparity may be related to low spatial resolution or to inclusion of patients partially treated by embolization, which can change local hemodynamics and obscure or attenuate the degree of steal [74].

Degree of steal. The degree of steal is related to the size of the AVM: the larger the AVM, the greater the likelihood of hypoperfusion in the peri-AVM tissue [92,97,98]. High-flow AVMs have also been found to be correlated with low CBF around an AVM [92].

Oxygen extraction. Peri-AVM oxygen extraction was noted to be higher with large AVMs, high-flow AVMs, and in patients with progressive neurological deficits [92]. However, severe hypoxia in peri-AVM tissue is unusual [28] and is probably related to compensatory responses (microcirculation, below).

Peri-AVM hypoperfusion. Hypoperfusion may not be uniform [98], which has the potential to complicate attempts to correlate hypoperfusion with the size of the shunt. This lack of uniformity may simply be a byproduct of the limitations of the methodology (e.g. lack of spatial resolution) used to measure CBF in the peri-AVM tissue. Hypoperfusion, however, was not correlated with focal neurological deficits in 152 patients, based on clinical information and data from MRI, CT, and transcranial Doppler [74]. In contrast, evaluation of 24 patients using oxygen-15 PET found a relationship between hypoperfusion and progressive neurological deficits [92].

Brain metabolism

There are a limited number of studies focused on metabolism of patients with AVMs. Some investigators suggest that there is impairment in metabolism (oxygen extraction, oxygen saturation [91,98] and glucose utilization in the peri-AVM tissue [89,99]), whereas others find normal conditions [28,67]. To some extent, this disparity may reflect technical limitations, different techniques, and/or the parameters analyzed. In addition, brain metabolism will be influenced by whether the patient is studied in the awake or anesthetized state.

Peri-AVM metabolic state. The metabolic state in the peri-AVM tissue may be the determinate factor in regulating flow in the microcirculation and in counter-acting the myogenic influence on CBF (see below, microcirculation).

Diaschisis. Brain metabolism and CBF distant from the shunt and the peri-AVM region may be abnormal. The underlying mechanisms for such changes are unclear, but they could be related to a primary neural mechanism of reciprocal innervation through transcallosal and intrahemispheric connections.

Microcirculation in tissue around arteriovenous malformations

Most studies suggest that flow in the peri-AVM tissue is, at a minimum, within the normal range because of compensatory mechanisms [7,95,98].

Capillary density. This is increased, perhaps as a reaction to hypoperfusion and to maintain oxygen availability [100]. Some animal models of AVM demonstrate changes in the microcirculation and the astrocytic foot plates and alteration in the blood–brain barrier [9]. As already noted, capillary density may be increased to maintain oxygen availability [100]. Elevated venous pressure delays microcirculatory transit time and potentially alters material transfer (including oxygen exchange). However, cerebral edema is rarely observed and the blood–brain barrier is usually intact in the patient pretreatment.

Capillary size. Capillaries become pathologically enlarged, which increases their surface area and may affect transfer processes (diffusion and ultrafiltration) unique to the microcirculation [41].

Blood volume and oxygen extraction. Both are increased in the peri-AVM area [98].

Vasomotor reserve. Xenon-enhanced CT has demonstrated impaired vascular reserve [93] with impairment related to large AVM volumes, venous congestion, and shared vascular territories. Use of MR angiography has identified differences in shared territorial and microvascular flows, which would account for perfusion impairment [63]. The mechanism for residual vasomotor reserve may be related to the competing influences of low arterial pressure (evoking vasodilatation) and high venous pressure (evoking vasoconstriction) and/or influence of metabolic factors.

Arteriolar reactivity. Peri-AVM arteriolar reactivity is intact. Although Spetzler hypothesized that arterioles in the peri-AVM tissue were maximally dilated and were in a state of vasoparalysis, CBF in the peri-AVM tissue can be increased with intravenous acetazolamide [57,97,101], hypercarbia [73], intra-arterial papavarine [70], calcium channel blockers (verapamil) [102], but not by nitric oxide-mediated vasodilators[102]. Therefore, these peri-AVM arterioles are not maximally dilated. Furthermore, an increase in systemic blood pressure induced by phenylephrine [50] or norepinephrine [28] does not result in a passive increase in CBF. In other words, the peri-AVM arterioles can also constrict. In contrast, some investigators in a small number of patients have not found a normal vasomotor response [97], which they attribute to a very low oxygen saturation and is perhaps characteristic of large AVMs.

Metabolic influences. Effects on the peri-AVM microcirculation have been shown using oxygen-enriched fluorocarbons in a setting of venous hypertension, which converted arteriolar vasodilatation to vasoconstriction [59]. Thus, metabolism appears to be the dominant factor regulating CBF. The early focus on the "plumbing" aspect of CBF and its measureable parameters such as pressure, flow, shunts, and steals may have obscured the role of metabolic factors in CBF regulation in the perinidal tissue. Evaluation of oxygen saturation in peri-AVM tissue showed that a decrease in feeding arterial flow did not reduce oxygen saturation, presumably related to compensatory or dominate metabolic influences on CBF [28]. Despite a paucity of studies designed to study peri-AVM brain metabolism, those that exist suggest that the peri-AVM tissue is metabolically challenged and adaptive signaling occurs in the vascular compartment to increase the flow of blood and oxygen [7].

Autoregulation. The relationship between systemic blood pressure and CBF (pressure autoregulation) in the peri-AVM region is intact, but the lower threshold is extended [7,30,50,97] and the autoregulation curve is shifted to the left. Metabolic factors, as outlined above, appear to be important in autoregulation. In the laboratory, low perfusion pressure even within the autoregulatory range [103,104] causes an increase in brain adenosine (a potent vasodilator). Furthermore, pressure autoregulation is impaired by adenosine receptor antagonists (theophylline) and in adenosine receptor knock-out animals [60].

References

1. Feindel W, Perot P. Red cerebral veins: a report on arteriovenous shunts in tumors and cerebral scars. *J Neurosurg* 1965;**22**:315–25.
2. Kulik T, Kusano Y, Aronhime S, *et al.* Regulation of cerebral vasculature in normal and ischemic brain. *Neuropharmacology* 2008;**55**:281–8.
3. Heistad D, Kontos H. Cerebral circulation. In Shepherd JT, Abboud FM, Geiger SR, eds. *Handbook of Physiology*, 2nd edn, Vol. **3**. Bethesda, MD: American Physiological Society, 1983, pp. 137–82.
4. Kobari M, Gotoh F, Fukuuchi Y, *et al.* Blood flow velocity in the pial arteries of cats, with particular reference to the vessel diameter. *J Cereb Blood Flow Metab* 1984;**4**:110–14.
5. Furchgott RF, Vanhoutte PM. Endothelium-derived relaxing and contracting factors. *FASEB J* 1989;**3**:2007–18.
6. Ngai AC, Winn HR. Modulation of cerebral arteriolar diameter by intraluminal flow and pressure. *Circ Res* 1995;**77**:832–40.
7. Quick CM, Leonard EF, Young WL. Adaptation of cerebral circulation to brain arteriovenous malformations increases feeding artery pressure and decreases regional hypotension. *Neurosurgery* 2002;**50**:167–73.
8. Bederson JB, Wiestler OD, Brustle O, *et al.* Intracranial venous hypertension and the effects of venous outflow obstruction in a rat model of arteriovenous fistula. *Neurosurgery* 1991;**29**:341–50.
9. Hai J, Ding M, Guo Z, *et al.* A new rat model of chronic cerebral hypoperfusion associated with arteriovenous malformations. *J Neurosurg* 2002;**97**:1198–202.
10. Morgan MK, Anderson RE, Sundt TM, Jr. A model of the pathophysiology of cerebral arteriovenous malformations by a carotid-jugular fistula in the rat. *Brain Res* 1989;**496**:241–50.
11. Spetzler RF, Wilson CB, Weinstein P, *et al.* Normal perfusion pressure breakthrough theory. *Clin Neurosurg* 1978;**25**:651–72.
12. Seok J, Warren HS, Cuenca AG, *et al.* Genomic responses in mouse models poorly mimic human inflammatory diseases. *Proc Natl Acad Sci USA* 2013;**110**:3507–12.
13. Mima A. Hemodialysis vascular access dysfunction: molecular mechanisms and treatment. *Ther Apher Dial* 2012;**16**:321–7.
14. Rubanyi GM, Freay AD, Kauser K, *et al.* Mechanoreception by the endothelium: mediators and mechanisms of pressure- and flow-induced vascular responses. *Blood Vessels* 1990;**27**:246–57.
15. Feigl EO. Coronary physiology. *Physiol Rev* 1983;**63**:1–205.
16. Quick CM, James DJ, Ning K, *et al.* Relationship of nidal vessel radius and wall thickness to brain arteriovenous malformation hemorrhage. *Neurol Res* 2002;**24**:495–500.
17. Stapf C, Mast H, Sciacca RR, *et al.* Predictors of hemorrhage in patients with untreated brain arteriovenous malformation. *Neurology* 2006;**66**:1350–5.
18. Pritz MB. Ruptured supratentorial arteriovenous malformations associated with venous aneurysms. *Acta Neurochir (Wien)* 1994;**128**:150–62.
19. Chuang YM, Guo W, Lin CP. Appraising the plasticity of the circle of Willis: a model of hemodynamic modulation in cerebral arteriovenous malformation. *Eur Neurol* 2010;**63**:295–301.
20. McGillicuddy JE, Kindt GW, Raisis JE, *et al.* The relation of cerebral ischemia, hypoxia, and hypercarbia to the Cushing response. *J Neurosurg* 1978;**48**:730–40.
21. Moftakhar P, Hauptman JS, Malkasian D, *et al.* Cerebral arteriovenous malformations. Part 1: cellular and molecular biology. *Neurosurg Focus* 2009;**26**:E10.
22. Zhu Y, Lawton MT, Du R, *et al.* Expression of hypoxia-inducible factor-1 and vascular endothelial growth factor in response to venous hypertension. *Neurosurgery* 2006;**59**:687–96.
23. Hashimoto T, Lam T, Boudreau NJ, *et al.* Abnormal balance in the angiopoietin-tie2 system in human brain arteriovenous malformations. *Circ Res* 2001;**89**:111–13.
24. Raisis JE, Kindt GW, McGillicuddy JE, *et al.* The effects of primary elevation of cerebral venous pressure on cerebral hemodynamics and intracranial pressure. *J Surg Res* 1979;**26**:101–7.
25. Giannotta SL, Raisis JE, McGillicuddy JE, *et al.* The effect of temperature on cerebrovascular resistance and cerebral metabolism in the primate. *J Surg Res* 1978;**25**:105–10.
26. Greitz T. A radiologic study of the brain circulation by rapid serial angiography of the carotid artery. *Acta Radiol Suppl* 1956;1–123.
27. Matsumoto K, Urano M, Hirai M, *et al.* Haemodynamic evaluation of cerebral arteriovenous malformations by quantification of transit time using high speed digital subtraction angiography: basic considerations. *J Clin Neurosci* 2000;7(Suppl 1):39–41.
28. Meyer B, Schaller C, Frenkel C, *et al.* Distributions of local oxygen saturation and its response to changes of mean arterial blood pressure in the cerebral cortex adjacent to arteriovenous malformations. *Stroke* 1999;**30**:2623–30.
29. Duong DH, Young WL, Vang MC, *et al.* Feeding artery pressure and venous drainage pattern are primary determinants of hemorrhage from cerebral arteriovenous malformations. *Stroke* 1998;**29**:1167–76.
30. Young WL, Kader A, Prohovnik I, *et al.* Pressure autoregulation is intact after arteriovenous malformation resection. *Neurosurgery* 1993;**32**:491–6.
31. Navari RM, Wei EP, Kontos HA, *et al.* Comparison of the open skull and cranial window preparations in the study of the cerebral microcirculation. *Microvasc Res* 1978;**16**:304–15.
32. Dacey RG, Jr., Duling BR. Effect of norepinephrine on penetrating arterioles of rat cerebral cortex. *Am J Physiol* 1984;**246**:H380–5.
33. Young WL, Kader A, Pile-Spellman J, *et al.* Arteriovenous malformation draining vein physiology and determinants of transnidal pressure gradients. The Columbia University AVM Study Project. *Neurosurgery* 1994;**35**:389–95.
34. Kontos HA, Wei EP, Navari RM, *et al.* Responses of cerebral arteries and arterioles to acute hypotension and hypertension. *Am J Physiol* 1978;**234**: H371–83.
35. Kee DB, Jr., Wood JH. Rheology of the cerebral circulation. *Neurosurgery* 1984;**15**:125–31.

36. Chien S, Usami S, Skalak R. Blood flow in small tubes. In Renkin EM, Michel CC, Geiger SR, eds. *Handbook of Physiology*: Vol. **IV**: *The Cardiovascular System*.Washington, DC: American Physiological Society, 1984, pp. 217–49.
37. Ngai AC, Winn HR. Estimation of shear and flow rates in pial arterioles during somatosensory stimulation. *Am J Physiol* 1996;**270**:H1712–17.
38. Segal SS, Damon DN, Duling BR. Propagation of vasomotor responses coordinates arteriolar resistances. *Am J Physiol* 1989;**256**:H832–7.
39. Xu HL, Mao L, Ye S, *et al.* Astrocytes are a key conduit for upstream signaling of vasodilation during cerebral cortical neuronal activation in vivo. *Am J Physiol Heart Circ Physiol* 2008;**294**:H622–32.
40. Ellison MD, Erb DE, Kontos HA, *et al.* Recovery of impaired endothelium-dependent relaxation after fluid-percussion brain injury in cats. *Stroke* 1989;**20**:911–17.
41. Attia W, Tada T, Hongo K, *et al.* Microvascular pathological features of immediate perinidal parenchyma in cerebral arteriovenous malformations: giant bed capillaries. *J Neurosurg* 2003;**98**:823–7.
42. Hamel E. Perivascular nerves and the regulation of cerebrovascular tone. *J Appl Physiol* 2006;**100**:1059–64.
43. Cohen Z, Molinatti G, Hamel E. Astroglial and vascular interactions of noradrenaline terminals in the rat cerebral cortex. *J Cereb Blood Flow Metab* 1997;**17**:894–904.
44. D'Alecy LG, Feigl EO. Sympathetic control of cerebral blood flow in dogs. *Circ Res* 1972;**31**:267–83.
45. Ibayashi S, Ngai AC, Howard MA, III, *et al.* Lack of sympathetic and cholinergic influences on cerebral vasodilation caused by sciatic nerve stimulation in the rat. *J Cereb Blood Flow Metab* 1991;**11**:678–83
46. Toda N, Tanaka T, Ayajiki K, *et al.* Cerebral vasodilatation induced by stimulation of the pterygopalatine ganglion and greater petrosal nerve in anesthetized monkeys *Neuroscience* 2000;**96**:393–8.
47. Bill A, Linder J. Sympathetic control of cerebral blood flow in acute arterial hypertension. *Acta Physiol Scand* 1976;**96**:114–21.
48. Heistad DD, Marcus ML, Gross PM. Effects of sympathetic nerves on cerebral vessels in dog, cat, and monkey. *Am J Physiol* 1978;**235**:H544–52.
49. Macfarlane R, Moskowitz MA, Sakas DE, *et al.* The role of neuroeffector mechanisms in cerebral hyperperfusion syndromes. *J Neurosurg* 1991;**75**:845–55.
50. Young WL, Pile-Spellman J, Prohovnik I, *et al.* Evidence for adaptive autoregulatory displacement in hypotensive cortical territories adjacent to arteriovenous malformations. Columbia University AVM Study Project. *Neurosurgery* 1994;**34**:601–10.
51. Miekisiak G, Kulik T, Kusano Y, *et al.* Cerebral blood flow response in adenosine 2a receptor knockout mice during transient hypoxic hypoxia. *J Cereb Blood Flow Metab* 2008;**28**:1656–64.
52. Ngai AC, Ko KR, Morii S, *et al.* Effect of sciatic nerve stimulation on pial arterioles in rats. *Am J Physiol* 1988;**254**:H133–9.
53. Joshi S, Young WL, Duong DH, *et al.* Intracarotid infusion of the nitric oxide synthase inhibitor, L-NMMA, modestly decreases cerebral blood flow in human subjects. *Anesthesiology* 2000;**93**:699–707.
54. Fogarty-Mack P, Pile-Spellman J, Hacein-Bey L, *et al.* Superselective intraarterial papaverine administration: effect on regional cerebral blood flow in patients with arteriovenous malformations. *J Neurosurg* 1996;**85**:395–402.
55. Bayliss WM. On the local reactions of the arterial wall to changes of internal pressure. *J Physiol* 1902;**28**:220–31.
56. Harder DR, Lange AR, Gebremedhin D, *et al.* Cytochrome P450 metabolites of arachidonic acid as intracellular signaling molecules in vascular tissue. *J Vasc Res* 1997;**34**:237–43.
57. Sullivan HG, Kingsbury TB, Morgan ME, *et al.* The rCBF response to Diamox in normal subjects and cerebrovascular disease patients. *J Neurosurg* 1987;**67**:525–34.
58. Wei EP, Kontos HA. Responses of cerebral arterioles to increased venous pressure. *Am J Physiol* 1982;**243**:H442–7.
59. Wei EP, Kontos HA. Increased venous pressure causes myogenic constriction of cerebral arterioles during local hyperoxia. *Circ Res* 1984;**55**:249–52.
60. Kusano Y, Echeverry G, Miekisiak G, *et al.* Role of adenosine A_2 receptors in regulation of cerebral blood flow during induced hypotension. *J Cereb Blood Flow Metab* 2010;**30**:808–15.
61. Norris JS, Valiante TA, Wallace MC, *et al.* A simple relationship between radiological arteriovenous malformation hemodynamics and clinical presentation: a prospective, blinded analysis of 31 cases. *J Neurosurg* 1999;**90**:673–9.
62. Essig M, Reichenbach JR, Schad LR, *et al.* High-resolution MR venography of cerebral arteriovenous malformations. *Magn Reson Imaging* 1999;**17**:1417–25.
63. Fiehler J, Illies T, Piening M, *et al.* Territorial and microvascular perfusion impairment in brain arteriovenous malformations. *AJNR Am J Neuroradiol* 2009;**30**:356–61.
64. Van Roost D, Schramm J, Solymosi L, *et al.* Presence and removal of arteriovenous malformation: impact of regional cerebral blood flow, as assessed with xenon/CT. *Acta Neurol Scand Suppl* 1996;**166**:136–8.
65. Batjer HH, Devous MD, Sr. The use of acetazolamide-enhanced regional cerebral blood flow measurement to predict risk to arteriovenous malformation patients. *Neurosurgery* 1992;**31**:213–17.
66. Hoshino T, Sakatani K, Yokose N, *et al.* Changes in cerebral blood oxygenation and hemodynamics after endovascular treatment of vascular malformation measured by time-resolved spectroscopy. *Adv Exp Med Biol* 2010;**662**:491–6.
67. Young WL, Kader A, Ornstein E, *et al.* Cerebral hyperemia after arteriovenous malformation resection is related to "breakthrough" complications but not to feeding artery pressure. The Columbia University Arteriovenous Malformation Study Project. *Neurosurgery* 1996;**38**:1085–93.
68. Ostapkovich ND, Baker KZ, Fogarty-Mack P, *et al.* Cerebral blood flow and CO2 reactivity is similar during remifentanil/N_2O and fentanyl/N_2O anesthesia. *Anesthesiology* 1998;**89**:358–63.
69. Gao E, Young WL, Pile-Spellman J, *et al.* Cerebral arteriovenous malformation feeding artery aneurysms: a theoretical

model of intravascular pressure changes after treatment. *Neurosurgery* 1997;**41**:1345–56.

70. Fogarty-Mack P, Pile-Spellman J, Hacein-Bey L, *et al.* The effect of arteriovenous malformations on the distribution of intracerebral arterial pressures. *AJNR Am J Neuroradiol* 1996;**17**:1443–9.
71. Ngai AC, Meno JR, Winn HR. Simultaneous measurements of pial arteriolar diameter and laser-Doppler flow during somatosensory stimulation. *J Cereb Blood Flow Metab* 1995;**15**:124–7.
72. Gutierrez-Gonzalez R, Gil A, Serna C, *et al.* Normal perfusion pressure breakthrough phenomenon: what still remains unknown. *Br J Neurosurg* 2012;**26**:403–5.
73. Young WL, Prohovnik I, Ornstein E, *et al.* The effect of arteriovenous malformation resection on cerebrovascular reactivity to carbon dioxide. *Neurosurgery* 1990;**27**:257–66.
74. Mast H, Mohr JP, Osipov A, *et al.* "Steal" is an unestablished mechanism for the clinical presentation of cerebral arteriovenous malformations. *Stroke* 1995;**26**:1215–20.
75. Kader A, Young WL, Pile-Spellman J, *et al.* The influence of hemodynamic and anatomical factors on hemorrhage from cerebral arteriovenous malformations. *Neurosurgery* 1994;**34**:801–7.
76. Miyasaka Y, Yada K, Kurata A, *et al.* Correlation between intravascular pressure and risk of hemorrhage due to arteriovenous malformations. *Surg Neurol* 1993;**39**:370–3.
77. Nornes H, Grip A. Hemodynamic aspects of cerebral arteriovenous malformations. *J Neurosurg* 1980;**53**:456–64.
78. Spetzler RF, Martin NA. A proposed grading system for arteriovenous malformations. *J Neurosurg* 1986;**65**:476–83.
79. Sadasivan B, Hwang PY. Large cerebral arteriovenous malformations: experience with 27 cases. *Surg Neurol* 1996;**45**:245–9.
80. Spetzler RF, Hargraves RW, McCormick PW, *et al.* Relationship of perfusion pressure and size to risk of hemorrhage from arteriovenous malformations. *J Neurosurg* 1992;**76**:918–23.
81. Pradhan N, Sadasivan PK, Arunodaya GR. Detection of seizure activity in EEG by an artificial neural network: a preliminary study. *Comput Biomed Res* 1996;**29**:303–13.
82. Fujii Y, Takeuchi S, Koike T, *et al.* Heparin administration and monitoring for neuroangiography. *AJNR Am J Neuroradiol* 1994;**15**:51–4.
83. Choi BY, Kim DH, Chung T, *et al.* Destabilization and mislocalization of POU3F4 by C-terminal frameshift truncation and extension mutation. *Hum Mutat* 2013;**34**:309–16.
84. Acerbi F, Genden E, Bederson J. Circumferential watertight dural repair using nitinol U-clips in expanded endonasal and sublabial approaches to the cranial base. *Neurosurgery* 2010;**67**:448–56.
85. Stefani MA, Porter PJ, terBrugge KG, *et al.* Large and deep brain arteriovenous malformations are associated with risk of future hemorrhage. *Stroke* 2002;**33**:1220–4.
86. Feindel W, Garretson H, Yamamoto L, *et al.* Blood flow patterns in the cerebral vessels and cortex in man studies by intracarotid injection of radioisotopes and Coomassie Blue dye. *J Neurosurg* 1965;**23**:12–22.
87. Albert P, Salgado H, Polaina M, *et al.* A study on the venous drainage of 150 cerebral arteriovenous malformations as related to haemorrhagic risks and size of the lesion. *Acta Neurochir (Wien)* 1990;**103**:30–4.
88. Yoon JH, Han JH, Jung JS, *et al.* Highly Improved Uniformity in the Resistive Switching Parameters of TiO2) Thin Films by Inserting Ru Nanodots. *Adv Mater* 2013;**25**:1987–92.
89. Fink GR. Effects of cerebral angiomas on perifocal and remote tissue: a multivariate positron emission tomography study. *Stroke* 1992;**23**:1099–105.
90. Brown RD, Jr., Wiebers DO, Forbes G, *et al.* The natural history of unruptured intracranial arteriovenous malformations. *J Neurosurg* 1988;**68**:352–7.
91. Asgari S, Rohrborn HJ, Engelhorn T, *et al.* Intraoperative measurement of cortical oxygen saturation and blood volume adjacent to cerebral arteriovenous malformations using near-infrared spectroscopy. *Neurosurgery* 2003;**52**:1298–304.
92. Iwama T, Hashimoto N, Hayashida K. Cerebral hemodynamic parameters for patients with neurological improvements after extracranial-intracranial arterial bypass surgery: evaluation using positron emission tomography. *Neurosurgery* 2001;**48**:504–10.
93. Van Roost D, Schramm J. What factors are related to impairment of cerebrovascular reserve before and after arteriovenous malformation resection? A cerebral blood flow study using xenon-enhanced computed tomography. *Neurosurgery* 2001;**48**:709–16.
94. Takeuchi S, Abe H, Nishimaki K, *et al.* Cerebral haemodynamic changes after endovascular treatment of arteriovenous malformations: evaluation by single-photon emission CT. *Acta Neurochir (Wien)* 1994;**127**:142–50.
95. Guo WY, Wu YT, Wu HM, *et al.* Toward normal perfusion after radiosurgery: perfusion MR Imaging with independent component analysis of brain arteriovenous malformations. *AJNR Am J Neuroradiol* 2004;**25**:1636–44.
96. Raisis JE, Kindt GW, McGillicuddy JE, *et al.* Cerebrospinal fluid lactate and lactate/pyruvate ratios in hydrocephalus. *J Neurosurg* 1976;**44**:337–41.
97. Hacein-Bey L, Nour R, Pile-Spellman J, *et al.* Adaptive changes of autoregulation in chronic cerebral hypotension with arteriovenous malformations: an acetazolamide-enhanced single-photon emission CT study. *AJNR Am J Neuroradiol* 1995;**16**:1865–74.
98. Iwama T, Hayashida K, Takahashi JC, *et al.* Cerebral hemodynamics and metabolism in patients with cerebral arteriovenous malformations: an evaluation using positron emission tomography scanning. *J Neurosurg* 2002;**97**:1314–21.
99. Tyler JL, Leblanc R, Meyer E, *et al.* Hemodynamic and metabolic effects of cerebral arteriovenous malformations studied by positron emission tomography. *Stroke* 1989;**20**:890–8.
100. Sekhon LH, Morgan MK, Spence I. Normal perfusion pressure breakthrough: the role of capillaries. *J Neurosurg* 1997;**86**:519–24.
101. Tarr RW, Johnson DW, Rutigliano M, *et al.* Use of acetazolamide-challenge

xenon CT in the assessment of cerebral blood flow dynamics in patients with arteriovenous malformations. *AJNR Am J Neuroradiol* 1990;**11**:441–8.

102. Joshi S, Young WL, Pile-Spellman J, *et al.* Intra-arterial nitrovasodilators do not increase cerebral blood flow in angiographically normal territories of arteriovenous malformation patients. *Stroke* 1997;**28**:1115–22.

103. Winn HR, Morii S, Berne RM. The role of adenosine in autoregulation of cerebral blood flow. *Ann Biomed Eng* 1985;**13**:321–8.

104. Winn HR, Welsh JE, Rubio R, *et al.* Brain adenosine production in rat during sustained alteration in systemic blood pressure. *Am J Physiol* 1980;**239**: H636–41.

Chapter 5

Natural history of arteriovenous malformations and indications for treatment

Aki Laakso and Juha Hernesniemi

Introduction

Arteriovenous malformations (AVMs) of the brain are developmental lesions, the formation of which is probably initiated during embryonic or fetal stages of development. Their exact etiology remains unknown. Despite their developmental origin, they are usually not hereditary lesions, although rare cases of familial occurrence have been reported [1]. Arteriovenous malformations are very heterogeneous and vary greatly in size and angioarchitecture. Considering their heterogeneity, it is somewhat surprising that multiple AVMs in one patient are very rare. Interestingly, AVMs have sometimes been observed to spontaneously disappear, or recur after angiographically complete obliteration [2–6]. The most serious and common clinical symptom of an AVM is hemorrhagic stroke, resulting from its rupture. As expected from a developmental lesion, an AVM may become symptomatic at any age, and it does so often during childhood, adolescence, and young adulthood, making it very different from most other cerebrovascular diseases, which are often acquired conditions and associated with multiple risk factors common to many other arterial diseases. An AVM may also cause symptoms by irritating the surrounding cortex with gliosis and hemosiderin, hence giving rise to epileptic seizures, or by bringing about chronic pathological hemodynamic changes in the brain, such as reversal of venous flow, venous hypertension, and hypoperfusion of regions surrounding the AVM. Sometimes progressive neurological deficits caused by the last are difficult to differentiate from symptoms possibly caused by a pulsating mass effect. This chapter reviews the natural history (including epidemiology, presenting symptoms, and risk of hemorrhage from untreated AVMs) and indications for treatment of AVMs.

Epidemiology

Prevalence

The true prevalence of brain AVMs is poorly known, and reported attempts to estimate it are scarce. A community-based retrospective study from Scotland reported a prevalence of 18 in 100 000 in the adult population (i.e., < 0.02%) [7]. A 10-fold higher prevalence estimate, 0.2% (95% confidence interval [CI], 0.07–0.49), was found in a German study including over 2500 healthy young men (applicants for the military service in German Air Force) undergoing cranial MRI [8]. Considering that the prevalence of intracranial aneurysms in adults is better established and is approximately 2–3% [9], the results from the first study would make AVMs more than 100 times rarer than aneurysms. In our population-based cerebrovascular neurosurgical practice, patients with aneurysms are approximately 10 times more prevalent than those with AVMs – a figure that seems to conform with many other high-volume cerebrovascular centers, and also very well with the German prevalence study. While the prevalence of AVMs is difficult to estimate reliably because of the rarity of the disease, the stability of these lesions over a carrier's lifetime makes them ideal candidates for prevalence analyses utilizing (very) large subject cohorts undergoing brain MRI for other indications. It is, therefore, likely that AVM prevalence will eventually be well established.

Incidence of newly diagnosed arteriovenous malformations

The incidence rate of newly diagnosed AVMs has been more readily studied – and with more uniform results – and is approximately 1 per 100 000 persons per year (varying from 0.89 to 1.34/100 000 person-years in different population-based studies) [10–13]. The incidence rate seems to be gradually increasing, obviously reflecting the increased availability of non-invasive brain imaging. This trend also inevitably leads to a shift in the AVM patient population, as the proportion of patients with unruptured and even asymptomatic, truly incidental, AVMs is growing. The increasing number of incidental AVMs in our practice will also continue to make our clinical decision making and patient counseling – to treat or not to treat – more challenging.

Mortality

Despite the fact that AVMs may remain asymptomatic for the duration of a patient's life, AVM carriers are predisposed to

Comprehensive Management of Arteriovenous Malformations of the Brain and Spine, ed. Robert F. Spetzler, Douglas S. Kondziolka, Randall T. Higashida, and M. Yashar S. Kalani. Published by Cambridge University Press.

significant morbidity and subsequent mortality caused by this pathology. Overall annual mortality rates have varied from 0.7 to 2.9% in different study populations [10,14–19], although most studies lack any comparison to a background population. We have reported that patients with AVMs have significant excess mortality compared with matched general population [20]. Our study population of 623 patients with AVMs from Finland also included a subset of 155 untreated patients, reflecting the effect of natural history of AVMs on patient survival. In these patients, the overall annual mortality rate was 3.4% during a median follow-up period of 18.9 years. The AVM-related annual mortality rate (either acute case fatality or chronic sequelae of AVM-related morbidity) in the same group was 1.6%; that is, almost 50% of mortality was explained by AVMs. The patients with AVMs were compared with the general population using the relative survival ratio (i.e., the survival of the patient population was compared with the expected survival of the whole population of Finland, matched for age, sex and historical era). Cumulative relative survival ratio in untreated patients with AVMs 30 years after presentation was 0.49 (i.e., approximately two-fold excess in mortality compared with matched general background population). In contrast, in patients with AVMs where the AVM had been completely eradicated, the cumulative relative survival ratio had decreased to only 0.87 after 30 years [20].

Clinical presentation

Hemorrhagic stroke

The increasing availability of neuroimaging is rapidly changing the pattern of symptomatology leading to AVM diagnosis. In the patient series published in the 1980s, over 70% of patients with AVMs presented with hemorrhage [15,19], whereas modern patient series from the late 1990s onwards typically report a hemorrhagic presentation rate of less than 50% [21,22]. Despite this, hemorrhagic stroke from AVM rupture still remains the most common presenting symptom, and 45–72% (median 52%) of patients suffered from hemorrhagic presentation at diagnosis in nine large AVM series [15,17,19,22–27].

Patients with AVM hemorrhage are younger than most other patients with stroke, and AVMs cause one-third of hemorrhagic strokes in young adults [28]. Typical age of presentation is in the third or fourth decade of life. Although AVM rupture is generally considered less dangerous than the rupture of an intracranial aneurysm or a spontaneous hypertensive intracranial hemorrhage (which both also clearly affect mostly older patients with other cardiovascular and systemic comorbidities, probably partially explaining worse outcomes), it still often results in significant neurological disability brought about by intracerebral hemorrhage within deep and/or eloquent structures. Reported case fatality and permanent disability rates after AVM hemorrhage are 5–25% and 10–40%, respectively [19,28–34].

Typical characteristics of AVMs that have been associated with hemorrhagic presentation in different studies include small size [21,22,25], deep venous drainage [21,22,25,35], and deep location [22,36]. Other, less consistently reported, features include non-borderzone (watershed) [22] and infratentorial [37] locations, associated aneurysms [22], hypertension [21], small number of draining veins [36], venous ectasias [36], and high feeding artery pressure [35]. However, it should be emphasized that factors associated with hemorrhagic presentation are not necessarily the same as independent risk factors predicting future hemorrhage. For example, small AVM size is one of the most constantly found "risk" factors for hemorrhagic presentation but it does not increase the risk of rupture of untreated AVM after diagnosis (see below). Many small AVMs probably remain completely unnoticed unless they bleed, whereas large AVMs may more often become symptomatic in a variety of ways, even in the absence of hemorrhage.

Epilepsy

The second most common presenting symptom of an AVM is epilepsy, with 18–35% (median 26%) of patients diagnosed because of seizures [15,17,19,22–27]. However, according to a Swedish prospective, population-based study, less than 1% of all first episodes of unprovoked seizures are caused by AVMs [38]. Reported anatomical AVM characteristics associated with epileptic presentation have included large size [39], cortical location of the nidus or the feeders [39,40], and temporal location of the AVM [41]. It is not yet well established how often AVM-related symptomatic epilepsy develops into medically refractory epilepsy prior to AVM treatment; in one recent series this had occurred in 18% of the patients [42].

Other

Less common presenting symptoms leading to AVM diagnosis are chronic headache (unrelated to bleeding) in 6–14% of patients and focal neurological deficit (temporary, fixed or progressive) resulting from a mass effect or hemodynamic disturbances in 3–10% [15,17,19,22–27]. As discussed above, the proportion of patients with incidentally found AVMs has been increasing, from less than 2% in early studies to 10% in contemporary series.

Risk of hemorrhage

Hemorrhagic stroke is both the most severe and the most frequent life-threatening complication of harboring an AVM. It is hence understandable that major efforts have been undertaken to identify risk factors predicting AVM rupture. Prevention of future hemorrhages should also be the primary aim of AVM treatment. Since the treatment of complex AVMs is associated with significant risks of morbidity and mortality, these should not exceed the estimated lifetime risk of harboring an untreated lesion. Establishing the probability of hemorrhage and evaluating possible anatomical and patient-related factors affecting this risk requires long-term follow-up studies in large cohorts of patients with untreated AVMs, collected with as little selection bias favoring the lack of treatment as possible. The average annual AVM rupture rate has been approximately 2–4% in most of the published cohorts, but it varies highly depending on various risk factors. As an example, in our natural history series, the risk of rupture from infratentorial AVM during the first five years after diagnosis was 11.6% per year, even though the overall average annual rupture rate in our cohort was 2.4% [43]. In a recent meta-analysis of AVM natural history studies, the average risk of rupture was 3.0% (95% CI, 2.7–3.4) [44]. When the lifetime risk of hemorrhage from an untreated AVM is estimated based on these figures, it is important to understand that the annual risk of rupture should not be multiplied by the (estimated) remaining years at risk; the proper formula for the cumulative probability of hemorrhage is $1 - (1 - p)^t$, where p is the annual probability of hemorrhage and t is the time at risk in years, given that the risk remains constant over time. Unfortunately, the risk estimation is made more complicated by the observation that the risk of rupture does not seem to remain stable over time. The hemorrhage rate has been highest during the first years after the diagnosis in many studies with sufficiently long follow-up times [17,22,27,43]. This observation also explains why studies with relatively short follow-up times generally report higher average annual rupture rates than those with longer follow-up periods. This phenomenon cannot be explained by dropout bias during long follow-ups, since it was observed also in our cohort with almost no patients lost to follow-up during the average observation period of 13.5 years (with the completeness of follow-up data of 98.7% in a cohort of 238 patients) [43]. One plausible explanation is that the AVM becomes hemodynamically unstable for some reason around the time it becomes symptomatic.

Previous rupture has been the most consistent factor found to predict AVM rupture during follow-up [15,16,22,24,26,27,43]. Although not a universal finding [18,36], it was also the most obvious risk factor in a recent meta-analysis, doubling the annual rupture rate from 2.2% (95% CI, 1.7–2.7) to 4.5% (95% CI, 3.7–5.5) [44]. In our series, hemorrhagic presentation tripled the risk of hemorrhage during the first five years after diagnosis compared with unruptured AVMs [43]. Deep and infratentorial AVM locations and exclusively deep venous drainage have also been consistently observed risk factors [22,23,27,36,43,44]. Associated aneurysms also seem to increase the risk of hemorrhage [44], although published reports are vague about whether the hemorrhages in patients with aneurysms are true nidal AVM hemorrhages or subarachnoid hemorrhages from – sometimes quite distant – aneurysms.

The effect of AVM size on the risk of hemorrhage remains an unresolved question. As discussed, small AVM size is undisputedly associated with hemorrhagic presentation, which does not automatically imply that it predicts future hemorrhage as well. In fact, small AVM size has not predicted hemorrhage in any study using multivariate models, and neither did it have any effect in the recent meta-analysis [44]. Many groups have not found AVM size to have any effect [15,22,24,26,27]. However, large AVM size has been a risk factor for subsequent rupture in four different cohorts [18,36,43,45]. So, either size really does not matter or there is some tendency for large AVMs to have a higher risk of rupture.

The effects of age and sex have been too inconsistent between different series to draw any conclusions [17,22,27,43,44].

Treatment indications

General principles

This section must commence by acknowledging that no AVM treatment has ever been proven safe and effective in a controlled trial that could be considered sufficient for class I evidence [46]. However, absence of evidence is not evidence for absence, and it would be nonsense to claim that there is no clear indication to eradicate, for example, a ruptured, Spetzler–Martin low-grade AVM in a young patient. It is also known from the largest AVM database in the world (in terms of duration of follow-up, >10 000 person-years) that, after complete cure, patients with AVMs attain close to normal life expectancy, whereas patients with untreated AVMs have approximately two-fold cumulative excess mortality at 30 years from diagnosis [20]. However, absence of hard evidence means that when talking about indications for AVM treatment, the practitioner has to interprete existing data and base opinions on those interpretations as well as personal experience, instead of being able to rely on evidence-based guidelines. This is the case also in this chapter, and the reader should understand that there simply cannot be an official treatment recommendation at present. We try here to simply convey the philosophy and basic principles used in our practice to treat these patients.

The main goal of brain AVM treatment is always to exclude it from circulation, thus preventing any future hemorrhage, while minimizing treatment-related morbidity. Current treatment modalities include microneurosurgical resection, endovascular embolization, and stereotactic radiosurgery. Although microsurgery can still be considered the most definite method to immediately and completely eradicate the whole lesion, there are circumstances under which the two other modalities are extremely useful and sometimes even the only feasible option. It is also common to employ more than one modality to effectively treat a single lesion. While it has been a matter of considerable debate whether partial occlusion can have any beneficial effect on the rupture risk or if it can be even potentially harmful, it is clear that complete eradication is the only way to completely eliminate the future risk of hemorrhage, and this should, therefore, always be the goal of treatment from the outset. In fact, particularly for complex AVMs, one should have a realistic and feasible plan with the aim of complete cure before even commencing treatment. Although unexpected situations will happen also in surgery, such as small hidden AVM remnants in postoperative angiograms, this principle is perhaps by nature more obvious to neurosurgeons, who know that AVM resection cannot really be stopped until the whole lesion is removed or the patient probably dies. Embolization and radiosurgery, by comparison, may seem less dangerous tools in a situation where the risk of not reaching the complete cure is tangible; however, there is really no convincing evidence that anything good is achieved by palliative embolization or radiosurgery. This is not to say that we oppose non-surgical treatments for AVMs; on the contrary, we often employ preoperative embolization – nowadays using a copolymer of ethylene and vinyl alcohol (Onyx; Covidien ev3 Neurovascular, Irvine, CA, USA) – particularly in larger and more complex AVMs, and use stereotactic radiosurgery for small, deep-seated unruptured AVMs. But multimodal treatment should only be used when it provides real synergy that makes the cumulative risks of multiple treatment sessions justifiable, and helps in reaching the ultimate goal of complete eradication. Furthermore, we strongly believe that AVM treatment should only take place in centers with all three modalities at disposal, because only then can the most appropriate modality/modalities be objectively chosen without secondary, non-medical incentives intervening in the decision-making process. Finally, we think that patients with AVMs should be treated only in centers with sufficiently high caseloads, as successful treatment requires considerable and continuous experience of a multidisciplinary team.

Ruptured arteriovenous malformations

Indication to treat AVMs that have already ruptured is, in general, uncontroversial and clear. As discussed above, prior rupture is the most significant risk factor for subsequent rupture, and cumulative rerupture risk reaches significant percentages rather rapidly (in a few years), usually justifying treatment even in elderly patients to prevent future hemorrhage. Hemorrhagic stroke from AVM very often presents with intracerebral hemorrhage, the surgical evacuation of which is often advisable and is often a life-saving procedure. Infrequently, a patient is encountered with a large and complex AVM that has caused a life-threatening hemorrhage; immediate evacuation of the hemorrhage is required with no time to perform digital subtraction angiography or possible preoperative embolization. In these rare patients, we plan the surgery based only on CT and CT angiography, evacuate only the intracerebral hemorrhage, and eradicate the AVM in a second operation after MRI, digital subtraction angiography, and preoperative embolization, usually within the next few days. However, smaller AVMs are usually amenable to resection in the first emergency operation, as modern CT angiography and intraoperative indocyanine green angiography usually provide enough information on the angioarchitecture in such less complex lesions. Even in patients with more complex AVMs, but where the hemorrhage does not require immediate evacuation, we usually plan the surgery within a few days after hemorrhage, preceded by the imaging and endovascular procedures. We believe that prompt elimination of the ruptured AVM facilitates rehabilitation and shortens the intensive care required, when "ultra-early" surgery is made feasible and safe by experienced microneurosurgeons and neuroanesthesiologists [47]. Microneurosurgery, preceded by preoperative embolization if necessary, is also always the preferred treatment modality in ruptured AVMs, because it eliminates the risk of a further rupture immediately. Of course, if the intracerebral hemorrhage does not require evacuation and the AVM can be completely embolized in a single session, surgery is not required, but complete cure by embolization in one session is not common. We do not recommend multistaged embolizations particularly in ruptured AVMs because we have experienced several peri- and postprocedural hemorrhagic complications after partial embolizations. Radiosurgery is far too slow in its action for ruptured AVMs and is the least preferred choice. In our practice, it is used only for those ruptured AVMs whose deep location makes them totally inaccessible for surgery. Even for many deep AVMs, the intracerebral hemorrhage may provide a safe corridor to the lesion, which can be used without inducing additional morbidity.

Despite the seemingly straightforward decision to treat ruptured AVMs, the issue becomes less clear in patients with the largest and most complex AVMs. Most of these fall into Spetzler–Martin grades IV and V, and are often called "high-grade" AVMs. In addition to their large size, they usually involve eloquent brain regions, deep venous drainage, and deep supplying perforators, and their treatment is known to carry very high risks of combined permanent morbidity and mortality [48]. Accordingly, many clinicians either do not recommend treatment at all for these lesions or reserve treatment for those patients with repeated hemorrhages and progressive deterioration [49]. However, our recent long-term follow-up study on patients with untreated high-grade AVMs demonstrated a very high rebleeding risk (6.0% per year) in patients with ruptured lesions [34]. Moreover, these subsequent hemorrhages carried an extremely high combined risk of permanent disability or death (65%). Therefore, once an AVM has ruptured, we aggressively treat these high-grade lesions if at all possible, particularly in younger patients. It also has to be remembered that while high-grade AVMs usually involve eloquent structures, hemorrhage has usually already caused neurological deficits and, therefore, surgery does not necessarily induce additional long-term disability in this difficult patient group.

Unruptured arteriovenous malformations

The treatment of unruptured AVMs is currently much more controversial [50]. It is true that most of the patients harboring an unruptured AVM are neurologically intact, although a small minority may have focal neurological symptoms without any evidence of previous hemorrhage. Since the purpose of AVM treatment is to eliminate the risk of hemorrhage, it is purely prophylactic in these patients. Prophylactic treatment is justified only if the treatment is likely to impose a risk that is lower than the risk associated with the untreated disease during the expected remaining lifetime of the patient. Although natural history studies provide a lot of information about the future hemorrhage risk of unruptured AVMs, it must be remembered that the vast majority of patients in these study cohorts have had symptomatic AVMs (e.g., epilepsy), and that purely incidental AVMs may have a rupture risk that is lower than that which could be estimated based on historical data.

Because of the unclear indications for treatment of unruptured AVMs, a randomized clinical trial is under way (A Randomized Trial of Unruptured Brain Arteriovenous malformations [ARUBA], www.arubastudy.org), with the objective of finding out whether intervention or watchful waiting is preferable for these lesions (see the Appendix, p. 327). However, the efficacy of prophylactic treatment, if present, probably requires decades rather than years of follow-up to become evident in this type of disease; consequently, there will be a long wait for a definite answer. Meanwhile, in situations where the patient and the treating physician are ambivalent on the treatment decision, the choice to enter the patient into the trial may just be the most appropriate one. In our experience, one of the key factors favoring prophylactic treatment after patient counseling has been the patient's strong wish to be treated, because the psychological burden of the possible risk of hemorrhage at uncertain point in future is often greater than the fear of the procedural complications, the timing of which can be decided by the patient. These issues may of course have great cultural variations. In addition, while the purpose of AVM treatment is always to prevent future hemorrhage, surgical excision of an AVM particularly may have a favorable effect on the associated epilepsy, even in medically refractory patients [41,42].

We usually recommend treatment for unruptured Spetzler–Martin grades I–III AVMs in children and young adults. While we have no fixed upper age limit for patients with unruptured AVMs, treatment is seldom rational in patients over approximately 60 years, unless the psychological burden is intolerable and the treatment risks very reasonable. Spetzler–Martin grade III is also rather heterogeneous in its associated treatment risks, and particularly eloquently located AVMs require careful patient counseling. Unruptured Spetzler–Martin grades IV–V AVMs are usually best left to careful conservative follow-up. The treatment for them may be carefully considered, particularly if the patient has progressive neurological deficits from hemodynamic disturbances. As a general rule, the younger the patient, the more aggressive our attitude is toward the lesion, because the cumulative natural history risk during the remaining lifetime is higher and the potential for recovery from possible complications better.

References

1. van Beijnum J, van der Worp HB, Schippers HM, *et al.* Familial occurrence of brain arteriovenous malformations: a systematic review. *J Neurol Neurosurg Psychiatry* 2007;**78**:1213–17.
2. Waltimo O. The change in size of intracranial arteriovenous malformations. *J Neurol Sci* 1973;**19**:21–7.
3. Pasqualin A, Vivenza C, Rosta L, *et al.* Spontaneous disappearance of intracranial arterio-venous malformations. *Acta Neurochir (Wien)* 1985;**76**:50–7.
4. Kader A, Goodrich JT, Sonstein WJ, *et al.* Recurrent cerebral arteriovenous malformations after negative postoperative angiograms. *J Neurosurg* 1996;**85**:14–18.
5. Lee SK, Vilela P, Willinsky R, *et al.* Spontaneous regression of cerebral arteriovenous malformations: clinical and angiographic analysis with review of the literature. *Neuroradiology* 2002;**44**:11–16.
6. Buis DR, van den Berg R, Lycklama G, *et al.* Spontaneous regression of brain arteriovenous malformations: a clinical study and a systematic review of the literature. *J Neurol* 2004;**251**:1375–82.
7. Al-Shahi R, Fang JS, Lewis SC, *et al.* Prevalence of adults with brain arteriovenous malformations: a community based study in Scotland using capture–recapture analysis. *J Neurol Neurosurg Psychiatry* 2002;**73**:547–51.
8. Weber F, Knopf H. Incidental findings in magnetic resonance imaging of the brains of healthy young men. *J Neurol Sci* 2006;**240**:81–4.
9. Vlak MH, Algra A, Brandenburg R, *et al.* Prevalence of unruptured intracranial aneurysms, with emphasis on sex, age, comorbidity, country, and time period: a systematic review and meta-analysis. *Lancet Neurol* 2011;**10**:626–36.
10. ApSimon HT, Reef H, Phadke RV, *et al.* A population-based study of brain arteriovenous malformation: long-term treatment outcomes. *Stroke* 2002;**33**:2794–800.
11. Brown RD, Jr., Wiebers DO, Torner JC, *et al.* Incidence and prevalence of intracranial vascular malformations in Olmsted County, Minnesota, 1965 to 1992. *Neurology* 1996;**46**:949–52.
12. Hillman J. Population-based analysis of arteriovenous malformation treatment. *J Neurosurg* 2001;**95**:633–7.
13. Stapf C, Mast H, Sciacca RR, *et al.* The New York Islands AVM Study: design, study progress, and initial results. *Stroke* 2003;**34**:e29–e33.
14. Abad JM, Alvarez F, Manrique M, *et al.* Cerebral arteriovenous malformations. Comparative results of surgical vs. conservative treatment in 112 cases. *J Neurosurg Sci* 1983;**27**:203–10.
15. Crawford PM, West CR, Chadwick DW, *et al.* Arteriovenous malformations of the brain: natural history in unoperated patients. *J Neurol Neurosurg Psychiatry* 1986;**49**:1–10.
16. Forster DM, Steiner L, Hakanson S. Arteriovenous malformations of the brain. A long-term clinical study. *J Neurosurg* 1972;**37**:562–70.
17. Itoyama Y, Uemura S, Ushio Y, *et al.* Natural course of unoperated intracranial arteriovenous malformations: study of 50 cases. *J Neurosurg* 1989;**71**:805–9.
18. Mine S, Hirai S, Ono J, *et al.* Risk factors for poor outcome of untreated arteriovenous malformation. *J Clin Neurosci* 2000;**7**:503–6.
19. Ondra SL, Troupp H, George ED, *et al.* The natural history of symptomatic arteriovenous malformations of the brain: a 24-year follow-up assessment. *J Neurosurg* 1990;**73**:387–91.
20. Laakso A, Dashti R, Seppanen J, *et al.* Long-term excess mortality in 623 patients with brain arteriovenous malformations. *Neurosurgery* 2008;**63**:244–53.
21. Langer DJ, Lasner TM, Hurst RW, *et al.* Hypertension, small size, and deep venous drainage are associated with risk of hemorrhagic presentation of cerebral arteriovenous malformations. *Neurosurgery* 1998;**42**:481–6.

22. Stapf C, Mast H, Sciacca RR, *et al.* Predictors of hemorrhage in patients with untreated brain arteriovenous malformation. *Neurology* 2006;**66**:1350–5.
23. Fults D, Kelly DL, Jr. Natural history of arteriovenous malformations of the brain: a clinical study. *Neurosurgery* 1984;**15**:658–62.
24. Halim AX, Johnston SC, Singh V, *et al.* Longitudinal risk of intracranial hemorrhage in patients with arteriovenous malformation of the brain within a defined population. *Stroke* 2004;**35**:1697–702.
25. Kader A, Young WL, Pile-Spellman J, *et al.* The influence of hemodynamic and anatomical factors on hemorrhage from cerebral arteriovenous malformations. *Neurosurgery* 1994;**34**:801–7.
26. Mast H, Young WL, Koennecke HC, *et al.* Risk of spontaneous haemorrhage after diagnosis of cerebral arteriovenous malformation. *Lancet* 1997;**350**:1065–8.
27. Yamada S, Takagi Y, Nozaki K, *et al.* Risk factors for subsequent hemorrhage in patients with cerebral arteriovenous malformations. *J Neurosurg* 2007;**107**:965–72.
28. Al-Shahi R, Warlow C. A systematic review of the frequency and prognosis of arteriovenous malformations of the brain in adults. *Brain* 2001;**124**:1900–26.
29. van Beijnum J, Lovelock CE, Cordonnier C, *et al.* Outcome after spontaneous and arteriovenous malformation-related intracerebral haemorrhage: population-based studies. *Brain* 2009;**132**:537–43.
30. da Costa L, Wallace MC, Ter Brugge KG, *et al.* The natural history and predictive features of hemorrhage from brain arteriovenous malformations. *Stroke* 2009;**40**:100–5.
31. Brown RD, Jr., Wiebers DO, Torner JC, *et al.* Frequency of intracranial hemorrhage as a presenting symptom and subtype analysis: a population-based study of intracranial vascular malformations in Olmsted Country, Minnesota. *J Neurosurg* 1996;**85**:29–32.
32. Choi JH, Mast H, Sciacca RR, *et al.* Clinical outcome after first and recurrent hemorrhage in patients with untreated brain arteriovenous malformation. *Stroke* 2006;**37**:1243–7.
33. Hartmann A, Mast H, Mohr JP, *et al.* Morbidity of intracranial hemorrhage in patients with cerebral arteriovenous malformation. *Stroke* 1998;**29**:931–4.
34. Laakso A, Dashti R, Juvela S, *et al.* Risk of hemorrhage in patients with untreated Spetzler–Martin grade IV and V arteriovenous malformations: a long-term follow-up study in 63 patients. *Neurosurgery* 2011;**68**:372–7.
35. Duong DH, Young WL, Vang MC, *et al.* Feeding artery pressure and venous drainage pattern are primary determinants of hemorrhage from cerebral arteriovenous malformations. *Stroke* 1998;**29**:1167–76.
36. Stefani MA, Porter PJ, terBrugge KG, *et al.* Large and deep brain arteriovenous malformations are associated with risk of future hemorrhage. *Stroke* 2002;**33**:1220–4.
37. Khaw AV, Mohr JP, Sciacca RR, *et al.* Association of infratentorial brain arteriovenous malformations with hemorrhage at initial presentation. *Stroke* 2004;**35**:660–3.
38. Forsgren L. Prospective incidence study and clinical characterization of seizures in newly referred adults. *Epilepsia* 1990;**31**:292–301.
39. Crawford PM, West CR, Shaw MD, *et al.* Cerebral arteriovenous malformations and epilepsy: factors in the development of epilepsy. *Epilepsia* 1986;**27**:270–5.
40. Turjman F, Massoud TF, Sayre JW, *et al.* Epilepsy associated with cerebral arteriovenous malformations: a multivariate analysis of angioarchitectural characteristics. *AJNR Am J Neuroradiol* 1995;**16**:345–50.
41. Hoh BL, Chapman PH, Loeffler JS, *et al.* Results of multimodality treatment for 141 patients with brain arteriovenous malformations and seizures: factors associated with seizure incidence and seizure outcomes. *Neurosurgery* 2002;**51**:303–9.
42. Englot DJ, Young WL, Han SJ, *et al.* Seizure predictors and control after microsurgical resection of supratentorial arteriovenous malformations in 440 patients. *Neurosurgery* 2012;**71**:572–80.
43. Hernesniemi JA, Dashti R, Juvela S, *et al.* Natural history of brain arteriovenous malformations: a long-term follow-up study of risk of hemorrhage in 238 patients. *Neurosurgery* 2008;**63**:823–9.
44. Gross BA, Du R. Natural history of cerebral arteriovenous malformations: a meta-analysis. *J Neurosurg* 2013;**118**:437–43.
45. Guidetti B, Delitala A. Intracranial arteriovenous malformations. Conservative and surgical treatment. *J Neurosurg* 1980;**53**:149–52.
46. Al-Shahi R, Warlow CP. Interventions for treating brain arteriovenous malformations in adults. *Cochrane Database Syst Rev* 2006;CD003436.
47. Kuhmonen J, Piippo A, Vaart K, *et al.* Early surgery for ruptured cerebral arteriovenous malformations. *Acta Neurochir Suppl* 2005;**94**:111–14.
48. Spetzler RF, Martin NA. A proposed grading system for arteriovenous malformations. *J Neurosurg* 1986;**65**:476–83.
49. Han PP, Ponce FA, Spetzler RF. Intention-to-treat analysis of Spetzler–Martin grades IV and V arteriovenous malformations: natural history and treatment paradigm. *J Neurosurg* 2003;**98**:3–7.
50. Stapf C, Mohr JP, Choi JH, *et al.* Invasive treatment of unruptured brain arteriovenous malformations is experimental therapy. *Curr Opin Neurol* 2006;**19**:63–8.

Chapter 6

Imaging evaluation of arteriovenous malformations

Matthew R. Amans and William P. Dillon

Introduction

Imaging is an essential component in the diagnosis, management, and follow-up of patients with arteriovenous malformations (AVM) and arteriovenous fistulae (AVF) in the brain and spine. This chapter will discuss the imaging characteristics; differential diagnosis, grading, and classification; and the imaging pitfalls when considering brain and spine AVMs and AVFs.

Vascular malformations present with a multitude of symptoms ranging from benign headaches and pulsatile tinnitus to progressive and debilitating neurological deficits and seizures. Non-contrast head CT is typically the study of choice for those presenting with non-specific symptoms. Intracranial hemorrhage is the most common pathological presentation (30–82%) for brain AVM, but other manifestations include encephalomalacia and ischemia [1–10]. Contrast-enhanced CT or CT angiography (CTA), MRI and MR angiography (MRA), or digital subtraction angiography (DSA) is often required for further evaluation.

Overview of imaging modalities

Imaging modalities available and their various permutations are summarized in Table 6.1.

CT

Nobel laureate Sir Godfrey Hounsfield developed CT for clinical use between 1972 and 1973. A tube that rotates around the patient generates X-ray beams/photons, and detectors collect the photons that pass through the patient. The amount of X-ray absorption by the body determines the intensity on a gray scale. The greater the attenuation of X-ray, the higher the density (whiter) on the CT image densities (bone is bright, air is black). Differences in density allow for differentiation of structures and pathology. Acute hemorrhage, for example, absorbs X-ray more than brain, which accounts for its higher density on CT (Fig. 6.1) [11].

Non-ionic contrast attenuates X-ray more than either blood or brain parenchyma and, therefore, appears more dense than either blood or brain parenchyma. Contrast-enhanced head CT (intravenous infusion of contrast followed by CT) demonstrates enhancement of structures lacking blood–brain barrier, and pathology that results in breakdown of the blood–brain barrier. Circulating contrast also increases the density in normal as well as pathological arteries and veins. Rapid thin section CT acquisition during intravenous contrast infusion is used for CTA and results in better visualization of the brain vascular system as well as of pathological entities such as AVMs and aneurysms.

Benefits of CT include nearly universal availability as well as rapid acquisition times. Improvements resulting in smaller, more portable CT scanners have allowed for reliable evaluation of hemorrhage and hydrocephalus in patients who are unable to travel to the radiology department (e.g., intubated patients in intensive care units). Portable CT scanners generally deliver greater radiation doses and produce images of limited spatial resolution compared with standard CT scanners [12].

Risks of CT and CTA are minimal and include those related to ionizing radiation in general (Tables 6.1 and 6.2), and those related to the administration of contrast material [13]. The latter include a small risk of allergic reactions and contrast-induced nephrotoxicity [14]. These complications have been minimized significantly with the use of non-ionic contrast media and proper hydration. Nonetheless, care should be taken when administering contrast to diabetic patients and to those with renal failure, multiple myeloma, or a history of atopy or prior allergic reactions to contrast media [14]. Those with allergic history may require premedication with steroids and antihistamines 12 and 2 hours prior to administration of contrast if CT is required. In these patients, MRI may be an alternative.

MRI

Nobel laureate Paul Lauterbur's imaging of distributions of H_2O and D_2O in a test tube originally published in *Nature* in 1973 [15] led to the development of modern MRI. Differing T_1 and T_2 relaxation parameters inherent to different soft tissues

Comprehensive Management of Arteriovenous Malformations of the Brain and Spine, ed. Robert F. Spetzler, Douglas S. Kondziolka, Randall T. Higashida, and M. Yashar S. Kalani. Published by Cambridge University Press.

Table 6.1. Imaging modalities available and their various permutations

Modality	Permutation	Details	Radiation dose (mSv)[a]
CT	Non-contrast	Imaging modality recommended for initial evaluation of acute onset of "worst headache" or thunderclap headache; initial imaging modality recommended for acute change in neurological status that may be secondary to acute hemorrhage or hydrocephalus	1–10
	Contrast enhanced	CT performed after intravenous administration of contrast material; particularly useful in evaluating venous thrombosis	1–10
	Angiography	CT performed during the arterial phase of contrast administration	1–10
	Perfusion	Multiple CT images obtained at a few sequences over the course of bolus administration of intravenous contrast; post-processing to determine mean transit time, cerebral blood volume, and cerebral blood flow	1–10
	Myelography	CT of the spine obtained after subarachnoid administration of contrast	10–30
MRI	Non-contrast	Typically acquired sequences include T_1- and T_2-weighted imaging, T_2 fluid-attenuated inversion recovery (FLAIR), diffusion-weighted imaging, multiplanar gradient-recalled	0
	Contrast enhanced	T_1-weighted images obtained after administration of contrast; structures external to the blood–brain barrier, or in breakdown of the blood–brain barrier, will enhance (become bright)	0
	Angiography	Both contrast-enhanced and non-contrast techniques are available; flow-related MRA such as time-of-flight MRI has the added ability to demonstrate relative velocity of blood flow such that fast flowing blood is bright; spatial resolution is typically improved with contrast-enhancement	0
	Myelography	MRI of the spine performed after administration of contrast in thecal sac	0
Digital subtraction angiography		Superior spatial and temporal resolution allows delineation of angioarchitecture and fluid dynamics of the brain/spine; embolization after angiography may treat lesions or decrease their vascularity, thus decreasing the risk profile of surgery	Variable

[a] Radiation dose is estimated adult effective dose.

allows for soft tissue spatial resolution in MRI. In general, the greater the water content, the longer the T_2 relaxation time and the brighter the signal on T_2-weighted sequences. Substances such as hemorrhage, fat, and protein have short T_1 relaxation times and show brighter signal on T_1-weighted sequences.

There are many advantages for MRI compared with CT, the main one being the lack of ionizing radiation. However, MRI is more expensive and more time consuming than CT. Imaging of patients who are unable to lie flat for at least 30 minutes typically results in uninterpretable images. Another safety consideration with MRI is the strong magnetic field employed, which can quickly turn ferromagnetic objects into missiles that may seriously injure patients.

While the contrast media used in MRI does not have the risk of nephrotoxicity that is associated with iodinated contrast, it may result in nephrogenic systemic fibrosis if given to patients with severe renal failure. Nephrogenic systemic fibrosis is a rare systemic fibrosing condition involving skin, subcutaneous tissues, and sometimes internal organs that occurs in patients with acute or severe chronic renal insufficiency who are administered gadolinium contrast agents. An association of this condition with gadolinium-based contrast agents, particularly at high doses, has led to the hypothesis that nephrogenic systemic fibrosis is a toxic reaction to free gadolinium [16].

Digital subtraction angiography

In comparison with CT and MRI, DSA has the advantages of increased spatial and temporal resolution. By obtaining sequential images over time during the injection of contrast into a vessel, the angiographer has the ability to observe the angioarchitecture of the brain or spine, as well as the vascular flow dynamics of the malformation in real-time. Consequently, DSA is the imaging modality of choice for diagnosis, classification, and treatment planning for vascular malformations of the brain and spine. It also allows a potential opportunity to treat (or embolize) a lesion as an alternative to, or to improve the risk profiles of, surgical interventions [17–19].

Risks of DSA include those from embolization during the procedure (e.g., non-target embolization), radiation exposure, access-related complications (e.g., bleeding and groin hematoma), and contrast-related complications (discussed above). The risk of permanent neurological deficit from catheter-related stroke is between 0.1% and 1% when performed by a reasonably experienced angiographer [18–20].

Imaging characteristics of brain arteriovenous malformations

CT features

Non-contrast CT has long been the imaging standard for identifying symptomatic intracranial hemorrhage [13]; however, T_2*-weighted imaging is more sensitive in the detection of intracranial hemorrhage. Nonetheless, CT is accurate in the detection of acute intracranial hemorrhage and has the added advantages of rapid acquisition times and nearly universal availability (Table 6.3) [21,22].

The diagnosis of AVM in the absence of hemorrhage can be difficult using non-contrast CT. Most brain AVMs have density similar to that of gray matter and the blood vessels and mass

Table 6.2. Relative radiation designation adapted from the American College of Radiology appropriateness criteria for headache

Relative radiation designation	Adult effective dose estimate (mSv)
0	0
*	<0.1
**	0.1–1.0
***	1–10
****	10–30
*****	30–100

mSv, millisieverts.
Source: from Strain *et al.*, 2000 [13].

effect from AVMs are minimal unless there is recent hemorrhage; this makes detection of small AVM near the gray matter difficult. Calcification, present in 20–25% of brain AVMs, and focal encephalomalacia around the AVM may alert the observer to the presence of an AVM. Arterialized pressures in the venous system may result in perinidal edema, visible on CT as low density, which may allow recognition of brain AVM on non-contrast CT (Fig. 6.2A,B).

Contrast administration enhances abnormal vascularity of AVMs (Fig. 6.2C,D) and CTA can identify enlarged feeding arteries, the vascular nidus, and the enlarged draining vein(s) typical of AVMs. It can also assist in surgical planning by demonstrating the relationship of the feeding arteries with the vascular nidus, the size of the nidus, and its location relative to eloquent areas of the brain [23–27]. Use of CTA may also identify architectural features of an AVM that increase the risk for hemorrhage, such as flow-related or dysplastic aneurysms of

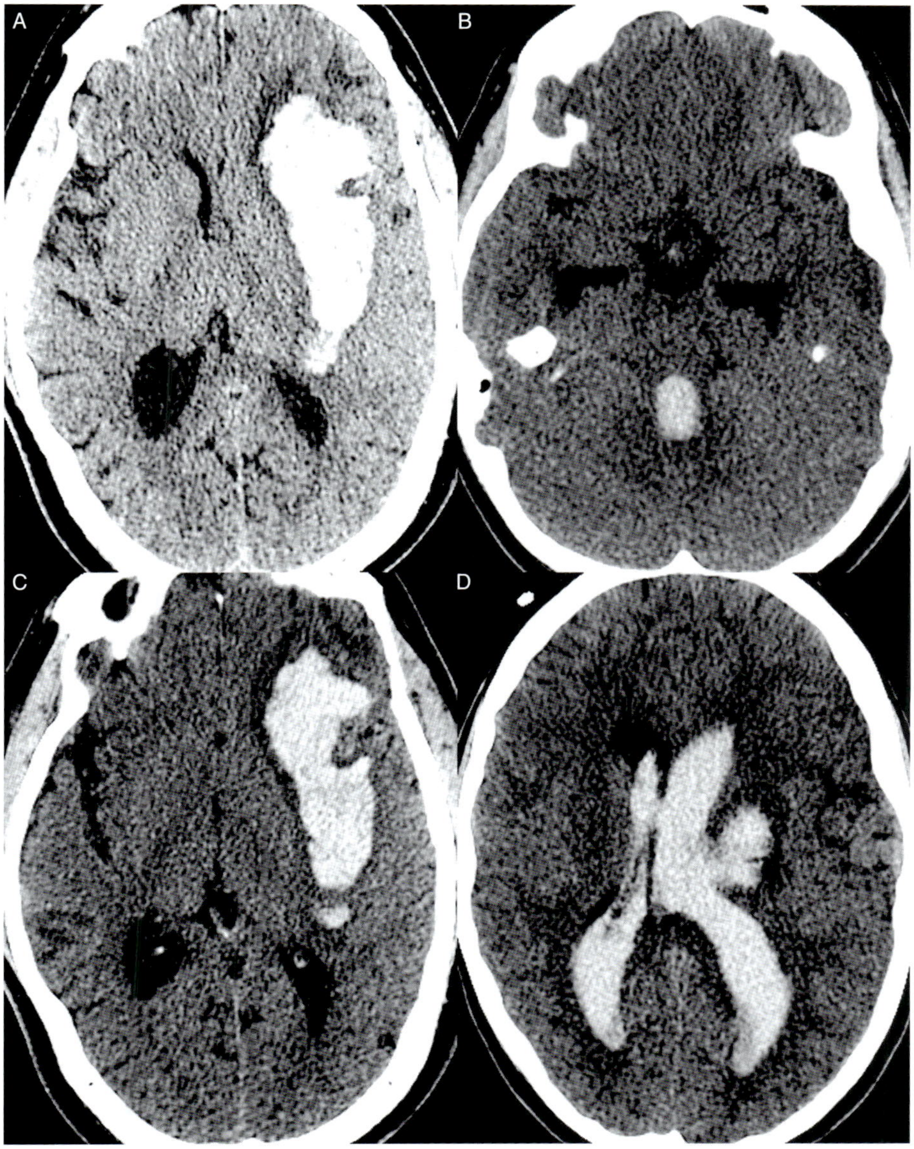

Fig. 6.1. Intracranial hemorrhage. (A) Non-contrast head CT demonstrating left basal ganglia parenchymal hemorrhage with effacement of regional sulci and the left lateral ventricle and minimal surrounding edema (low density) caused by hemorrhage from an arteriovenous malformations (AVM). (B) Hemorrhage in the fourth ventricle and hydrocephalus (note enlargement of temporal horns of lateral ventricles) caused by a pial AVM. (C) Left parenchymal hemorrhage with surrounding edema and effacement of sulci and lateral ventricle. (D) Left corona radiata AVM with hemorrhage and dissection of the hemorrhage into the lateral ventricles.

Table 6.3. Adaptation of the American College of Radiology appropriateness criteria for imaging of headache

Imaging modality	Appropriate rating[a]	Comments	Radiation dose (mSv)[b]
Non-contrast head CT	9	Recommended initial imaging study for new-onset "worst headache"	1–10
CT angiography head	8	Further evaluation for vascular etiology of abnormality demonstrated on non-contrast head CT; evaluation with MRI may be a suitable alternative	1–10
MR angiography, head with or without contrast	8	May be useful alternative to CT angiography; additionally, time-of-flight MR angiography can provide velocity of flow information in suspected dural AVF	0
Digital subtraction angiography	7	Required for full demonstration of vascular anatomy and for treatment planning of AVF and AVM of brain and spine	1–10
MRI head without contrast	7	Demonstration of abnormal vascular architecture; provides anatomical information for surgical staging of AVMs	0
MRI head without and with contrast	6	Particularly useful in evaluating for alternative diagnoses of intracerebral and subarachnoid hemorrhages and hematomyelia	0
CT head without and with contrast	6		1–10

AVF, arteriovenous fistula; AVM, arteriovenous malformations.
[a] American College of Radiology rating scale: 1–3, usually not appropriate; 4–6, may be appropriate; 7–9, usually appropriate.
[b] Radiation dose is estimated adult effective dose.
Source: adapted from Strain *et al.*, 2000 [13].

the feeding arteries, venous varices, or stenosis of the draining veins. Intranidal ectasias, which may be either arterial or venous, are more difficult to identify on CTA than with DSA [18].

Small brain AVMs can be difficult to identify even on contrast-enhanced CT. Identification of early contrast enhancement of a venous structure during the arterial phase of imaging, indicative of arterial venous shunting, may be the only clue that a small AVM is present. Mass effect from recent hemorrhage can also limit detection of AVM by compressing the abnormal vasculature, limiting inflow of contrast material.

Patients in the postoperative period with acute changes in their neurological examination are best initially evaluated with CT to assess for intracranial hemorrhage or acute hydrocephalus. Evaluation for small infarctions is limited on early postoperative CT examinations, usually because of the presence of concomitant edema and a streak artifact induced by metallic surgical clips [7].

MRI features

The best cross-sectional technique to depict the presence and location of an AVM is MRI. Brain AVMs have a variable signal intensity on T_1-weighted images because of the presence of hemorrhage and calcification, as well as the velocity of blood flow in the vessels (Fig. 6.2 E–I). Typically, the nidus is identified as a focal area of low intensity flow voids seen on both T_1- and T_2-weighted images. This appearance has often been referred to as a "bag of worms." Normal brain is not present within the interstices of a vascular nidus. Adjacent dysplastic vessels near the vascular nidus may contribute to overestimation of the size of the nidus on MRI.

Susceptibility-weighted imaging (SWI) using gradient echo sequences demonstrates a variable amount of blooming depending on the presence of extravascular blood products. This is important as even subclinical hemorrhage seen on SWI may indicate a higher propensity for future clinical hemorrhage [28,29]. Diffusion-weighted sequences are usually normal unless there is concomitant surrounding infarction or hemorrhage. Perinidal edema resulting from high pressure in the venous system is visualized as hyperintensity on T_2-weighted imaging and hypointensity on T_1-weighted imaging.

Use of MRA can demonstrate the vessels feeding or draining an AVM and may depict flow-related or dysplastic aneurysms or stenosis of veins draining the AVM, two common risk factors for hemorrhage.

Arterial spin labeled (ASL) is an MR technique in which water protons in arterial blood in the neck vessels are tagged electromagnetically and allowed to move into the brain, where their volume is a reflection of arterial cerebral blood flow. Under normal circumstances, the tagged water decays to normal signal intensity during the parenchymal or capillary phase of blood flow, and the signal is no longer visualized in the veins. If there is shunting, which is associated with both AVMs and AVFs, the tagged water can be identified in the veins receiving the shunted arterial blood [30]. While DSA remains the standard to identify residual AVM post-treatment, ASL improves MRI effectiveness in identifying and measuring shunting in AVMs and AVFs [31]. Comparison of ASL with DSA in the post-gamma knife follow-up of AVMs showed that the techniques were comparable, but DSA was slightly more sensitive for the detection of residual AVM [32]. Changes in the hemodynamics of an AVM or AVF after embolization may also be quantified using ASL [33].

Smaller (micro) AVMs, and particularly small AVMs in the setting of hereditary hemorrhagic telangiectasias, have a different imaging appearance to the classical AVM. Micro-AVMs may be occult on imaging and are often poorly demonstrated on

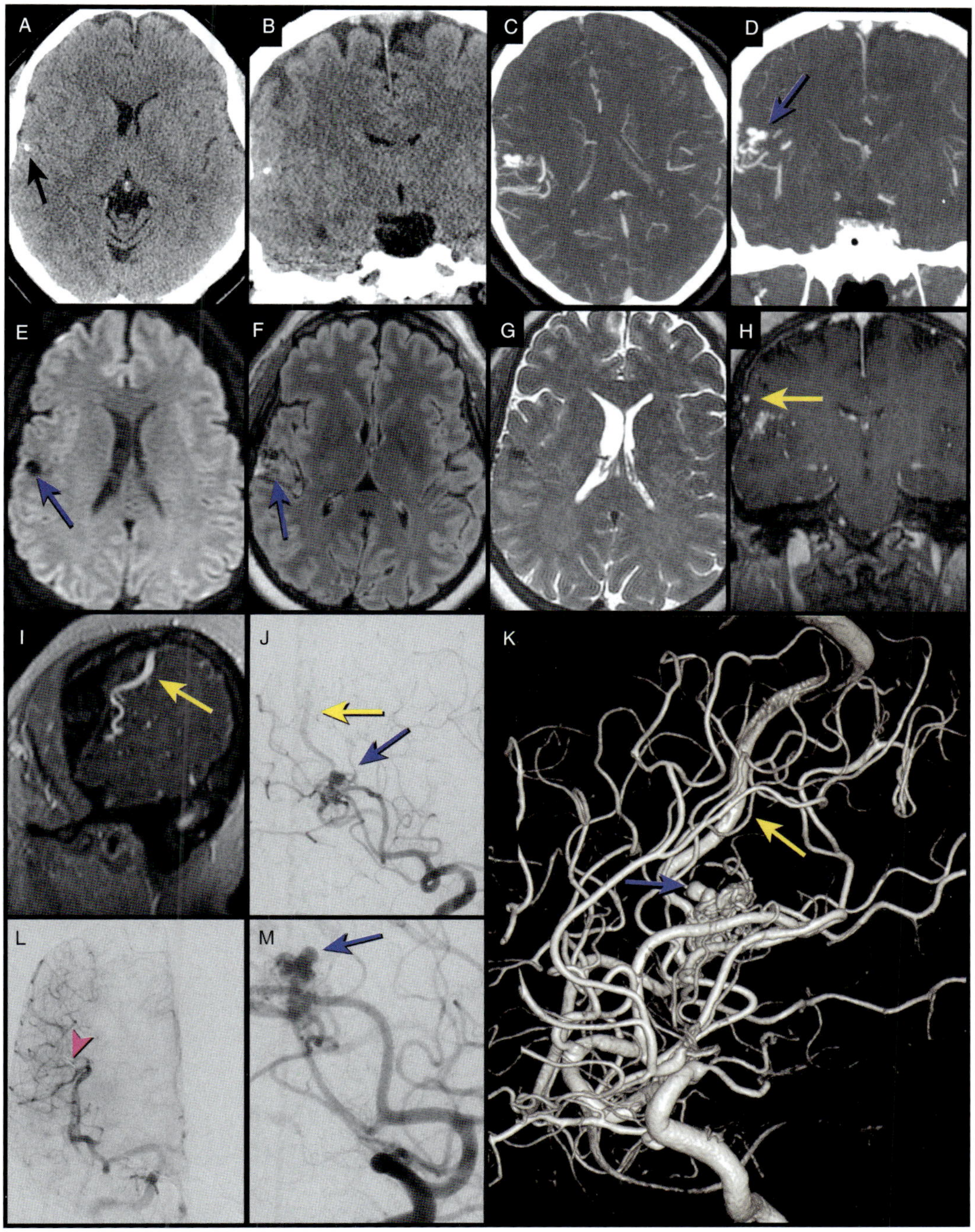

Fig. 6.2. Brain arteriovenous malformations in a 52-year-old woman who presented with new onset of seizures. (A,B) Non-contrast CT demonstrated parenchymal calcification (black arrow) in the right frontal lobe with abnormal contour of the adjacent parenchyma (non-eloquent territory). Maximum intensity projections (5 mm thickness) from CT angiography. (C D) A <3 cm vascular nidus with an intranidal aneurysm (blue arrow). (E) MRI demonstrated magnetic susceptibility secondary to calcification (blue arrow) on diffusion-weighted imaging. (F,G). Flow voids (arrow) in the right frontal lobe corresponding to the AVM nidus seen with T_2 FLAIR (F) and T_2-weighted imaging (G). (H) Contrast-enhanced coronal SPGR (spoiled gradient echo recalled, a T_1-weighted imaging modality) demonstrated enhancing tangle of vessels consistent with the vascular nidus and an enlarged draining vein extending laterally (yellow arrow). (I) Sagittal reconstruction of the isovoxel acquisition SPGR demonstrated the enlarged draining vein to better advantage (yellow arrow). (J–M) Preoperative digital subtraction angiography demonstrated the <3 cm AVM supplied by right middle cerebral artery branches with an intranidal aneurysm (blue arrow), which is a risk factor for hemorrhage. The early draining vein is best appreciated on the early arterial phase image (J) as an enlarged vessel draining away from the AVM (yellow arrow). No deep drainage could be demonstrated in this AVM. Grading was Spetzler–Martin grade I (<3 cm, non-eloquent territory, superficial drainage only). (L) Postoperative angiography demonstrated the surgical clip (pink arrowhead) and no evidence of residual AVM.

T_1- and T_2-weighted imaging. Administration of gadolinium contrast agents intravenously may result in hazy enhancement, appreciated as high signal (T_1 shortening) on T_1-weighted imaging, of a small AVM.

Spetzler and Martin [34] demonstrated that certain angioarchitectural features of AVMs predict neurological outcome from surgery. These include the size of the nidus, the eloquence of the involved brain, and the location of draining veins. Eloquent areas include brainstem, thalamus, hypothalamus, cerebellar peduncles, and sensorimotor, language, or primary visual cortex. These locations are best delineated on MRI.

Gliosis of the brain adjacent to AVM can also be demonstrated with MRI. The pathophysiology behind the gliosis of the peri-AVM brain is controversial, but it may relate to venous pulsations or vascular steal phenomenon [11,18,35]. In the setting of postoperative decline in mental status, CT may best demonstrate intervening hydrocephalus or hemorrhage; however, MRI with diffusion weighting is most sensitive in the demonstration of postoperative infarction.

Digital subtraction angiography features

Diagnostic cerebral angiography, typically using DSA, is the study of choice for preoperative evaluation of brain AVMs. Sequential images over time during the injection of contrast into a vessel allow the angiographer to observe the angioarchitecture of the AVM as well as the vascular flow dynamics (including the identification of vascular shunting) of the AVM in real-time.

Vascular shunting is the hallmark of AVM detection. Vascular shunt from artery to vein (with or without an intervening nidus) is seen as opacification of a vein during the arterial or capillary phases of an angiogram. While shunting is the hallmark of an AVM, vascular shunting can be seen in a wide variety of other etiologies including venous malformations, stroke, seizures, and tumors.

Use of DSA offers the highest resolution for the preoperative evaluation of feeding arteries, the AVM nidus, and its drainage pathway. Hemorrhagic risk factors such as arterial enlargement, arterial variations, and arterial aneurysms are best seen with DSA, particularly during the early arterial phase of the injection. Arterial aneurysms, in particular, increase the risk of hemorrhage and have a variable reported incidence in patients with brain AVM, ranging from 2.7% to 46% (Fig. 6.2 J,M).

Additional feeding vessels are not always appreciated on CTA or MRA as well as they are on DSA. For example, dural supply to brain AVMs is identified in 27% of patients using angiography but is difficult to appreciate on cross-sectional imaging [36]. Dural supply is particularly prominent in patients with previous surgery, possibly resulting from adhesions between dural layers, or after prior partial embolization, possibly caused by angiogenesis as a response to ischemia. Dural supply may be either direct to the AVM via dural leptomeningeal anastomosis or indirect via anastomosis to cortical arteries feeding the AVM [18].

Micro-AVMs consist of a normal-sized feeding artery, a nidus <1 cm in size, and a normal-sized draining vein. These are often quite difficult to appreciate on any modality other than DSA. Early venous shunting may be the first indication of the presence of a micro-AVM. High-magnification imaging, fast-filming, and superselective techniques may be required to identify micro-AVMs [18].

Venous drainage of an AVM should be analyzed for its own characteristics, as well as its relationship to the venous drainage pattern of the regional brain [18]. The draining vein(s) should be evaluated for their location and the presence of pseudoaneurysm, varix, or stenosis, which are associated with increased risk of AVM rupture [19]. Deep venous drainage has been identified as a prognostic factor for hemorrhage [21]. Venous drainage is considered deep if any or all of the venous drainage is through the deep veins such as internal cerebral veins or basal veins of Rosenthal. In the posterior fossa, deep venous drainage is any pathway other than via direct drainage into the straight sinus or transverse sinus [34].

Partial surgical resection of an AVM is not thought to change the natural history of brain AVM and in fact may increase the risk of hemorrhage [37]. Use of DSA is recommended in the early postoperative period to facilitate early revision resection. However, abnormal angioarchitecture of surgically ligated arteries and abnormal parenchymal blush patterns from parenchymal injury in the early postoperative period may be difficult to distinguish from a small residual AVM nidus. Additionally, postoperative parenchymal injury can result in vascular shunting, which may further complicate evaluation for a residual nidus. In such patients, repeat angiography after surgical changes have resolved (6 to 8 weeks) may be required for definitive evaluation.

Imaging characteristics of intracranial arteriovenous fistulae

An AVF is an abnormal communication between an artery and vein, without an intervening nidus. It can be either congenital or acquired. Because of marked differences in the pathophysiology of acquired and congenital intracranial AVF, this chapter will focus on the imaging of acquired adult and pediatric AVFs [18]. Intracranial AVFs most commonly occur within the dura, hence the terminology dural arteriovenous fistula (DAVF). While DAVFs may occur anywhere within the dura, they are most commonly associated with a dural venous sinus. The arterial supply is typically from adjacent branches of the dural arteries (less frequently osseous branches; pial supply even more rare) and the venous drainage may include any combination of dural venous sinus, osteodural veins, and leptomeningeal veins, including the cerebral, cerebellar, or perimedullary veins (Fig. 6.3) [18].

A DAVF can present with a wide variety of neurological symptoms. Common neurological symptoms include tinnitus and bruit, cranial nerve palsy, exophthalmos, focal neurological deficits, global neurological deficits, symptoms related to increased intracranial pressure, intracranial hemorrhage, and hydrocephalus. Apart from the cranial nerve symptoms, which are commonly attributed to vascular steal phenomenon, the majority of symptoms occur secondary to venous hypertension [38].

The classification schemes for DAVF published by Cognard *et al.* in 1995 [39], and Borden *et al.* in 1995 [40] highlighted the importance of venous outflow in clinical symptomatology and its relationship to risk of intracranial hemorrhage (Table 6.4). Both schemes were validated by Davies *et al.* in 1996 [41]; however, both schemes ignored changes in DAVF fluid dynamics (i.e., development of venous outflow stenosis) over time and

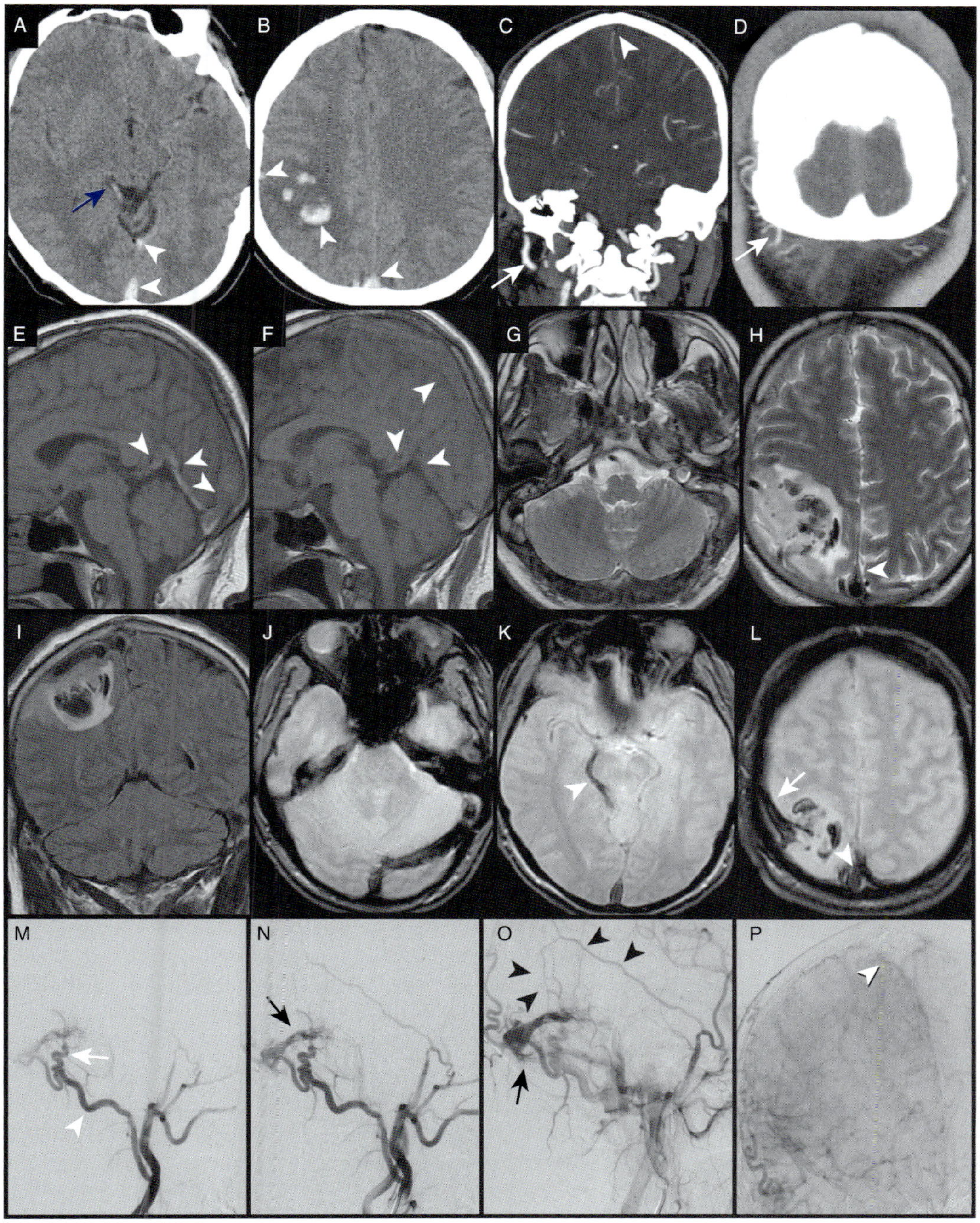

Fig. 6.3. Intracranial arteriovenous fistula (AVF) in a 42-year-old woman with history of pulse synchronous pulsatile tinnitus who presented to the emergency department with acute onset of left-sided weakness. (A,B) Non-contrast head CT demonstrated high density in the right basal vein of Rosenthal (A, blue arrow) as well as the straight sinus (A, top white arrowhead) and torcula (A, bottom white arrowhead). Hemorrhage in the right posterior frontal lobe and anterior parietal lobe was demonstrated as high density in (B, arrowheads). Note the "fluffy" appearance of the hemorrhage suggestive of venous etiology. Low density surrounding the hemorrhage is consistent with edema. Lateral to the hemorrhage is high density in the vein of Labbé (white arrowhead). The bottom white arrowhead again demonstrates high density in the torcula. (C,D) CT angiography demonstrated the "empty delta sign" of contrast surrounding the thrombus within the superior sagittal sinus on the coronal CT (C), the arrow indicating the asymmetrically enlarged right occipital artery. Intraparenchymal hemorrhage indicates that this fistula is "high risk". (E,F) Sagittal T_1-weighted imaging visualized the T_1 shortening (bright signal) within the vein of Galen, straight sinus, and superior sagittal sinus. (G–I) The T_2-weighted and FLAIR sequences showed sinuses with T_2 hypointensity that could easily be mistaken for flow voids. The T_2 sequence through the level of the posterior fossa (G) demonstrated a tangle of vessels in the region of the left transverse sinus. (J–L) Blooming of the thrombus within the sinuses was demonstrated on the gradient recall echo sequence as well as within the basal vein of Rosenthal (K, arrowhead), and a prominent cortical vein (L, arrow). (M) Diagnostic angiography with selective injection of the left external carotid artery in the early arterial phase showed transmastoid perforator artery (arrow) arising from the abnormally enlarged occipital artery (arrowhead) and draining into the transverse sinus. (N,O) Later arterial phase imaging better demonstrated the transverse sinus (black arrows) as well as the additional supply to the fistula via the middle meningeal artery (arrowheads). (P) Late venous phase from the right common carotid injection showed lack of contrast filling the superior sagittal sinus (white arrowhead) and right transverse sinus. Note the angiographic correlate of the "empty delta sign" on this image. The deep venous system is not visible on any angiographic injection, consistent with thrombosis.

Table 6.4. Classifications of cerebral dural arteriovenous fistulae by Cognard *et al.* and Borden *et al.*

Cognard classification	Borden classification
Type I: drainage into sinus or meningeal vein with only anterograde drainage through sinus and cortical veins	Type I: drainage into sinus or meningeal vein directly
Type IIa: drainage into sinus or meningeal vein with insufficient anterograde flow capacity, resulting in retrograde flow into dural venous sinus only (anterograde flow in meningeal vein)	
Type IIb: drainage into sinus or meningeal vein with insufficient anterograde flow capacity, resulting in retrograde flow into meningeal vein only (anterograde flow in venous sinus)	Type II: drainage into sinus or meningeal vein directly but also retrograde flow into cortical veins
Type IIa+b: drainage into sinus or meningeal vein with insufficient anterograde flow capacity, resulting in retrograde flow into both dural venous sinus and cortical vein	
Type III: drainage into cortical vein without venous ectasia	Type III: drainage into cortical veins and no dural sinus or mengingeal venous drainage
Type IV: drainage into cortical vein with venous ectasia >5 mm in diameter and three times larger than the diameter of the draining vein	
Type V: drainage (of intracranial arteriovenous fistula) into spinal perimedullary veins	

Sources: adapted from Cognard *et al.*, 1995 [39] and Borden *et al.*, 1995 [40]

also ignored anatomical predispositions [42]. Therefore, each patient with DAVF should be individually examined with a strong emphasis placed on defining the angioarchitecture of venous drainage and fluid dynamics [18]. Because of the ability to demonstrate venous drainage and shunting in DAVF on DSA, it is the diagnostic imaging modality of choice for full characterization of DAVF prior to intervention (Fig. 6.3M–P). Nonetheless, because of the wide variety of presenting neurological symptoms, many patients with DAVF are initially evaluated using CT or MRI. This section will first focus on the cross-sectional imaging characteristics of DAVF and will then turn to its angioarchitectural features on DSA.

CT features

It may be very difficult to identify DAVF on CT as the dural vessels shunting into a dural sinus are quite small and unless there is dural sinus thrombosis these vessels may appear normal on CT. Increased pressure in the recipient vein or sinus may lead to retrograde flow into parenchymal veins, which may become dilated and visible on contrast-enhanced CT or MRI. Above a certain pressure level, parenchymal edema ensues, which is demonstrated on CT as low density edema. Continued increase in pressure in the veins, which is subsequently transmitted to the capillaries, can even result in hemorrhage, identified on CT as fluffy areas of high density (Fig. 6.3B). If the fistula empties directly into a normal venous sinus, without retrograde filling of parenchymal veins, it may be very difficult to identify. It can be difficult to identify DAVF even on contrast-enhanced CT where early contrast enhancement of a venous structure during the arterial phase of imaging, indicative of arterial venous shunting, may be the only clue that a DAVF is present.

A DAVF may also result in enlargement of the feeding dural arteries. If the middle meningeal artery is involved, there may be enlargement of the foramen spinosum over time. Subtle enlargement of the occipital artery may also be a clue to an underlying DAVF (Fig. 6.3C,D). Similarly, subtle enlargement of veins can be a clue to the altered venous pressures secondary to the DAVF. Asymmetric enlargement of the superior ophthalmic vein secondary to increased pressure in the cavernous sinus in the setting of indirect cavernous carotid fistula is a classic example of DAVF.

Occasionally, a DAVF may result in subarachnoid or intraparenchymal hemorrhage. Non-contrast CT is typically the first modality used in symptomatic intracranial hemorrhage [13]. Subarachnoid hemorrhage in a pattern atypical for aneurysm rupture, or intraparenchymal hemorrhage in a younger patient or in a patient without a history of hypertension, should raise concern for an underlying vascular malformations such as AVM or DAVF. In these patients, evaluation with CTA, MRI with MRA, or DSA should also be considered [13].

Contrast-enhanced CT or CTA can identify enlarged feeding arteries or enlarged draining veins, but DAVFs may still remain quite difficult to identify. Use of CTA may demonstrate early filling of the involved veins [43,44] and may also be able to identify DAVF characteristics that increase the risk for hemorrhage, such as stenosis of the recipient vein or sinus, aneurysms on the feeding arteries (either extradural or subarachnoid in location), or parenchymal venous collateral drainage [18].

Sometimes, DAVFs are associated with venous sinus thrombosis [18]. Thrombosis of the dural venous sinus is seen as high density on non-contrast CT (Fig. 6.3A,B). Care must be taken in diagnosing venous sinus thrombosis on non-contrast CT because a patient's hemodynamic status may affect the density of their blood. For example, patients with anemia have lower blood density and those with hemoconcentration from dehydration or elevated hematocrits have high-density vessels. Sinus thrombosis on contrast-enhanced CT is seen as a filling defect or sometimes as an unanticipated low density relative to the other veins of the cerebral venous complex (Fig. 6.3C).

MRI features

Features of intracranial AVF using MRI parallel those seen in CT. Enlarged venous structures, without a visible nidus, such as

Table 6.5. Imaging intracranial hemorrhage by modality

Stage[a]	CT density	T_1 intensity	T_2 intensity	Hemoglobin configuration
Hyperacute (<6 h)	Increased	=	Increased	Intracellular oxyhemoglobin
Acute (6 h to first couple of days)	Increased	Decreased	Decreased	Intracellular deoxyhemoglobin
Early subacute (first couple of days to about 1 or 2 weeks)	Increased	Increased	Decreased	Intracellular methemoglobin
Late subacute (1 or 2 weeks to several months)	=	Increased	Increased	Extracellular methemoglobin
Chronic (as early as 2 weeks and may be visible for several years)	Decreased	Decreased	Decreased	Extracellular hemosiderin/ferritin

[a] The time frame for the stages of hemorrhage is provided only as a rough guideline. The exact timing depends on the patient's hematocrit, local oxygen tension, local pH, and local glucose concentrations. This also helps to account for why various stages of hemorrhage can be demonstrated in a hematoma, particularly why the edges of the hemorrhage are often at a more advanced stage than the center.

a dilated superior ophthalmic vein in the setting of a cavernous carotid fistula or dilated parenchymal veins in the setting of retrograde flow via vein of Labbé, are clues to shunt physiology of an AVF. Edema resulting from venous hypertension is seen as hyperintensity on T_2-weighted imaging and hypointensity on T_1-weighted imaging. Abnormal and asymmetric flow voids can occasionally be identified on T_1- or T_2-weighted imaging near a dural sinus.

Gradient echo imaging with T_2*-weighting or SWI may demonstrate blood products from prior petechial hemorrhage secondary to venous hypertension. The imaging appearance of hemorrhage on T_1- and T_2-weighted imaging depends on the status of the hemoglobin (Table 6.5).

Time-of-flight MRA has improved the diagnostic accuracy of MRI in identifying high-velocity vascular shunting [45]. In this method, the signal intensity of venous structures is usually suppressed by saturation bands placed superior to the time-of-flight MRA slabs. Hyperintensity in a venous structure on time-of-flight MRA should suggest arterialization of that structure, and is analogous to early contrast filling of a venous structure in CTA or DSA.

Diagnostic accuracy for DAVF is improved with ASL, particularly for small fistulae with slower shunt velocities where time-of-flight MRA may not be as sensitive [30].

Similar to identifying dural sinus thrombosis on contrast-enhanced CT by absence of enhancement, MRI demonstrates sinus thrombosis by absence of a flow void, best seen on T_1-weighted imaging (Fig. 6.3E,F). The superior sagittal sinus, straight sinus, and other midline sinuses are usually best depicted on sagittal T_1-weighted imaging. The T_2 hypointensity of deoxyhemoglobin in acute sinus thrombosis should not be confused with a patent flow void (Fig. 6.3G–I). In T_2*-weighted sequences (such as SWI or gradient recalled echo) will demonstrate prominent hypointense signal that may extend beyond the normal lumen (so-called blooming) (Fig. 6.3J–L). Similarly, cortical vein thrombosis may be seen as a short, linear, or serpentine hypointense structure along the surface of the brain on SWI or T_2*-weighted sequences, with a loss of the flow void best depicted with T_1-weighted imaging.

Contrast-enhanced MRI may show blushing, indistinct contrast enhancement, or even solid enhancement in areas of parenchyma where there is venous congestion from an AVF (Fig. 6.4D). Central pontine enhancement and spinal cord enhancement have both been reported in DAVF [46,47]. Particular care should be taken in differentiating enhancing lesions, such as an expansile T_2-hyperintense cord, with enhancement from neoplasm. Lack of flow voids in such patients does not ensure the diagnosis of neoplasm, and prior to biopsy DAVF should be considered as a possible etiology.

Despite the presence of symptoms of AVF, CT and MRI can appear normal [47]. If there is strong suspicion for DAVF, imaging workup is incomplete without DSA, which is recommended to exclude DAVF particularly in patients with a suggestive history such as pulse-synchronous tinnitus in the presence of a normal otoscopic examination [48].

Digital subtraction angiography features

The imaging modality of choice for diagnosis, classification, and treatment planning of DAVF is DSA because of its superior spatial and temporal resolution compared with cross-sectional techniques. Generally, CT and MRI are unable to provide enough information pertaining to the angioarchitecture of DAVFs for therapeutic planning, even if the diagnosis is initially made on cross-sectional imaging [18]. In addition, DSA is the modality best suited to evaluate hemodynamics and angioarchitecture in and around the brain, allowing full identification of the fistulous site, contributing arteries, and venous drainage pathways [18].

There is a common pathology in DAVFs and AVMs of direct connection of arteries with veins, resulting in arterialized pressures in the venous system; however, the site of connection is markedly different in an AVM and AVF. In AVMs, a vascular nidus, or tangle of vessels, is typically located within the brain or cord parenchyma and is usually easily identified. In AVFs, typically a dural artery connects directly to a cortical vein or dural sinus without an intervening capillary nidus. This, usually small, connection is not easily identified on cross-sectional imaging. On DSA, the AVF site is seen as an abrupt transition in vessel caliber between the smaller artery and the larger vein [44,49]. As with AVMs, DAVFs may have arterial contributions from multiple feeding arteries.

Similar to AVMs, identification of risk factors for hemorrhage in AVFs is best demonstrated on DSA. Arterial aneurysms can be on either extradural or subarachnoid feeding arteries. Arterial aneurysms are slightly more common in

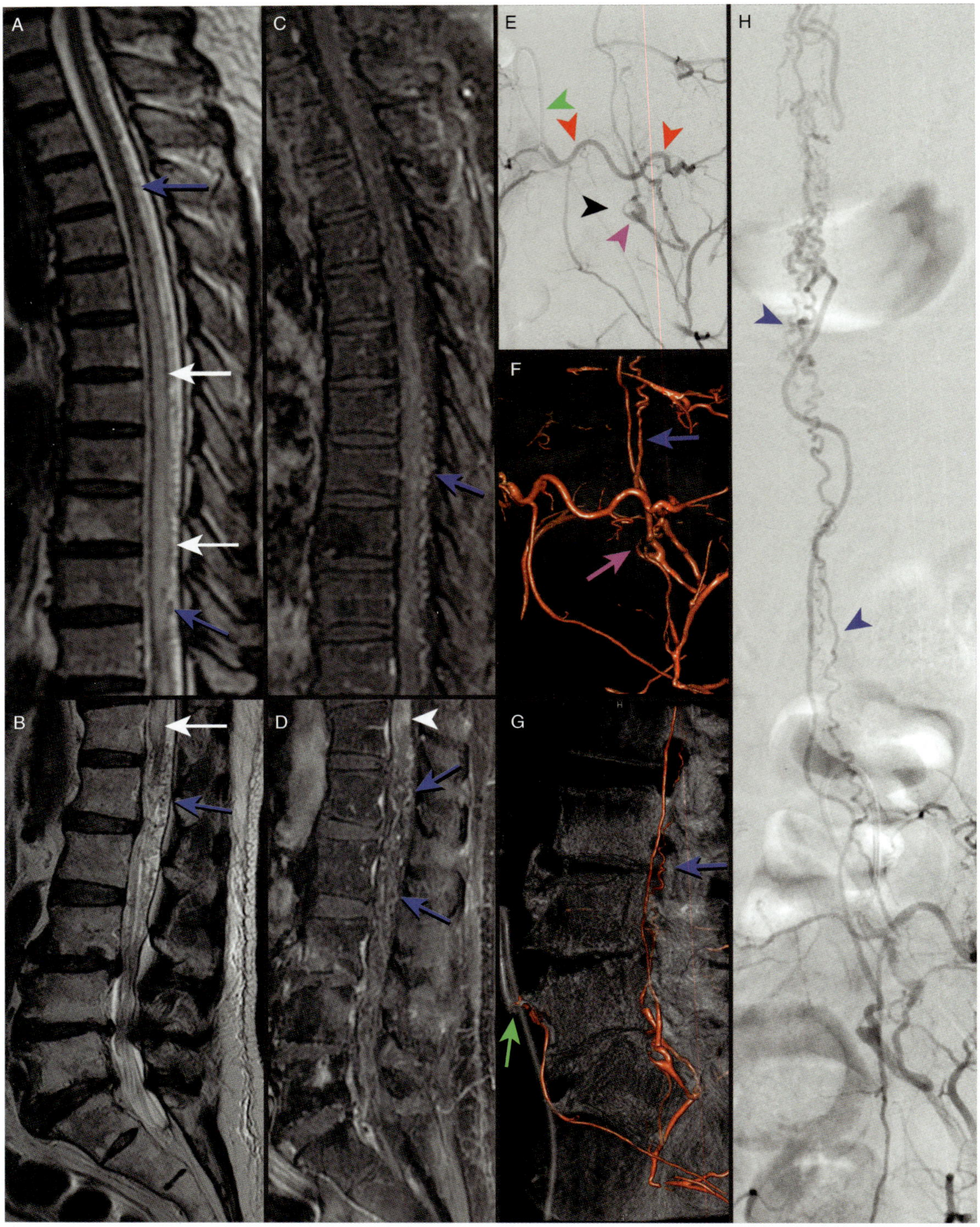

Fig. 6.4. Spine arteriovenous fistula (AVF) in a 65-year-old man presenting with progressive bilateral lower extremity weakness as well as bladder and bowel incontinence. (A–D) MRI demonstrated cord expansion with central T_2 hyperintensity consistent with edema (white arrows). The edema extended from the conus medullaris cranially to T4 level. Marked flow voids were noted around the conus medullaris and superior cauda equine (B) and extending up the dorsal surface of the cord (A), indicated by blue arrows, which also enhance (C,D). The conus medullaris was also mildly and diffusely enhanced (D, white arrowhead), not to be mistaken for neoplastic enhancement. (E) The high magnification angiographic projection demonstrated the radicular artery of left L5 (red arrowhead) to supply the fistula site (purple arrowhead). (F,G) Three-dimensional reconstructions of the angiogram with dual volume technique also helped to illustrate the course of the vessels involved. (H) The serpentine nature of the superficial venous ectasia can be seen in this low-magnification left L5 injection angiographic projection as well as in the contrast images.

pediatric AVFs and are rarely symptomatic [50]. Because the venous drainage pattern determines the natural history of DAVFs [38], angiographic analysis for therapeutic planning is focused on the venous drainage pattern.

Moderate- and high-flow DAVFs in adults may result in global neurological deficits such as abnormal mentation, particularly when associated with venous sinus thrombosis or severe stenosis [18,38,43]. Sinus venous hypertension can result

Table 6.6. Adaptation of the American College of Radiology appropriateness criteria for imaging of sudden onset of myelopathy

Imaging modality	Appropriate rating[a]	Comments	Radiation dose (mSv)[b]
MRI spine without contrast	9	Recommended initial imaging modality in non-traumatic myelopathy in a patient without infectious disease	0
MRI spine without and with contrast	8	Primary imaging modality recommended in a patient with infectious disease presenting with myelopathy	0
Myelography and postmyelography CT spine	6	For problem solving, or if MRI is unavailable or contraindicated	10–30
CT spine without contrast	5	Recommended initial imaging in traumatic myelopathy for evaluation of spine stability; otherwise of limited appropriateness	1–10
X-ray myelography	4		1–10
CT angiography spine	4	When vascular pathology is suspected.	1–10
Arteriography spine	4	Recommended whenever vascular pathology identified with MRI or CT; problem-solving tool to help in differentiating vascular and neoplastic spinal lesions when MRI is equivocal	Varies
MR angiography spine without and with contrast	4	When vascular pathology is suspected	0
X-ray spine	3	Useful as follow-up imaging study for stability or fracture progression	1–10
CT spine with contrast	3		1–10
CT spine without and with contrast	1		10–30
X-ray discography	1		1–10

[a] American College of Radiology rating scale: 1–3, usually not appropriate; 4–6, may be appropriate; 7–9, usually appropriate.
[b] Radiation dose is estimated adult effective dose.
Source: adapted from Seidenwurm *et al.*, 2012 [53].

in chronic impairment of absorption of cerebrospinal fluid, resulting in increased intracranial pressure, papilledema, and hydrocephalus [51]. Care must be taken not to prematurely diagnose dural sinus thrombosis until full angiographic analysis has been performed, as unopacified blood from a high-flow shunt can mimic sinus thrombosis.

Synchronous and metachronous DAVFs in separate anatomical locations in the same patient have a reported frequency of about 8%, necessitating full angiographic analysis of all major arteries even when one DAVF is identified in a patient. Use of DSA is also made after therapy to evaluate any residual shunting [52].

Imaging characteristics of spinal arteriovenous fistulae

Unlike intracranial AVMs and AVFs, which often present with a non-specific symptom of headache, AVFs of the spinal cord most often present with signs of myelopathy. Early recognition and treatment of spinal AVFs can result in improved patient outcomes and often reverse the presenting neurological deficit [17]. The best modality to depict the spinal cord and location of pathology is MRI and it is the recommended initial imaging modality in atraumatic myelopathy (Table 6.6) [53].

Spinal AVFs are characterized by abnormal connections between the arteries and veins that drain the cord parenchyma, which results in increased pressure within the capillaries of the spinal cord. Increased venous pressure within the coronal venous plexus, which has no valves, results in interstitial edema within the center of the spinal cord; if left untreated, hemorrhagic or bland infarction of the spinal cord will occur. Cord edema, intramedullary hemorrhage, and enlarged dilated veins are most accurately identified on MRI; however, DSA is required for complete understanding of the involved anatomy as well as to determine management [17,54,55].

Spinal dural AVF (SAVF) is the most common vascular lesion of the spine and accounts for 70% of all AVMs in the spine [54]. Saraf-Lavi *et al.* subdivided SAVFs into extradural and intradural types, with intradural lesions categorized as either dorsal or ventral [56]. The most common SAVF is the intradural dorsal type. In this type, a (most often single) radicular branch of the dorsospinal artery fistulizes with a single draining vein within the dura of a nerve root sleeve [56,57]. This results in arterialized pressures in the vein that are transmitted retrograde to the spinal cord, leading to increased capillary pressure and ultimately edema in the center of the spinal cord. Dorsal intradural SAVF most commonly occur in the lower thoracic or upper lumbar spine, and as such the most common myelopathic symptoms arise from venous congestion in the lower cord and conus medullaris. Symptoms range from gradual leg weakness to urinary and bowel incontinence [18]. These intradural SAVFs may rarely also occur at the level of the sacrum or the cervical spine, fed by branches of the iliac arteries and vertebral artery, respectively. Rarely, a fistula at the skull base, fed by branches of the external carotid artery, drains inferiorly to the venous plexus of the cervical spinal cord, resulting in cervical spine cord edema.

MRI features

Physiological effects of increased pressure in the venous vasculature such as cord edema, cord enlargement, and dilated veins along the pial surface can be demonstrated with MRI. However, MRI is often unable to identify the specific site of the SAVF and, consequently, is not the most accurate imaging modality for characterization. Nonetheless, MRI is the most appropriate initial imaging modality for evaluating patients in whom the diagnosis of SAVF is suspected, as venous congestion and dilated veins are easily detected on T_2-weighted images (Fig. 6.4).

Venous congestion results in vasogenic edema in the central area of the spinal cord, which appears on MRI as central T_2 hyperintensity that spares the peripheral spinal cord. The cranial and caudal margins of the edema are usually ill-defined and have been described as flame shaped. The cord is often expanded where edematous. Mild enhancement secondary to venous congestion may be seen, particularly in delayed imaging times, but unless infarction occurs, marked enhancement is typically absent (Fig. 6.4D) [55].

Hemorrhage may accompany cord edema if venous hypertension persists untreated. This condition of progressive spinal cord infarction, referred to as Foix–Alajouanine syndrome, results from increased venous pressure caused by blockage of outflow in the greatly distended venous convolutions and obstructed radicular arteries. On MRI, hemorrhage has varying degrees of T_1 hyperintensity and T_2 hypointensity. Use of T_2*-weighted imaging demonstrates low signal "blooming" depending on amount of hemorrhage.

Using the inherent T_2 hyperintensity of cerebrospinal fluid as contrast, MRI can often demonstrate the prominent serpentine flow voids of the arterialized coronal venous plexus of the spinal cord in SAVF. In a retrospective blinded review of patients with myelopathy, Toossi *et al.* [57] showed that MRI was sensitive in identifying SAVF as the primary diagnosis in up to 94%. The sensitivity of spinal cord T_2 hyperintensity for flow voids was 100% and the specificity was 97%.

The cranial and caudal extent of flow voids is variable and may extend along the entire length of the cord. Flow voids in the engorged and ectatic veins can also be observed on T_1-weighted imaging before and following contrast, as well as on myelography. An MR myelogram (injection of gadolinium-based contrast in the subarachnoid space and subsequently performing T_1-weighted imaging) will also demonstrate enlarged tubular structures as filling defects in the gadolinium-enhanced subarachnoid space.

Importantly, MRI is able to suggest alternative diagnoses in patients with myelopathy, such as neoplastic, demyelinating, or infectious etiologies. Marked expansion of the cord, dense or heterogeneous enhancement, enhancement with little edema, and peripheral cord signal abnormalities should raise concern for etiologies other than AVF for a patient's myelopathy.

The study of choice for the full characterization of SAVF remains DSA. Advances in MRA, particularly time-resolved contrast-enhanced MRA and ASL, allow for more reliable identification of the metameric level of an arteriovenous shunt but as yet does not reliably categorize the type of fistula [56,58].

CT features

Non-contrast CT has little use in the workup of spinal AVM or AVF. Rare findings that might be seen, however, include subarachnoid hemorrhage, seen as high density in the subarachnoid space on non-contrast CT, and remodeling of the cortical bone, which can be seen in long-standing vascular enlargement. Metameric types of spinal fistula (e.g., Cobb syndrome) can demonstrate large channels within the vertebral body or erosions of the caudal rib margins [59].

Contrast enhancement on CT or CTA may demonstrate enhancement of the abnormal veins draining a SAVF. While engorged veins can often be seen on CTA, lack of temporal resolution and more dynamic imaging limits the evaluation of a fistula site with CTA.

Use of CT myelography (injection of contrast in the subarachnoid space and then performing CT examination of the spine) can demonstrate the pial-based engorged and tortuous draining veins along the surface of the spinal cord, but it does not assess venous or fistula patency.

Digital subtraction angiography features

Spinal angiography using DSA is the study of choice for evaluating SAVF prior to therapy as this allows for the most accurate identification of the feeding artery, location of the fistula, and the drainage pathway, as well as providing opportunities for embolization [59–62].

Use of DSA most accurately identifies the spinal arteries contributing to SAVF. In cervical myelopathy, the entire spinal axis should be examined to establish the origin of the anterior spinal artery. Origin of the anterior spinal artery at the same level as the radicular supply to a dural AVF generally precludes endovascular treatment of the SAVF [18].

Full angiographic analysis of the entire spine as well as the intracranial and extracranial circulation is recommended, particularly when no shunt can be identified at the thoracic, lumbar, or sacral levels. Multiple DAVFs in the same patient at the same time have been reported but occur much less often with SAVF than with intracranial DAVFs [18,49].

The vasculature of the spinal column can be divided into the following five territories: upper cervical regions (C1–C4), mid-cervical region, (C5–C7), upper thoracic region (T1–T4), thoracic and upper lumbar region (T5–L3), and lower lumbar region (L3–L4). As a midline structure, the spine also has bilateral vascular supply. Therefore, each side should be systematically studied.

Evaluation of the upper cervical region (C1–C4) should include evaluation of bilateral vertebral arteries, occipital arteries, ascending pharyngeal arteries, thyrocervical trunks, and costocervical trunks. Evaluation of the midcervical region (C5–C7) should include bilateral vertebral arteries, thyrocervical trunks, costocervical trunks, supreme intercostal arteries, and the ascending pharyngeal arteries. Evaluation of the upper thoracic region (T1–T4) should include evaluation of the supreme intercostal arteries and thyrocervical trunks. Evaluation of the thoracic and upper lumbar regions (T5–L3) should include systematic evaluation of bilateral intercostal lumbar arteries of the involved level, intercostal arteries of two levels above and below a fistula or tumor site, and the lower lumbar and sacral region (L4–sacrum). Lower lumbar region (L3–L4) should include systematic bilateral evaluation of the iliolumbar arteries, lateral sacral arteries, and medial sacral artery [18].

Spinal arteriovenous malformations

A spinal AVM (SAVM) and a SAVF share shunt physiology but differ in that a nidus is present in SAVMs. Additionally, the intramedullary anastomoses of the arteries of the spinal cord make it possible for SAVM to be angiographically visualized via different sources (as opposed to a more common single radiculomedullary branch in SAVF). Because of the complexity of the axial and longitudinal, intrinsic and extrinsic, arterial anastomosis, angiographic diagnosis of intramedullary versus extramedullary location can be difficult to extrapolate on DSA and MRI is complementary in its ability to spatially localize SAVM in relation to the cord tissue and the meningeal spaces [17,18].

Also in contrast to SAVF, SAVM-induced myelopathy is most commonly associated with hemorrhage. Hemorrhage secondary to SAVM may be either subarachnoid or within the spinal cord proper (hematomyelia). Hematomyelia is seen frequently in cervical AVM and is often associated with onset of new, significant, and often devastating neurological deficits (Fig. 6.5) [18]. While an SAVM is a frequent source of hematomyelia, the differential diagnosis of hematomyelia also includes cavernous malformations, mycotic and other spinal artery aneurysms, neoplasms (e.g., ependymoma, astrocytoma, meningeal sarcoma, hemangioblastoma), polyarteritis nodosa, and coagulopathy [11,17,18,55].

Symptomatology associated with spinal hemorrhage typically starts as severe back pain (often between the scapulae and/or at the site of rupture) and then rapidly spreads to the rest of the back, neck, and into the legs. If hemorrhage is diffuse, or begins in the upper cervical spine, intracranial subarachnoid hemorrhage may cause severe headaches or altered consciousness [18].

MRI features

The MRI features of SAVMs are similar in most ways to the appearance of SAVFs (see above), but typically the SAVM includes dilated venous flow voids in the subarachnoid space corresponding to dilated perimedullary veins, which may be seen most readily on T_2 sequences, and cord edema (demonstrated by T_2 hyperintensity within the cord substance, sparing the periphery with mild expansion and minimal or no enhancement) (Fig. 6.5).

However, imaging findings on MRI may be much more extensive with SAVM than with SAVF. The vascular nidus can be seen as a “bag of worms” or flow void, similar to the intracranial AVM described above. The nidus may be within the cord substance (intramedullary), external to the cord (extramedullary), or even partially within the cord [58].

Findings for hematomyelia using MRI vary depending on the age of the hemorrhage and can range from T_2 hyperintensity to markedly T_2 hypointensity. Typically, there is associated T_1 shortening with the hemorrhage (Fig. 6.5A). Gradient-weighted or SWI sequences will demonstrate blooming. A SAVM should not have enhancement on post-gadolinium T_2 sequences.

Metameric and other congenital types of AVM may have multiple sites, including extraspinal components. Identifying these types of AVM may necessitate altering standard imaging protocols to widen fields of view if the pathology is not imaged completely.

Often, MRI is the only modality required to make the diagnosis of SAVM; however, full characterization of feeding arteries, draining vessels, and the nidus requires DSA; MRI provides complementary information to DSA in its enhanced ability to localize the vascular nidus relative to the cord parenchyma.

Use of MRA may be helpful in both diagnosis of SAVM and in suggesting the level of primary arterial supply; however, DSA continues to be required for full characterization of a SAVM and for complete evaluation of the feeding and draining vessels.

A retrospective 2007 study of 34 spinal fistula patients comparing MRA with DSA found MRI/MRA to be as accurate as DSA in diagnosing a spinal fistula. Use of MRA was also able to correctly identify the feeding spinal artery for SAVF in 14 of 19 patients with SAVFs, and MRA was within one vertebral level of the feeding artery in the remaining five. In 10 of 11 patients with SAVM, MRA was able to correctly identify the main feeding artery. The largest margin of error was found to occur when differentiating sacral SAVF from conus SAVM; only two of five were correctly differentiated [58].

CT features

Non-contrast CT has limited utility in the workup of SAVM or SAVF, possibly identifying hemorrhage or bony changes [59].

Contrast-enhanced CT may demonstrate enhancement of the abnormal veins draining an SAVM, the vascular nidus, and occasionally can help to identify the main feeder. Use of CT myelography can demonstrate the enlarged cord and pial-based engorged and tortuous draining veins. Distinguishing SAVF from SAVM is markedly limited on CT myelography, and it is not considered a primary imaging for the workup for SAVFs.

Digital subtraction angiography features

Because DSA allows the angiographer to selectively image each possible feeding artery separately, it is particularly useful in SAVMs. Superselection of individual feeding arteries allows for detangling the complex network of collateralization normally present in the arterial vasculature of the spine in order to delineate the angioarchitecture and to plan the treatment course for an SAVM (Fig. 6.5G,I) [17].

Use of DSA identifies the main feeding artery as well as smaller vessels that supply the vascular nidus. Feeding artery

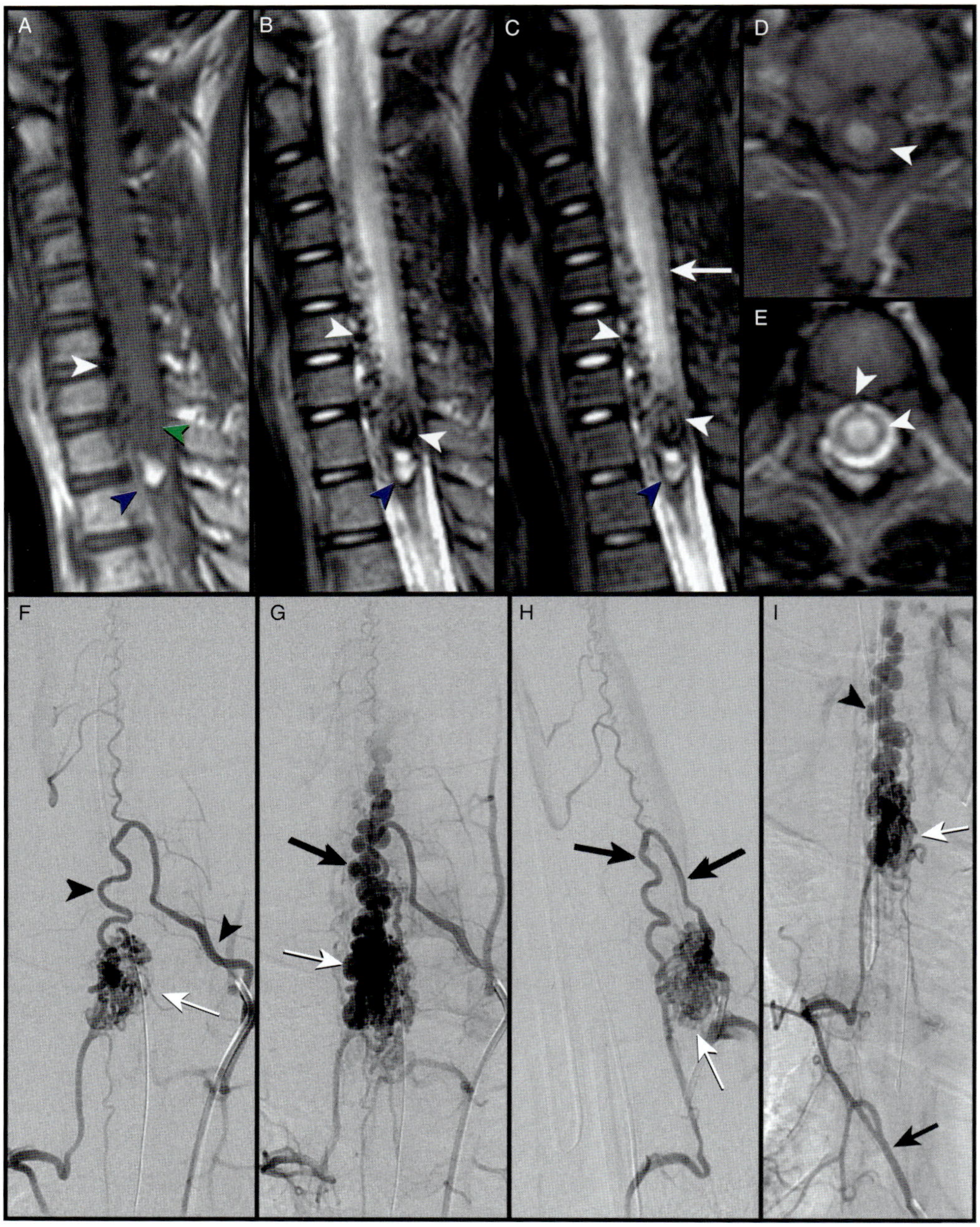

Fig. 6.5. Spine arteriovenous malformations (AVM) in a 9-year-old child who presented with bilateral upper and lower extremity weakness over the previous 2 months. (A–E) MRI demonstrated dilated veins on the pial surface as flow voids (white arrowheads) on T_1-weighted imaging (A), T_2-weighted imaging (B and E), and diffusion-weighted imaging (C). (F–I) Angiographic projections best showed the flow voids within the expanded cord, indicating the vascular nidus, which are also demonstrated in A–E (white arrows). The T_1-hyperintense, T_2-hyperintense lobule inferior to the nidus is consistent with hematomyelia (blue arrow). Expansion of the cord with central T_2 hyperintensity and mild T_1 hypointensity indicates edema (A, green arrowhead). The axial T_2-weighted image (E) particularly illustrates the central cord edema. Multiple feeding arteries were identified on the angiographic study, including from bilateral thyrocervical trunks. Venous ectasia extended both cephalad and caudal in this example.

aneurysms are much more rare in SAVM than with intracranial AVMs, likely secondary to differences in hemodynamic conditions between the spine and brain [18].

The preferred modality for definitive documentation and characterization of aneurysms associated with SAVMs is DSA. Demonstrating an intranidal or flow-related aneurysm on DSA increases the risk profile of the AVM. Documenting changing size or shape of an aneurysm or pseudoaneurysm (sometimes formed from a ruptured aneurysm) indicates an unstable hemodynamic situation requiring treatment. On occasion, rupture of an aneurysm may incite thrombosis of the aneurysm that is only identified on later DSA after recanalization. Flow-related aneurysms might resolve spontaneously after curing an SAVM [18].

Venous ectasias or varices should be differentiated from arterial aneurysms. The venous ectasias are seen at, or downstream from, the arteriovenous junction. The arteriovenous junction is identified by the abrupt caliber change between the smaller artery and the slightly larger dilated veins. The veins of SAVMs are typically smaller than those in brain AVMs, except in hereditary hemorrhagic telangiectasia. One of the proposed causes for relative lack of venous dilatation in SAVM is that the predominantly subarachnoid location of the veins limits the anatomical hindrance to venous outflow, thus limiting the intravenous pressure and decreasing the incidence of markedly dilated veins in SAVMs [18].

Dural supply to an SAVM is rare but can be seen more commonly in spinal dural adhesions either from surgical intervention or repeated hemorrhage. In such patients, the dural recruitment occurs at the level of the adhesions. Otherwise, the radicular arteries supplying the myelomere level will be the predominant feeder for the SAVM [18].

Extensive axial, transmedullary, arterioarterial, and venovenous anastomoses as well as complex intrinsic and extrinsic longitudinal anastomoses limits angiographic ability to fully delineate the extent of the vascular nidus [18]. Planar imaging with DSA often limits evaluation of the boundaries of the spinal cord, medulla, and the subarachnoid space. Use of three-dimensional spinal angiography does offer some additional benefit; however, full appreciation of nidus involvement in multiple compartments requires additional imaging with MRI (Fig. 6.5) [17]

Evaluation of patterns of venous outflow can indirectly provide clues as to the compartment involved, and SAVMs are most often single-compartment lesions. In all five spine territories (delineated above), a single anterior or posterior venous drainage corresponds to nidus involvement of the ventral or dorsal aspect of the cord, respectively. Since central cord venous drainage is via dorsal perforating veins, which drain into the posterior venous drainage system, isolated posterior venous drainage may also be seen with central location of the vascular nidus [18].

Conclusions

To summarize, a multimodality approach to imaging of intracranial and spinal AVMs and AVFs provides the highest level of information required for the classification and treatment planning of these complex structures. While CT is the initial study of choice for screening patients for intracranial hemorrhage and hydrocephalus with the ubiquitous symptom of headache, MRI best depicts the parenchymal real estate involved by these lesions. However, DSA remains the gold standard for diagnosis, therapeutic planning, and possibly treatment for vascular lesions of the brain and spine; non-invasive imaging is markedly improving with the additions of newer sequences such as time-of-flight MRA and ASL.

References

1. Arteriovenous Malformation Study Group. Arteriovenous malformations of the brain in adults. *N Engl J Med* 1999;**340**:1812–18.
2. Al-Shahi R, Bhattacharya JJ, Currie DG, *et al.* Prospective, population-based detection of intracranial vascular malformations in adults: the Scottish Intracranial Vascular Malformation Study SIVMS). *Stroke* 2003;**34**:1163–9.
3. da Costa L, Wallace MC, terBrugge KG, *et al.* The natural history and predictive features of hemorrhage from brain arteriovenous malformations. *Stroke* 2009;**40**:100–5.
4. Hartmann A, Mast H, Mohr JP, *et al.* Morbidity of intracranial hemorrhage in patients with cerebral arteriovenous malformation. *Stroke* 1998;**29**:931–4.
5. Hofmeister C, Stapf C, Hartmann A, *et al.* Demographic, morphological, and clinical characteristics of 1289 patients with brain arteriovenous malformation. *Stroke* 2000;**31**:1307–10.
6. Hoh BL Chapman PH, Loeffler JS, *et al.* Results of multimodality treatment for 141 patients with brain arteriovenous malformations and seizures: factors associated with seizure incidence and seizure outcomes. *Neurosurgery* 2002;**51**:303–9.
7. Ogilvy CS, Stieg PE, Awad I, *et al.* AHA Scientific Statement: recommendations for the management of intracranial arteriovenous malformations: a statement for healthcare professionals from a special writing group of the Stroke Council, American Stroke Association. *Stroke* 2001;**32**:1458–71.
8. Stapf C, Labovitz DL, Sciacca RR, *et al.* Incidence of adult brain arteriovenous malformation hemorrhage in a prospective population-based stroke survey. *Cerebrovasc Dis* 2002;**13**:43–6.
9. Stapf C, Mast H, Sciacca RR, *et al.* The New York Islands AVM Study: design, study progress, and initial results. *Stroke* 2003;**34**:e29–e33.
10. Stapf C, Mast H, Sciacca RR, *et al.* Predictors of hemorrhage in patients with untreated brain arteriovenous malformation. *Neurology* 2006;**66**:1350–5.
11. Yousem DM, Grossman RI. *Neuroradiology*. Philadelphia, PA: Mosby, 2010.
12. Rumboldt Z, Huda W, All JW. Review of portable CT with assessment of a dedicated head CT scanner. *AJNR Am J Neuroradiol* 2009;**30**:1630–6.
13. Strain JD, Strife JL, Kushner DC, *et al.* American College of Radiology appropriateness criteria: headache. *Radiology* 2000;**215**(Suppl 1):855–60.
14. Davenport MS, Khalatbari S, Dillman JR, *et al.* Contrast material-induced nephrotoxicity and intravenous low-osmolality iodinated contrast material. *Radiology* 2013;**267**:94–105.
15. Lauterbur PC. Image formation by induced local interactions. Examples employing nuclear magnetic resonance. *Nature* 1973;**242**:190–1.
16. Zou Z, Zhang HL, Roditi GH, *et al.* Nephrogenic systemic fibrosis: review of 370 biopsy-confirmed cases. *JACC Cardiovasc Imaging* 2011;**4**:1206–16.
17. Caragine LP, Jr., Halbach VV, Ng PP, *et al.* Vascular myelopathies-vascular malformations of the spinal cord: presentation and endovascular surgical management. *Semin Neurol* 2002;**22**:123–32.
18. Lasjaunias PL, Berenstein A, terBrugge KG. *Surgical Neuroangiography*. New York: Springer, 2001.
19. Morris P. *Practical Neuroangiography*, 2nd edn. Philadelphia, PA: Lippincott, Williams, & Wilkins, 2006.
20. Hadizadeh DR, von FM, Gieseke J, *et al.* Cerebral arteriovenous malformation: Spetzler–Martin classification at subsecond-temporal-resolution

four-dimensional MR angiography compared with that at DSA. *Radiology* 2008;**246**:205–13.

21. Kidwell CS, Chalela JA, Saver JL, *et al.* Comparison of MRI and CT for detection of acute intracerebral hemorrhage. *JAMA* 2004;**292**:1823–30.
22. NINDS t-PA Stroke Study Group. Intracerebral hemorrhage after intravenous t-PA therapy for ischemic stroke. *Stroke* 1997;**28**:2109–18.
23. Kokkinis C, Vlychou M, Zavras GM, *et al.* The role of 3D-computed tomography angiography (3D-CTA) in investigation of spontaneous subarachnoid haemorrhage: comparison with digital subtraction angiography (DSA) and surgical findings. *Br J Neurosurg* 2008;**22**:71–8.
24. Kano H, Kondziolka D, Flickinger JC, *et al.* Stereotactic radiosurgery for arteriovenous malformations. Part 3: outcome predictors and risks after repeat radiosurgery. *J Neurosurg* 2012;**116**:21–32.
25. Kano H, Kondziolka D, Flickinger JC, *et al.* Stereotactic radiosurgery for arteriovenous malformations. Part 4: management of basal ganglia and thalamus arteriovenous malformations. *J Neurosurg* 2012;**116**:33–43.
26. Kano H, Lunsford LD, Flickinger JC, *et al.* Stereotactic radiosurgery for arteriovenous malformations. Part 1: management of Spetzler–Martin grade I and II arteriovenous malformations. *J Neurosurg* 2012;**116**:11–20.
27. Mikami T, Hirano T, Sugino T, *et al.* Presurgical planning for arteriovenous malformations using multidetector row CT. *Neurosurg Rev* 2012;**35**:393–9.
28. Yousem DM, Flamm ES, Grossman RI. Comparison of MR imaging with clinical history in the identification of hemorrhage in patients with cerebral arteriovenous malformations. *AJNR Am J Neuroradiol* 1989;**10**:1151–4.
29. Hasan DM, Amans M, Tihan T, *et al.* Ferumoxytol-enhanced MRI to image inflammation within human brain arteriovenous malformations: a pilot investigation. *Transl Stroke Res* 2012;**3**:166–73.
30. Le TT, Fischbein NJ, Andre JB, *et al.* Identification of venous signal on arterial spin labeling improves diagnosis of dural arteriovenous fistulas and small arteriovenous malformations. *AJNR Am J Neuroradiol* 2012;**33**:61–8.
31. Wolf RL, Wang J, Detre JA, *et al.* Arteriovenous shunt visualization in arteriovenous malformations with arterial spin-labeling MR imaging. *AJNR Am J Neuroradiol* 2008;**29**:681–7.
32. Amponsah K, Ellis TL, Chan MD, *et al.* Retrospective analysis of imaging techniques for treatment planning and monitoring of obliteration for gamma knife treatment of cerebral arteriovenous malformation. *Neurosurgery* 2012;**71**:893–9.
33. Suazo L, Foerster B, Fermin R, *et al.* Measurement of blood flow in arteriovenous malformations before and after embolization using arterial spin labeling. *Interv Neuroradiol* 2012;**18**:42–8.
34. Spetzler RF, Martin NA. A proposed grading system for arteriovenous malformations. *J Neurosurg* 1986;**65**:476–83.
35. Morris P. *Practical Neuroangiography.* Baltimore, MD: Williams & Wilkins, 1997.
36. Newton TH, Cronqvist S. Involvement of dural arteries in intracranial arteriovenous malformations. *Radiology* 1969;**93**:1071–8.
37. Hoh BL, Carter BS, Ogilvy CS. Incidence of residual intracranial AVMs after surgical resection and efficacy of immediate surgical re-exploration. *Acta Neurochir (Wien)* 2004;**146**:1–7.
38. Lasjaunias P, Chiu M, ter Brugge K, *et al.* Neurological manifestations of intracranial dural arteriovenous malformations. *J Neurosurg* 1986;**64**:724–30.
39. Cognard C, Gobin YP, Pierot L, *et al.* Cerebral dural arteriovenous fistulas: clinical and angiographic correlation with a revised classification of venous drainage. *Radiology* 1995;**194**:671–80.
40. Borden JA, Wu JK, Shucart WA. A proposed classification for spinal and cranial dural arteriovenous fistulous malformations and implications for treatment. *J Neurosurg* 1995;**82**:166–79.
41. Davies MA, terBrugge K, Willinsky R, *et al.* The validity of classification for the clinical presentation of intracranial dural arteriovenous fistulas. *J Neurosurg* 1996;**85**:830–7.
42. Lasjaunias P. Editorial comment on Davies' papers. Angioarchitecture and natural history of dural arteriovenous shunts. *Interv Neuroradiol* 1997;**3**:313–17.
43. Morris JM. Imaging of dural arteriovenous fistula. *Radiol Clin North Am* 2012;**50**:823–39.
44. Singh V, Smith WS, Lawton MT, *et al.* Risk factors for hemorrhagic presentation in patients with dural arteriovenous fistulae. *Neurosurgery* 2008;**62**:628–35.
45. Akiba H, Tamakawa M, Hyodoh H, *et al.* Assessment of dural arteriovenous fistulas of the cavernous sinuses on 3D dynamic MR angiography. *AJNR Am J Neuroradiol* 2008;**29**:1652–7.
46. Versari PP, D'Aliberti G, Talamonti G, *et al.* Progressive myelopathy caused by intracranial dural arteriovenous fistula: report of two cases and review of the literature. *Neurosurgery* 1993;**33**:914–18.
47. Brunereau L, Gobin YP, Meder JF, *et al.* Intracranial dural arteriovenous fistulas with spinal venous drainage: relation between clinical presentation and angiographic findings. *AJNR Am J Neuroradiol* 1996;**17**:1549–54.
48. Weissman JL, Hirsch BE. Imaging of tinnitus: a review. *Radiology* 2000;**216**:342–9.
49. Barnwell SL, Halbach VV, Dowd CF, *et al.* Multiple dural arteriovenous fistulas of the cranium and spine. *AJNR Am J Neuroradiol* 1991;**12**:441–5.
50. Lasjaunias PL, Berenstein A, Raybaud C. *Surgical Neuroangiography.* New York: Springer, 1987.
51. Lamas E, Lobato RD, Esperarza J, *et al.* Dural posterior fossa AVM producing raised sagittal simus pressure. Case report. *J Neurosurg* 1977;**46**:804–10.
52. van Dijk JM, terBrugge KG, Willinsky RA, *et al.* Clinical course of cranial dural arteriovenous fistulas with long-term persistent cortical venous reflux. *Stroke* 2002;**33**:1233–6.
53. Seidenwurm DJ, Wippold FJ, Cornelius RS, *et al.* American College of Radiology appropriateness criteria: myelopathy. *J Am Coll Radiol* 2012;**9**:315–24.
54. Krings T, Thron AK, Geibprasert S, *et al.* Endovascular management of

spinal vascular malformations. *Neurosurg Rev* 2010;**33**:1–9.

55. Rodesch G, Lasjaunias P. Spinal cord arteriovenous shunts: from imaging to management. *Eur J Radiol* 2003;**46**:221–32.
56. Saraf-Lavi E, Bowen BC, Quencer RM, *et al.* Detection of spinal dural arteriovenous fistulae with MR imaging and contrast-enhanced MR angiography: sensitivity, specificity, and prediction of vertebral level. *AJNR Am J Neuroradiol* 2002;**23**:858–67.
57. Toossi S, Josephson SA, Hetts SW, *et al.* Utility of MRI in spinal arteriovenous fistula. *Neurology* 2012;**79**:25–30.
58. Mull M, Nijenhuis RJ, Backes WH, *et al.* Value and limitations of contrast-enhanced MR angiography in spinal arteriovenous malformations and dural arteriovenous fistulas. *AJNR Am J Neuroradiol* 2007;**28**:1249–58.
59. Cullen S, Krings T, Ozanne A, *et al.* Diagnosis and endovascular treatment of pediatric spinal arteriovenous shunts. *Neuroimaging Clin N Am* 2007;**17**:207–21.
60. Kim LJ, Spetzler RF. Classification and surgical management of spinal arteriovenous lesions: arteriovenous fistulae and arteriovenous malformations. *Neurosurgery* 2006;**59**(Suppl):S195–201.
61. Spetzler RF, Detwiler PW, Riina HA, *et al.* Modified classification of spinal cord vascular lesions. *J Neurosurg* 2002;**96**:145–56.
62. Hetts SW, Moftakhar P, English JD, *et al.* Spinal dural arteriovenous fistulas and intrathecal venous drainage: correlation between digital subtraction angiography, magnetic resonance imaging, and clinical findings. *J Neurosurg Spine* 2012;**16**:433–40.

Chapter 7

Intraoperative evaluation of blood flow with indocyanine green videoangiography

Francesco Acerbi, Morgan Broggi, Marco Schiariti, Giovanni Broggi, and Paolo Ferroli

Introduction

Fluorescence angiography was first applied during neurosurgical procedures in the late 1960s by Feindel *et al.*[1], who used fluorescein to examine the anatomical aspects of the epicerebral circulation in five patients undergoing craniotomy and outlined the specific advantages during surgery for angiomas and aneurysms. Interestingly, they recognized the possibility for fluorescence angiography to identify the feeding arteries to an arteriovenous malformations (AVM), allowing for a planned resection [1].

Indocyanine green (ICG) fluorescence angiography was initially developed in ophthalmology to evaluate retinal microcirculation in a variety of disorders. Indocyanine green is a near-infrared fluorophore with absorption and emission peaks of 805 and 835 nm, respectively; it provides high-quality vascular images by using a special optical setup for near-infrared light [2]. After intravenous injection, ICG is bound to globulins within 2 seconds and remains intravascular when vessel permeability is normal [2]. It is not metabolized by the body and is excreted by the liver. There is no reabsorption by the intestine and no enterohepatic recirculation. It has a plasma half-life of 3–4 minutes [2].

Fluorescence angiography with ICG was first applied in neurosurgery in 2001 by Kuroiwa *et al.* [3], who evaluated venous sinuses and the course of superficial veins before dural opening by adding a filter adapted for the wavelength of ICG to a Zeiss surgical microscope [3]. Two years later, Raabe *et al.* reported the first standard use of ICG videoangiography during vascular procedures, mainly aneurysm clipping [2]. They suggested that the use of ICG videoangiography could influence surgical strategy, because they were able to evaluate the perfusion of the residual aneurysm and the patency of parent, branching, and small vessels (which were not visible with intraoperative digital subtraction angiography [DSA]) after clipping. However, they also recognized that the angiographic view was restricted to the angle of the surgical approach and that vessels covered by blood clots, aneurysm, or brain tissue could not be visualized.

Raabe *et al.* further developed ICG videoangiography in neurosurgery by integrating the technology into a Zeiss surgical microscope for treatment of 20 patients with intracranial aneurysms [4]. A prospective two-center trial at the Johann Wolfgang Goethe University, Germany, and the Barrow Neurological Institute, USA, included 114 patients with 124 aneurysms and compared surgical microscope-based ICG videoangiography with intraoperative or postoperative DSA. In 90% of patients, ICG videoangiography corresponded with intraoperative DSA, and provided relevant information for the surgical strategy in 9% [5]. On the basis of this prospective study, ICG videoangiography during aneurysm surgery has become standard practice in many neurosurgical centers. In addition, its application now includes other vascular neurosurgical procedures such as AVM removal [6–13], arteriovenous fistula occlusion [14–16], extracranial–intracranial bypass surgery [17] and, more recently, tumor removal [18]. It is also a useful adjunct to study venous flow dynamic intraoperatively in pathological veins [18,19] and normal veins [20]; this application is suggested for the evaluation of venous sacrifice during surgical approaches for different pathologies [20,21].

One limitation of ICG videoangiography is that it cannot demonstrate a quantitative, time-dependent, and spatially precise analysis of intravascular blood flow. However, new software integrated in the Zeiss Pentero microscope (FLOW 800 software; Carl Zeiss Meditec, Oberkochen, Germany) allows for a direct, semiquantitative analysis of intravascular blood flow. Several authors have reported the use of FLOW 800 to assess the dynamics of blood flow during neurosurgery [10–13,20]. In addition, Kamp *et al.* have suggested that the parameters derived by quantitative ICG videoangiography with FLOW 800 may improve intraoperative evaluation of the pathophysiology of cerebral perfusion and ischemia in patients with vascular pathology [22].

Indocyanine green videoangiography in surgery for arteriovenous malformations

In 2007, Takagi *et al.* reported the use of ICG videoangiography in a child with a diffuse Spetzler–Martin grade III AVM; ICG videoangiography identified a residual nidus, left from a

Comprehensive Management of Arteriovenous Malformations of the Brain and Spine, ed. Robert F. Spetzler, Douglas S. Kondziolka, Randall T. Higashida, and M. Yashar S. Kalani. Published by Cambridge University Press.

previous operation, which was not revealed with standard DSA [6].

The first prospective evaluation of ICG videoangiography during AVM surgery was performed in 10 patients by Spetzler and coworkers in 2009 [7] In this study, surgeons found ICG videoangiography useful in 9 out of 10 patients; ICG videoangiography clearly revealed arteriovenous shunting and helped the surgeon to discern the AVM arteries, draining veins, and cortical en passage veins, distinctions not obvious with conventional intraoperative microscopic magnification. In one patient, ICG videoangiography was used to identify a small ruptured AVM hidden within a hematoma cavity. However, ICG videoangiography was less helpful in identifying persistent early venous drainage and residual AVM. Furthermore, in one patient with an AVM located in the third ventricle, the quality of the ICG videoangiography was poor because of the deep and narrow surgical corridor and it was not helpful for AVM resection.

Hänggi *et al.* studied 15 patients with AVMs using intraoperative ICG videoangiography before, during, and at the end of resection [8]. Pre-resection ICG videoangiography, performed on 12 of the 15 patients produced excellent images with clear spatial resolution for analysis of the arterial, early venous, capillary, and venous phases. This analysis provided the location of the nidus and differentiated between terminal and en passage feeders in superficial AVMs. Pre-resection ICG videoangiography was not used in three patients because the deep location of the AVM was considered a contraindication. Use of ICG videoangiography during resection provided information regarding the location of en passage feeders, the integrity of adjacent arteries, and the location of AVM compartments in 12 patients (77%). In two patients, this information modified the surgical strategy. In addition, in both of these patients the planned ICG videoangiography performed after the resection (which was assumed to be complete) demonstrated residual shunting into the major draining vein. The postoperative DSA corresponded to the terminal ICG videoangiography control in all but one patient. In that patient, a small residual nidus close to the brainstem, which was missed by ICG videoangiography, was found with DSA. Additionally, in one patient with a deep thalamic AVM, the final ICG videoangiography evaluation was inconclusive, probably because of the depth of the surgical field and insufficient illumination.

Our group reported in 2010 intraoperative diagnosis of a micro-AVM of the trigeminal root aided by ICG videoangiography [9]. In 2012, Takagi *et al.* published the first study that compared ICG videoangiography and intraoperative DSA during AVM surgery [13]. In their series of 11 patients, ICG videoangiography was performed in 9 before resection, in 7 after clipping of the main feeders, and in all 11 at the end of the resection. In each patient, DSA was performed before resection, after clipping of the main feeders, and after total resection to check for alterations of flow. The authors found a significant difference in terms of duration of the two techniques (4.7 ± 1.4 minutes for ICG videoangiography compared with 16.6 ± 3.8 minutes for intraoperative DSA). With pre-resection ICG videoangiography, surgeons identified the feeders in only three patients (33%), the nidus in all nine (100%), and the draining veins in eight (89%). With intraoperative DSA, surgeons visualized the feeders, nidus, and draining veins in all patients. After clipping of feeders, both ICG videoangiography and intraoperative DSA showed a flow reduction of the nidus in all patients. After total resection of the nidus, ICG videoangiography and intraoperative DSA confirmed the absence of early venous drainage in all patients. The authors concluded that ICG videoangiography is useful for visualizing the nidus and superficial draining veins during AVM surgery; however, they questioned its efficacy for identifying the main feeders of the nidus before resection [13].

The FLOW 800 software is the latest manifestation of the ICG videoangiography technique. The software improves differentiation of feeding arteries, normal cortical arteries, and draining veins by producing a visual map of the dynamics of vascular blood flow in the operative field. This map uses a gradient color scale to instantly identify the direction and sequence of blood flow; for example, arteries are shown as red, arterialized veins as orange or yellow, and normal veins as violet. In patients where multiple doses of ICG are administered, residual dye may cause false-positive findings. In these patients, an intensity diagram, which displays flow variation over time, may help to differentiate feeders from normal vessels.

Jhawar *et al.* described the use of FLOW 800 in a patient with a large complex right parietal AVM [12] and noted its utility in identifying feeders to the malformations. The same group reported the use of FLOW 800 in three other patients with AVMs [10], further supporting the use of this technique in identifying components of the vascular malformations. Faber *et al.* [11] used the technique in two patients with AVMs. They confirmed that FLOW 800 enables intraoperative, real-time analysis of arterial and venous vessel architecture and concluded that it may increase the efficacy and safety of neurovascular surgery in a select subset of patients with superficial AVMs. Finally, in a larger study, Kamp *et al.* assessed the usefulness of FLOW 800 in 30 patients with cerebrovascular problems [22], including two with AVMs in which quantitative ICG videoangiography helped to identify feeders and draining veins by their flow latencies. This technique allowed the normalization of flow to be identified after removal of the shunt. In addition, in one patient, a region of interest in the parenchyma adjacent to the AVM indicated a possible impaired perfusion that seemed to return to normal after AVM removal.

The primary limitation of ICG videoangiography is that it captures only what is visible within the field of the microscope and, as a consequence, it requires that vessels be clear of any obstructing tissue or blood clots (e.g., such as may be present after AVM rupture) [7,8]. In addition, calcifications within the vessels can impede a correct evaluation of the flow. This meticulous and sometimes difficult dissection of AVM-related vessels, which is a precondition to the use of ICG videoangiography, can be a time-consuming surgical process. Moreover, experience has demonstrated that ICG videoangiography is of limited use for deep-seated AVMs that must be approached through a long, narrow corridor. In these patients, the signal and illumination can be low and the limited depth of field can make interpretation of ICG videoangiography data difficult [7,8].

Furthermore, the classic ICG videoangiography method was qualitative and based on the subjective impression of the operating neurosurgeon [8]. Only with the FLOW 800 software has ICG videoangiography become a quantitative method for evaluating vascular and regional cerebral cortical blood flow during surgery [22]. However, at this time, most measures that can be obtained with ICG videoangiography are derived from postprocessing analysis and depend on various local and systemic parameters; they are, therefore, still difficult to interpret in real-time during neurosurgical procedures.

Institutional experience

Patients

We have used ICG videoangiography routinely in patients with cerebrovascular problems and selectively in patients with neuro-oncological pathology since 2006 [9,18,20,23]. This chapter retrospectively analyzes the last 25 consecutive patients (17 women and 8 men; mean age, 39.6 years; age range, 7–67 years) with cerebral AVMs where ICG videoangiography was used during surgery between January 2010 and October 2012. The AVMs were classified by the Spetzler–Martin scale [24]: 9 were grade I, 5 were grade II, 6 were grade III, 2 were grade IV, and 1 was grade V. One patient presented with a direct arteriovenous fistula without a clear nidus (patient 16), and one patient presented with radionecrosis after radiosurgery on a grade II AVM in the rolandic area (patient 8). Presenting symptoms included headache in 12 patients, seizure in 6, and focal neurological deficit caused by hemorrhage or ischemic vascular steal in 3. The AVMs were partially embolized before surgery in eight patients (32%) (Table 7.1).

Methods

All operations were performed using the OPMI Pentero surgical microscope with integrated ICG technology (Carl Zeiss) as described in previous reports [9,18–20]. The recommended dose for intravenous ICG injection is 0.2–0.5 mg/kg with a maximum daily dose of 5 mg/kg. Because ICG administration may be repeated several times during surgery, our institution uses a standard dose of 12.5 mg in 2.5 mL saline for each injection. Vessel fluorescence showing real-time arterial, capillary, and venous filling is apparent within seconds of administration and clears within 10 minutes, at which time additional injections are possible. The resultant video can be played and replayed in real-time or slow motion and paused with controllers on the handle of the microscope.

In 2010, FLOW 800 software integrated in the Zeiss Pentero microscope was used for patients with vascular pathology and selected patients with tumors. This software measures fluorescence intensities in arbitrary intensity units corresponding to the intensity detected by the camera. In addition, it automatically calculates maps of maximal fluorescence intensities and delay times (the interval between 0 and 50% of maximum fluorescence intensity). These maps are shown on the screen as grayscale for maximal fluorescence intensities and as colorscale for delay times according to time to half-maximal fluorescence (Figs. 7.1–7.3). In addition, the course of fluorescence can be further analyzed in any area of the exposed brain by using freely definable regions of interest (Figs. 7.1–7.3).

During the procedure, ICG videoangiography is usually performed at two stages: before and after resection of the AVM. Before the AVM resection, a primary superficial survey is performed to obtain information about the site of the nidus, superficial angioarchitecture, and flow dynamics of AVM-related vessels. After the resection, a terminal assessment is performed to identify residual AVM nidus or residual arteriovenous shunt and to check the patency of adjacent arteries and veins. In selected patients, a progress analysis is performed during the resection with one or more clips on main feeders to evaluate hemodynamic changes.

For the 25 patients discussed here, the surgical reports, videos, and images were reviewed to obtain data about intraoperative ICG videoangiography including duration, type of study, and utility. The utility of ICG videoangiography was defined as useful or not useful based on the subjective judgment of the operating surgeons and the cerebrovascular team. In addition, a more detailed judgment was made regarding what information ICG videoangiography had provided. All but six patients underwent early postoperative DSA examination (i.e., within the first three postoperative days).

Results

Overall 53 ICG videoangiographies were performed (including 32 FLOW 800 assessments) during 25 procedures. Each ICG videoangiography and its evaluation by the surgeon took 5 minutes or less (usually 3 minutes for injection and registration and 2 minutes for interpretation of data). Use of ICG videoangiography with FLOW 800 analysis required additional time: data collection by the microscope required 1 to 2 minutes; interpretation of the visual maps (maximal fluorescence intensities and delay times) and analysis of the course of fluorescence by positioning regions of interest required 2 to 10 minutes. This process was completed by at least the two surgeons who performed the procedure and usually a third member of the cerebrovascular team, all of whom were experienced in the use of ICG videoangiography. In total, classic ICG videoangiography added 8.5 ± 1.05 minutes to the procedure, and ICG videoangiography with FLOW 800 analysis added 16.7 ± 2.15 minutes (Table 7.1).

Of the 25 patients, a primary superficial survey was performed on 21 patients (Table 7.1) In three of the other four patients (patients 5, 14, and 17), it was not performed because of the deep location of the AVM and in the other patient (patient 20) there was a superficial AVM with relative clarity of its architecture under microscopic view. For the 21 patients where it was performed, it was considered useful in 17 (81%). In 16 patients, ICG videoangiography helped to identify the nidus and en passage feeders and to distinguish between AVM arteries and veins (Fig. 7.4B). In one patient (patient 8), the primary survey confirmed the absence of residual arteriovenous shunt in the context of radionecrosis after AVM radiosurgery. In addition, in one patient (patient 16), ICG videoangiography

Table 7.1. Summary of patient characteristics, indocyanine green use, and outcome

Patient	Age (years)/sex	Date of surgery	Arteriovenous malformations location	Spetzler–Martin grade	Preoperative embolization, no.	No. standard ICG	FLOW 800	Time for ICG and interpretation min (s)	Use of ICG helpful?	Postoperative digital subtraction angiography, result	Glasgow Outcome Scale
1	32/F	19/01/2010	L deep temporal	III	No	2 (pre, post)	No	9 (30)	Yes, final check only	Yes, neg	5
2	29/F	21/01/2010	L frontobasal	III	No	2 (pre, post)	No	11	Yes, AV dist. + final check	No, CTA neg	5
3	39/F	26/02/2010	L superficial occipital	I	Yes, 1	2 (pre, post)	No	9 (45)	Yes, AV dist. + final check	Yes, neg	5
4	44/F	11/05/2010	R superficial temporal	I	No	2 (pre, post)	No	10	Yes, AV dist. + final check	Yes, neg	5
5	54/M	29/06/2010	R mesial occipital	III	Yes, 1	1 (post)	No	4 (45)	Yes, final check only	Yes, neg	5
6	60/M	23/07/2010	L frontobasal	I	No	2 (pre, post)	No	10 (15)	Yes, final check only	No, CTA neg	5
7	46/F	01/11/2010	L frontal	IV	Yes, 3	2 (pre, post)	No	12 (40)	Yes, final check only (difficulty in interpretation of pre-resection scan due to dimension of AVM)	Yes, neg	3
8[a]	46/M	15/12/2010	R frontal	/	/	1 (pre)	No	2 (15)	Yes, confirmed the absence of AV shunt	–	3
9	57/F	24/02/2011	R superficial temporal	I	No	2 (pre, post)	No	9	Yes, AV dist. + final check	No, CTA neg	5
10	33/F	09/06/2011	R occipital	IV	Yes, 1	3 (1 pre, 2 post)	Yes	21	Yes, AV dist. + final check	Yes, neg	5
11	62/M	28/07/2011	L superficial frontal	II	No	1 (post)	No	2 (40)	Yes, final check only	Yes, neg	5
12	43/F	25/08/2011	L cerebellar	V	Yes, 1	2 (pre, post)	No	12 (15)	No	Yes, neg	2
13	14/F	19/09/2011	L superficial parieto-occipital	II	No	2 (pre, post)	No	10	Yes, AV dist. + final check	Yes, neg	5
14	7/F	05/10/2011	L mesial occipital	II	No	1 (post)	Yes	2 (30)	Yes, final check	Yes, neg	5
15	35/F	25/01/2012	R superficial temporal	I	Yes, 3	3 (1 pre, 2 post)	Yes	17 (20)	Yes, AV dist. + final check	Yes, neg	5

Table 7.1. (cont.)

Patient	Age (years)/sex	Date of surgery	Arteriovenous malformations location	Spetzler–Martin grade	Preoperative embolization, no.	No. standard ICG	FLOW 800	Time for ICG and interpretation min (s)	Use of ICG helpful?	Postoperative digital subtraction angiography, result	Glasgow Outcome Scale
16[b]	48/F	29/03/2012	R occipital	/	/	2 (pre, post)	Yes	13 (30)	Identification of the AV shunt in the context of hema-toma, final check	Yes, neg	5
17	67/M	12/04/2012	Midline cerebellar	II	No	1 (post)	Yes	5 (15)	Yes, final check	No, CTA neg	5
18	33/F	20/04/2012	R superficial temporal	I	No	3 (pre, prog, post)	Yes	24 (45)	Yes, AV dist., hemo-dynamic effect of clipping of the main feeders, final check	Yes, neg	5
19	40/F	10/05/2012	L superficial parieto-occipital	III	Yes, 1	3 (pre, prog, post)	Yes	20 (30)	Yes, AV dist., hemo-dynamic effect of clipping of the main feeders, final check	Yes, neg	5
20	37/F	15/05/2012	R superficial frontal	I	No	1 (post)	Yes	5	Yes, final check	Yes, neg	5
21[c]	42/F	13/06/2012	R mesial frontal	I	No	3 (1 pre, 2 post)	Yes	18 (30)	Yes, AV dist. + final check	Yes, neg	5
22	17/M	04/07/2012	R superficial occipital	III	No	3 (pre, prog, post)	Yes	23 (30)	Yes, AV dist., hemo-dynamic effect of clipping of the main feeders, final check	No, CTA neg	5
23	29/M	12/07/2012	R superficial frontal	II	No	3 (pre, prog, post)	Yes	22(20)	Yes, AV dist., hemo-dynamic effect of clipping of the main feeders, final check	Yes, neg	5
24	32/F	01/10/2012	L superficial occipital	III	No	3 (pre, prog, post)	Yes	21 (30)	Yes, AV dist., hemo-dynamic effect of clipping of the main feeders, final check	Yes, neg	5
25	43/M	24/10/2012	R superficial temporal	I	Yes, 3	3 (pre, prog, post)	Yes	23 (15)	Yes, AV dist., hemo-dynamic effect of clipping of the main feeders, final check	No, CTA neg	5

L, left; R, right; AV, arteriovenous; AVM, arteriovenous malformations; S-M, Spetzler–Martin (grade); AV dist., ability to distinguish AVM arteries and veins; ICG, indocyanine green; neg, negative for residual AVM; pre, pre-resection; prog, progress analysis; post, post-resection; postop, postoperative; CTA, CT angiography.

[a] Patient 8 was previously submitted to radiosurgery for a right frontal AVM in rolandic area; indication for surgery was to evaluate the significance of edema, likely attributable to radionecrosis; intraoperative ICG confirmed the absence of arteriovenous shunt in the area of radionecrosis that was removed en bloc.

[b] Patient 16 presented with a hematoma in the occipital region caused by a direct arteriovenous fistula without a clear nidus on preoperative digital subtraction angiography.

[c] Patient 21 is the only patient who had already undergone surgery for her AVM; she underwent partial resection in 1984.

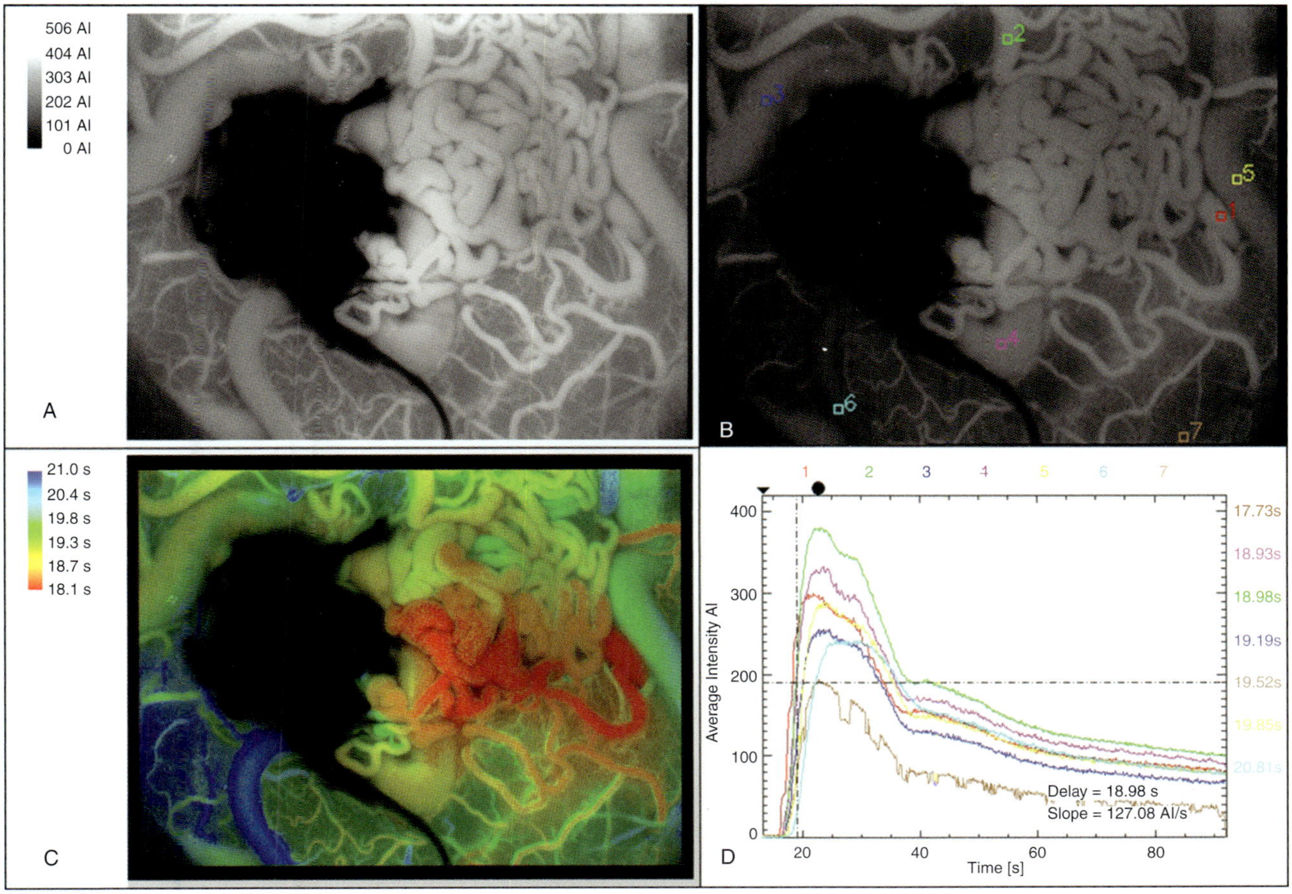

Fig. 7.1. Indocyanine green videoangiography with FLOW 800 software (primary superficial survey) for Case 2 (patient 19). (A) Map of maximal fluorescence intensity. (B) Multiple regions of interest: two each in two feeders, one from the middle cerebral artery (red) and one from the posterior cerebral artery (green); three each in three main draining veins (blue, pink, and yellow); one in a vein apparently not involved in the arteriovenous malformations (AVM) flow (pale blue); and one in the peri-AVM brain parenchyma (brown). (C) Map of delay times, with a gradient color scale according to time to half-maximal fluorescence, was better able to delineate differences between superficial feeders (red and yellow) and arterialized drainage veins (green). (D) Evaluation of the time course of fluorescence and the time to half-maximal fluorescence in each region of interest as positioned in (B). This helped to distinguish the superficial feeders flow (one faster with 17.73 seconds and the other slower with 18.98 seconds) from the main drainage veins (18.93, 19.19 and 19.85 seconds) and from normal veins (20.91 seconds).

helped to identify the arteriovenous shunt in the context of previous hematoma. The primary superficial survey was not considered useful in four patients. In two patients, the deep location of the AVM (patient 1) or the long surgical corridor (patient 6) made it difficult to retrieve any useful information at the beginning of the surgery. In two patients, the complexity of the AVM (patient 7 with a grade IV and patient 12 with a grade V) made it difficult to obtain useful information for surgical strategies; both of these patients had classic ICG without FLOW 800 analysis. Overall, ICG FLOW 800 was used in 10 of the 21 patients. In all patients, the new software allowed a simpler understanding of the angioarchitecture, particularly regarding the ability to differentiate between AVM arteries and veins using colored maps of time to half-maximal fluorescence (Fig. 7.1C). In addition, in one patient, (patient 16), ICG videoangiography helped to identify the arteriovenous shunt in the context of a previous hematoma.

A progress analysis was performed in six patients aided by FLOW 800 software; ICG videoangiography allowed for real-time evaluation of the hemodynamic effects of clipping the main feeders of the AVM (Fig. 7.2).

A terminal assessment was completed in 24 patients. In 21 patients, ICG videoangiography confirmed the absence of an arteriovenous shunt and normalization of arterial and venous flow in the exposed area (Figs. 7.3 and 7.4D). The terminal assessment showed a small portion of unexpected residual nidus in one patient (patient 10) and unexpected residual arteriovenous shunt in two patients (patients 15 and 21). In these three patients, surgery was continued, and a second terminal assessment confirmed the absence of an arteriovenous shunt. Analysis with DSA angiography or CT angiography confirmed total AVM removal in all patients.

Illustrative cases

Case 1 (patient 9): classic indocyanine green videoangiography

A 57-year-old woman presented after a previous episode of right superficial temporal hematoma (Fig. 7.5A,B). She was diagnosed with a small right temporal AVM (Spetzler–Martin grade I). The patient was neurologically intact. She underwent

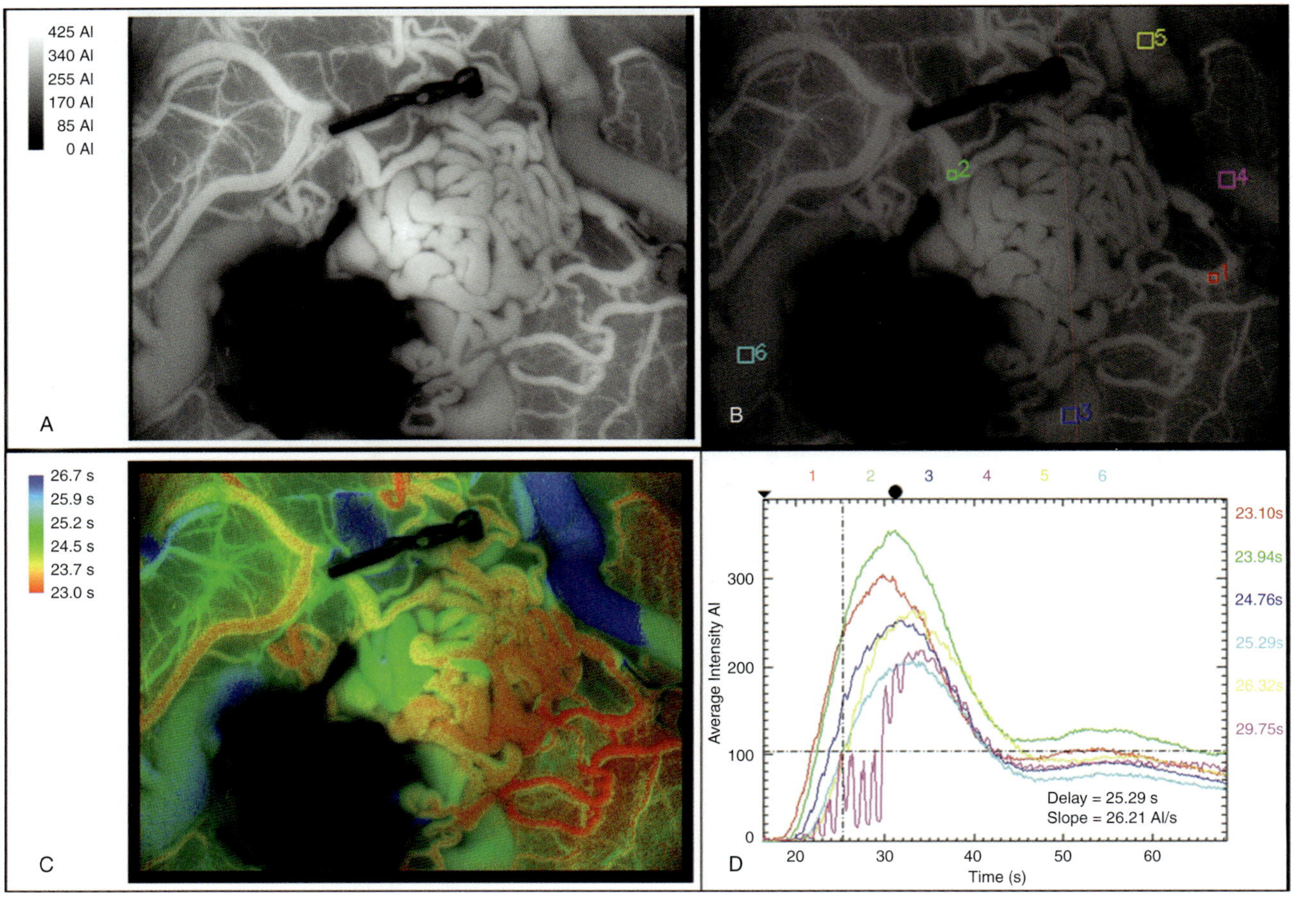

Fig. 7.2. Indocyanine green videoangiography with FLOW 800 software (progress analysis with clipping of the two main superficial feeders) for Case 2 (patient 19). (A) Map of maximal fluorescence intensity did not allow a clear definition of hemodynamic changes before and after temporary clipping but showed the absence of flow perturbation in normal brain parenchyma around the arteriovenous malformations (AVM) (see also Fig. 7.5A). (B) Two regions of interest were again positioned in two feeders after the clip (red and green), and four regions of interest were positioned in three main draining veins (blue, pale blue, pink, and yellow). (C) Map of delay time allowed a better understanding of the change of AVM flow after clipping, particularly in the area fed by the posterior cerebral artery, with a slowing down of the flow in the lateral inferior draining vein (now blue). (D) Evaluation of the time course of fluorescence and the time to half-maximal fluorescence in each region of interest (see also Fig. 7.3D) showed a clear modification of the hemodynamic of the AVM, with a slowing down of the flow in the venous site, particularly in the lateral inferior vein (pink and yellow), and with an increase in the arteriovenous difference of time to half-maximal fluorescence from 2.12 seconds (19.85-17.73 seconds) to 6.65 seconds (29.75-23.10 seconds).

a right mini-invasive, image-guided temporal approach to remove her AVM. After the dura was opened, a small sulcal temporal AVM and arterialization of the distal part of the vein of Labbé could be visualized under microscopic view (Fig. 7.4A).

The primary superficial survey revealed rapid flow in the two main feeders to the AVM, depicted the nidus more clearly, and sharply delineated the arterialized flow inside the efferent vein (Fig. 7.4B). After the AVM was removed (Fig. 7.4C), a terminal assessment ICG videoangiography confirmed total removal of the nidus, restoration of homogeneous flow in the arteries exposed under the dura, and slower venous flow in the vein of Labbé (Fig. 7.4D). Total ICG videoangiography time was 9 minutes (Table 7.1).

The patient's postoperative course was uneventful, and she was discharged home on postoperative day 4. In this case, DSA was not performed because of the clear videoangiographic picture and the small dimension of the nidus with clear vessel architecture; CT angiography showed the absence of residual nidus.

Case 2 (patient 19): indocyanine green videoangiography with FLOW 800 analysis

A 40-year-old woman presented with a long history of headache. An MRI suggested the presence of a left parieto-occipital Spetzler–Martin grade III AVM (Fig. 7.6), which was confirmed by DSA (Fig. 7.6B–D). The feeders came from branches of the middle cerebral artery (Fig. 7.6B) and from the posterior cerebral artery (Fig. 7.6C), and drainage was only superficial toward the sagittal and transverse sinuses (Fig. 7.6D). The patient was neurologically intact. Preoperative embolization was performed, and a small feeder from the middle cerebral artery was closed with Onyx. A left image-guided parieto-occipital approach was used to remove the AVM. After the dura was opened, the microscopic view confirmed the presence of the superficial nidus of the AVM with multiple, partially embolized feeders (Fig. 7.7).

A primary superficial survey with ICG videoangiography with FLOW 800 analysis was then performed. A map of maximal fluorescence intensity (Fig. 7.1A) was used because the

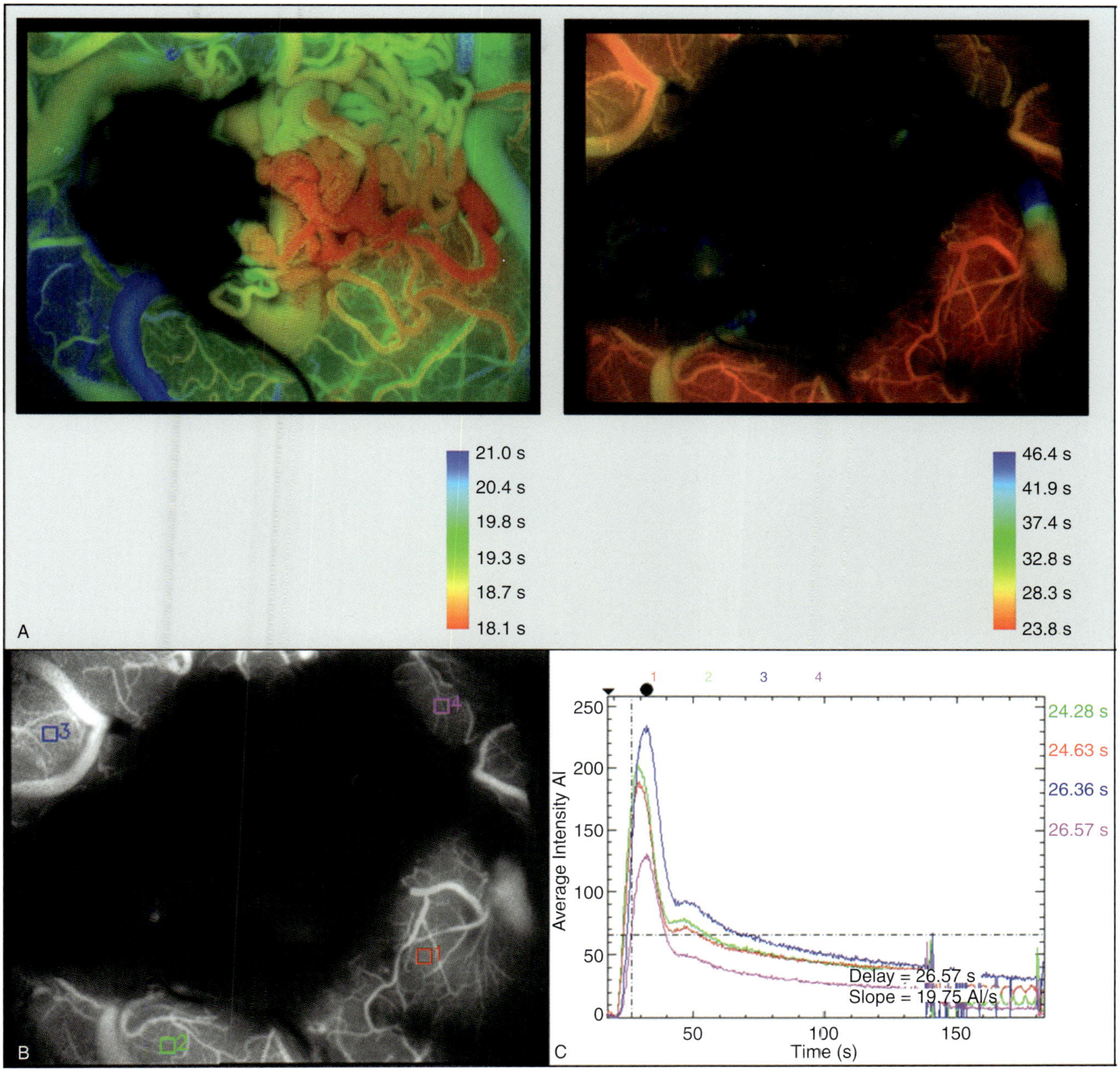

Fig. 7.3. Indocyanine green videoangiography with FLOW 800 software (terminal assessment) for Case 2 (patient 19). (A) After removal of the arteriovenous malformations (AVM), the map of delay time confirmed the absence of residual nidus or arteriovenous shunt (upper right). (B) Four regions of interest were placed in the brain parenchyma near the surgical cavity. (C) The time course of fluorescence and time to half-maximal fluorescence were studied in these four regions of interest and demonstrated similar flows in all four regions.

complexity of the AVM with multiple feeders and the dimension of the nidus made classic ICG videoangiography difficult to interpret. In contrast, the map of delay times (Fig. 7.1C), with a gradient color scale according to time to half-maximal fluorescence, better delineated the differences between superficial feeders and draining veins. In addition, the specific pattern of fluorescence was evaluated in multiple regions of interest: two each were positioned in two feeders, one from the middle cerebral artery and one from the posterior cerebral artery; three each were positioned in three main draining veins; one was positioned in a vein that was apparently not involved in the AVM flow; and one was placed in the peri-AVM brain parenchyma (Fig. 7.1B). It was then possible to evaluate a graph of the time course of fluorescence and the time to half-maximal fluorescence in each region of interest (Fig. 7.1D), thus distinguishing the flow of the superficial feeders (one faster with 17.73 seconds and the other slower with 18.98 seconds) from the main draining veins (18.93, 19.19, and 19.85 seconds) and from normal veins (20.91 seconds).

To better understand the hemodynamics of this AVM, a progress analysis was performed after dissection of the nidus and clipping of the main superficial feeders (Fig. 7.2). Two temporary clips were placed in the two main superficial feeder vessels (which had been identified from the previous ICG videoangiography). The map of maximal fluorescence intensity did not clearly show the hemodynamic changes before and after

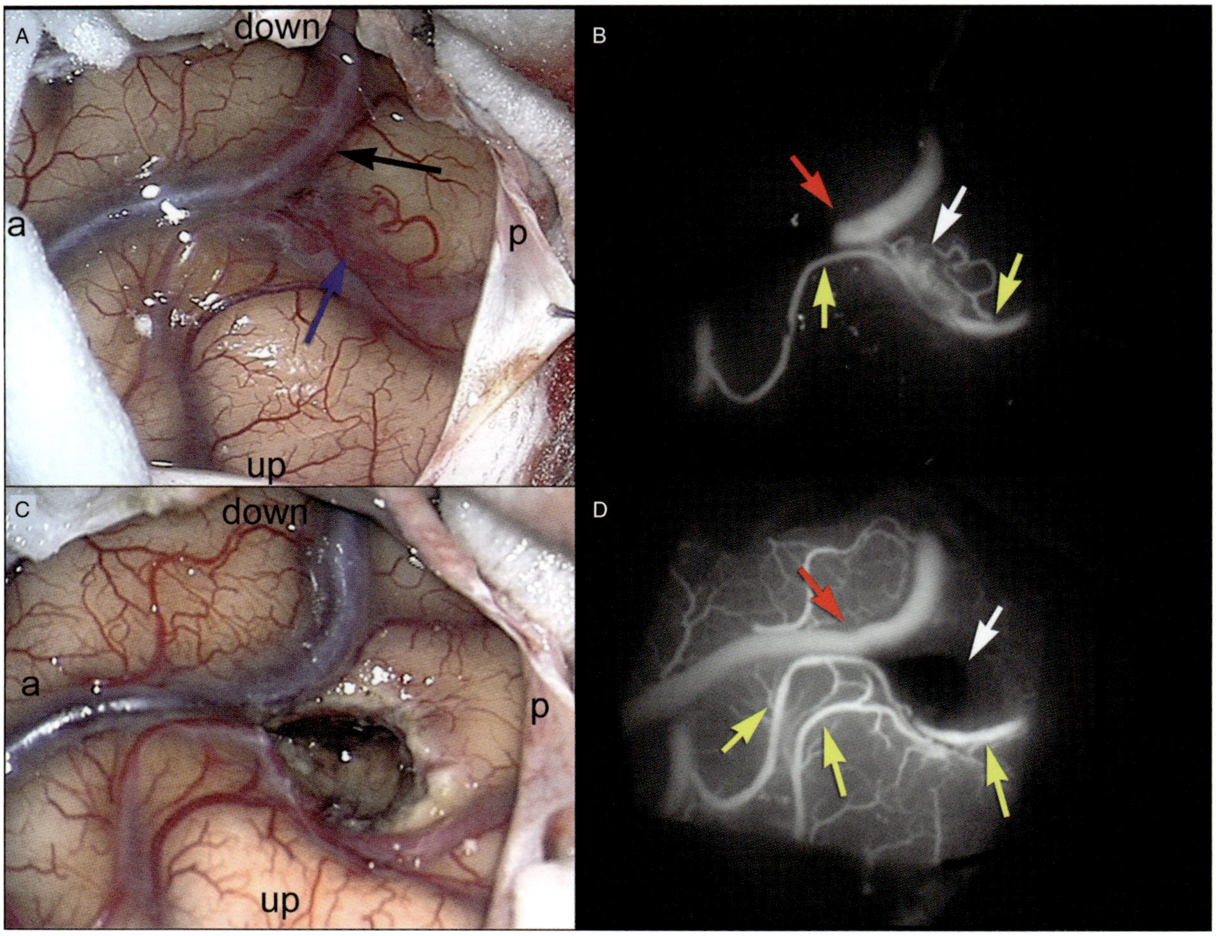

Fig. 7.4. Intraoperative pictures for Case 1 (patient 9). The patient underwent a right mini-invasive, image-guided temporal approach to remove her arteriovenous malformations (AVM). (A) After dural opening, microscopic view confirmed the presence of a small sulcal temporal AVM (blue arrow) and the arterialization of the distal part of the vein of Labbé (black arrow). (B) The primary superficial survey showed a fast flow in the two main feeders of the AVM (yellow arrows), clearly depicted the nidus (white arrow), and allowed a sharp delineation of the arterialized flow inside the efferent vein (red arrow). (C) Microscopic view after AVM removal. (D) Terminal assessment with indocyanine green videoangiography confirmed total removal of the nidus (white arrow), restoration of homogeneous flow in the arteries exposed under the dura (yellow arrows), and a normal homogeneous venous flow inside the vein of Labbé (red arrow). a, anterior; p, posterior.

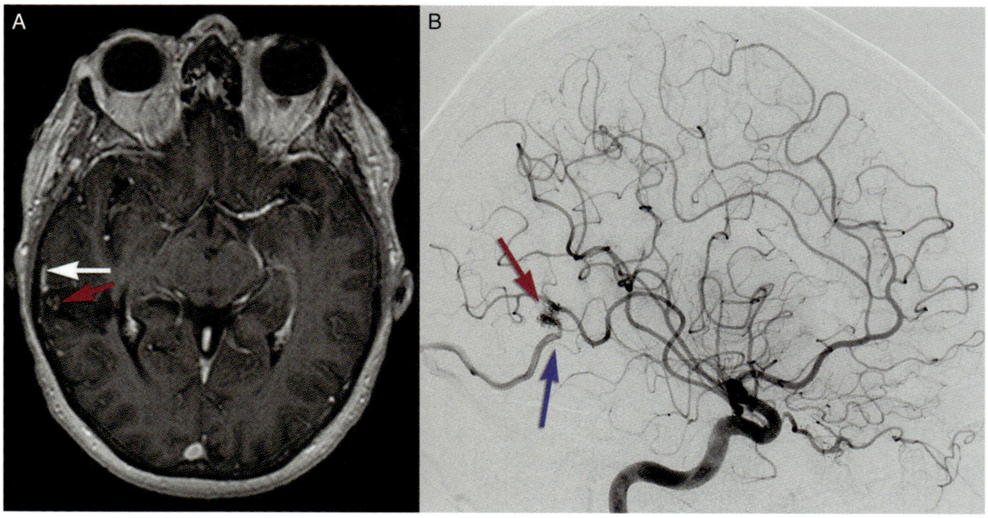

Fig. 7.5. Preoperative neuroradiological evaluation for Case 1 (patient 9). Preoperative MRI with intravenous gadolinium administration used for neuronavigation (A) and digital subtraction angiography (B) showed the small temporal nidus of the arteriovenous malformations (red arrows, A and B) and the drainage into the vein of Labbé (white arrow, A; blue arrow, B).

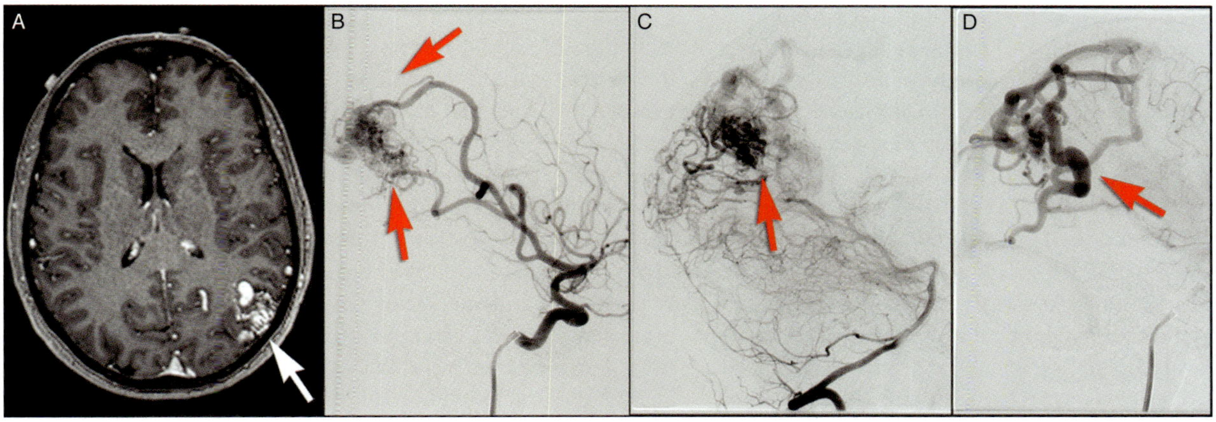

Fig. 7.6. Preoperative neuroradiological evaluation for Case 2 (patient 19). Preoperative MRI with intravenous gadolinium administration used for neuronavigation (A) and digital subtraction angiography (B–D) showed a left parieto-occipital arteriovenous malformations with feeders coming from branches of the middle cerebral artery (B, red arrows) and from the posterior cerebral artery (C, red arrow), and draining only superficial toward sagittal and transverse sinus (D, red arrow).

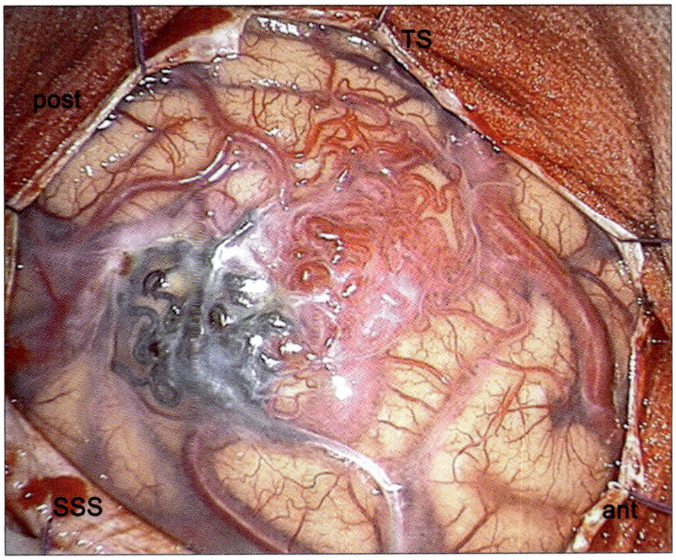

Fig. 7.7. Intraoperative microscopic picture for Case 2 (patient 19). The patient underwent a left image-guided, parieto-occipital approach to remove her arteriovenous malformations. After dural opening, microscopic view confirmed the presence of the superficial nidus with multiple partially embolized feeders.

temporary clipping but did show the absence of flow perturbation in normal peri-AVM brain parenchyma (Fig. 7.1A vs. 7.2A). In contrast, the map of delay time allowed a better understanding of the changes in blood flow after clipping, particularly in the area fed by the posterior cerebral artery (Fig. 7.1C vs. 7.2C). In this progress analysis, the specific pattern of fluorescence was also studied in different regions of interest: two each in two feeders after clipping and four each in three main draining veins (Fig. 7.2B). The evaluation of the time course of fluorescence and the time to half-maximal fluorescence in each region of interest (Fig. 7.1D vs. 7.2D) showed a clear modification of the hemodynamics of the AVM, with a reduced rate of flow in the venous phase, particularly in the lateral inferior vein, and with an increase in the difference of time to half-maximal fluorescence between the arterial and venous phases from 2.12 seconds (19.85 vs. 17.73 seconds) to 6.65 seconds (29.75 vs. 23.10 seconds). The AVM was then completely removed starting from the two superficial feeders that had been identified on ICG videoangiography.

A terminal assessment ICG videoangiography confirmed total removal of the AVM (Fig. 7.3A). In addition, the time course of fluorescence and time to half-maximal fluorescence was evaluated in four regions of interest placed in the brain parenchyma near the surgical cavity; these showed a comparable flow in the area, suggesting the absence of ischemic lesions in the superficial area exposed during surgery. Total ICG videoangiography time in this patient was 20 minutes and 30 seconds (Table 7.1). Total removal of the AVM was confirmed with DSA. The patient was neurologically intact at the time of discharge on postoperative day 6.

Discussion

This retrospective analysis of 25 patients confirms the utility of ICG videoangiography during surgery for AVM, as already suggested in previously published series [6–13]. Addition of ICG videoangiography is relatively quick and inexpensive and requires only a dedicated surgical microscope. The dye clears within 10 minutes, allowing multiple injections to be used. In our series, up to three injections are used during the operation and the standard dose for each administration is reduced to 12.5 mg in order to avoid exceeding the suggested maximum daily dose. No morbidity or mortality related to ICG injection was recorded in this series of AVM surgeries or in more than 300 patients at our institution.

Apart from ease of use, ICG videoangiography has many advantages over a simple microscopic view. Specifically, the primary superficial survey provides additional information, including the orientation of the primary angioarchitecture of the AVM in 17 of the 21 patients (81%), helping to identify the nidus and en passage feeders and allowing AVM arteries and veins to be distinguished. In addition, in one patient, ICG videoangiography identified an arteriovenous shunt in the context of a hematoma, a finding also reported by Killory *et al.* [7]. However, the primary survey seemed to be advantageous only for superficial AVMs. The more deeply located AVMs in our series were either not considered good candidates for initial ICG videoangiography or resulted in poor quality videos and images. In addition, classic ICG videoangiography, used in the beginning of our series, was considered difficult to interpret in large AVMs. In these patients, it was not possible to differentiate arteries and veins or to identify en passage feeders.

The application of the new FLOW 800 software appears to overcome these limits and we began using this technique in selected patients with vascular pathology and tumors in 2010 and in AVM surgery in 2011. To date, we have used this tool in 13 patients with AVMs, the highest number of reported AVM surgeries studied with this tool. During the primary superficial survey, the delay times visual map (time to half-maximal fluorescence displayed as a gradient color scale) was particularly useful in differentiating AVM arteries and veins (Fig. 7.1C and Case 2). In addition, a better understanding of the AVM hemodynamics could be gained by studying the time course of fluorescence and the time to half-maximal fluorescence in multiple regions of interest within one graph (Fig. 7.1D and Case 2). This advantage was particularly useful when a progress analysis with clipping of the main feeders of the AVM was performed (Fig. 7.2 and Case 2).

As previously described by Hänggi *et al.* [8] and Takagi *et al.* [13], terminal assessment ICG videoangiography was particularly important for confirming the complete removal of the AVM and normalization of arterial and venous flow. In addition, more rarely, it could indicate the persistence of part of the AVM, as demonstrated in three of our patients (one unexpected residual nidus and two unexpected residual arteriovenous shunts).

Despite its many advantages, there are limits to this new technique of intraoperative cerebral blood flow study. One of the most important limitations is that it can only show what is exposed in the surgical approach. Hence, when dealing with deep-seated AVMs through a narrow or long surgical corridor, ICG videoangiography may not be indicated, at least as a primary superficial survey. In addition, even though the introduction of FLOW 800 allows a semiquantitative and more objective evaluation of the vessel and parenchymal flows, it requires more time to be performed and interpreted (in our series a mean of 8.2 minutes more than the total time for classic ICG videoangiography), it must be completed with the microscope fixed in position to analyze cerebral blood flow (this is more problematic for aneurysm surgery than for AVM surgery), and it has a steep learning curve. In our experience, two to three surgeons with ICG videoangiography expertise should be present in the operating room. We waited almost one year before using FLOW 800 during AVM surgery to familiarize our team with the technique and to be able to perform the evaluation of cerebral blood flow during surgery.

Intraoperative DSA was not used in this study and so no comparison of the two techniques is possible. While we recognize that intraoperative DSA should still be considered the "gold standard" [7,13] for evaluating vascular flow in AVM surgery, particularly in more complex situations, we believe that ICG videoangiography, particularly with the aid of FLOW 800 software, is a reliable and simple adjunct for evaluating AVM hemodynamics intraoperatively, particularly in institutions where intraoperative DSA is not readily available or to reduce the need to perform multiple DSA during surgery.

References

1. Feindel W, Yamamoto YL, Hodge CP. Intracarotid fluorescein angiography: a new method for examination of the epicerebral circulation in man. *Can Med Assoc J* 1967;**96**:1–7.
2. Raabe A, Beck J, Gerlach R, *et al.* Near-infrared indocyanine green video angiography: a new method for intraoperative assessment of vascular flow. *Neurosurgery* 2003;**52**:132–9.
3. Kuroiwa T, Kajimoto Y, Ohta T. Development and clinical application of near-infrared surgical microscope: preliminary report. *Minim Invasive Neurosurg* 2001;**44**:240–2.
4. Raabe A, Beck J, Seifert V. Technique and image quality of intraoperative indocyanine green angiography during aneurysm surgery using surgical microscope integrated near-infrared video technology. *Zentralbl Neurochir* 2005;**66**:1–6.
5. Raabe A, Nakaji P, Beck J, *et al.* Prospective evaluation of surgical microscope-integrated intraoperative near-infrared indocyanine green videoangiography during aneurysm surgery. *J Neurosurg* 2005;**103**:982–9.
6. Takagi Y, Kikuta K, Nozaki K, *et al.* Detection of a residual nidus by surgical microscope-integrated intraoperative near-infrared indocyanine green videoangiography in a child with a cerebral arteriovenous malformation. *J Neurosurg* 2007;**107**:416–18.
7. Killory BD, Nakaji P, Gonzales LF, *et al.* Prospective evaluation of surgical microscope-integrated intraoperative near-infrared indocyanine green angiography during cerebral arteriovenous malformation surgery. *Neurosurgery* 2009;**65**:456–62.
8. Hänggi D, Etminan N, Steiger HJ. The impact of microscope-integrated intraoperative near-infrared indocyanine green videoangiography on surgery of arteriovenous malformations and dural arteriovenous fistulae. *Neurosurgery* 2010;**67**:1094–103.
9. Ferroli P, Acerbi F, Broggi M, *et al.* Arteriovenous micromalformation of the trigeminal root: intraoperative diagnosis with indocyanine green videoangiography: case report. *Neurosurgery* 2010;**67**:ons309–10.
10. Chen SF, Kato Y, Oda J, *et al.* The application of intraoperative near-infrared indocyanine green videoangiography and analysis of fluorescence intensity in cerebrovascular surgery. *Surg Neurol Int* 2011;**2**:42.
11. Faber F, Thon N, Fesl G, *et al.* Enhanced analysis of intracerebral arterioveneous malformations by the intraoperative use of analytical indocyanine green videoangiography: technical note. *Acta Neurochir (Wien)* 2011;**153**:2181–7.
12. Jhawar SS, Kato Y, Oda J, *et al.* FLOW 800-assisted surgery for arteriovenous malformation. *J Clin Neurosci* 2011;**18**:1556–7.
13. Takagi Y, Sawamura K, Hashimoto N, *et al.* Evaluation of serial intraoperative

surgical microscope-integrated intraoperative near-infrared indocyanine green videoangiography in patients with cerebral arteriovenous malformations. *Neurosurgery* 2012;**70**:34–42.

14. Oh JK, Shin HC, Kim TY, *et al.* Intraoperative indocyanine green video-angiography: spinal dural arteriovenous fistula. *Spine (Phila Pa 1976)* 2011;**36**: E1578–80.

15. Misra BK, Purandare HR. Application of indocyanine green videoangiography in surgery for spinal vascular malformations. *J Clin Neurosci* 2012;**19**:892–6.

16. Killory BD, Nakaji P, Maughan PH, *et al.* Evaluation of angiographically occult spinal dural arteriovenous fistulae with surgical microscope-integrated intraoperative near-infrared indocyanine green angiography: report of 3 cases. *Neurosurgery* 2011;**68**:781–7.

17. Woitzik J, Horn P, Vajkoczy P, *et al.* Intraoperative control of extracranial-intracranial bypass patency by near-infrared indocyanine green videoangiography. *J Neurosurg* 2005;**102**:692–8.

18. Ferroli P, Acerbi F, Albanese E, *et al.* Application of intraoperative indocyanine green angiography for CNS tumors: results on the first 100 cases. *Acta Neurochir Suppl* 2011;**109**:251–7.

19. Ferroli P, Tringali G, Albanese E, *et al.* Developmental venous anomaly of petrous veins: intraoperative findings and indocyanine green video angiographic study. *Neurosurgery* 2008;**62**:ons418–21.

20. Ferroli P, Acerbi F, Tringali G, *et al.* Venous sacrifice in neurosurgery: new insights from venous indocyanine green videoangiography. *J Neurosurg* 2011;**115**:18–23.

21 Ferroli P, Nakaji P, Acerbi F, *et al.* Indocyanine green ICG) temporary clipping test to assess collateral circulation before venous sacrifice. *World Neurosurg* 2011;**75**:122–5.

22. Kamp MA, Slotty P, Turowski B, *et al.* Microscope-integrated quantitative analysis of intraoperative indocyanine green fluorescence angiography for blood flow assessment: first experience in 30 patients. *Neurosurgery* 2012;**70**:65–73.

23. Ferroli P, Acerbi F, Tringali G, *et al.* Self-closing Nitinol U-clips for intracranial arterial microanastomosis: a preliminary experience on seven cases. *Acta Neurochir (Wein)* 2009;**151**:969–76.

24. Spetzler RF, Martin NA. A proposed grading system for arteriovenous malformations. *J Neurosurg* 1986;**65**:476–83.

Chapter 8

Neuromonitoring for arteriovenous malformations surgery

Christian Musahl and Nikolai J. Hopf

Introduction

Intraoperative neurophysiological monitoring (IONM) has become an increasingly important and invaluable addition to neurosurgical procedures. Neurovascular surgeons, in particular, rely more and more on the continuous feedback provided by IONM. Monitoring of sensory and motor function, speech, and memory function as well as locating and monitoring of cranial nerves has become possible through applying the respective techniques, thus improving patient outcome and making neurosurgical procedures safer [1–3]. The primary goal of IONM is to recognize and prevent structural damage to the brain by mechanical or vascular means and provide functional guidance to the surgeon.

The use of IONM makes it possible to identify the individual patterns of neural function, thus facilitating the location of the patient's individual distribution of eloquent areas such as the motor cortex, Broca's area, and so on. Cranial nerve motor nuclei or their fiber tracts can be located at the floor of the fourth ventricle or within their course through the skull base and around vascular lesions. Continuous monitoring of sensory, motor, and auditory pathways can directly influence the operative strategy and thereby prevent complications such as the impairment or loss of neural function. Neurological deficits can be reduced, or even avoided, only if the evoked potentials identified mirror the current state of surgery (time equivalence), meaning that changes must correlate with surgical steps and the change in potentials must be reversible if it has a cause that can be eliminated. This technical accuracy has only been made possible by the advent of modern computer technology, which has allowed procedures to be followed that demand averaging of (evoked potential) data and comparison with a baseline study. Current monitoring machines are about five times faster than their predecessors and are capable of recording 16 different signals at the same time. This results in much faster feedback to the surgeon and opens up the possibility of monitoring complex procedures such as brainstem monitoring.

The term IONM covers a large variety of different methods that need to be selected according to the pathology at hand [4,5]. There are two two major subgroups. The first group provides the surgeon with continuous intraoperative information about the function and integrity of certain brain regions or fiber tracts, which can be analyzed immediately by comparing the data with the initial values at the start of surgery. In this way IONM can provide critical, decision-guiding information right when it is needed. Techniques of this category are evoked potentials (somatosensory [SEP], motor [MEP], auditory [AEP], and visual [VEP]), electromyography (EMG), D-wave, electroencephalography (EEG), the bulbospongiosus reflex, and monitoring of speech function during awake craniotomies. The second category, mapping, includes direct cortical stimulation, phase reversal, and navigated transcranial magnetic stimulation (nTMS).

Our neurosurgical department uses IONM during every surgery for cerebral and spinal arteriovenous malformations (AVMs). Depending on the location of the AVM, monitoring will be more or less extensive, containing at the very minimum the continuous monitoring of SEPs and MEPs.

Methods

Anesthesiology

To have the full benefit of IONM, an experienced neuroanesthesiologist is mandatory since its successful use is highly dependent on anesthesia. Ideally, there should be sufficient analgesic sedation with precise controllability combined with a marginal but predictable effect on neuronal activity. Short-acting muscle relaxants such as pancuronium should be used, so that their effect has washed out once the critical steps of the surgery are being performed. In the case of MEPs or EMG registration, muscle relaxants are prohibited. Since inhalational anesthetics lead to a reduction of amplitudes and a delay of latency in SEP monitoring, as well as a significant elevation of the motor threshold above an inhalation concentration of 0.5 of minimum alveolar concentration, total intravenous anesthesia should be applied. Barbiturates and benzodiazepines have a similar suppressing effect on MEPs. Opioids have very little effect on MEPs but can lead to a misleading reduction of amplitude if applied as a bolus injection.

Comprehensive Management of Arteriovenous Malformations of the Brain and Spine, ed. Robert F. Spetzler, Douglas S. Kondziolka, Randall T. Higashida, and M. Yashar S. Kalani. Published by Cambridge University Press.

Therefore, total intravenous anesthesia is recommended using propofol in combination with an opioid. Bolus injections should be avoided. Inhalational anesthetics can be used only with a maximum alveolar concentration below 0.5 if necessary.

The depth of anesthesia may be monitored with the bispectral index, which is standard in all cerebrovascular procedures in many neurovascular centers. Bispectral index monitoring is a non-invasive, continuous measurement of the effect of anesthetics on brain function. The strip-like sensor is placed on the patient's forehead and provides values from 0 (equivalent to EEG silence) to 100 (equivalent to fully awake) derived from EEG data. A bispectral index value of 40–60 is ideal. It has been reported that bispectral index monitoring can significantly reduce the risk of anesthesia awareness during surgery [6].

Monitoring

Evoked potentials

Evoked potentials are specific responses from any part of the nervous system that follow an electrical stimulation. The latency and size of the amplitude of these potentials carry important information about the monitored system. Evoked potentials present a functional testing of the respective neuronal pathways and allow conclusions about their integrity. A precise analysis of these specific responses has only been made possible through the introduction of monitoring computers that sum up and average the evoked potentials, eliminate additional "noise" from baseline EEG and muscles, and amplify the naturally low nerve potentials.

Somatosensory evoked potentials

Acquisition of SEPs follows stimulation of a peripheral nerve, in general the median nerve for the upper extremity and the tibial nerve for the lower extremity. They provide an objective functional observation of the somatosensory system. The bipolar stimulation probe is firmly placed above the nerve at the typical location (carpal tunnel for the median nerve and posterior to the medial malleolus for the tibial nerve). If the acquired potentials are of poor quality, it is advisable to lower the frequency of stimulation and prolong the single stimuli. The intensity of stimulation can be as high as 50 mA, and 250 repetitions per averaging cycle are sufficient for the acquisition of adequate potentials with a good signal to noise ratio.

The action potential spreads along the ascending pathways of the dorsal column and leads to electrical activation in the primary sensory cortex of the contralateral postcentral gyrus, where it can be recorded through electrodes in the scalp [7,8].

Influencing factors that may lead to changes in SEPs independent from surgical manipulations are a decrease in body temperature or blood pressure, pneumocephalus, and changes in anesthesia.

Motor evoked potentials

MEPs can be recorded after direct or transcranial magnetic or electrical stimulation of the motor cortex. For intraoperative monitoring, transcranial electrical MEPs with a multipulse or train stimulation have become a standard procedure in vascular neurosurgery. Corkscrew electrodes for stimulation are placed over C3 and C4 (international 10–20 EEG system). The intensity of stimulation should not exceed 200 mA, while usually 100 mA is sufficient to receive adequate potentials. If surgically exposed motor cortex is stimulated, significantly less current is required (only 10–20 mA).

The stimulation leads to neuron activation of the pyramidal tract with descending activity along the corticospinal tract. To record muscle MEPs, subdermal needle electrodes are recommended. Suitable muscles for stimulation are the abductor pollicis brevis or forearm flexors for the upper extremities, and the abductor hallucis brevis and anterior tibial muscle for the lower extremities. Changes in latency of the response and its amplitude as well as motor threshold suggest structural damage of the motor system.

Halogenated anesthetics such as enflurane, flurane, and isoflurane as well as muscle relaxants are influencing factors that may lead to changes in or loss of MEPs. Other factors include blood pressure changes and compression of peripheral nerves caused by poor patient positioning.

Auditory evoked potentials

An electrode placed in front of the tragus is used to record AEPs. These are generated by repetitive click sounds of 95 dB applied through an earplug, while deafening the other ear with a continuous noise of 65 dB. Clinical evaluation is based on the amplitude and latency of the AEPs. These potentials have a very low amplitude (<1 μV) and a short latency (<6 millisecond). Due to the low amplitude, amplification should be as high as possible. The frequency of stimulation should be high enough to allow fast detection of pathological change while conserving single impulse discrimination.

The evoked signal runs from the cochlea through the cochlear nerve and cochlear nucleus, crosses to the contralateral lateral lemniscus, the inferior colliculus in the midbrain, and the medial geniculate body to reach the primary auditory cortex. Within 1 second after stimulation about 20 evoked waves are generated, although only waves I through V are of clinical relevance (Fig. 8.1). These five waves can be correlated quite well to anatomical landmarks within the auditory pathway. Wave I has its origin in the distal cochlear nerve, wave II in the junction between the nerve and cochlear nucleus, wave III arises from the caudal part of the pons, wave IV represents the medial lemniscus, and wave V projects to the inferior colliculus.

Factors that can influence the potentials are a sudden fall in patient temperature or blood pressure, loud noises within the operating room (drill), cerebellar retractors, cold irrigation, and heat generation within the surgical field.

Visual evoked potentials

The introduction of powerful light-emitting diodes has made a stable stimulation of the visual system possible [9]. However, an exact anatomical correlation of changes in amplitude or latency is not possible at the moment.

Amplitude and latency are highly influenced by anesthesia. Consequently, VEP monitoring is not yet considered a standard procedure during vascular neurosurgery.

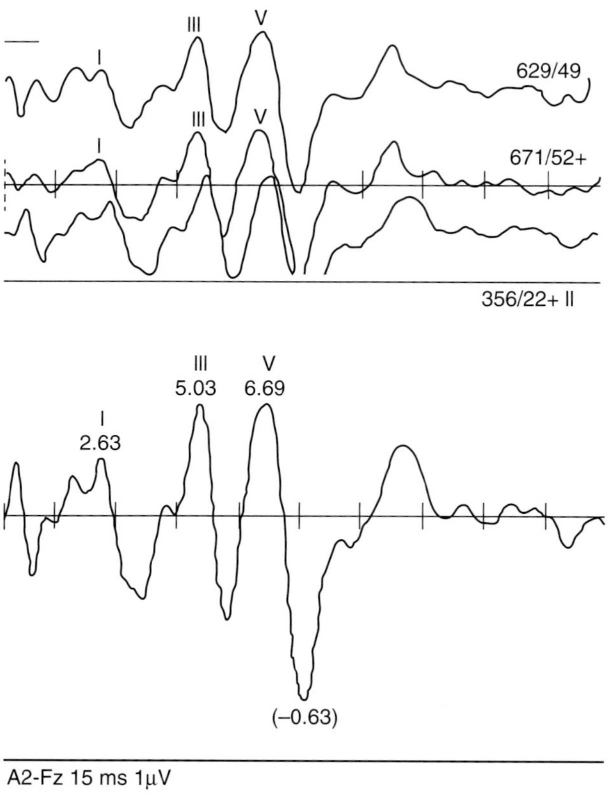

Fig. 8.1. Regular auditory evoked potential recorded during surgical procedure with baseline measurement at the bottom and continuous intraoperative measurements (3) at the top. Waves I, II, III, and V are marked. (With permission from Nikolai Hopf.)

Epidural motor evoked potentials (D-wave)

Epidural MEPs or D-waves are evoked by transcranial electrical stimulation as described above. With the single stimulus technique, recordings are obtained from the spinal cord by an epidurally inserted strip electrode. The primary monitored parameter is the amplitude of the D-wave since it is a relative measure for the number of fast conducting fibers in the corticospinal tract. An intraoperative reduction of the D-wave amplitude usually happens gradually. In general, an irreversible injury to the spinal cord correlates with an amplitude reduction of more than 50%. In combination with muscle MEPs, it allows a fairly precise prediction of the neurological outcome. Patients showing an intraoperative loss of muscle MEPs but preservation of the D-wave usually have an immediate postoperative motor deficit that gradually improves, whereas an additional reduction of 50% or even loss of the D-wave predicts a permanent or at least long-term motor deficit [10].

In contrast to ordinary MEPs, anesthetics or muscle relaxants hardly influence the recording of the D-wave at all.

Electromyography of cranial nerves

Two different kinds of EMG monitoring techniques have to be differentiated: direct stimulation of the exposed motor nerve in order to identify and monitor nerve function and free-running EMG for monitoring spontaneous cranial nerve activity. Both will be discussed in this chapter.

The idea behind the monitoring of cranial nerves was initially developed for surgery of the cerebellopontine angle [11]. Identification of the facial nerve within the operating field was achieved through simultaneously stimulating the nerve and observing the patient's face. Delgado *et al.* [12] were the first to report that EMG potentials derived from facial muscles following stimulation of the intracranial aspect of the facial nerve could demonstrate preserved nerve function after surgery of vestibular schwannomas. Mono- or bipolar stimulation of cranial nerves and the recording of potentials from the corresponding muscles by needle electrodes has now become a standard procedure [11]. With the introduction of multimodal IONM, this technique has been extended to all motor cranial nerves [13,14]. In addition, direct stimulation of exposed central neural structures (e.g., at the floor of the fourth ventricle) and identification and discrimination of cranial nerves, nuclei or tracts are possible [15,16].

For stimulation of cranial nerve nuclei, a bipolar stimulation probe is used with 0.05–2 mA. Signal registration is carried out by paired needle electrodes within the corresponding muscle. During and at the end of surgery, nerve function can be controlled by sequential stimulation of the nerve in different locations (proximal and distal). The latency of the potential after distal stimulation should be lower than after proximal stimulation in an intact nerve. If only distal stimulation results in a potential, a discontinuation within the nerve must be present and a postoperative deficit is likely.

Cerebrospinal fluid can influence the result by shortcutting the current. If proximal and distal latencies are identical, transmission through the cerebrospinal fluid and not the nerve is probable and the measurement should be repeated in a dry setting.

Recording of free-running EMG for monitoring of spontaneous cranial nerve activity is possible using the same needle electrodes within the respective muscles (Fig. 8.2) [13,15]. Inappropriate manipulation or injury (e.g., stretching of a cranial nerve by retraction) can be recognized and even made audible to the surgeon. The feedback provided occurs simultaneously with surgical action and thus supports the safety of the procedure. There are two kinds of EMG potential: contact activity describes an electrical activity that takes place simultaneously to surgical manipulation (contact) and ceases directly after manipulation is stopped; pathological activity or pathological spontaneous activity exceeds surgical manipulation and, in contrast to contact activity, indicates impairment of the neural structure and postoperative deficit. Additional indicators for postoperative deficit are long-lasting activities with high frequencies and amplitudes, which indicate a loss of nerve fibers.

Electroencephalography

Intraoperative EEG monitoring provides information about cortical and direct subcortical function. It does not provide any information about the function of deeper lying structures such as sensory–motor tracts, cranial nerves or the spinal cord. The recordings present a summation of excitatory and inhibitory potentials, with an amplitude of 10–100 μV generated

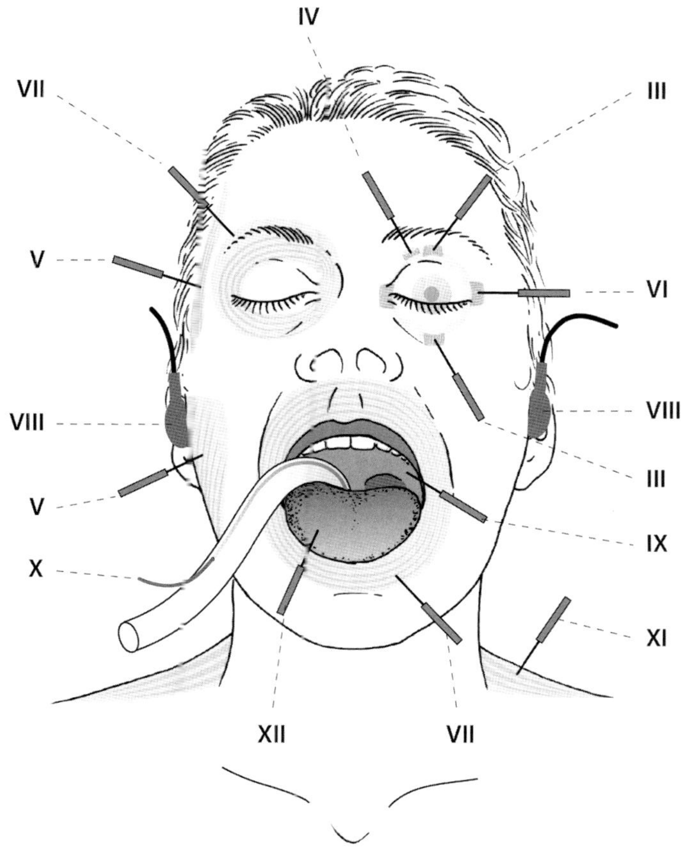

Fig. 8.2. Standard needle positioning for electromyography monitoring of cranial nerves. Note that the electrode for monitoring of cranial nerve X is located within the respiratory tube. (With permission from Nikolai Hopf.)

in the cerebral cortex. In order to achieve a standardized placement of scalp electrodes that enables the reproducibility of measurements, the internationally recognized 10–20 system was developed. The recorded waves provide information about the state of electric activity in the brain. Delta waves (up to 4 Hz) are present in "slow wave sleep," deep anesthesia, and as a pathological finding during ischemic events. During general anesthesia, theta waves (4–7 Hz) are most commonly seen. Similar to delta waves, these can also be registered during ischemic events, intoxication, and severe metabolic imbalance. Alpha wave activity (8–12 Hz) is seen most frequently over the occipital lobe in an awake patient with closed eyes. Beta waves (12–30 Hz) are recorded under mental activity or concentration, or can be provoked with small doses of barbiturates and benzodiazepines. During surgery under deep anesthesia, neither alpha nor beta wave activity will be visible.

The cortical electric activity, which is registered by an EEG, requires approximately 50% of the brain's oxygen demand. The other 50% is needed to maintain the cellular integrity of the brain. If the oxygen supply decreases, for example during occlusion of a major vessel, this balance shifts to benefit cellular integrity. This results in reduced cerebral EEG activity, thus showing the surgeon that there is tissue at risk.

In clinical practice, two recording electrodes per hemisphere, one for the anterior cerebral artery territory and one for the middle cerebral artery territory, have proven to be sufficient.

The bulbospongiosus reflex

The bulbospongiosus reflex (previously called the bulbocavernosus reflex) is a polysynaptic reflex that is used for monitoring anal sphincter function. Stimulation of the dorsal penile/clitoral nerve is achieved through a ring electrode around the penis or two surface electrodes over the clitoris and labium. A short train of five stimulations has proven to be most effective for optimal stimulation [17]. The recording of potentials is obtained from the external anal sphincter muscle with two needle electrodes. Preservation of the bulbospongiosus reflex during surgery indicates intact postoperative sphincter control. An intraoperative loss of the bulbospongiosus reflex indicates an at least transient loss of sphincter control.

Influencing factors are the same as for regular MEP monitoring and so the same anesthetic regimen is recommended.

Mapping

Intraoperative mapping

Direct cortical stimulation

An AVM around or directly within eloquent areas might alter normal anatomy to such an extent that it becomes difficult for the surgeon to identify these areas correctly [18]. Functional mapping with intraoperative direct cortical stimulation is the "gold standard" in these patients. After cortical exposure, short trains of five stimuli with a pulse width of 0.5 milliseconds and an interstimulus interval of 4 milliseconds are applied. Stimulation intensity is increased in steps of 1 mA with an upper intensity limit of 25 mA until an EMG response is recorded (Fig. 8.3). Motor potentials are recorded from limb muscles through needle electrodes and positive and negative answers are noted. Every stimulated area is marked with a number creating an individual map of motor function [19]. During removal of the lesion, integrity of these areas as well as subcortical fiber tracts can be checked repeatedly until the end of surgery through direct stimulation. Intact potentials correlate with a good neurological outcome.

Influencing factors that may lead to false negative stimulation results are changes in anesthesia and the use of muscle relaxants.

Phase reversal

Phase reversal is a method of identifying the central sulcus through cortical recording of SEPs of the median or tibial nerve [20]. Localization is based on the observation that the polarity of the recorded potentials from the sensory and the motor gyri are reversed (phase reversal). While stimulating the median or tibial nerve in the same way as for recording SEPs, the exposed surface of the cerebral cortex is mapped by placing a strip electrode for recording orthogonally across the assumed central sulcus. The strip contains four or more separately recording electrodes. Potentials recorded directly from the somatosensory cortex are of large amplitude and an

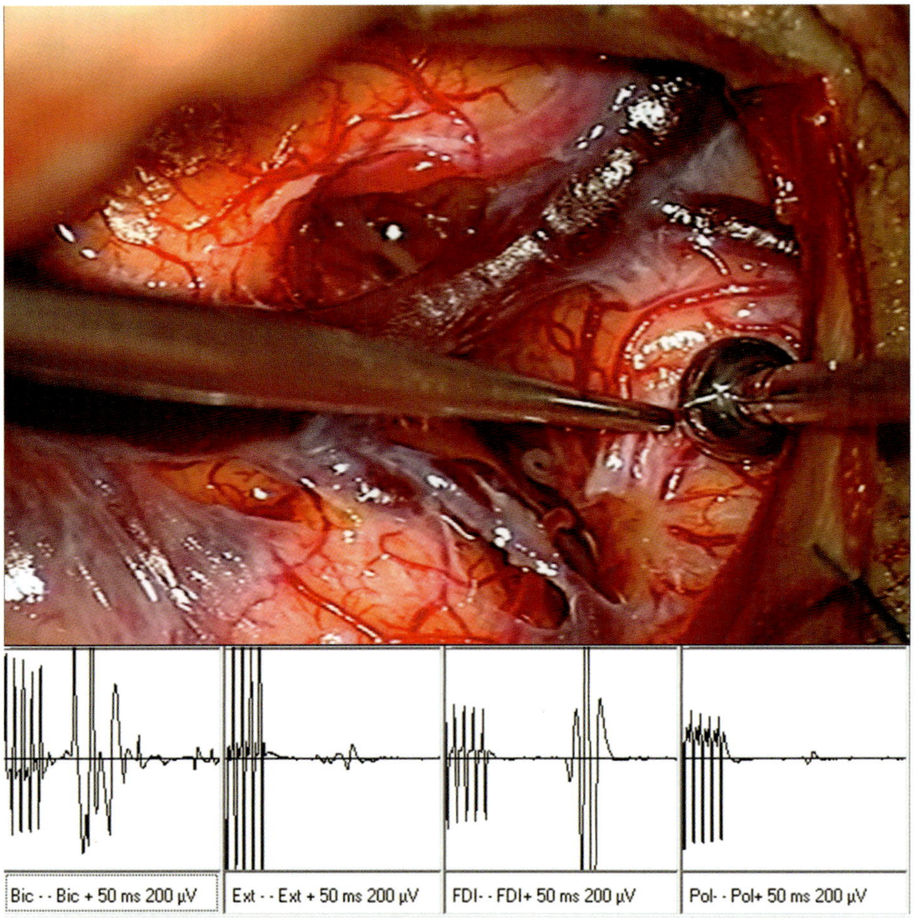

Fig. 8.3. Intraoperative direct cortical stimulation. The intraoperative image of direct cortical stimulation after localizing the supposed motor cortex by neuronavigation (left). At the bottom are the direct cortical stimulation responses from the upper extremity with large response from biceps (1) and the small hand muscles (3). (With permission from Nikolai Hopf.)

interpretable response can be obtained by direct observation of the potentials or after averaging only a few responses, thus requiring less than 10 seconds. Recording from an electrode on the sensory cortex will lead to a prominent negative peak with a latency of about 20 milliseconds for the median nerve, and a positive peak after 40 milliseconds for the tibial nerve. Recording from an electrode on the motor cortex will lead to a positive peak (Fig. 8.4). The central sulcus is located between the positive and negative peaks. Influencing factors are the same as for regular SEP monitoring.

Speech monitoring

For AVMs around Broca's and Wernicke's areas, monitoring of speech function is extremely useful but demands the cooperation of an awake patient. An experienced surgical and anesthesiological team as well as a speech therapist is essential. The modern regimen of propofol and remifentanil allows the anesthesiologist to closely control a patient's level of analgesia and sedation. The advantage of this combination is that it ensures patient comfort while also allowing rapid return to consciousness intraoperatively for awake cortical mapping and speech function control.

Intraoperatively, patients are positioned comfortably on their elevated back with the head turned slightly to the right and fixed in the Mayfield clamp. Following craniotomy and the opening of the dura, the patient regains consciousness. The patient now has to continuously recognize and name out loud the objects presented by the speech therapist on specific cards or a computer screen. At the same time, the surgeon applies bipolar stimulation over 4 seconds at 5–20 mA to the cortical structures. As a result of the stimulation, epileptic seizures may occur; consequently, continuous EEG monitoring during the procedure is required. Stimulation of Broca's or Wernicke's area results in transient aphasia. Points of stimulation are marked by numbers, creating an individual cortical map with respect to speech function [19]. After mapping, resection of the AVM can either be completed under general anesthesia if eloquent areas prove to be a safe distance from the lesion, or in a fully awake patient performing repetitive speech monitoring.

Preoperative mapping

Navigated transcranial magnetic stimulation

Functional MRI (fMRI) for preoperative non-invasive localization of brain functions is the gold standard. In order to detect the motor cortex, the patient has to perform a standardized motor paradigm. Since the resolution is highly dependent on the patient's motor task performance, the method has limitations in non-compliant or severely paretic patients [21]. Additionally, AVMs traditionally pose a

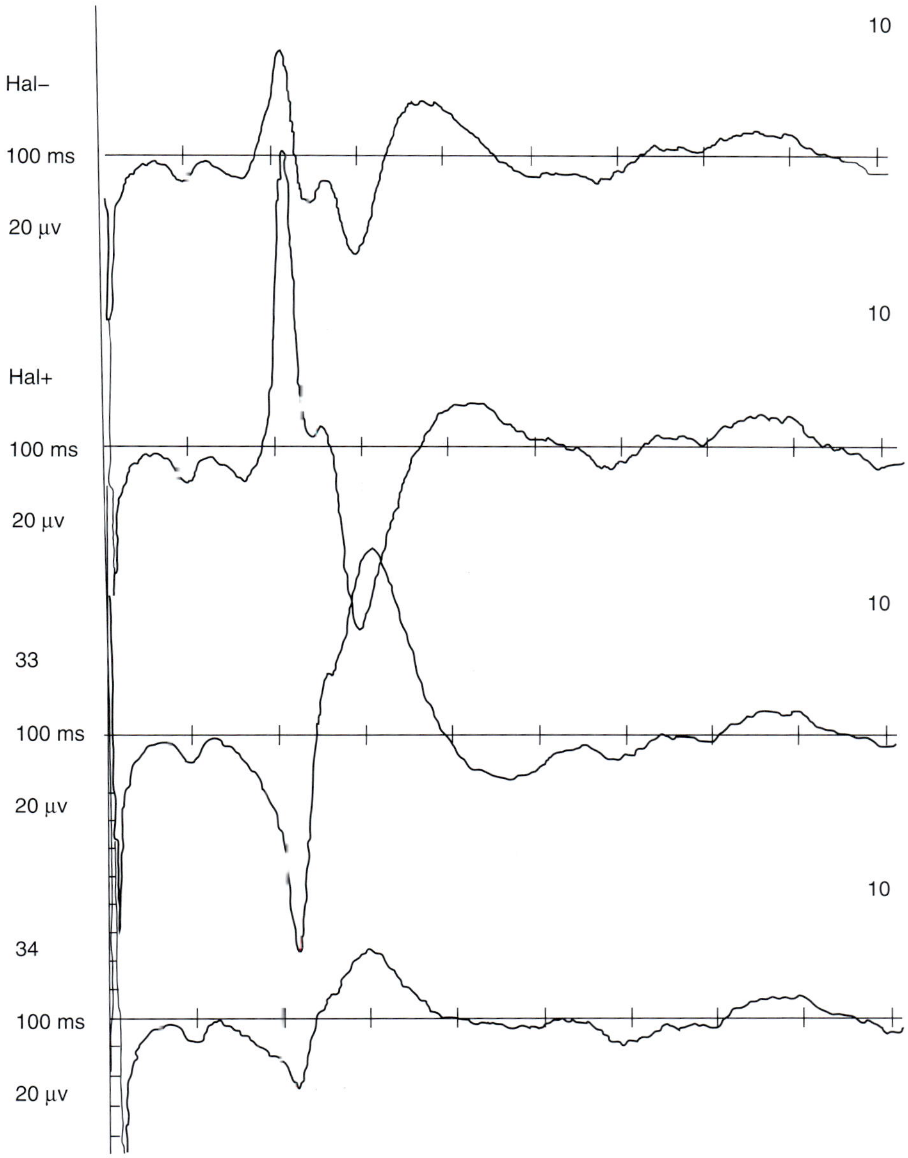

Fig. 8.4. Cortical recording of somatosensory evoked potentials of the median nerve for localization of the central sulcus. Phase reversal can be observed between electrodes two and three. (With permission from Nikolai Hopf.)

problem for fMRI because of their unusual hemodynamics [22]. Use of nTMS is a novel alternative for preoperative functional mapping. It detects eloquent cortical areas directly, comparable to intraoperative direct cortical stimulation [23].

The first commercially available system for nTMS was the NBS System 4 (Nexstim, Helsinki, Finland). It is equipped with an optical tracking system as a base for a non-invasive frameless neuronavigation, combined with a navigated magnetic coil. The system is connected to a computer interface for calculating the distribution of the electrical field depending on individual anatomy and coil position. A previously obtained MP-RAGE (magnetization-prepared rapid acquisition gradient echo) sequence is necessary for neuronavigation in order to yield accurate localizing results. The patient is registered in the nTMS neuronavigation system using the integrated protocol of surface and landmark registration. A magnetically induced current inside a tissue is applied by TMS, thus eliciting a direct electrical stimulation as used in the intraoperative direct cortical stimulation. As described above, EMG is recorded from the limb muscles of interest. Positive responses reflecting the motor cortex are integrated via DICOM import (Digital Imaging and Communications in Medicine) in the intraoperative neuronavigation software iPlan 2.0 (Brainlab, Feldkirchen, Germany), fused to the MP-RAGE images, and exported to the operating room (Fig. 8.5).

We use nTMS for preoperative localization of the motor cortex in all patients with lesions adjacent to or within the motor cortex. The technique requires only a minimum level of compliance. Aphasic patients and those suffering from dementia or severe frontal lobe syndrome are barely able to perform a specific fMRI motor paradigm but can be examined accurately with nTMS [24]. It is particularly useful in patients with AVMs where fMRI often is not feasible, and in small children where it may be the only option for preoperative functional testing.

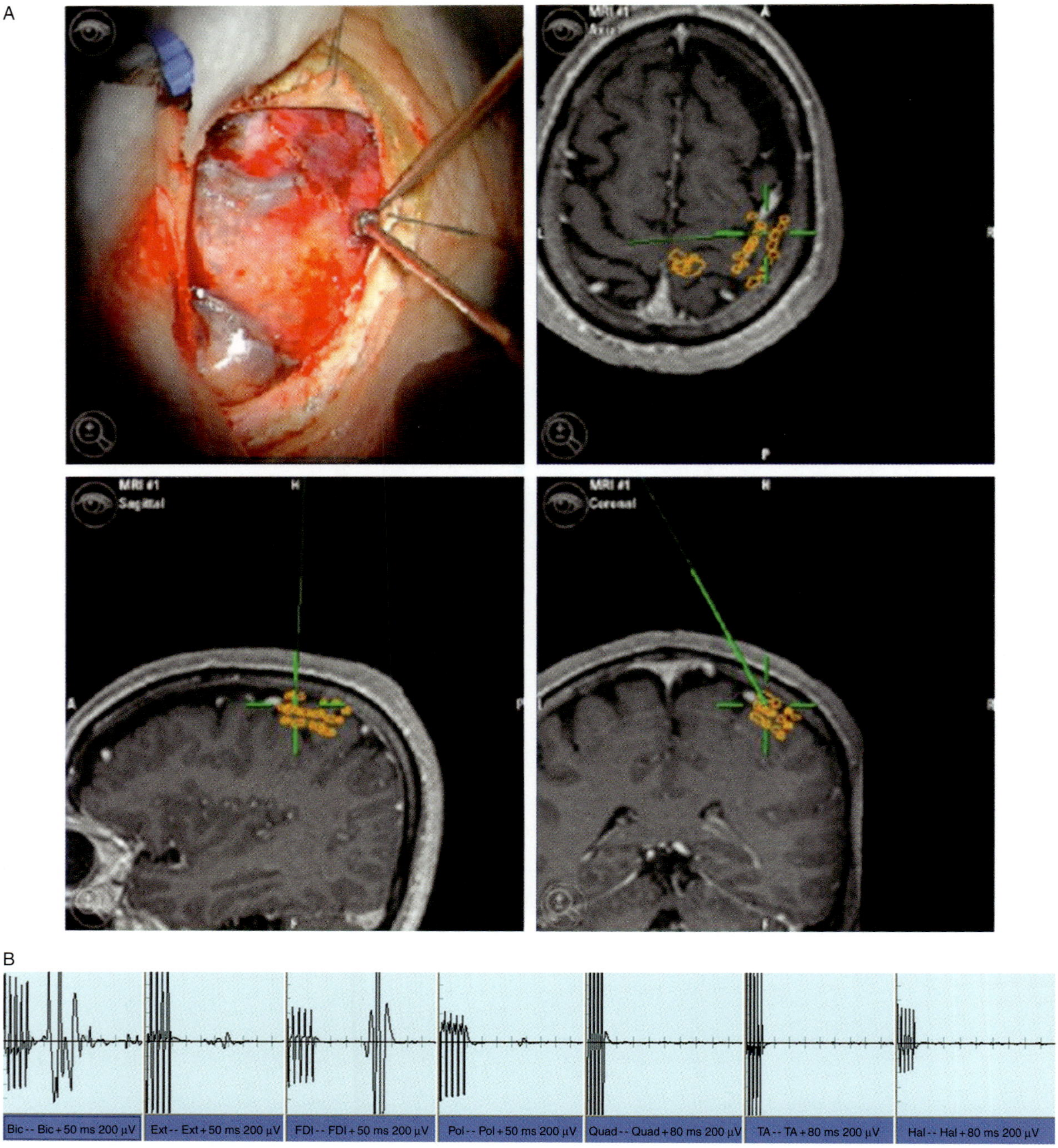

Fig. 8.5. Intraoperative neurophysiological monitoring. (A) An intraoperative screenshot of the MR neuronavigation during direct cortical stimulation. (B) The motor response during direct cortical stimulation. The orange dots within the MRI represent the spots of motor response after preoperative transcranial magnetic stimulation, showing good correlation with direct cortical stimulation. (With permission from Nikolai Hopf.)

Clinical implications of intraoperative neurophysiological monitoring

Supratentorial arteriovenous malformations

Supratentorial AVMs are a very heterogeneous group. Depending on the size and location of the AVM, monitoring might be minimal or very extensive. A patient with a right frontal AVM, Spetzler–Martin grade I, might be operated on without any monitoring at all. We tend to use at least continuous SEP and MEP monitoring as well as bispectral index monitoring for safety measures. This also applies to deeper locations with close relation to the sensory and motor tracts where monitoring of SEPs and MEPs is essential. For cortical AVMs around the central sulcus, we recommend preoperative localizing of the motor cortex using nTMS, particularly if fMRI is not feasible. The data can be used intraoperatively to detect the motor cortex using a navigation system. Additionally, or if neither of the above methods are available, direct cortical stimulation and/or phase reversal should be used for the exact location of the motor cortex.

An AVM adjacent to Broca's or Wernicke's area should receive similar treatment with an extensive preoperative workup. If possible, nTMS or fMRI should be used to identify the exact location of these areas to minimize postoperative neurological deficit. If preoperative localization is not possible or the AVM is located directly within one of these regions, an awake craniotomy should be considered for resection of the AVM. During awake craniotomy, EEG monitoring should be applied for early recognition of epileptic activity.

Infratentorial arteriovenous malformations

Infratentorial AVMs can be roughly divided into two groups with regard to the extent of intraoperative monitoring required: purely hemispheric AVMs and AVMs around the brainstem and the cranial nerves. Purely hemispheric AVMs demand a minimum of IONM. In many neurosurgical departments, these AVMs are resected without any monitoring at all. For safety measures we use SEP, MEP, and bispectral index monitoring during surgery.

Any AVMs around the cerebellopontine angle and the brainstem demand a lot more attention concerning IONM. Additionally to SEP, MEP, and bispectral index monitoring, a free-running EMG of cranial nerves III–XI (depending on the exact location of the AVM) should be used when operating within the cerebellopontine angle and around the brainstem in order to prevent damage to the cranial nerves and their nuclei. Direct stimulation of the cranial nerves as well as their nuclei should be utilized for identifying these structures within the cerebellopontine angle or at the floor of the fourth ventricle when treating an AVM of the brainstem. An experienced neuro-anesthesiologist and neurophysiological technician are mandatory during AVM surgery in that region. A well-trained and experienced team can significantly lower morbidity and mortality of these complex procedures.

Spinal arteriovenous malformations

Monitoring for spinal AVMs usually consists of MEP and SEP monitoring. For lesions around the spinal cord, D-wave monitoring is very useful since it offers a much more valid prognosis of the expected neurological deficit in combination with MEPs than achieved with MEP monitoring alone. To prevent post-operative loss of anal sphincter control, monitoring of the bulbospongiosus reflex should be used for all intramedullary AVMs as well as for AVMs around the conus medullaris and the cauda equina. Preservation of the bulbospongiosus reflex during surgery indicates intact postoperative sphincter control.

Conclusions

Use of IONM is a valuable addition to neurosurgical practice. It includes several different monitoring and mapping modalities, which can be selected depending on the size and location of the AVM. Use of IONM has made neurosurgical procedures safer and the outcome more predictable. It has, therefore, become a standard procedure to use IONM for practically all neurovascular procedures and particularly in AVM surgery.

References

1. Sala F, Bricolo A, Faccioli F, *et al.* Surgery for intramedullary spinal cord tumors: the role of intraoperative neurophysiological) monitoring. *Eur Spine J* 2007;**16**(Suppl 2):S130–9.
2. Sala F, Lanteri P. Brain surgery in motor areas: the invaluable assistance of intraoperative neurophysiological monitoring. *J Neurosurg Sci* 2003;**47**:79–88
3. Sala F, Krzan MJ, Deletis V. Intraoperative neurophysiclogical monitoring in pediatric neurosurgery: why, when, how? *Childs Nerv Syst* 2002;**18**:264–87.
4. Deletis V, Sala F. Intraoperative neurophysiological monitoring of the spinal cord during spinal cord and spine surgery: a review focus on the corticospinal tracts. *Clin Neurophysiol* 2008;**119**:248–64.
5. Moller AR. *Intraoperative Neurophysiological Monitoring*, 2nd edn. Totowa, NJ: Humana Press, 2006.
6. Myles PS, Leslie K, McNeil J, *et al.* Bispectral index monitoring to prevent awareness during anaesthesia: the B-Aware randomised controlled trial. *Lancet* 2004;**363**:1757–63.
7. Grundy BL. Monitoring of sensory evoked potentials during neurosurgical operations: methods and applications. *Neurosurgery* 1982;**11**:556–75.
8. Grundy BL, Nelson PB, Doyle E, *et al.* Intraoperative loss of somatosensory-evoked potentials predicts loss of spinal cord function. *Anesthesiology* 1982;**57**:321–2.
9. Kodama K, Goto T, Sato A, *et al.* Standard and limitation of intraoperative monitoring of the visual evoked potential. *Acta Neurochir (Wien)* 2010;**152**:643–8.
10. Deletis V, Sala F. Intraoperative neurophysiological monitoring of the spinal cord during spinal cord and spine surgery: a review focus on the corticospinal tracts. *Clin Neurophysiol* 2008;**119**:248–64.
11. Moller AR, Jannetta PJ. Monitoring of facial nerve function during removal of acoustic tumor. *Am J Otol* 1985; Suppl:27–9.
12. Delgado TE, Bucheit WA, Rosenholtz HR, *et al.* Intraoperative monitoring of facila muscle evoked responses obtained by intracranial stimulation of the facila nerve: a more accurate technique for facila nerve dissection. *Neurosurgery* 1979;**4**:418–21.
13. Eisner W, Schmid UD, Reulen HJ, *et al.* The mapping and continuous monitoring of the intrinsic motor nuclei during brain stem surgery. *Neurosurgery* 1995;**37**:255–65.
14. Romstock J, Strauss C, Fahlbusch R. Continuous electromyography monitoring of motor cranial nerves during cerebellopontine angle surgery. *J Neurosurg* 2000;**93**:586–93.
15. Strauss C, Romstock J, Nimsky C, *et al.* Intraoperative identification of motor areas of the rhomboid fossa using direct stimulation. *J Neurosurg* 1993;**79**:393–9.
16. Fritschi JA, Reulen HJ, Spetzler RF, *et al.* Cavernous malformations of the brain

stem. A review of 139 cases. *Acta Neurochir (Wien)* 1994;**130**:35–46.

17. Deletis V, Vodusek DB. Intraoperative recording of the bulbocavernosus reflex. *Neurosurgery* 1997;**40**:88–92.
18. Ebeling U, Reulen HJ. Space-occupying lesions of the sensori-motor region. *Adv Tech Stand Neurosurg* 1995;**22**:137–81.
19. Ojemann G, Ojemann J, Lettich E, *et al.* Cortical language localization in left-dominant hemisphere. An electrical stimulation mapping investigation in 117 patients. *J Neurosurg* 1989;**71**:316–26.
20. Cedzich C, Taniguchi M, Schafer S, *et al.* Somatosensory evoked potential phase reversal and direct motor cortex stimulation during surgery in and around the central region. *Neurosurgery* 1996;**38**:962–70.
21. Stippich C, Kress B, Ochmann H, *et al.* [Preoperative functional magnetic resonance tomography (FMRI) in patients with rolandic brain tumors: indication, investigation strategy, possibilities and limitations of clinical application.] *Rofo* 2003;**175**:1042–50.
22. Juenger H, Ressel V, Braun C, *et al.* Misleading functional magnetic resonance imaging mapping of the cortical hand representation in a 4-year-old boy with an arteriovenous malformation of the central region. *J Neurosurg Pediatr* 2009;**4**:333–8.
23. Picht T, Schmidt S, Brandt S, *et al.* Preoperative functional mapping for rolandic brain tumor surgery: comparison of navigated transcranial magnetic stimulation to direct cortical stimulation. *Neurosurgery* 2011;**69**:581–8.
24. Coburger J, Musahl C, Henkes H, *et al.* Comparison of navigated transcranial magnetic stimulation and functional magnetic resonance imaging for preoperative mapping in rolandic tumor surgery. *Neurosurg Rev* 2013;**36**:65–76.

Chapter 9

Neuroanesthesia for treatment of arteriovenous malformations

Alana M. Flexman and Adrian W. Gelb

Introduction

Anesthesia for neurovascular procedures must integrate the patient's comorbid conditions, the effect of anesthesia on the patient's neurophysiology, and considerations unique to the proposed procedure. This chapter will provide an overview of the basic principles of clinical neurophysiology, the interactions between anesthesia and the brain, and the specific anesthetic considerations for patients undergoing treatment of arteriovenous malformations (AVMs).

Cerebrovascular physiology

Cerebral blood flow (CBF) is regulated through several physiological mechanisms during anesthesia. These mechanisms include (1) cerebral autoregulation, (2) arterial carbon dioxide and oxygen tension alterations, (3) coupling of CBF to cerebral metabolism, and (4) intrinsic neural control.

Cerebral autoregulation is an adaptive mechanism through which the brain maintains a constant CBF over a wide range of systemic perfusion pressures (Fig. 9.1). In the typical healthy adult brain, CBF is constant for a mean arterial pressure ranging approximately from 60 to 160 mmHg (cerebral perfusion pressure of 50–150 mmHg), although the boundaries of autoregulation vary depending on patient factors and there is normally a very wide interindividual variation in the autoregulatory range. Factors such as chronic uncontrolled hypertension and anemia may shift the autoregulatory curve to the right [1,2]. Outside the range of autoregulation, CBF becomes linearly related to cerebral perfusion pressure and the brain may be vulnerable to hypo- or hyperperfusion. Furthermore, cerebral autoregulation may be globally or regionally disrupted in proximity to an intracranial hematoma or an AVM (see also Chapter 4).

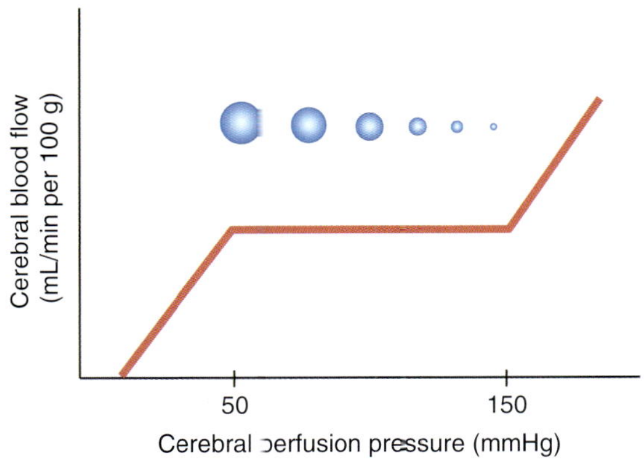

Fig. 9.1. The cerebral autoregulatory curve. Cerebral blood flow is maintained at a constant level through a wide range of systemic blood pressures through alterations in blood vessel diameter (circles).

Under anesthesia, several factors can be manipulated to influence CBF and, by extension, cerebral blood volume (CBV) as well as intracranial pressure (ICP) and intraoperative brain swelling. These include arterial partial pressure of carbon dioxide ($Paco_2$), arterial partial pressure of oxygen (Pao_2), cerebral metabolic rate (CMR) of oxygen ($CMRo_2$), and temperature. Reducing the $Paco_2$ through hyperventilation is common practice during neurosurgical procedures to reduce CBF, CBV, brain bulk, and ICP. The effects of hyperventilation are immediate; it reduces CBF by 3–4% per 1 mmHg change in $Paco_2$ in a linear fashion between 20 and 80 mmHg [1]. Alterations in $Paco_2$ modulate CBF through changes in the pH of the perivascular cerebrospinal fluid. These effects result from increases in the bicarbonate levels of the cerebrospinal fluid; they are transient and and last approximately 6 to 8 hours [3]. Reductions in the Pao_2 to approximately <50 mmHg lead to dramatic increases in CBF.

Changes in $CMRo_2$ effect changes in regional CBF through flow–metabolism coupling. When intact, this physiological mechanism ensures that CBF is proportional to metabolic demands; however, it may be disrupted by anesthetic agents and severe intracranial pathology. In addition, it may cause excessive CBF during periods of seizure activity because of the significant increase in $CMRo_2$. Similarly, decreases in temperature reduce $CMRo_2$ and, therefore, CBF. Cerebral blood flow decreases 7% for every 1°C decrease in body temperature below 37°C [4].

Comprehensive Management of Arteriovenous Malformations of the Brain and Spine, ed. Robert F. Spetzler, Douglas S. Kondziolka, Randall T. Higashida, and M. Yashar S. Kalani. Published by Cambridge University Press.

Table 9.1. The effect of selected anesthetic agents on cerebral blood flow, cerebral metabolic rate for oxygen, and intracranial pressure

Agent	Cerebral blood flow	Cerebral metabolic rate for oxygen	Intracranial pressure
Propofol	↓↓	↓↓	↓↓
Opioids	↓	↓	–/↓
Benzodiazepines	↓	↓	↓
Volatile anesthetics	↑	↓	–/↑[a]
Nitrous oxide	↑	↑	↑
Ketamine[b]	↓	↓	↓
Etomidate	↓	↓	↓

[a] Volatile anesthetics may increase ICP at high doses (0.7–1.0 minimum alveolar concentration for desflurane, and isoflurane, >1 for sevoflurane).
[b] In the presence of general anesthesia.

Anesthesia and cerebrovascular physiology

Anesthetic agents influence cerebrovascular physiology through direct effects on the vasculature and indirect alterations of CMR. The effects of different anesthetic agents on cerebrovascular physiology are summarized in Table 9.1. Intravenous anesthetic agents such as propofol potently suppress $CMRo_2$ and vasoconstrict the cerebral vessels via flow–metabolism coupling. Propofol has been shown to preserve cerebral autoregulation in both low and high doses [5]. Benzodiazepines and opioid anesthetic agents cause a similar, but much less significant, reduction in CBF and $CMRo_2$. Propofol given together with an opioid agent such as remifentanil produces a predictable reduction in CBF, $CMRo_2$, and ICP while preserving cerebral autoregulation, and it is therefore considered an ideal agent for patients with decreased intracranial compliance or increased ICP [6].

In contrast, volatile agents such as desflurane and sevoflurane are direct cerebral vasodilators and can potentially increase ICP, particularly at greater than 0.7 minimum alveolar concentration (MAC). Volatile anesthetics impair cerebral autoregulation and flow–metabolism coupling in a dose-dependent fashion, with desflurane having this effect at <1 MAC and sevoflurane at >1 MAC [7]. The cerebral vasodilation induced by volatile anesthetics is partially offset by vasoconstriction induced by $CMRo_2$ suppression at low doses; however, the vasodilatory effect predominates at high doses. The generally accepted order of vasodilating potency is desflurane > isoflurane > sevoflurane [5].

The use of nitrous oxide in neurosurgery is controversial because of several theoretical disadvantages. Nitrous oxide is associated with vasodilation of the cerebral vessels and an increase in CMR [8]. Furthermore, nitrous oxide is known to increase the size of enclosed gas spaces, including pneumocephalus, which is universally seen after open craniotomy [9]. Despite these theoretical concerns, there is no convincing evidence that the use of nitrous oxide, in conjunction with other anesthetic agents, is associated with worse outcomes in neurosurgical patients [10].

Opioids cause a reduction in both CBF and $CMRo_2$, but to a much lesser degree than agents such as propofol. In addition, opioids preserve cerebral autoregulation and minimize the hemodynamic response to surgical stimulation. For these reasons, opioids are commonly used as adjuncts to either volatile agents or propofol for maintenance of anesthesia. Benzodiazepines (e.g., midazolam) similarly cause a mild degree of cerebral vasoconstriction and reduction in $CMRo_2$.

The use of ketamine and etomidate in neurosurgical patients is controversial. Ketamine has traditionally been avoided in patients with decreased intracranial compliance because of earlier evidence that ketamine resulted in elevations in ICP. Previous data demonstrated an increase in CBF, $CMRo_2$, and ICP associated with high doses of ketamine used in isolation [11,12]. However, several more recent studies have demonstrated that ketamine reduces ICP when used in conjunction with other anesthetic agents and controlled ventilation [13]. Similarly, the role of etomidate in the neurosurgical setting is the subject of debate. Unlike many other anesthetic agents, etomidate is associated with less hypotension during induction and reductions in CBF, $CMRo_2$, and ICP. Despite these benefits, further research has suggested that etomidate may exacerbate cerebral ischemia in experimental animal models and may not be appropriate for neurosurgical patients [14]. Furthermore, even a single dose of etomidate has been associated with adrenal suppression and mortality in critically ill patients [15].

Intracranial hypertension and management

Patients undergoing treatment for AVMs may present with increased ICP, particularly if they present with an intracranial bleed. In addition, these patients frequently experience intraoperative brain swelling and further neurological injury during resection of an AVM. Patients with evidence of increased ICP preoperatively (i.e., midline shift or increased ICP) have been found to be at increased risk of intraoperative brain swelling after opening of the dura mater [16]. An anesthetic approach can be used to manage increased ICP and intraoperative brain swelling.

Brain tissue, cerebrospinal fluid, and CBV make up the intracranial compartment; reduction of ICP must target one of these components. Brain tissue volume can be modified through the administration of hyperosmotic solutions such as mannitol or hypertonic saline. Osmotic agents are very effective and work by drawing fluid out of brain cells and into the intravascular compartment. At high doses, mannitol may be associated with adverse effects such as hyper- or hypokalemia, significant intravascular volume loss, and congestive heart failure immediately following administration [17,18]. Furosemide, a loop diuretic, is occasionally given together with mannitol to reduce brain water, although the clinical efficacy of this drug in humans is not well established [19,20]. Steroids such as dexamethasone are commonly given to reduce tissue swelling induced by intracranial lesions or surgery; however, the beneficial effects may be delayed.

Many strategies to reduce ICP aim to reduce the CBV. Hyperventilation, for example, effectively reduces CBF and improves ICP. Intraoperative brain swelling and ICP was significantly lower in hyperventilated patients ($Paco_2$, 25 ± 2 mmHg) than in normal ventilated patients ($Paco_2$, 37 ± 2 mmHg) [21]. Intravenous anesthetic agents such as propofol are potent vasoconstrictors as a result of flow–metabolism coupling, in contrast to the volatile anesthetic agents (e.g., desflurane, sevoflurane) that dilate the cerebral vessels. For this reason, propofol-based anesthetics are often preferred in patients with decreased intracranial compliance. Despite the theoretical benefits, the evidence is conflicting about whether intravenous anesthesia reduces intraoperative brain swelling more effectively than volatile anesthetic agents [21].

Cerebral venous drainage also influences CBV. For example, improving cerebral venous drainage by placing the patient in a head-up position can significantly reduce brain swelling and ICP [22]. In addition, constriction around the neck should be minimized (e.g., endotracheal tube ties, collars) to improve venous outflow.

Anesthesia and cerebral protection

Neuroprotection with anesthetic agents has been the subject of intense research. Several potential pathways involved in secondary ischemic injury have been targeted, including apoptosis, inflammation, oxidative stress, and inhibition of protein synthesis [23]. In controlled animal models of cerebral injury and ischemia, many anesthetic agents, including both volatile and intravenous anesthetic agents, have been shown to have neuroprotective effects [10]. Most anesthetics significantly reduce $CMRo_2$ and, theoretically, should reduce cerebral injury during periods of oxygen deprivation. Unfortunately, the benefits seen in experimental animal models of cerebral ischemia do not correlate well with clinical observations in humans [10]. A large clinical trial (GALA) randomized patients undergoing carotid endarterectomy to either general or local anesthesia and did not find any differences in stroke or neurological status postoperatively [24]. Similarly, a post hoc analysis from the Intraoperative Hypothermia Aneurysm Surgery Trial (IHAST) found no benefit from pharmacological agents given with or without hypothermia [25].

Hypothermia has also been investigated extensively for neuroprotection. Similar to anesthetic agents, experimental animal models of focal and global ischemia have demonstrated beneficial effects of hypothermia in reducing cerebral infarct size and deficit, but human data are conflicting. Positive neurological outcomes with hypothermia have been seen in clinical trials on patients with cardiac arrest, adult cardiovascular surgery, and neonatal asphyxia [26–29]. A large, randomized clinical trial comparing mild hypothermia to normothermia in aneurysm surgery failed to demonstrate a benefit in any of the short- or long-term neuropsychological parameters, and hypothermic patients had an increased incidence of bacteremia [25,30]. Studies in traumatic brain injury provide conflicting evidence, and a Cochrane review did not support routine use of hypothermia [31]. Hyperthermia, in contrast, is strongly associated with poor neurological outcome, and it should be avoided when possible [32,33].

Fluid management

The current literature on fluid administration in neurosurgical patients is limited. Hypotonic fluids are typically avoided due to the movement of free water from the intravascular compartment into brain tissue, with resultant cerebral edema [17]. In contrast, hyperosmolar solutions such as mannitol and hypertonic saline are commonly used to draw water out of brain tissue and reduce ICP. Intravenous solutions containing glucose are usually avoided due to the detrimental neurological effects of hyperglycemia.

Colloid solutions containing albumin or synthetic starches are commonly used in the operating room, although the safety of these products in neurosurgical patients is not clear. A subgroup analysis of patients with traumatic brain injury included in a randomized trial compared albumin with saline and demonstrated worse outcomes in patients who received albumin [34]. In addition, the increased risk of coagulopathy associated with synthetic starch solutions may precipitate intracranial bleeding in neurosurgical patients [35].

The existing evidence provides limited guidance on the appropriate transfusion threshold for patients with neurosurgical pathology or brain injury [36]. Patients undergoing resection of AVMs are at risk for sudden, massive blood loss. In a retrospective review, approximately one-third of patients undergoing embolization followed by resection of AVMs required a blood transfusion [37]. The decision to transfuse a patient must take into account the patient's comorbid disease, severity of neurological compromise, and degree of ongoing bleeding. Both transfusion and anemia are repeatedly associated with worse neurological outcomes in observational studies of brain-injured patients [38,39]. A recent study showed that hemoglobin levels <9 g/dL were associated with increased evidence of cerebral tissue hypoxia in patients with subarachnoid hemorrhage [40].

Perioperative evaluation

The preoperative evaluation of patients with AVMs must focus on not only the AVM but also on the patient's coexisting disease. In addition to a typical anesthetic evaluation, the anesthesiologist assesses the patient's presenting complaint, current neurological status, complications such as seizure activity, and evidence of elevated ICP if the AVM has ruptured. Comorbid conditions are also evaluated, including cardiovascular and respiratory illnesses that may alter both the anesthetic management and perioperative risk assessment of patients. Rare diseases and hereditary disorders (e.g., hereditary hemorrhagic telangiectasia) associated with intracranial or spinal AVMs should be noted. On examination, the patient's baseline vital signs will be documented, with specific attention to blood pressure as this will guide intraoperative management.

Investigations typically include blood work to determine the patient's hemoglobin, electrolytes, and renal function, particularly if contrast administration is planned. In addition, a blood group and antibody screen should be done in all patients, given the potential for significant blood loss. Neurological imaging may be reviewed by the anesthesiologist to assess for evidence of raised ICP. Occasionally, the anesthesiologist will review the imaging with the neurosurgeon to better understand the intraoperative risks and surgical plan.

The anesthesiologist will advise the patient or nursing staff on medications that will be administered preoperatively. Some medications, such as hypoglycemic agents and diuretics, are withheld once the patient is fasting. Most antihypertensives, with the exception of angiotensin-converting enzyme inhibitors (e.g., ramipril) and angiotensin receptor blockers (e.g., candesartan), are continued up until surgery. Antiepileptic medications should be continued throughout the perioperative period to reduce the risk of seizures. Premedication with a benzodiazepine may be offered to anxious patients, although excessive sedation should be avoided preoperatively in patients with increased ICP.

Perioperative monitoring

Hemodynamic monitoring

Provision of anesthesia for neurosurgical procedures requires increased monitoring of hemodynamic and neurological parameters. Careful monitoring and control of hemodynamic parameters is essential for patients with AVMs because of potential hyper- and hypoperfusion states. These patients may have significant hemodynamic changes during induction of anesthesia, laryngoscopy and intubation, pinning, and surgical stimulation. Close hemodynamic monitoring is also warranted in the early postoperative period given the potential risk of intracranial hemorrhage following resection. In addition, these patients may require intraoperative blood sampling. Neuroanesthesiologists must accurately determine $Paco_2$ as hyperventilation may be required to facilitate surgical exposure. Furthermore, patients undergoing treatment of AVMs may experience significant intraoperative blood loss and require serial blood hematocrit determinations. Finally, these patients may require correction of electrolyte abnormalities and hyperglycemia, both common in this population. For these reasons, invasive hemodynamic monitors such as intra-arterial and central venous catheters are commonly inserted in addition to standard ASA (American Society of Anesthesiologists) monitors (inspired oxygen sensor, end-tidal carbon dioxide, noninvasive blood pressure monitors, electrocardiography, pulse oximetry, and temperature).

Neurological monitoring

In addition to hemodynamic monitors, many centers employ intraoperative neurological monitoring. These monitors include cerebral oximetry, jugular bulb saturation, and processed electroencephalography to monitor the patient's level of consciousness. Although there is no current consensus on the use of these monitors during neurosurgical procedures, many institutions use them to guide anesthetic management.

Anesthesia and neurophysiological monitoring

Intraoperative neurophysiological monitoring is commonly used for resection of intracranial and spinal AVMs. A combination of sensory and motor evoked potentials, electroencephalography, and electromyelography monitoring is often used, particularly when surgery is done in eloquent or ischemically vulnerable areas in the brain or spinal cord [41]. Anesthetic factors can have a significant impact on the quality of the monitoring, and excellent communication between the neurophysiologists, surgeons, and anesthesiologists is essential. (See Chapter 8 for a detailed discussion on neurophysiological monitoring.)

Several intraoperative physiological variables can influence neurophysiological monitoring, including hypotension, hypothermia, anemia, and electrolyte imbalances. Mean arterial blood pressure is likely the most important modifiable factor influencing neurophysiological monitoring, and inadequate cerebral or spinal perfusion pressure may result in suppression of evoked potentials [42]. Augmentation of systemic blood pressure with vasoactive drugs may be required if evoked potentials become depressed.

Anesthetic agents can profoundly alter electrophysiological monitoring. Volatile anesthetics can significantly increase the latency and amplitude of evoked potentials, particularly at doses >0.7 MAC. Sensory and motor evoked potentials are minimally suppressed by opioids (e.g., fentanyl, remifentanil, and sufentanil) and benzodiazepines (e.g., midazolam, diazepam, and lorazepam). Muscle relaxants should be avoided when motor evoked potential and/or electromyelography monitoring is used.

Anesthetic considerations for specific procedures

In order to provide optimal care, neuroanesthesiologists must consider the specific proposed procedure as well as individual patient factors. The basic principles of cerebral physiology must be followed, although the choice of specific anesthetic agents or monitors may vary with familiarity and institutional preference in the absence of concrete outcome data. Communication between the neuroanesthesiologists, neurosurgeons, neurointerventionalists, and nurses on the healthcare team is essential for the best patient outcome.

Resection of intracranial arteriovenous malformations

Several common considerations apply to patients undergoing craniotomy and resection of AVMs. These considerations include (1) maintaining adequate cerebral perfusion pressure and preventing secondary neurological injury, (2) providing optimal operating conditions including a "slack" brain, (3) facilitating rapid neurological assessment postoperatively, and (4) ensuring a safe position for prolonged procedures.

The anesthesiologist must anticipate and mitigate hemodynamic instability throughout the perioperative period to ensure adequate cerebral perfusion pressure and to minimize both secondary injury and the risk of intracranial bleeding as a result of excessive hypertension. Hemodynamic alterations typically occur during induction of anesthesia, laryngoscopy, pinning of the head frame, surgical stimulation of opening the cranium, and emergence from anesthesia. Patients undergoing resection in close proximity to vital brainstem structures may also experience bradycardia, hypertension, or hypotension. The "slack" brain is optimal for the neurosurgeon as it reduces retraction pressure and facilitates exposure. Typically this is accomplished with mild to moderate hyperventilation and 0.5–1 g/kg mannitol. Further interventions such as head-up positioning, hyperventilation, and total intravenous anesthesia may be used if significant brain edema is encountered during the procedure. Neurological assessment of the patient is ideally done immediately after extubation. Although many anesthetic regimens are used successfully, the ultra-short-acting opioid remifentanil is often used intraoperatively to facilitate early neurological assessment of patients postoperatively.

In addition, the anesthesiologist will prepare for several possible perioperative complications. Given the vascular nature of the lesion, an important complication is intraoperative hemorrhage. Typically, large-bore peripheral and/or central intravenous access will be obtained following induction, and blood products should be immediately available. Another important potential complication is intraoperative venous air embolism. Air may be entrained through open venous structures and obstruct cardiac output in the heart and gas exchange in the lungs. Anesthetic management is primarily supportive by providing 100% oxygen, fluid resuscitation, and hemodynamic support. The most important factor is prevention of further entrainment of air, and additional monitors (e.g., precordial Doppler) may be used for early detection of air. Procedures on the posterior fossa are associated with an increased risk of venous air embolism [43].

Finally, a carefully controlled emergence from anesthesia is critical. Ideally, the patient will have minimal coughing and gagging, which can precipitate increased intracranial and vascular pressures. Hemodynamics must be carefully controlled, typically with titrated doses of antihypertensive agents such as labetalol and hydralazine.

Endovascular treatment of arteriovenous malformations

Interventional neuroradiology procedures are the fastest growing neurosurgical procedure and pose unique challenges for the anesthesiologist [44]. The anesthetic considerations are similar to those for surgical procedures, with the additional considerations of (1) remote location of the radiology suite, (2) requirement for a motionless patient during radiological imaging, and (3) potential complications of intracranial vessel rupture or occlusion within a closed cranium.

The patients who undergo embolization of AVMs or dural arteriovenous fistulae range from healthy outpatients to critically ill patients following rupture of their AVM or fistula. These procedures are typically performed in a location remote from the operating room, and potential delays in urgently obtaining additional equipment and personnel must be considered. In addition, the patient may require prolonged time in transfer to the postanesthesia recovery room or intensive care unit, with full monitoring and resuscitation equipment available. During the procedure, the anesthesiologist has limited access to the patient, including the airway, in the event that intervention is required, such as in the case of oversedation, seizure, or rupture of the malformations. Finally, anticoagulation (heparin) is often required for these procedures; clear communication between the interventionalist and anesthesia teams is essential to avoid excessive or inadequate anticoagulation.

Either general or local anesthesia with sedation may be used for these procedures, and the choice of anesthesia is often guided by a discussion between the interventionalist and anesthesia teams. The advantages of local anesthesia are the ability to monitor the neurological status of the patient throughout the procedure and the avoidance of the risks of general anesthesia, although there is a risk of adverse respiratory complications with an unsecured airway [45]. General anesthesia is often chosen for long complex procedures, and this technique has other advantages, including providing a motionless patient with reduced imaging artifact. General anesthesia is preferred by many patients, as these procedures can be long and uncomfortable [46].

The management of anesthesia for interventional neuroradiology procedures is similar to that for surgical management of AVMs. Premedication, as well as induction and maintenance of anesthesia, is administered on a case-by-case basis. The use of invasive monitors is typically less common than in the operating room, although intra-arterial blood pressure monitoring is useful during periods of hemodynamic instability and in the event of rupture of the AVM [47]. In addition, beat-to-beat blood pressure monitoring is valuable if induced hypotension and reduced flow in the feeding artery of an intracranial AVM are required during glue injection [48]. If required urgently, invasive arterial pressure monitoring can be quickly obtained from the femoral sheath used for the procedure.

Experienced neuroanesthesiologists are prepared for rare but disastrous complications of intracranial vessel occlusion or rupture. In the event of occlusion of a cerebral vessel, the blood pressure may be augmented to increase collateral flow until perfusion is restored. If rupture of an intracranial vessel occurs, rapid reversal of heparin with protamine is required (1 mg protamine for each 100 U heparin given) [48]. These decisions should only be implemented after discussion with the interventionalist. As the patient may require surgical management, the anesthesiologist must rapidly prepare for safe transfer to the operating room.

Awake surgery

Occasionally, patients may undergo "awake" resection of AVMs to facilitate neurophysiological mapping and preservation of eloquent areas. These patients pose a particular challenge because the neuroanesthesiologist must carefully balance patient comfort and intermittent sedation with ensuring adequate ventilation and oxygenation in patients fixed in surgical pins. Although the specific anesthetic technique varies by institution and patient, "awake" craniotomies typically involve an asleep/awake/asleep method in which the patient is sedated during the opening of the cranium and resection of the lesion with a period of minimal sedation in between to allow for neurological testing. Potential pitfalls of awake neurosurgery include airway obstruction, hypoxia, and hypercarbia associated with oversedation as well as patient intolerance and anxiety during the procedure. In addition, the anesthesiologist must be prepared to treat seizures induced by direct brain stimulation during mapping. Significant hemorrhage in an awake patient can be very challenging as patients become apprehensive and anxious while hypotension results in agitation and restless behavior.

Children with arteriovenous malformations

Children form a significant subset of patients who require treatment of AVMs. The general anesthetic principles are similar to those for adults, with some additional considerations. Children, particularly infants and small children, have unique anatomical and physiological features that must be taken into account. The infant brain is proportionally larger and receives an increased fraction of cardiac output compared with the adult brain. In addition, the absolute systemic blood volume is smaller than that of adults. For these reasons, anesthetic providers must be vigilant about intraoperative blood loss and consider using invasive hemodynamic monitors and large-bore intravenous access. In addition, awake children will often not tolerate insertion of an intravenous line and require an inhalational induction. Very young infants and those with persistent fetal shunts are at increased risk of intraoperative paradoxical air embolism. Neuroanesthesiologists should carefully de-air intravenous lines and take steps to minimize the risk of air entrainment. Finally, children with an AVM may shunt a large portion of their cardiac output through the vascular malformations. Shunting can lead to inadequate systemic perfusion and perioperative hemodynamic instability and hypoxia.

Conclusions

Patients undergoing treatment of AVMs of the brain and spine present several unique considerations for the neuroanesthesiologists. Clear communication between the neurosurgery, neurointerventionalist, and anesthesiology teams about the management plan and potential complications is essential to providing safe care.

References

1. Dagal A, Lam AM. Cerebral autoregulation and anesthesia. *Curr Opin Anaesthesiol* 2009;**22**:547–52.
2. Vavilala MS, Lee LA, Morris GP, *et al.* Cerebral autoregulation before and after blood transfusion in a child. *J Neurosurg Anesthesiol* 2001;**13**:233–6.
3. Andrews RJ, Bringas JR, Alonzo G. Cerebrospinal fluid pH and PCO_2 rapidly follow arterial blood pH and PCO_2 with changes in ventilation. *Neurosurgery* 1994;**34**:466–70.
4. Polderman KH. Mechanisms of action, physiological effects, and complications of hypothermia. *Crit Care Med* 2009;**37**:S186–202.
5. Strebel S, Lam AM, Matta B, *et al.* Dynamic and static cerebral autoregulation during isoflurane, desflurane, and propofol anesthesia. *Anesthesiology* 1995;**83**:66–76.
6. Cole CD, Gottfried ON, Gupta DK, *et al.* Total intravenous anesthesia: advantages for intracranial surgery. *Neurosurgery* 2007;**61**:369–77.
7. Engelhard K, Werner C. Inhalational or intravenous anesthetics for craniotomies? Pro inhalational. *Curr Opin Anaesthesiol* 2006;**19**:504–8.
8. Dinsmore J. Anaesthesia for elective neurosurgery. *Br J Anaesth* 2007;**99**:68–74.
9. Saidman LJ, Eger EI. Change in cerebrospinal fluid pressure during pneumoencephalography under nitrous oxide anesthesia. *Anesthesiology* 1965;**26**:67–72.
10. Todd MM. Outcomes after neuroanesthesia and neurosurgery: what makes a difference. *Anesthesiol Clin* 2012;**30**:399–408.
11. Takeshita H, Okuda Y, Sari A. The effects of ketamine on cerebral circulation and metabolism in man. *Anesthesiology* 1972;**36**:69–75.
12. Shaprio HM, Wyte SR, Harris AB. Ketamine anaesthesia in patients with intracranial pathology. *Br J Anaesth* 1972;**44**:1200–4.
13. Himmelseher S, Durieux ME. Revising a dogma: ketamine for patients with neurological injury? *Anesth Analg* 2005;**101**:524–34.
14. Drummond JC, McKay LD, Cole DJ, *et al.* The role of nitric oxide synthase inhibition in the adverse effects of etomidate in the setting of focal cerebral ischemia in rats. *Anesth Analg* 2005;**100**:841–6.
15. Chan CM, Mitchell AL, Shorr AF. Etomidate is associated with mortality and adrenal insufficiency in sepsis: a meta-analysis. *Crit Care Med* 2012;**40**:2945–53.
16. Rasmussen M, Bundgaard H, Cold GE. Craniotomy for supratentorial brain tumors: risk factors for brain swelling after opening the dura mater. *J Neurosurg* 2004;**101**:621–6.
17. Tommasino C. Fluids and the neurosurgical patient. *Anesthesiol Clin North America* 2002;**20**:329–46.
18. Manninen PH, Lam AM, Gelb AW, *et al.* The effect of high-dose mannitol on serum and urine electrolytes and osmolality in neurosurgical patients. *Can J Anaesth* 1987;**34**:442–6.
19. Thenuwara K, Todd MM, Brian JE, Jr. Effect of mannitol and furosemide on plasma osmolality and brain water. *Anesthesiology* 2002;**96**:416–21.
20. Todd MM, Cutkomp J, Brian JE. Influence of mannitol and furosemide, alone and in combination, on brain water content after fluid percussion injury. *Anesthesiology* 2006;**105**:1176–81.
21. Gelb AW, Craen RA, Rao GS, *et al.* Does hyperventilation improve operating condition during supratentorial craniotomy? A multicenter randomized crossover trial. *Anesth Analg* 2008;**106**:585–94.
22. Tankisi A, Cold GE. Optimal reverse Trendelenburg position in patients undergoing craniotomy for cerebral tumors. *J Neurosurg* 2007;**106**:239–44.
23. Fukuda S, Warner DS. Cerebral protection. *Br J Anaesth* 2007;**99**:10–17.
24. Gough MJ, Bodenham A, Horrocks M, *et al.* GALA: an international multicentre randomised trial comparing general anaesthesia versus local

anaesthesia for carotid surgery. *Trials* 2008;**9**:28.

25. Hindman BJ, Bayman EO, Pfisterer WK, *et al.* No association between intraoperative hypothermia or supplemental protective drug and neurologic outcomes in patients undergoing temporary clipping during cerebral aneurysm surgery: findings from the Intraoperative Hypothermia for Aneurysm Surgery Trial. *Anesthesiology* 2010;**112**:86–101.
26. Bernard SA, Gray TW, Buist MD, *et al.* Treatment of comatose survivors of out-of-hospital cardiac arrest with induced hypothermia. *N Engl J Med* 2002;**346**:557–63.
27. Grigore AM, Murray CF, Ramakrishna H, *et al.* A core review of temperature regimens and neuroprotection during cardiopulmonary bypass: does rewarming rate matter? *Anesth Analg* 2009;**109**:1741–51.
28. Augoustides JG, Floyd TF, McGarvey ML, *et al.* Major clinical outcomes in adults undergoing thoracic aortic surgery requiring deep hypothermic circulatory arrest: quantification of organ-based perioperative outcome and detection of opportunities for perioperative intervention. *J Cardiothorac Vasc Anesth* 2005;**19**:446–52.
29. Tagin MA, Woolcott CG, Vincer MJ, *et al.* Hypothermia for neonatal hypoxic ischemic encephalopathy: an updated systematic review and meta-analysis. *Arch Pediatr Adolesc Med* 2012;**166**:558–66.
30. Todd MM, Hindman BJ, Clarke WR, *et al.* Mild intraoperative hypothermia during surgery for intracranial aneurysm. *N Engl J Med* 2005;**352**:135–45.
31. Sydenham E, Roberts I, Alderson P. Hypothermia for traumatic head injury. *Cochrane Database Syst Rev* 2009; CD001048.
32. Hajat C, Hajat S, Sharma P. Effects of poststroke pyrexia on stroke outcome: a meta-analysis of studies in patients. *Stroke* 2000;**31**:410–14.
33. Todd MM, Hindman BJ, Clarke WR, *et al.* Perioperative fever and outcome in surgical patients with aneurysmal subarachnoid hemorrhage. *Neurosurgery* 2009;**64**:897–908.
34. Myburgh J, Cooper DJ, Finfer S, *et al.* Saline or albumin for fluid resuscitation in patients with traumatic brain injury. *N Engl J Med* 2007;**357**:874–84.
35. Hartog CS, Bauer M, Reinhart K. The efficacy and safety of colloid resuscitation in the critically ill. *Anesth Analg* 2011;**112**:156–64.
36. McEwen J, Huttunen KH. Transfusion practice in neuroanesthesia. *Curr Opin Anaesthesiol* 2009;**22**:566–71.
37. Ledezma CJ, Hoh BL, Carter BS, *et al.* Complications of cerebral arteriovenous malformation embolization: multivariate analysis of predictive factors. *Neurosurgery* 2006;**58**:602–11.
38. Naidech AM, Jovanovic B, Wartenberg KE, *et al.* Higher hemoglobin is associated with improved outcome after subarachnoid hemorrhage. *Crit Care Med* 2007;**35**:2383–9.
39. Smith MJ, Le Roux PD, Elliott JP, *et al.* Blood transfusion and increased risk for vasospasm and poor outcome after subarachnoid hemorrhage. *J Neurosurg* 2004;**101**:1–7.
40. Oddo M, Milby A, Chen I, *et al.* Hemoglobin concentration and cerebral metabolism in patients with aneurysmal subarachnoid hemorrhage. *Stroke* 2009;**40**:1275–81.
41. Jameson LC, Sloan TB. Neurophysiologic monitoring in neurosurgery. *Anesthesiol Clin* 2012;**30**:311–31.
42. Miller C, Mirski M. Anesthesia considerations and intraoperative monitoring during surgery for arteriovenous malformations and dural arteriovenous fistulas. *Neurosurg Clin N Am* 2012;**23**:153–64.
43. Mirski MA, Lele AV, Fitzsimmons L, *et al.* Diagnosis and treatment of vascular air embolism. *Anesthesiology* 2007;**106**:164–77.
44. Hughey AB, Lesniak MS, Ansari SA, *et al.* What will anesthesiologists be anesthetizing? Trends in neurosurgical procedure usage. *Anesth Analg* 2010;**110**:1686–97.
45. Metzner J, Posner KL, Domino KB. The risk and safety of anesthesia at remote locations: the US closed claims analysis. *Curr Opin Anaesthesiol* 2009;**22**:502–8.
46. Schulenburg E, Matta B. Anaesthesia for interventional neuroradiology. *Curr Opin Anaesthesiol* 2011;**24**:426–32.
47. Lai YC, Manninen PH. Anesthesia for cerebral aneurysms: a comparison between interventional neuroradiology and surgery. *Can J Anaesth* 2001;**48**:391–5.
48. Lee CZ, Young WL. Anesthesia for endovascular neurosurgery and interventional neuroradiology. *Anesthesiol Clin* 2012;**30**:127–47.

Chapter 10

Classification of brain and spinal arteriovenous malformations and fistulae

Robert M. Koffie, Bradley A. Gross, and Rose Du

Introduction

Several classification systems for arteriovenous shunts of the neuroaxis have been proposed [1–5, 57]. Formally, these shunts are often stratified into arteriovenous malformations (AVMs), defined as having a nidus between shunted arterial and venous blood, and arteriovenous fistulae (AVFs), referring to a direct fistula between an artery and a vein. Typically, the term cerebral AVM implicates a parenchymal AVM with pial and sometimes dural arterial supply. Although the term pial fistula can be used to denote a fistula between a pial artery and vein, fistulae of the brain are more commonly dural AVFs (DAVFs) – a term often used synonymously with dural AVMs – to describe vascular shunts fed by meningeal arteries with drainage into either a major sinus or the leptomeningeal veins. Herein, we describe classification schemes for these lesions. Interestingly, those for cerebral AVMs are largely based on the risk of a particular intervention (e.g., surgery, radiosurgery or embolization); those for cerebral DAVFs are largely based on the natural history of the lesions, and those for spinal arteriovenous shunts are largely descriptive, correlating in part to both natural history and risk/indications for intervention.

Cerebral arteriovenous malformations

Patients with AVMs can be managed expectantly or actively treated with radiosurgery, endovascular embolization, or microsurgical resection [1,3,4]. Classification schemes have been developed to correlate with the risk of particular interventions along with the likelihood of a successful outcome [1,3]. Most of these classification schemes combine specific anatomical properties of the lesion, particularly nidus size, venous drainage pattern, and eloquence of the brain affected, as well as the number of feeding arteries, shunt flow, and clinical characteristics such as patient age and presentation modality.

Natural history

Despite the preponderance of AVM grading schemes for various treatment modalities [1,3,6], grading schemes for AVM hemorrhage risk or natural history are relatively rare and infrequently cited. The oft-cited overall annual hemorrhage rate for cerebral AVMs is reported to range from 2 to 4% per year [7–10]. However this is an overall rate derived from an exceedingly heterogeneous group of AVMs and, therefore, it has little meaning for individual AVMs unless specific risk factors for hemorrhage are considered. Several large natural history studies have underscored prior hemorrhage, deep location, deep venous drainage, and associated aneurysms as significant risk factors increasing the risk of hemorrhage in AVMs [7–10]. Pregnancy is another generally accepted risk factor [11], although it has not been well validated in prospective natural history studies, likely because of intuitive ethical limitations of carrying out such a study.

In the study of Stapf *et al.*, patients with unruptured superficial AVMs without exclusive deep venous drainage had an overall annual hemorrhage rate of 0.9% [12]. This rate increased significantly to 34% for ruptured deep AVMs with exclusively deep venous drainage. In a prospective study of 678 patients with AVMs, the annual hemorrhage rate was 4.6% per year for the entire cohort, increasing to 6.9% per year for patients with AVMs with associated aneurysms, and to 7.5% per year for patients with initial hemorrhagic presentation [13].

In an attempt to provide an AVM grading scheme correlating to natural history/hemorrhage risk, one study found that a history of prior bleed (relative risk [RR], 9.09), a single draining vein (RR, 1.66), and/or a diffuse AVM morphology (RR, 1.64) significantly increased the risk of AVM hemorrhage [14]. They proposed an AVM grading scheme stratifying patients into four risk groups (Table 10.1) [15]. Although this study highlighted an important characteristic that was not underscored by most other natural history studies (single draining vein), this grading scheme is infrequently employed. In the light of modern studies [13,16–18], most neurosurgeons focus on prior hemorrhage as a cardinal risk factor, with secondary factors including associated aneurysms, deep location, and deep venous drainage.

A statistical estimate for the lifetime risk of hemorrhage based on a multiplicative law of probability has been developed

Comprehensive Management of Arteriovenous Malformations of the Brain and Spine, ed. Robert F. Spetzler, Douglas S. Kondziolka, Randall T. Higashida, and M. Yashar S. Kalani. Published by Cambridge University Press.

Table 10.1. Natural history grading scheme according to Pollock *et al.*

Group (No. risk factors)	Annual hemorrhage rate (%)
Low risk (0)	0.99
Intermediate–low risk (1)	2.22
Intermediate–high risk (2)	3.72
High risk (3)	8.94

Modified from Pollock *et al.*, 1996 [14].

[19] and posits that if n is number of years left in life, and p is the annual risk of hemorrhage, then lifetime risk of hemorrhage R is:

$$R = (1 - [1 - p]^n)$$

Fundamental to this equation is the assumption that a constant yearly risk of hemorrhage occurs independent of behavior of the lesion over all years, which is likely inaccurate [17,20]. In addition, the equation is not very simple and clinically useful at the bedside and has, therefore, been simplified such that the risk of rupture is merely equal to 105 minus the patient's age [19,21]. While all these formulations and percentages are extensively reported in the literature [14,19], it is very likely that, as our understanding of AVMs increases over the years, factors such as genetics, hemodynamics, inflammation, intranidal angiogenesis, as well as the anatomical characteristics highlighted above will all be incorporated to generate a simple, applicable, and accurate natural history classification scheme for cerebral AVMs.

Surgical grading schemes

Luessenhop and Gennarelli [22] were among the first to formulate a popularized grading scheme for cerebral AVMs in 1977. They assigned grades I through IV, corresponding to the number of feeding arteries and the vascular territory origin of these feeders. An AVM supplied by multiple territories was graded based on the vascular territory with the largest number of feeders. Those AVMs with more than four feeding arteries were excluded from the grading scheme. The scheme was studied in a series of 49 patients where it became clear that grade I AVMs were associated with low risk, while higher-grade AVMs were associated with increased surgical morbidity, with grade III and IV AVMs being too risky to manage operatively, with a morbidity and mortality of 30% and 20%, respectively[22].

A subsequent grading scheme by Luessenhop and Rosa in 1984 [67] was based on the angiographic size of the AVM. Grade I denoted an AVM <2 cm, grade II denoted 2–4 cm, grade III 4–6 cm, and grade IV >6 cm. This grading system was evaluated in a series of 90 patients after surgical treatment of grades I and II AVMs and low morbidity (0 and 6%, respectively) and mortality (0% for both) was seen. High-grade lesions had a surgical morbidity and mortality of 44% and 12%, respectively, encouraging more conservative management of these AVMs. This classification system was quickly followed by that of Shi and Chen in 1986 [23], which was based on four main factors: AVM size, location and depth, arterial supply, and venous drainage. In this scheme, these four factors were divided into four grades as outlined in Table 10.2.

The grading scheme was explored in a surgical series of 100 patients; patients with AVMs grade I and II had excellent outcomes whereas those with grade III and IV AVMs had much higher morbidity/mortality (Table 10.2) [23]. While the Shi and Chen grading system was very effective at predicting surgical outcomes, its complexity made it difficult to implement clinically, precluding its widespread application.

The most widely cited and well-known classification scheme in the neurosurgical literature was published in 1986: the Spetzler–Martin grading scheme for surgical risk of AVM resection [1]. Like the Shi and Chen classification system, AVMs are classified anatomically into grades I–V, but only based on the size (points 1–3 for a size of 0–3, 3–6, and >6 cm, respectively), location (eloquent brain, 1 point; non-eloquent brain, 0 point), and venous drainage (superficial, 0 point; deep, 1 point) as outlined in Table 10.3. Radiological examples of Spetzler–Martin graded AVMs are shown in Fig. 10.1.

Grade VI is assigned to AVMs that are inoperable (e.g., intrinsic brainstem AVMs), which are not assigned categorical scores. In a clinical series of 100 patients, patients with Spetzler–Martin grade I AVMs had no minor deficits (defined as temporary worsening of neurological function, mild ataxia, or mild increase in brainstem deficit) or major deficits (defined as aphasia, hemianopsia, or hemiparesis) after surgery. Only 1 out of 21 patients with grade II AVMs had minor deficits, and none had major deficits. Of the 25 patients in the study with grade III AVMs, three had minor deficits and one had a major deficit postoperatively. Patients with grade IV and V AVMs did comparatively poorly with higher minor (grade IV, 20%; grade V, 19%) and major (grade IV, 7%; grade V, 12%) deficits. Other studies exploring the Spetzler–Martin grading scheme also confirmed these outcomes [24–27] and showed that the grading scheme was accurate at predicting operative morbidity and mortality in patients with cerebral AVMs.

To address the potential heterogeneity among grade III AVMs, Lawton *et al.* further stratified this subclass based on surgical results in 76 patients [28]. Patients with small grade III AVMs (3 cm) had a 3% surgical morbidity compared with those with medium-sized AVMs (3–6 cm), who had an intermediate surgical morbidity of 7%. Based on these findings, Lawton *et al.* proposed further subdividing Spetzler–Martin grade III AVMs into four subtypes: grade III– (representing those with size score of 1), grade III (representing those with size score 2 but located in non-eloquent brain), grade III+ (representing those with size score 2 but located in eloquent brain), and grade III* (representing AVMs with a size score of 3, which are rarely seen). Lawton posited that grade III– AVMs should be managed as though they were Spetzler–Martin grade II whereas grade III+ and III* should be managed similar to Spetzler–Martin grade IV lesions.

In 2011, Spetzler *et al.* modified their original classification scheme, grouping operable AVMs (grades I and II) into class A

Table 10.2. Shi and Chen classification scheme for arteriovenous malformations

Grade	Size (cm)	Location and depth	Arterial Supply	Venous drainage	Morbidity (%), mortality (%)
I	<2.5	Superficial and non-crucial	Single superficial branch of MCA or ACA	Single, emptying into superficial dural sinuses	0, 0
II	2.5–5.0	Superficial but in functional areas	Multiple superficial MCA or ACA branches	Multiple drainage into superficial dural sinuses	0, 0
III	5–7.5	Deep (e.g., interhemispheric deep cerebellum or cerebrum, corpus collosum, basal ganglia)	PCA branches, deep branches of MCA or ACA, or branches of vertebral artery	Deep cerebral vein emptying into vein of Galen, straight sinus; possible superficial venous drainage	20, 0
IV	>7.5	Deep, involving vital structures (e. g., brainstem, diencephalon)	Main branches of all three major cerebral arteries or the vertebrobasilar artery	Deep cerebral vein with huge dilatation or aneurysm-like structures	80, 20

MCA, middle cerebral artery; ACA, anterior cerebral artery; PCA, posterior cerebral artery.
Modified from Shi and Chen, 1986 [23].

Table 10.3. Spetzler–Martin grading system of arteriovenous malformations

Grade	Class	Characteristics[a]	Treatment
I	A	S1E0V0	Surgery
II	A	S1E0V1 S1E1V0 S2E0V0	Surgery
III	B	S1E1V1 (III–)[b] S2E0V1 (III)[b] S2E1V0 (III+)[b] S3E0V0 (III*)[b]	Multidisciplinary: endovascular, radiosurgery, surgery
IV	C	S2E1V1 S3E0V0 S3E1V0	Conservative management
V	C	S3E1V1	Conservative management

[a] S, size (S1, <3 cm; S2, 3–6 cm; S3, >6 cm); E, eloquence (E1, eloquent area; E0, non-eloquent); V, venous drainage (V1, deep; V0, only superficial).
[b] Grade III subdivisions based on Lawton: III–, akin to surgical risk of grade II; III+ and III*, akin to grade IV [28].
Data from Spetzler and Martin, 1986 [1] and Spetzler and Ponce, 2011 [2].

and inoperable AVMs (grades IV and V) into class C, leaving grade III AVMs as class B [2]. In a study of 1476 patients comparing the new three-tier system with the original five-tier scheme, the authors found that the predictive power of the two classification schemes was identical (0.713 vs. 0.711, respectively, for calculated area under the receiver operating characteristics curve). The modified three-tier Spetzler–Martin classification of cerebral AVMs simplifies the original classification scheme, provides a practical guide to treatment, and provides statistical power for comparisons in newer studies.

While the Spetzler–Martin AVM grading scheme remains the most widely used, others have been proposed since its introduction. Tamaki *et al.* proposed a new grading system in which points were assigned for size (small or large), number of feeding artery systems (1–2 or >3), and location (superficial or deep), separating AVMs into five grades with a strong correlation to surgical difficulty [29]. Tamaki *et al.* noted that age is a significant predictor of outcome among patients with AVMs but did not include it in their proposed classification scheme in part to obtain a more simplified scheme. Pertuiset *et al.* proposed perhaps the most comprehensive grading system reported so far, incorporating age, previous hemorrhage, and angiographic features such as AVM location and feeding artery supply (points assigned for caliber of feeding arteries, nidus volume, circulatory velocity, cerebral steal, etc.), leading to an elaborate point system with possible scores ranging from 3 to 69 points [30]. The University of Toronto Brain AVM Study Group developed a classification using three variables, weighted with a rounded odds ratio: eloquence (4 possible points), nidus diffuseness (3 possible points), and deep venous drainage (2 possible points); this resulted in 9 points stratified [31]. These two systems probably have not gained widespread clinical application because of their complexity.

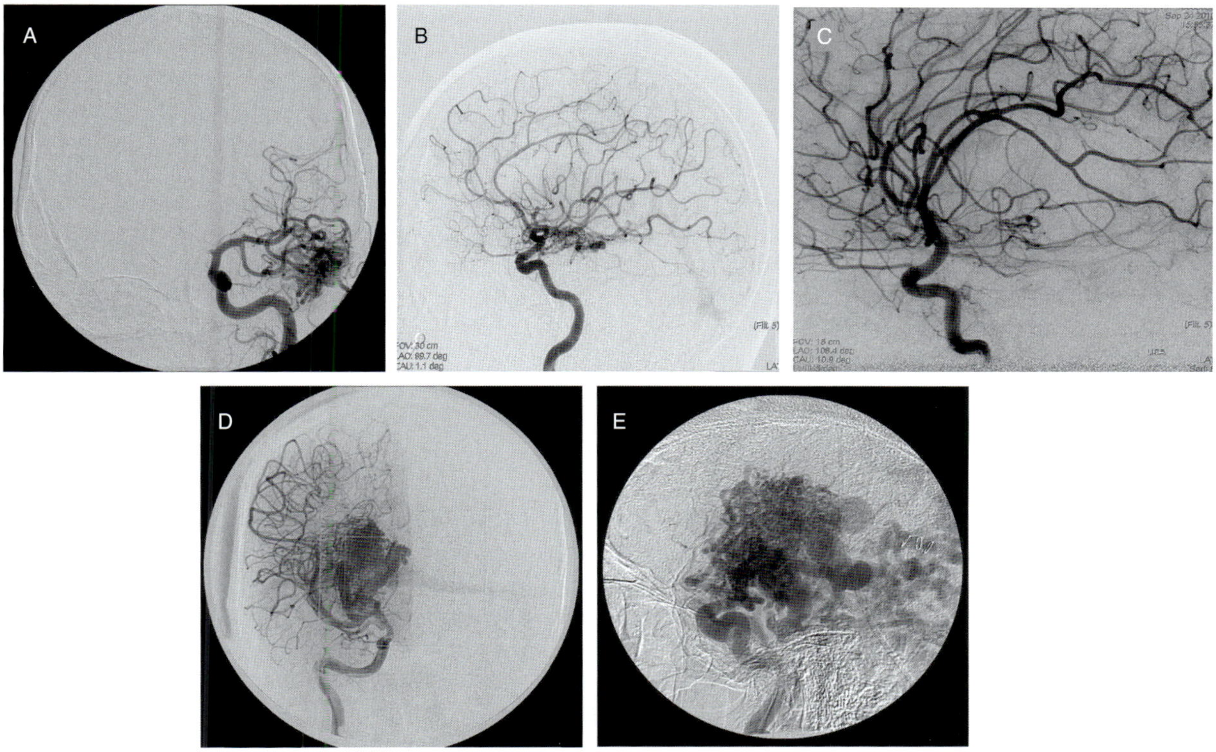

Fig. 10.1. Selected arteriovenous malformations (AVMs). (A) Spetzler–Martin grade I AVM in the anterior left temporal lobe supplied by middle cerebral artery branches with drainage into the vein of Labbé (anteroposterior view of left common carotid injection). (B) Spetzler–Martin grade II AVM in the right mesial temporal lobe supplied by the anterior choroidal and small perforating branches of the posterior communicating artery with drainage into the basal vein of Rosenthal (lateral view of right internal carotid artery injection). (C) Spetzler–Martin grade III AVM in the right basal ganglia supplied by lenticulostriate arteries with drainage into the sphenoparietal sinus and the basal vein of Rosenthal (lateral projection of right common carotid artery injection). (D) Spetzler–Martin grade IV AVM in the basal ganglia supplied by lenticulostriate arteries with deep drainage into the right internal cerebral and basal veins (anteroposterior projection of internal carotid artery injection). (E) Spetzler–Martin grade V frontoparietal AVM supplied by lenticulostriate and M2 branches with deep venous drainage (lateral projection of internal carotid artery injection).

Table 10.4. The supplementary classification point system of Lawton *et al.*

Variable	Definition	Points
Age (years)	<20	1
	20–40	2
	>40	3
Unruptured presentation	No	0
	Yes	1
Diffuse	No	0
	Yes	1

Modified from Lawton *et al.*, 2010 [34].

Although the Spetzler–Martin grading system remains the most simple and practical to apply, it does not take into account well-known critical features of AVMs such as a history of prior hemorrhage, AVM nidus morphology (compact vs. diffuse), and patient age [32,33]. In an attempt to incorporate these important factors, Lawton and colleagues proposed a classification scheme to supplement the Spetzler–Martin grade based on a point system, as outlined in Table 10.4 [34].

Supplementary grades were determined by summing up all the points in Table 10.4 with scores ranging from 1 to 5. Lawton *et al.* investigated their approach in a study of 300 surgical patients comparing the predictive accuracy of using the Spetzler–Martin scale with the supplementary scale outlined above [34]. They found that the supplementary scale had higher predictive accuracy and more evenly stratified surgical risk. Taken together, they posited that the supplementary grading system can be added to the Spetzler–Martin score to obtain an overall score ranging from 2 to 10, with a combined score of <6 corresponding to potentially acceptable surgical morbidity and a score ≤4 corresponding to minimal morbidity. The supplementary grade played largely a confirmatory role when it was consistent with the Spetzler–Martin score (i.e., both high or low). When there is a mismatch between the supplementary score and the Spetzler–Martin grade, however, the supplementary score was found to be crucial in clarifying treatment plans, in some cases even altering management decisions. For example, Lawton *et al.* reported that of the 84 of patients who had Spetzler–Martin grades I and II cerebral AVM and a supplementary score >3, 41% were neurologically worse after surgery, which was worse than the morbidity of Spetzler–Martin grade IV patients (31%). Conversely, of the patients with Spetzler–Martin grade IV and V AVMs with low supplementary scores, only 29% (compared with 35% for all patients irrespective of supplementary score) had worse neurological outcomes postoperatively. Taken together, these findings suggest that high overall supplementary scores correlate with worse morbidity with surgery. As surgical approaches to treating AVMs continue to evolve, there is likely to be further optimization of current classification systems to better manage patients with cerebral AVMs.

Radiosurgery grading schemes

Multiple grading schemes have been devised to evaluate risks and outcomes when treating patients with AVMs using radiosurgery [15,35,36]. One of the first of these methods was that proposed by Inoue *et al.* based on the observation that size, morphology, and hemodynamics are key factors for predicting radiosurgical outcome [35]. They classified AVMs based on size and the above factors in the following way: AVM hemodynamics was categorized as either Moya-type (i.e., small-caliber feeding arteries, compact nidus, and veins that drain in the venous phase of the angiogram), shunt type (large-caliber feeding arteries, indistinct nidus, and veins that drain early in the arterial phase), or mixed; morphology was categorized as either homogeneous or heterogeneous. By implementing this approach in a radiosurgical series of 330 patients, they were able to show that patients with small homogeneous Moya-type cerebral AVMs had the highest obliteration rate (87%), while those with shunt and mixed hemodynamics benefited from radiosurgery only after pretreatment with endovascular embolization [35].

Pollock and Flickinger [15] proposed an alternative and more quantitative radiosurgical scheme for classifying cerebral AVMs. By carrying out a multivariate analysis of data from 220 patients, they were able to demonstrate that the most important factors for determining optimal clinical outcome after radiosurgery are AVM volume, age, location, previous embolization, and number of draining veins, with the last two factors adding little to the predictive accuracy. They then developed a quantitative equation incorporating key factors:

$$\text{AVM score} = 0.1 \times \text{Volume (cm}^3\text{)} + 0.02 \times \text{Age (years)} + 0.3 \times \text{Location of lesion (points 0–2)}$$

where a frontal or temporal lesion is 0 points, parietal, occipital, intraventricular, corpus callosum, or cerebellar lesion is 1 point; and basal ganglia, thalamic, or brainstem lesion is 2 points. In their study, they demonstrated that patients with a composite AVM score <1 had excellent outcomes (80–95%), whereas only 29% of patients with scores >2 had excellent outcomes, defined as complete nidus obliteration without new or worsening neurological deficits. The Pollock and Flickinger equation was validated at a different institution using a cohort of 136 patients, but the equation was slightly modified by changing the location variable to two tiers (i.e., lesions in hemispheres, corpus callosum, and cerebellum were assigned 0 points, whereas those in the basal ganglia, thalamus, and brainstem were assigned 1 point) [36]. Radiosurgical treatments typically require long-term follow-up to ensure that repeat procedures are not necessary; consequently, the patients involved in the above studies will need a longer follow-up period to determine the true effectiveness of these radiosurgery classification schemes.

Table 10.5. Neuroendovascular classification scheme of cerebral arteriovenous malformations

Points	No. feeding arteries	Eloquence of adjacent area	Presence of arteriovenous fistula
0	None	Non-eloquent	No
1	<3	Eloquent	Yes
2	3 to <6		
3	≥6		

Modified from Feliciano *et al.*, 2010 [38].

Endovascular grading schemes

Unlike radiosurgery, which is usually carried out as a treatment modality independent of open surgery, endovascular procedures for treating cerebral AVMs are typically surgical or radiosurgical adjuncts rather than independent curative treatments. Therefore, there have been comparably fewer studies aimed at devising endovascular classification schemes for cerebral AVMs. The main endovascular-specific classification scheme for AVMs is that reported by Viñuela *et al.* [37]. This scheme is based on AVM size, number of feeding arteries, and presence of pial versus perforating feeding arteries. They defined low-grade AVMs as those that are small (<2 cm), have fewer than two feeding arteries, and are not supplied by perforators; high-grade lesions are those that are >4 cm in size, have at least four feeders, and are supplied by perforators. From their experience, the authors reported that high-grade AVMs required multimodal treatment in addition to endovascular embolization; however, a large study looking at actual morbidities and mortalities is yet to be reported [37].

Feliciano and colleagues in 2010 proposed another endovascular classification scheme for AVMs analogous to the Spetzler–Martin grading scheme (Table 10.5) [38]. Their classification scheme is currently being implemented in a clinical study to evaluate its accuracy and to quantify outcomes as a function of points [38]. While the results of this study are yet to be published, it is worth noting that factors that predict unfavorable outcome during endovascular procedures such as deep venous drainage, Spetzler–Martin grade III–V (odds ratio, 10.6), and periprocedural hemorrhage (odds ratio, 17) [39] were not included in the above classification scheme, which may decrease its clinical utility.

Cerebral dural arteriovenous fistulae

The DAVFs are abnormal communications between meningeal arteries and veins within a venous space contained within the dura mater. Patients with DAVFs can remain asymptomatic or present with symptoms ranging from mild tinnitus to intracranial hemorrhage. In contrast to cerebral AVMs, where most classification schemes are dedicated to predicting the risk of an intervention, those for DAVFs are more commonly designed to predict their natural history.

The DAVFs can remain asymptomatic, spontaneously involute, or progressively become more aggressive. Several studies have shown that the natural history of DAVFs depends on various factors, including pattern of venous drainage, presence of varices, and mode of presentation (asymptomatic, minimally symptomatic, non-hemorrhagic neurological deficit, or hemorrhage) [40–42]. Common to all reported classification schemes is the concept that DAVFs with leptomeningeal venous drainage are more aggressive [40–45]. Although infrequent, a number of reports indicate that relatively benign fistulae (i.e., asymptomatic lesions) can evolve into malignant lesions with leptomeningeal venous reflux [44,46,47]. Changes in drainage pattern may be induced by changes in the volume of the arteriovenous shunt and/or the development of venous flow impairment (venous stenosis or thrombosis).

One of the first classification schemes for DAVFs was proposed by Djindjian *et al.* in 1978 [49] and was later modified as the Merland-Cognard classification scheme [44]. The scheme was based on the clinical presentation of 205 patients followed over 18 years [48]. In this scheme, DAVFs were classified into five types (I–V) with type II lesions further subdivided into types IIa, IIb, and IIa+b, as outlined in Table 10.6.

In a study by Djindjian *et al.*, 83 of 84 patients with type I DAVFs presented with non-aggressive symptoms, which included headaches, bruit, minimal vertigo, and ocular symptoms not related to intracranial hypertension. Patients with higher-grade lesions were more likely to present with intracranial hemorrhage, intracranial hypertension, focal neurological deficit, and seizures: 37% of patients with type IIa, 30% with type IIb, 86% with type IIa + b, 76% with type III, 97% with type IV, and 100% with type V [49]. A similar, albeit slightly simpler scheme was proposed by Borden *et al.* at a similar time, dividing DAVFs into three main types (I–III) (Figs. 10.2–10.4) as outlined in Table 10.6 [43]. Borden *et al.* further subclassified DAVFs into two groups with subtype A assigned to fistulae with a direct, single connection between the feeding artery and draining vein or sinus, and subtype B ascribed to complex lesions with multiple fistulous connections.

These schemes for classifying DAVFs [40–43,49] are designed primarily based on the rate of hemorrhagic presentation. From these schemes, it is evident that leptomeningeal

Table 10.6. Classification schemes for dural arteriovenous fistulae

Borden	Cognard	Description	Hemorrhage rate (%)
I	I	Anterograde flow into dural venous sinus	0
I	IIa	Retrograde flow into dural venous sinus	0
II	IIb	Anterograde flow into dural venous sinus with cortical drainage	6
II	IIa+b	Retrograde flow into dural venous sinus with cortical drainage	6
III	III	Cortical venous drainage only without venous ectasia	10
III	IV	Cortical venous drainage only with venous ectasia (>5 mm diameter or three times larger than the diameter of the draining vein)	21
	V	Cranial dural arteriovenous fistula draining into spinal perimedullary veins	Not well established; some cite as high as 75% [50]

Data from Borden *et al.* [43] and Cognard *et al.* [44].

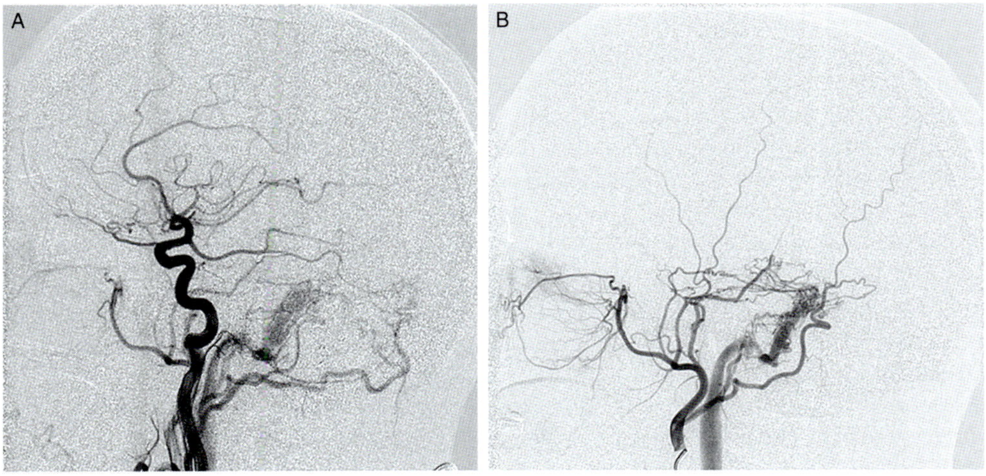

Fig. 10.2. Borden I, Cognard I cerebral dural arteriovenous fistula in a 47-year-old man with a history of traumatic brain injury and pulsatile tinnitus. (A,B) The fistula was supplied by the occipital, posterior auricular, middle meningeal, and ascending pharyngeal arteries (A; lateral projection of injection into the common carotid artery) as well as the tentorial artery (B; lateral projection of injection into the external carotid artery). Drainage was antegrade into the left sigmoid sinus.

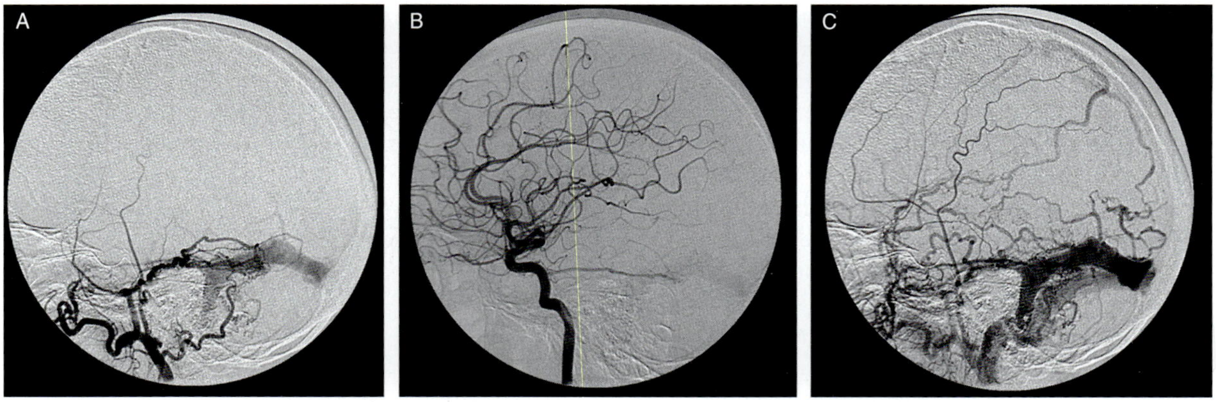

Fig. 10.3. Borden II, Cognard IIa+b dural arteriovenous fistula in a 62-year-old woman with tinnitus. (A,B) A fistula of the left transverse sinus was supplied by the occipital, middle meningeal, ascending pharyngeal arteries (A; lateral projection of injection into the external carotid artery), and the tentorial arteries (B; lateral projection of injection into the internal carotid artery). (C) Retrograde leptomeningeal reflux was seen (lateral projection of injection into the external carotid artery).

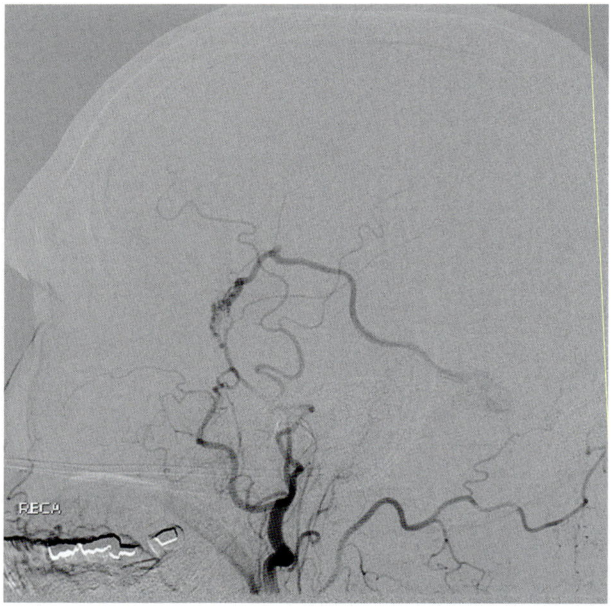

Fig. 10.4. Incidental Borden III, Cognard III dural arteriovenous fistula. It was supplied by the middle meningeal artery with direct leptomeningeal venous drainage (lateral projection of injection into the external carotid artery).

venous drainage and venous ectasia are significant risk factors for hemorrhage [40–42]. According to one modern natural history study incorporating data from one institution in a pooled analysis with previously published data from other natural history studies, the annual hemorrhage rate for DAVFs with leptomeningeal venous reflux was 6%, increasing to 21% for those with venous ectasia (Table 10.6) [46]. Furthermore, as strongly suggested by the study of Strom *et al.*, symptomatic DAVF with leptomeningeal venous drainage had a notably greater risk of hemorrhage [41]. These studies support timely intervention for symptomatic DAVF with leptomeningeal venous drainage. Even asymptomatic lesions in medically fit patients deserve treatment. Those without leptomeningeal venous drainage should be treated if symptoms are debilitating. Otherwise, they merit observation with non-invasive imaging to monitor for the potential of regression or possible progression to develop leptomeningeal venous drainage.

Table 10.7. Classification scheme for spinal shunts

Classic scheme	Kim–Spetzler scheme	Description
Type I	Intradural dorsal AVF	Radicular artery communicates directly with a dural vein
Type II	Intramedullary AVM	Pial arteriovenous malformations fed by anterior or posterior spinal arteries
Type III	Extradural–intradural AVM	Complex juvenile metameric lesions occurring along discrete somite levels
Type IV	Intradural ventral AVF	Pial AVF fed by anterior spinal artery and drained by the coronal venous plexus

AVM, arteriovenous malformations; AVF, arteriovenous fistula.
Data from Kim and Spetzler [53].

Spinal arteriovenous shunts

Spinal arteriovenous shunts are a heterogeneous group of vascular anomalies in which an abnormal communication occurs between a radicular/pial artery and spinal vein. Although a wide variety of classification schemes have been proposed for these lesions, the simplest are descriptive and essentially segregate spinal DAVFs, spinal pial AVMs, and spinal pial AVFs [51]. Spinal metameric AVMs are typically classified as their own separate subclass [52]. Classically, spinal arteriovenous shunts are classified into four main types. Kim and Spetzler [53] proposed a new scheme in which lesions are classified based on their anatomical location (extradural, extradural–intradural, or intradural). In the classic type I–IV classification scheme of spinal vascular anomalies, type I lesions are DAVFs (i.e., a radicular artery communicates directly with a dural vein at the nerve root sleeve, leading to arterialization of the perimedullary coronal venous plexus). Kim and Spetzler [53] group these lesions in their intradural category (Table 10.7).

Type I spinal AVMs (Fig. 10.5) can be subclassified into IA and IB based on whether one or more radicular feeding arteries are present, respectively. Type I lesions represent

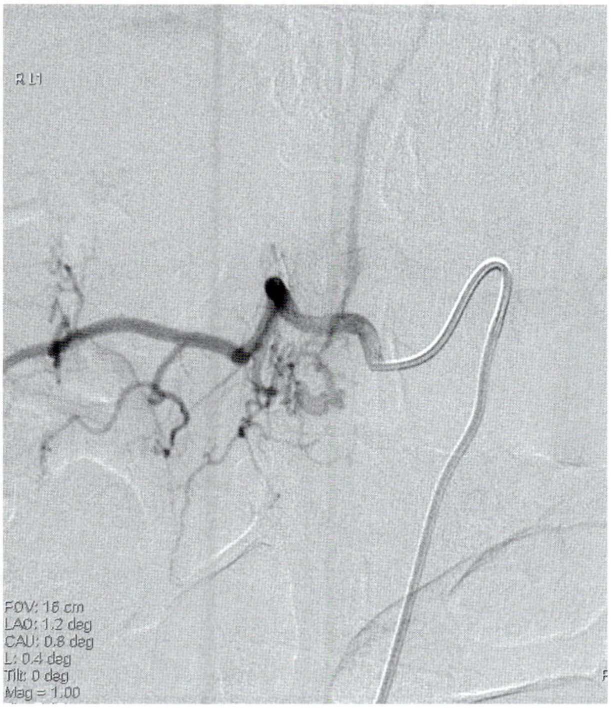

Fig 10.5. Type 1 spinal arteriovenous shunt. This 53-year-old patient with progressive myelopathy was found to have a dural arteriovenous fistula supplied by an L1 radicular artery (AP projection of right L1 segmental artery injection).

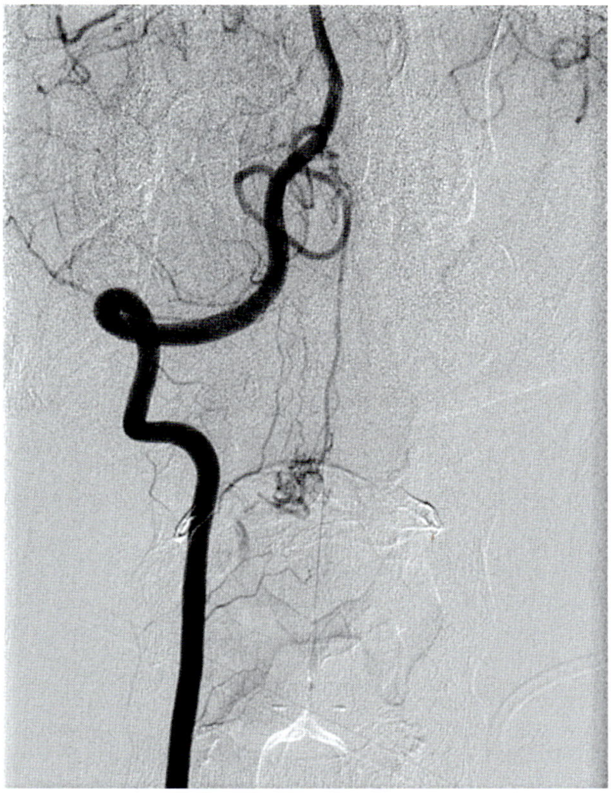

Fig 10.6. Type II spinal arteriovenous shunt. This 20-year-old patient presented with spinal hemorrhage from this pial arteriovenous malformations, supplied by the anterior spinal artery (AP projection of right vertebral artery injection).

approximately 60–80% of all spinal arteriovenous shunts, and patients with these lesions typically present with myelopathy secondary to venous hypertension [5,54,55]. The natural history of type I spinal arteriovenous shunts evolves with progressively worsening symptoms, with significant impairment in neurological function observed in 19% of patients at 6 months and severe disability reported in 50% of patients within three years [53].

Although embolization may be successful if embolic material (typically Onyx in modern series) can reach the fistula point, this approach may be relatively contraindicated in patients where there are difficulties of access because of arterial tortuosity or small caliber as well as where feeding radicular arteries also supply the spinal cord itself. The latter places the spinal cord at risk for infarction with embolization. In contrast, surgical disconnection of the fistula is often relatively simple, with post-operative improvement in neurological symptoms seen in the majority of patients [5]. Hence, the designation of "type I" to a spinal arteriovenous shunt connotes a lesion with a potentially progressive natural history as a result of myelopathy with a generally good prognosis because of its low-risk and generally highly successful treatment options [56].

Type II lesions are spinal pial AVMs akin to their cerebral AVM counterparts (Fig. 10.6). Kim and Spetzler [53] classified type II lesions as "intramedullary" AVMs [56,57]. They can have single or multiple feeding arteries originating from the anterior or posterior spinal arteries and can have a compact or diffuse nidus. These lesions typically present with myelopathy or hemorrhage. Conus medullaris lesions, considered separately in the Kim and Spetzler [53] classification scheme, typically have multiple feeders with direct arteriovenous shunts and large dilated veins, inducing neurological dysfunction through venous hypertension, ischemia, and mass effect from venous dilatation [58].

Type II spinal AVMs are amenable to both endovascular and surgical treatment approaches. Although the latter is associated with greater obliteration rates, it generally does not approach the rates seen with surgical treatment of cerebral AVMs [59–62]. Endovascular treatment of type II spinal AVMs has been reported to achieve obliteration in 45–53% of patients with a permanent complication rate of 6–10.6% [59–62]. Surgical treatment of type II spinal AVMs is associated with a morbidity of 5% and an angiographically confirmed obliteration rate of 75–90% [56,57,59]. Therefore, while these lesions may be cured if compact, they are more challenging treatment targets with a generally more unfortunate natural history because of their proclivity to hemorrhage and/or cause myelopathy [51,63].

Type III spinal arteriovenous shunts are complex juvenile metameric lesions that occur along discrete somite levels and typically involve the spinal canal, nerve roots, bone, muscle, and skin. Kim and Spetzler classify these lesions as spinal extradural–intradural arteriovenous shunts [53]. They carry a more guarded and poor prognosis given the difficulty of treating them [66]. While some have reported successful obliteration of these shunts [64], management of these lesions typically involves palliative embolization.

Type IV spinal AVMs are pial AVFs, elegantly described by Heros *et al.* in 1986 [65]. They contrast with their

DAVF/type I counterparts in both their pial arterial supply as well as their greater risk of hemorrhage. They are usually fed by the anterior spinal artery and are therefore ventrally located and are drained by the coronal venous plexus. They are further subclassified based on the Anson and Spetzler nomenclature of A–C [66]. Type IVA spinal AVMs are small simple AVFs fed by the anterior or posterior spinal arteries without associated vessel dilatation and have low flow. These lesions are best treated surgically given the difficulty of catheterizing the small caliber vessels that feed them [66]. Type IVB spinal AVMs are those fed by one or two dilated medium-sized vessels and typically have higher flow, with consequent dilatation of the draining veins. These lesions are typically treated with preoperative endovascular embolization followed by surgery [66]. Type IVC AVMs are giant fistulae with very high shunt volumes and large dilated draining veins. They are best treated with endovascular embolization, which has been associated with successful obliteration in 68% of patients [66].

Conclusions

Classification schemes are essential for the proper communication of surgical results, studies of natural history, and reports of morbidity and mortality associated with treatment. With advances in imaging and in our understanding of the biology of vascular malformations, these tools are likely to add to existing classification schemes.

References

1. Spetzler RF, Martin NA. A proposed grading system for arteriovenous malformations. *J Neurosurg* 1986;**65**:476–83.
2. Spetzler RF, Ponce FA. A 3-tier classification of cerebral arteriovenous malformations. *J Neurosurg* 2011;**114**:842–9.
3. Spetzler RF, Zabramski JM. Grading and staged resection of cerebral arteriovenous malformations. *Clin Neurosurg* 1990;**36**:318–37.
4. Gross BA, Du R. Surgical and radiosurgical results of the treatment of cerebral arteriovenous malformations. *J Clin Neurosci* 2012;**19**:1001–4.
5. Ropper AE, Gross BA, Du R. Surgical treatment of type I spinal dural arteriovenous fistulas. *Neurosurg Focus* 2012;**32**:E3.
6. Martin NA, King WA, Wilson CB, *et al.* Management of dural arteriovenous malformations of the anterior cranial fossa. *J Neurosurg* 1990;**72**:692–7.
7. Jane JA, Kassell NF, Torner JC, *et al.* The natural history of aneurysms and arteriovenous malformations. *J Neurosurg* 1985;**62**:321–3.
8. Graf CJ, Perret GE, Torner JC. Bleeding from cerebral arteriovenous malformations as part of their natural history. *J Neurosurg* 1983;**58**:331–7.
9. Michelsen WJ. Natural history and pathophysiology of arteriovenous malformations. *Clin Neurosurg* 1979;**26**:307–13.
10. Fults D, Kelly DL, Jr. Natural history of arteriovenous malformations of the brain: a clinical study. *Neurosurgery* 1984;**15**:658–62.
11. Gross BA, Du R. Hemorrhage from arteriovenous malformations during pregnancy. *Neurosurgery* 2012;**71**:349–55.
12. Stapf C, Mohr JP, Pile-Spellman J, *et al.* Epidemiology and natural history of arteriovenous malformations. *Neurosurg Focus* 2001;**11**:E1.
13. da Costa L, Wallace MC, terBrugge KG, *et al.* The natural history and predictive features of hemorrhage from brain arteriovenous malformations. *Stroke* 2009;**40**:100–5.
14. Pollock BE, Flickinger JC, Lunsford LD, *et al.* Factors that predict the bleeding risk of cerebral arteriovenous malformations. *Stroke* 1996;**27**:1–6.
15. Pollock BE, Flickinger JC. A proposed radiosurgery-based grading system for arteriovenous malformations. *J Neurosurg* 2002;**96**:79–85.
16. Stapf C, Mast H, Sciacca RR, *et al.* Predictors of hemorrhage in patients with untreated brain arteriovenous malformation. *Neurology* 2006;**66**:1350–5.
17. Hernesniemi JA, Dashti R, Juvela S, *et al.* Natural history of brain arteriovenous malformations: a long-term follow-up study of risk of hemorrhage in 238 patients. *Neurosurgery* 2008;**63**:823–9.
18. Laakso A, Dashti R, Juvela S, *et al.* Natural history of arteriovenous malformations: presentation, risk of hemorrhage and mortality. *Acta Neurochir Suppl* 2010;**107**:65–9.
19. Kondziolka D, McLaughlin MR, Kestle JR. Simple risk predictions for arteriovenous malformation hemorrhage. *Neurosurgery* 1995;**37**:851–5.
20. Gross BA, Du R. Rate of re-bleeding of arteriovenous malformations in the first year after rupture. *J Clin Neurosci* 2012;**19**:1087–8.
21. Brown RD, Jr. Simple risk predictions for arteriovenous malformation hemorrhage. *Neurosurgery* 2000;**46**:1024.
22. Luessenhop AJ, Gennarelli TA. Anatomical grading of supratentorial arteriovenous malformations for determining operability. *Neurosurgery* 1977;**1**:30–5.
23. Shi YQ, Chen XC. A proposed scheme for grading intracranial arteriovenous malformations. *J Neurosurg* 1986;**65**:484–9.
24. Hamilton MG, Spetzler RF. The prospective application of a grading system for arteriovenous malformations. *Neurosurgery* 1994;**34**:2–6.
25. Deruty R, Pelissou-Guyotat I, Mottolese C, *et al.* The combined management of cerebral arteriovenous malformations. Experience with 100 cases and review of the literature. *Acta Neurochir (Wien)* 1993;**123**:101–12.
26. Heros RC, Tu YK. Is surgical therapy needed for unruptured arteriovenous malformations? *Neurology* 1987;**37**:279–86.

27. Steinmeier R, Schramm J, Muller HG, *et al.* Evaluation of prognostic factors in cerebral arteriovenous malformations. *Neurosurgery* 1989;**24**:193–200.

28. Lawton MT. Spetzler–Martin grade III arteriovenous malformations: surgical results and a modification of the grading scale. *Neurosurgery* 2003;**52**:740–8.

29. Tamaki N, Ehara K, Lin TK, *et al.* Cerebral arteriovenous malformations: factors influencing the surgical difficulty and outcome. *Neurosurgery* 1991;**29**:856–61.

30. Pertuiset B, Ancri D, Kinuta Y, *et al.* Classification of supratentorial arteriovenous malformations. A score system for evaluation of operability and surgical strategy based on an analysis of 66 cases. *Acta Neurochir (Wien)* 1991;**110**:6–16.

31. Arteriovenous Malformation Study Group. Arteriovenous malformations of the brain in adults. *N Engl J Med* 1999;**340**:1812–18.

32. Du R, Keyoung HM, Dowd CF, *et al.* The effects of diffuseness and deep perforating artery supply on outcomes after microsurgical resection of brain arteriovenous malformations. *Neurosurgery* 2007;**60**:638–46.

33. Lawton MT, Du R, Tran MN, *et al.* Effect of presenting hemorrhage on outcome after microsurgical resection of brain arteriovenous malformations. *Neurosurgery* 2005;**56**:485–93.

34. Lawton MT, Kim H, McCulloch CE, *et al.* A supplementary grading scale for selecting patients with brain arteriovenous malformations for surgery. *Neurosurgery* 2010;**66**:702–13.

35. Inoue HK, Kohga H, Kurihara H, *et al.* Classification of arteriovenous malformation for radiosurgery. Neuroimaging, histopathology and radiobiologic effects. *Stereotact Funct Neurosurg* 1995;**64**(Suppl 1):110–17.

36. Pollock BE, Flickinger JC. Modification of the radiosurgery-based arteriovenous malformation grading system. *Neurosurgery* 2008;**63**:239–43.

37. Viñuela F, Duckwiler T, Guglielmi G. *Intravascular Embolization of Brain Arteriovenous Malformations*. Rolling Meadows, IL: Association of Neurological Surgeons, 1995.

38. Feliciano CE, de Leon-Berra R, Hernandez-Gaitan MS, *et al.* A proposal for a new arteriovenous malformation grading scale for neuroendovascular procedures and literature review. *P R Health Sci J* 2010;**29**:117–20.

39. Ledezma CJ, Hoh BL, Carter BS, *et al.* Complications of cerebral arteriovenous malformation embolization: multivariate analysis of predictive factors. *Neurosurgery* 2006;**58**:602–11.

40. Soderman M, Pavic L, Edner G, *et al.* Natural history of dural arteriovenous shunts. *Stroke* 2008;**39**:1735–9.

41. Strom RG, Botros JA, Refai D, *et al.* Cranial dural arteriovenous fistulae: asymptomatic cortical venous drainage portends less aggressive clinical course. *Neurosurgery* 2009;**64**:241–7.

42. Gross BA, Ropper AE, Du R. Cerebral dural arteriovenous fistulas and aneurysms. *Neurosurg Focus* 2012;**32**:E2.

43. Borden JA, Wu JK, Shucart WA. A proposed classification for spinal and cranial dural arteriovenous fistulous malformations and implications for treatment. *J Neurosurg* 1995;**82**:166–79.

44. Cognard C, Gobin YP, Pierot L, *et al.* Cerebral dural arteriovenous fistulas: clinical and angiographic correlation with a revised classification of venous drainage. *Radiology* 1995;**194**:671–80.

45. Malik GM, Pearce JE, Ausman JI, *et al.* Dural arteriovenous malformations and intracranial hemorrhage. *Neurosurgery* 1984;**15**:332–9.

46. Gross BA, Du R. The natural history of cerebral dural arteriovenous fistulae. *Neurosurgery* 2012;**71**:594–602.

47. Satomi J, van Dijk JM, terBrugge KG, *et al.* Benign cranial dural arteriovenous fistulas: outcome of conservative management based on the natural history of the lesion. *J Neurosurg* 2002;**97**:767–70.

48. Gobin YP, Rogopoulos A, Aymard A, *et al.* Endovascular treatment of intracranial dural arteriovenous fistulas with spinal perimedullary venous drainage. *J Neurosurg* 1992;**77**:718–23.

49. Djindjian R, Merland JJ, Theron J. *Super-selective Arteriography of the External Carotid Artery*. New York: Springer, 1978.

50. Davies MA, TerBrugge K, Willinsky R, *et al.* The validity of classification for the clinical presentation of intracranial dural arteriovenous fistulas. *J Neurosurg* 1996;**85**:830–7.

51. Rodesch G, Hurth M, Alvarez H, *et al.* Classification of spinal cord arteriovenous shunts: proposal for a reappraisal: the Bicêtre experience with 155 consecutive patients treated between 1981 and 1999. *Neurosurgery* 2002;**51**:374–9.

52. Ferch RD, Morgan MK, Sears WR. Spinal arteriovenous malformations: a review with case illustrations. *J Clin Neurosci* 2001;**8**:299–304.

53. Kim LJ, Spetzler RF. Classification and surgical management of spinal arteriovenous lesions: arteriovenous fistulae and arteriovenous malformations. *Neurosurgery* 2006;**59**:S195–201.

54. Huffmann BC, Gilsbach JM, Thron A. Spinal dural arteriovenous fistulas: a plea for neurosurgical treatment. *Acta Neurochir (Wien)* 1995;**135**:44–51.

55. Lee TT, Gromelski EB, Bowen BC, *et al.* Diagnostic and surgical management of spinal dural arteriovenous fistulas. *Neurosurgery* 1998;**43**:242–6.

56. Connolly ES, Jr., Zubay GP, McCormick PC, *et al.* The posterior approach to a series of glomus (type II) intramedullary spinal cord arteriovenous malformations. *Neurosurgery* 1998;**42**:774–85.

57. Velat GJ, Chang SW, Abla AA, *et al.* Microsurgical management of glomus spinal arteriovenous malformations: pial resection technique: clinical article. *J Neurosurg Spine* 2012;**16**:523–31.

58. Wilson DA, Abla AA, Uschold TD, *et al.* Multimodality treatment of conus medullaris arteriovenous malformations: 2 decades of experience with combined endovascular and microsurgical treatments. *Neurosurgery* 2012;**71**:100–8.

59. Boström A, Krings T, Hans FJ, *et al.* Spinal glomus-type arteriovenous malformations: microsurgical treatment in 20 cases. *J Neurosurg Spine* 2009;**10**:423–9.

60. Patsalides A, Knopman J, Santillan A, *et al.* Endovascular treatment of spinal arteriovenous lesions: beyond the dural fistula. *AJNR Am J Neuroradiol* 2011;**32**:798–808.

61. Niimi Y, Berenstein A, Setton A, *et al.* Embolization of spinal dural arteriovenous fistulae: results and follow-up. *Neurosurgery* 1997;**40**:675–82.

62. Morgan MK. Outcome from treatment for spinal arteriovenous malformation. *Neurosurg Clin N Am* 1999;**10**:113–19.

63. Rodesch G, Lasjaunias P. Spinal cord arteriovenous shunts: from imaging to management. *Eur J Radiol* 2003;**46**:221–32.

64. Fairhall JM, Reddy R, Sears W, *et al.* Successful endovascular and surgical treatment of spinal extradural metameric arteriovenous malformations. Case report. *J Neurosurg Spine* 2010;**13**:784–8.

65. Heros RC, Debrun GM, Ojemann RG, *et al.* Direct spinal arteriovenous fistula: a new type of spinal AVM. Case report. *J Neurosurg* 1986;**64**:134–9.

66. Anson JA, Spetzler RF. Surgical resection of intramedullary spinal cord cavernous malformations. *J Neurosurg* 1993;**78**:446–51.

67. Luessenhop AJ, Rosa L. Cerebral arteriovenous malformations: Indications for and results of surgery, and the role of intravascular techniques. *J Neurosurg* 1984;**60**:14–22.

Chapter 11

Surgical approaches and nuances for supratentorial arteriovenous malformations

Mohammed Ali Aziz-Sultan, Mohamed Samy Elhammady, and Roberto C. Heros

Introduction

An arteriovenous malformations (AVM) is an abnormal collection of blood vessels consisting of direct fistulous connections between arteries and veins without a normal intervening capillary bed or functional neural tissue. They are generally believed to be congenital lesions developing during the fourth and eighth weeks of gestation. Although the incidence and prevalence of cerebral AVMs is not known with certainty, autopsy data suggest that their frequency of detection is approximately 4.3% [1,2]. Cerebral AVMs are most commonly discovered in the third or fourth decade of life. Intracerebral hemorrhage remains the most common presentation and can be seen in more than 70% of patients [3,4]. They account for 2% of all strokes and 38% of intracerebral hemorrhages in patients between 15 and 45 years of age [5–7]. The other common presentations include seizures (25–50% of patients), progressive neurological deficit from mass effect or steal, and chronic headaches.

A thorough understanding of the natural history of cerebral AVMs is paramount to forming a proper treatment plan. A number of series have evaluated the natural history of AVMs with regard to the risk of hemorrhage (Table 11.1) [3,4,8–13]. Although a detailed discussion of these studies is beyond the scope of this chapter, it has been shown that in the majority of these series the overall annual risk of rupture is approximately 2–4%. Furthermore, several factors have been suggested to influence the rate of rupture, including hemorrhagic presentation, AVM size and location.

Once an AVM is suspected, a number of diagnostic imaging modalities can help to define the lesion. Computed tomography is a good initial screening test and may demonstrate the location of the AVM as well as the presence of acute hemorrhage, calcifications, or hydrocephalus. In order to further visualize the nidus, contrast must be administered to delineate the vasculature and here MRI is superior to CT in delineating the macroarchitecture and the anatomical relationship of the AVM to surrounding brain. It can help in understanding the size, proximity to eloquent areas, and three-dimensional structure of the nidus, feeding vessels, and draining veins. Cerebral digital subtraction angiography is still considered the gold standard to assess a patient with an AVM. This study can provide valuable information regarding size, location, and configuration of the AVM nidus as well as the pattern and location of feeding arteries and draining veins. In addition, it may detect the presence of angioarchitectural features associated with an increased risk of hemorrhage, such as feeding artery or intranidal aneurysms [14–18], deep venous drainage [19], venous aneurysm or outflow compromise [20], perforating feeding vessels [21], and deep or periventricular location. Other adjunctive tests such as positron emission tomography, functional MRI, and the Wada test (intracarotid amobarbital procedure) can be used to assess the functionality of the cortical structures adjacent to the AVM.

In his writings about the treatment of cerebrovascular malformations, Harvey Cushing in 1928 wrote, "It would be nothing less than foolhardy to attack one of the deep-seated racemose lesions.… The surgical history of most of the reported cases shows not only the futility of an operative attack upon one of these angiomas but the extreme risk of serious cortical damage which it entails…" [22]. Since the initial discouraging surgical experience of Cushing and his contemporaries, tremendous advances have been made in our understanding of the pathogenesis, clinical presentation, and natural history of cerebral AVMs. Furthermore, major developments have been made in microsurgical, endovascular, and radiosurgical treatment of these lesions. This chapter discusses the various factors that influence decision making as well as the surgical technique and nuances of supratentorial AVM resection.

Decision making

The management of patients with cerebral AVMs is based on a thorough understanding of the natural history and the risk of intervention. In our opinion, the risk of intervention is best made by a neurosurgeon with experience in AVM surgery and preferably in endovascular therapy. Decisions regarding the management of cerebral AVMs are complex. There is no magic formula or specific protocol where a patient can be fitted

Comprehensive Management of Arteriovenous Malformations of the Brain and Spine, ed. Robert F. Spetzler, Douglas S. Kondziolka, Randall T. Higashida, and M. Yashar S. Kalani. Published by Cambridge University Press.

Table 11.1. Natural history studies for arteriovenous malformations

Study	Type of study	No. patients	Average follow-up (years)	Annual hemorrhage rate
Graf *et al.* (1983) [8]	Retrospective	191	4.8	2–3% in patients without hemorrhage; 6% at first year after hemorrhage, then 2% in patients with hemorrhage
Crawford *et al.* (1986) [4]	Retrospective	217	10.4	2%; 36% cumulative risk at 10 years in patients with hemorrhage, 17% in patients without hemorrhage
Brown *et al.* (1988) [9]	Retrospective	168 (all unruptured)	8.2	2.2%
Ondra *et al.* (1990) [3]	Retrospective	160	23.7	4% overall; 3.9% in patients with hemorrhage, 4.3% with seizure, 3.9% with other symptoms
Mast *et al.* (1997) [10]	Prospective	281	1.0	2.2% in patients without hemorrhage, 17.8% in patients with hemorrhage
Halim *et al.* (2004) [11]	Retrospective	790	4.0	7% for first year, then 3%
Stapf *et al.* (2006) [12]	Prospective database	622	102 days	1.3% for unruptured arteriovenous malformations, 5.9% for ones presenting with hemorrhage
Hernesniemi *et al.* (2008) [13]	Retrospective	238	13.5 years	2.4% overall; three times higher in the first 5 years (4.6%) than in subsequent years (1.6%)

to automatically make a decision for the clinician. On the contrary, as will be discussed, there are several factors specific to each patient that must be taken into consideration in order to formulate an individualized treatment plan.

Arteriovenous malformations-related factors

Grading systems

One of the most important factors to consider in the treatment paradigm is the AVM itself. Although several classification schemes have been proposed, the Spetzler–Martin grading system has become the most widely accepted for both communication of information regarding cerebral AVMs and prediction of the technical difficulty and risks associated with surgical resection [23]. In this system, AVMs receive a grade from I through V that corresponds to a point scale depending on the size of the AVM, its proximity to eloquent neural tissue, and whether the AVM drains into the deep venous system.

Size. Size is scored by measuring the greatest diameter of the AVM nidus on digital subtraction angiography, CT, or MRI. The AVM nidus is subsequently rated as small (<3 cm), medium (3–6 cm), or large (>6 cm). The size of the AVM serves as a surrogate for the number of feeding arteries, the amount of flow through the AVM, and the degree of hemodynamic effect on the adjacent brain.

Eloquence of adjacent brain. Eloquent neural tissue is defined as a region of the brain that harbors easily identifiable neurological function and can result in a disabling neurological deficit if injured. These regions include the sensory, motor, language, and visual cortex; the hypothalamus and thalamus; the internal capsule; brainstem; cerebellar peduncles; and deep cerebellar nuclei. Other regions of the brain with function that can be easily compensated for or that result in subtle non-disabling neurological deficits when injured, such as the frontopolar or cerebellar cortex, are considered non-eloquent.

Pattern of venous drainage. Venous drainage is scored as "superficial" if all the draining veins are components of the cortical venous system and as "deep" if any or all of the drainage is through the internal cerebral veins or Galenic system. The presence of deep venous drainage is an indirect indicator of the fact that the AVM involves the ventricular wall or is located or extends to the deeper regions of the brain. These features render surgical resection more technically challenging as they are difficult to access and are invariably supplied by deep penetrating arteries even if they are not visualized angiographically.

The higher the AVM grade, the greater the difficulty and risk associated with surgical resection. Low-grade AVMs (grades I and II) have low morbidity rates (0–5%) associated with their resection and are, therefore, typically treated surgically, whereas high-grade AVMs (grades IV and V) have high morbidity rates (12–38%) associated with their resection and are frequently managed conservatively [24,25]. Grade III AVMs represent a heterogeneous group of lesions with variable surgical risk. Lawton suggested subdividing Spetzler–Martin grade III AVMs into three subgroups based on size (S1, 3 cm; S2, 3–6 cm; S3, >6 cm), brain area affected (E1, eloquent area; E0, non-eloquent), and venous drainage (V1, deep; V0, only superficial; see Table 10.3): grade III– (S1V1E1), which has a surgical risk similar to that of low-grade AVMs and can be safely treated with microsurgical resection; grade III+ (S2V0E1), which has a surgical risk similar to that of high-grade AVMs and is best managed conservatively; and grade III (S2V1E0), which has intermediate surgical risks and requires judicious selection for surgery [25]. A similar modification was proposed by de Oliveira and colleagues [26]; grade III AVMs were subdivided into IIIA if they were large and IIIB if they were small but had deep venous drainage and/or were located in eloquent areas. They generally recommended embolization followed by surgical resection for grade IIIA and radiosurgery for grade IIIB.

Although many experienced surgeons have confirmed the validity of the Spetzler–Martin grading system in predicting surgical morbidity and mortality, the classification fails to directly address several important factors such as the pattern of arterial supply (superficial vs. deep perforating), the configuration of the nidus (compact vs. diffuse), and the presence of feeding artery aneurysms, direct arteriovenous fistulae, and stenosis or occlusion of the venous draining system. Furthermore, it does not take into consideration the influence of size, location, and pattern of venous drainage on the natural history.

Size

The influence of size on future hemorrhage has been controversial. In a series of 168 patients followed after presentation without a prior hemorrhage, the size of the AVM was not found to be predictive of future hemorrhage in a multivariate statistical analysis [9]. However, other studies have found small AVMs to be at higher risk of hemorrhage. Spetzler *et al.* [27] reported a significantly higher incidence of hemorrhagic presentation with small (<3 cm) AVMs compared with large (>6 cm) AVMs (82% vs. 21%). They compared intraoperative feeding artery pressure measurements in small and large AVMs [27]. They found significantly higher feeding artery pressures in small AVMs and suggested that differences in arterial feeding pressures may be responsible for the observed relationship between size of AVMs and the frequency and severity of hemorrhage. The same institution calculated an overall annual hemorrhage rate of 1.5% for large AVMs (grades IV and V) [28]. However, newer natural history studies have shown that large size is an independent factor for hemorrhage on multivariate analysis [13].

Location

Deep and infratentorial location has been shown to be associated with a higher risk of bleeding than with supratentorial AVMs. In addition, the morbidity rate associated with these hemorrhages is significant, with 85.5% of patients suffering hemiparesis or hemiplegia [29]. Although resection of these lesions may be more challenging, surgery may be considered, as the worse natural history associated with these lesions may outweigh the risk of observation or treatment with another modality such as radiosurgery.

Pattern of venous drainage

Deep venous drainage has also been thought to be an important risk factor for AVM hemorrhage. Nataf *et al.* [30] reported a strong correlation between the frequency of hemorrhages and the presence of deep drainage. Similarly, AVMs with a single draining vein [31] or with impairment of venous drainage caused by stenosis or kinking [20] may have a higher risk of bleeding. This can be explained by impaired venous outflow from the AVM nidus, resulting in hemodynamic overload and eventual rupture. In our opinion, AVMs with these features should be strongly considered for surgical resection even when the risk of surgical excision may be relatively high.

Patient-related factors

The patient's age, general health and clinical condition, occupation, and lifestyle must be considered in the decision-making process. The patient's age is most important in determining the cumulative risk of AVM rupture during the remainder of the patient's life expectancy. Assuming an annual hemorrhage rate of 2–4% and an average life expectancy of 70 years, the cumulative risk (in percentage) of AVM rupture may be estimated by the following formula: 105 – patient's age in years [32,33]. Hence, a more aggressive approach for surgical treatment can be justified in younger patients, as their cumulative risk of hemorrhage is so high. In addition, neurological deficit caused at a young age is generally better tolerated and has a greater chance of recovery. The general health of the patient is important as severe comorbid conditions may preclude surgery as a reasonable treatment option. The clinical presentation and neurological condition of a patient will often dictate timing of surgery; for example, as indicated above, the patient may need emergency evacuation of a hematoma caused by a ruptured AVM, or it may be best to wait until the patient has improved to a neurological plateau when AVM resection can be approached electively. Patients with AVMs who present with major hemorrhage, progressive neurological deterioration, uncontrolled epilepsy, or intractable headaches should be considered for surgical resection. The occupation and lifestyle of a patient are important considerations as the neurosurgeon begins to weigh the risks and benefits of treatment of an AVM in a critical area of the brain. For example, a patient who is a pilot and is dependent on perfect vision presenting with an occipital AVM may feel differently about surgical resection with a >50% chance of causing a postoperative hemianopsia than a patient with an AVM in the same location who is a housewife.

Surgeon-related factors

As discussed above, a surgeon's personal experience with AVM management is an important factor to be considered. Ethical considerations related to surgeon's experience come into play at a point where the surgeon determines if an AVM is operable or inoperable. Most competent neurosurgeons can remove safely a small AVM located in non-eloquent brain. However, with more complex lesions, the decision should preferably be made by an experienced cerebrovascular neurosurgeon at a referral center that specializes in AVM surgery. The surgeon should be familiar with the literature as well as his or her own personal experience and should be able to explain to the patient all treatment options with their associated risks and benefits. Importantly, the surgeon should inform the patient clearly and unambiguously of what, in his or her opinion, is the best treatment option, which in certain patients may be no treatment at all.

Management

The main goal of treatment of a cerebral AVM is aimed at prevention of future hemorrhage and possible neurological deterioration. Currently, the treatment options for AVMs include microsurgical resection only, preoperative endovascular embolization followed by microsurgical resection, stereotactic radiosurgery only, preprocedural endovascular embolization followed by radiosurgical treatment, endovascular embolization only, and observation only. Each treatment modality has its specific advantages and disadvantages. The following section will discuss the surgical technique and nuances of supratentorial AVM resection in various locations. Endovascular embolization and radiosurgical treatment as well as the surgical management of infratentorial AVMs will be addressed in other chapters in this book.

Microsurgical resection

Timing of surgery

Surgery for an AVM is generally an elective procedure. For a ruptured AVM that leads to intracranial hemorrhage but no significant neurological deficits, our policy is to operate in a delayed fashion (4–6 weeks). During this period, the risk of early rebleeding is relatively low, yet it allows time for the hematoma to liquefy, the associated surrounding edema to resolve, and the dysautoregulated brain tissue to recover. In the setting of life-threatening hemorrhage necessitating urgent surgery, we generally recommend only gentle evacuation of the clot without disturbing the AVM. Only for an AVM of small surface area that can easily be removed with the clot do we attempt to excise the AVM on an emergency basis. Although some authors have reported good outcomes with acute surgical resection [34], it is important to recognize that significant neurological deficits following AVM rupture are not necessarily permanent. Frequently, the deficit observed in these situations occurs as a result of a hematoma exerting pressure on critical brain structures rather than actual destruction of functional neural tissue. It is, therefore, in our opinion a mistake to operate on an AVM acutely believing that surgery could not worsen an already existing complete neurological deficit. Following a reasonable delay to allow such potential recovery to occur, the surgeon will be in a better situation to judge whether, given the degree of the recovery, it may not be preferable to treat the patient with an alternative treatment modality (i.e., radiosurgery) or to recommend conservative therapy. We prefer to repeat cerebral angiography near the time of surgery to make sure that AVM configuration has not changed since the time of hemorrhage.

General surgical technique

Intraoperative angiography should be used for all AVM surgery unless the position of the patient makes it impractical. In such instances, immediate postoperative angiography should be performed. A radiolucent three-pin head-holder frame is used for patients for whom intraoperative angiography is contemplated. A femoral arterial sheath is placed at the start of the procedure particularly if the final position of the patient for surgery makes access to the groin region difficult. Alternatively, the groin can be prepared for intraoperative femoral access following AVM resection to minimize sheath-related complications caused by prolonged arterial access. The head position varies according to the location of the AVM. For convexity lesions, the head is positioned so that the cortical representation of the AVM is uppermost in the operative field.

For cortical AVMs, we prefer a large craniotomy with a margin of a few centimeters around the lesion. The main advantage of a large exposure is the ability to easily identify the cortical vascular anatomy for comparison with the cerebral angiogram. Occasionally, feeding arteries are seen on the cortical surface at some distance from the AVM prior to their descent into a sulcus to reach the malformations and these would not be apparent through a smaller craniotomy. Similarly, the change in color of arterialized draining veins to blue, an indicator that the arterial supply to the AVM has been interrupted, may only be seen several centimeters away from the lesion as the veins receive normal cortical drainage. Finally, it may be more difficult to control bleeding from the surrounding parenchyma through a smaller craniotomy.

The dura is carefully opened to avoid injury to adherent superficial draining veins. Excision of an AVM generally proceeds through several well-defined stages. First, the cortical surface anatomy is correlated with the preoperative angiogram. If the AVM is not visible on the cortical surface, a useful technique is to follow a superficial arterialized draining vein back to the malformation, although this has the potential risk of injuring the vein. The best alternative, when available, is to follow a superficial feeding artery into a sulcus. Intraoperative ultrasound and frameless stereotactic guidance may also aid in identifying the malformations. Next, the sulci around the AVM are opened and the feeding arteries are identified, coagulated, and sectioned. It is more difficult to coagulate a high-flow AVM feeder than a normal artery of the same diameter. Interruption of flow through a large feeding artery with a temporary AVM or weck clip will facilitate coagulation of the artery. We have found that irrigating bipolar forceps are extremely useful during AVM surgery. Our bipolar forceps technique consists of intermittent coagulation for 1–2 seconds under constant irrigation while avoiding complete closure of the forceps to prevent adherence of the cauterized vessel to the bipolar tips. Furthermore, we continuously maintain cleanliness of the bipolar tips, which also prevents sticking. It is important to divide arterial feeders close to the nidus and only after ensuring that they do not supply normal brain tissue after passing through the malformations (vessels en passage). Although draining veins are generally larger and have thinner walls, it is occasionally difficult to differentiate whether a particular vessel is a feeding artery or a draining arterialized vein. A useful technique is to place a temporary clip on the vessel in question; a draining vein will become less turgid and frequently bluer distal to the clip whereas an artery will continue to pulsate against the clip. Alternatively a microvascular flow probe or a microscope equipped with indocyanine green videoangiography may be used to determine the direction of flow.

After all visible superficial feeders have been sacrificed, a circumferential cortical incision is made immediately adjacent to the AVM. The corticectomy is then carried to the depth of the sulci and further occlusion of the remaining superficial feeding arteries is performed. Although, an attempt is made to preserve all arterialized veins until the end of the resection, it is occasionally necessary to sacrifice one or more superficial veins to facilitate dissection. This is generally well tolerated as long as the main venous drainage is left intact. If early sacrifice of a vein is contemplated, it may be wise to first occlude it temporarily to ensure that the nidus does not swell or bleed.

Dissection of the AVM continues circumferentially in a spiral fashion. Where the AVM is located in non-eloquent regions of the brain, the cortical incision can be made several millimeters away from the AVM to facilitate dissection of the AVM. However, where the AVM is located within or immediately adjacent to eloquent areas, the surgeon must work directly on the AVM loops. A useful technique is gentle coagulation of the AVM loops in an attempt to shrink the nidus away from eloquent cerebral tissue. However, this technique should only be attempted after the main arterial supply to the AVM has been interrupted and the turgor of the nidus has diminished significantly. Early coagulation of the AVM nidus, while the internal pressure and flow are high, may result in increased AVM pressure and subsequent rupture through diminution of nidus volume without a decrease in arterial inflow. If bleeding from the AVM occurs, it can usually be controlled by placement of a cotton pad over the bleeding point and application of gentle pressure with a self-retaining retractor. Bleeding from the brain, away from the AVM, should not be packed as this may result in serious intraparenchymal hemorrhage. In such instances, the bleeding usually occurs from a vessel that has retracted into the surrounding brain tissue or from a remnant of the AVM that has been disconnected from the main nidus. The surgeon must resist the temptation to "pack" the bleeding and be diligent in finding and coagulating the offending vessel(s).

Circumferential dissection is carried down to the deepest aspect of the AVM near or within the ventricular ependymal surface. Coagulation and sectioning of the small friable subependymal or perforating feeding arteries in this location can be very challenging. Once injured, these deep vessels have a tendency to retract, and occasionally bipolar coagulation is completely ineffective. In such instances, control of these fine vessels can only be achieved by placement of Sundt microclips, which were specifically designed for this purpose. Frequently with AVMs that reach the ventricle, the bleeding will not cease until the ependyma has been reached and the small remaining ependymal feeding arteries, which can be more easily coagulated, have been occluded.

After the nidus has been dissected from the surrounding brain and all the apparent arterial feeders have been sacrificed, the color of the large draining veins should become darker and eventually change from red to blue. If the vein remains arterialized, the surgeon should search for residual feeders, which are frequently located beneath or in close proximity to the vein. Only after these final arterial vessels have been interrupted can the non-arterialized draining vein be taken.

The final stage is inspection of the resection cavity for residual AVM nidus. Once hemostasis has been achieved, the patient's mean arterial pressure is raised by 15–20 mmHg above baseline and maintained for approximately 10 minutes. Any bleeding during this period is highly suspicious for residual AVM nidus and should be inspected thoroughly. If no bleeding occurs, the surgical cavity is lined with a single layer of Surgicel and the patient's blood pressure is kept at or slightly below normal and maintained at this level for 24 hours. Intraoperative angiography is then performed to confirm complete AVM resection.

Surgical considerations for specific locations

The technique of AVM resection is modified for lesions in certain locations to take into account the location of arterial supply and venous drainage as well as to minimize the risk of brain injury.

Convexity location

Frontal AVMs are primarily supplied by branches of the anterior and middle cerebral arteries (ACA and MCA, respectively). Temporal lesions receive supply from branches of the MCA, posterior cerebral artery (PCA), and anterior choroidal artery. Parietal malformations can receive supply from all three major supratentorial arteries. Occipital AVMs are fed primarily by PCA branches with contribution from the MCA and ACA for larger lesions that extend medially. Convexity AVMs are often wedge shaped, with the apex directed toward and frequently reaching the ventricle. They can have both superficial and deep venous drainage.

Surgical resection of convexity AVMs follows the same techniques described above. Performing a large craniotomy and use of stereotactic guidance is helpful in understanding the anatomy. Special care should be exercised in lesions with arterial supply from external carotid arteries as serious bleeding may occur during the craniotomy. Preoperative embolization, although very useful in such patients, carries the risk of skin necrosis particularly if the scalp flap is not based on a different arterial pedicle. If embolization is not performed, then multiple burr holes and careful stripping and coagulation of the dura are necessary.

Peri-sylvian location

Peri-sylvian AVMs include lesions that involve the frontal and temporal operculum or the insular cortex. One of the key features that must be kept in mind during resection of sylvian AVMs is the fact that they are primarily supplied by branches of the MCA en passage to normal brain tissue. Venous drainage is usually into the superficial and deep sylvian veins.

Anteriorly located lesions are approached through a standard frontotemporal (pterional) craniotomy. The sylvian fissure may be opened either in a medial-to-lateral or a lateral-to-medial direction. The MCA branches are identified and carefully skeletonized by coagulating or clipping and dividing all side branches to the malformations. Temporary clipping of the MCA may be used to facilitate dissection of an arterial branch or control excessive bleeding. An AVM located in the middle or posterior portions of the sylvian fissure is approached through a temporal craniotomy. In these patients, it is not necessary to open the horizontal (medial) stem of the sylvian fissure (Fig. 11.1).

An AVM located entirely within the insula is approached through the sylvian fissure followed by skeletonization of the MCA branches to control the medially directed feeders. The presence of lenticulostriate perforator supply signifies deep extension of the AVM, which usually makes it inoperable. Occasionally these AVMs can be more extensive and involve the temporal lobe stem, the medial temporal lobe, and reach the atrium (Fig. 11.2).

Medial temporal location

Anterior medial temporal lesions are supplied by branches of the anterior choroidal and posterior communicating arteries as well as anterior temporal branches of the MCA and PCA (Fig. 11.3). Venous drainage is usually into the basal vein of Rosenthal and occasionally into the sphenoparietal sinus and vein of Labbé. Anterior medial temporal AVMs involve the uncus, amygdala, and anterior hippocampus and are best approached through a pterional trans-sylvian approach. Once the sylvian fissure has been opened and the arterial feeders sacrificed, the AVM can be removed by working from a medial to lateral direction. It is important to follow feeders from early anterior temporal MCA branches to ensure that they do not give rise to lenticulostriate arteries.

Posterior medial temporal AVMs are fed by branches of the anterior choroidal artery and PCA (Fig. 11.4). They involve the hippocampus, parahippocampus, and fusiform gyrus and can be approached through a temporal craniotomy by working either subtemporally or through the inferior temporal gyrus. Exposure through the inferior temporal gyrus avoids the

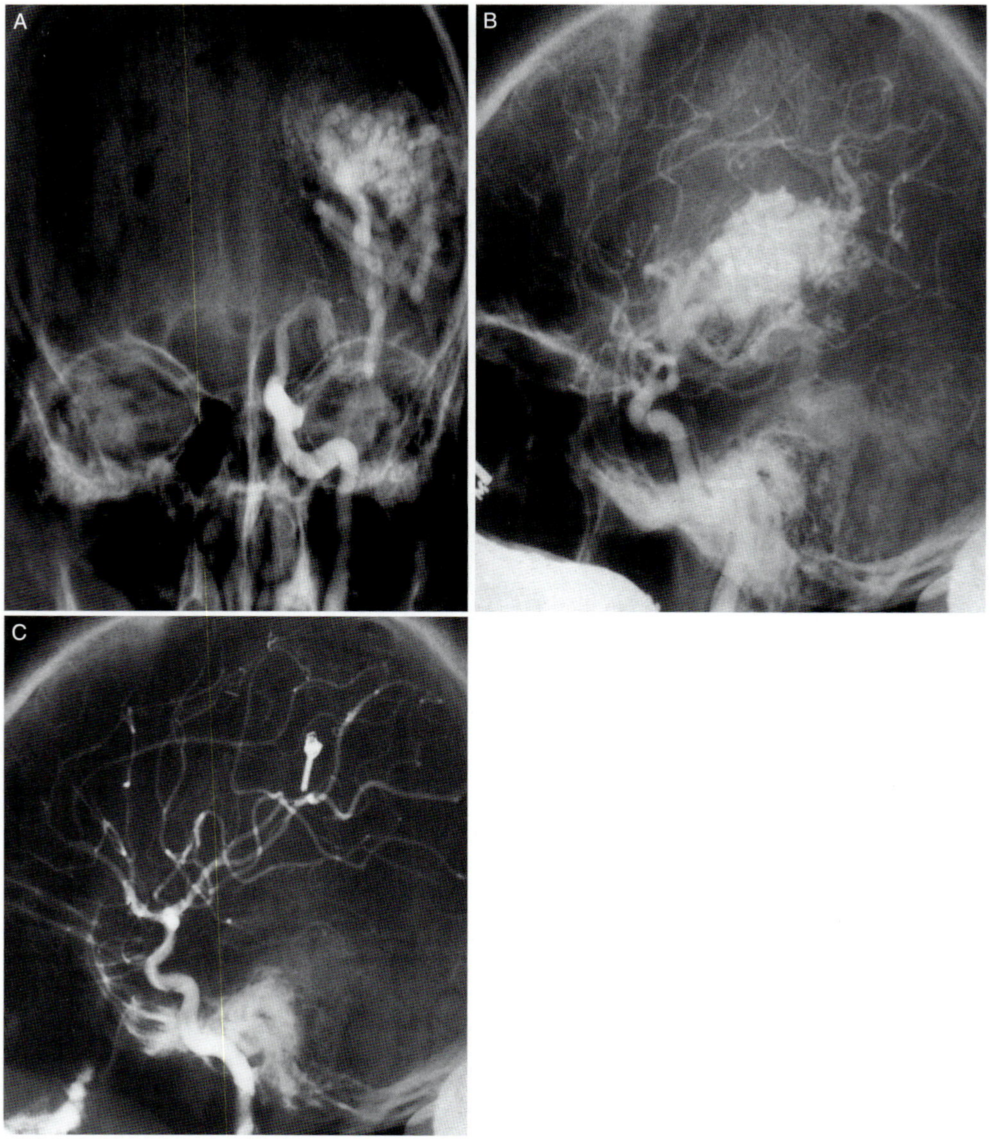

Fig. 11.1. Sylvian arteriovenous malformations (AVM). (A) Anteroposterior left carotid injection. (B) Lateral left carotid injection. (C) Postoperative left carotid injection showing complete removal of the AVM and preservation of the middle cerebral arteries.

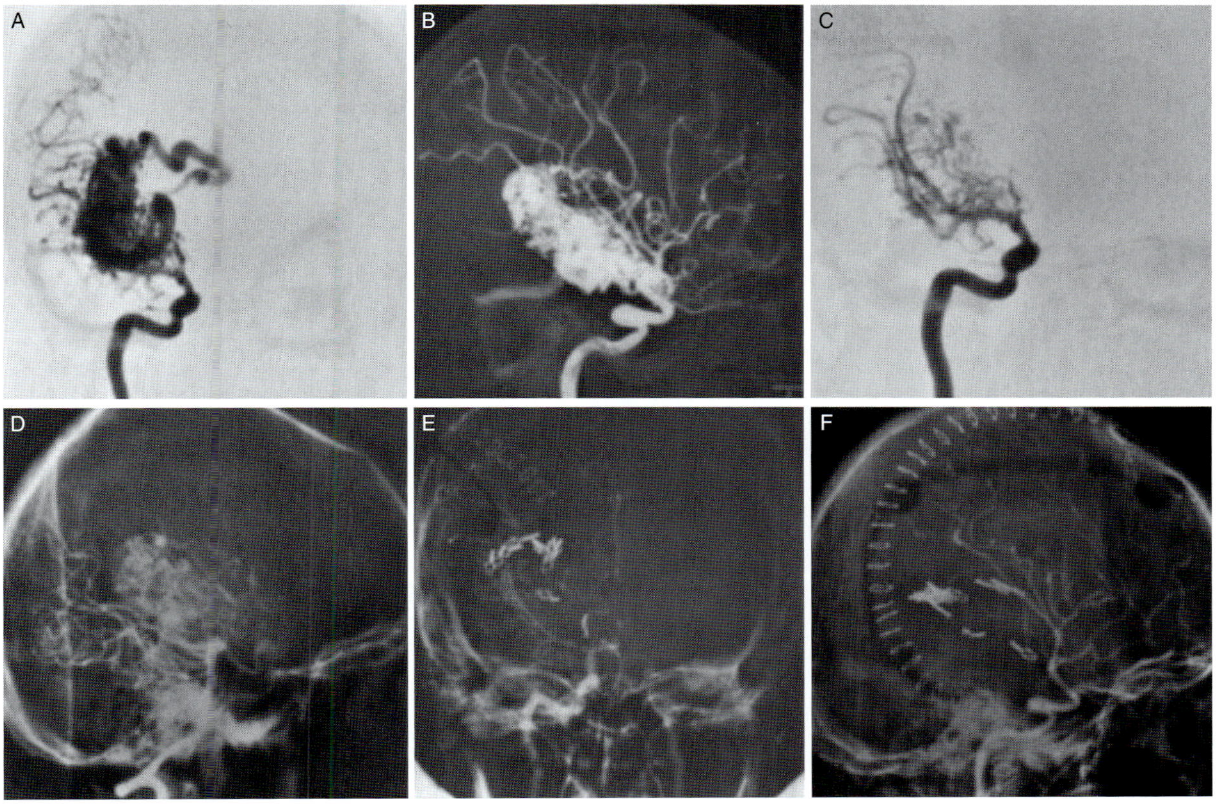

Fig. 11.2. Large insular/medial temporal arteriovenous malformations (AVM). (A) Right anteroposterior carotid injection. (B) Right lateral carotid injection. (C) Early anteroposterior carotid injection demonstrating lenticulostriate feeders. (D) Lateral vertebral injection demonstrating posterior cerebral feeders. (E) Postoperative anteroposterior carotid injection demonstrating complete removal of the AVM. (F) Postoperative lateral carotid injection.

temporal lobe retraction and stretching of the vein of Labbé that is frequently associated with the subtemporal approach; however, it is more likely to cause a superior quadrantanopia. Once the temporal horn has been accessed, the anterior choroidal feeders can be controlled through the choroidal fissure. The PCA feeders can then be reached either subtemporally or through the inferior temporal gyrus.

Trigonal location

Trigonal malformations are supplied by branches of the PCA and lateral posterior choroidal artery and usually drain into the deep venous system via the basal vein of Rosenthal (Fig. 11.5). Surgical approaches to these lesions are largely based on where the bulk of the AVM nidus is located.

Laterally and inferiorly located malformations involving the floor and lateral wall of the trigone can be approached transtemporally either through the inferior or middle temporal gyrus on the non-dominant side or through the inferior temporal gyrus on the dominant hemisphere to avoid speech deficits. Early control of PCA feeders can be achieved through an initial subtemporal approach prior to attacking the nidus transtemporally.

Medially and superiorly located malformations involving the roof of the trigone and occasionally the pulvinar can be approached either through a posterior interhemispheric approach or transcortically through the superior parietal lobule. Although the posterior interhemispheric trans-isthmus approach permits early access to PCA feeders and avoids injury to the optic radiation, it requires significant retraction of the occipital lobe, and potential visual field deficits, because the trigone is approximately 3 cm lateral to the midline. Furthermore, the surgical working view through this approach is tangential to the AVM. For these reasons, we prefer to use a transcerebral approach through the superior parietal lobule. The approach is carried between the parietal sensory association fibers and the occipital visual association fibers and offers a direct view to trigonal lesions. The cortical incision is made approximately 7 cm from the tentorium, which corresponds to an external landmark of 9 cm above the inion and 3 cm from the midline. The cortisectomy is then deepened toward the trigone using ultrasound or frameless stereotactic guidance. We have used this approach routinely without resulting sensory or visual deficits, particularly if the AVM is small, although with larger AVMs, it is occasionally impossible to prevent some visual field loss from damage to the visual radiations along the tapetum.

Parasagittal location

Parasagittal lesions are primarily supplied by branches of the PCA and pericallosal and callosomarginal arteries, with contribution from the MCA particularly in patients where the malformations reaches the convexity. Venous drainage is usually into superior and inferior sagittal sinuses. The challenge in surgical resection of parasagittal AVMs lies in the ability to control the interhemispheric feeders. The operative position is dictated by the arterial supply to the malformations and whether it reaches

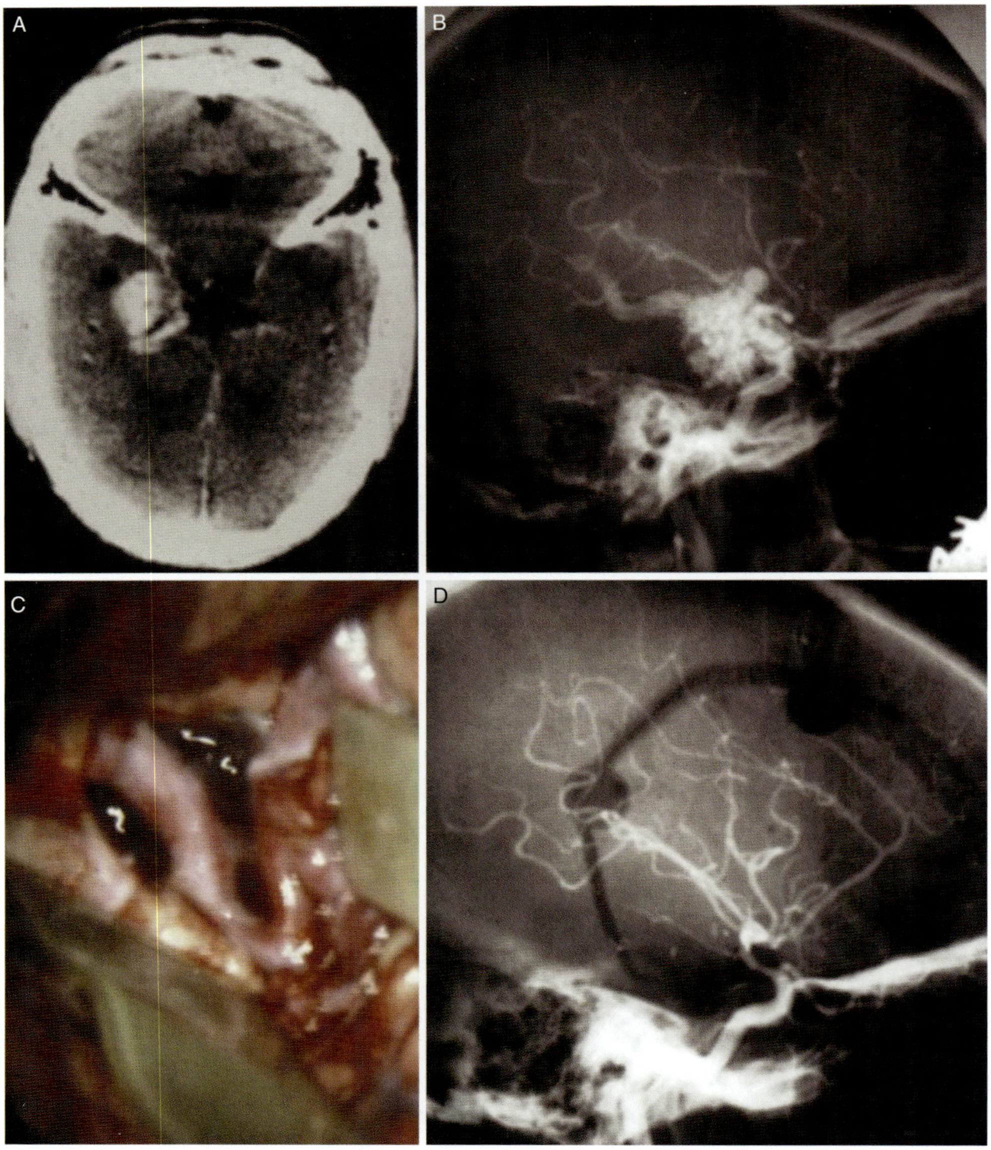

Fig. 11.3. Anteromedial temporal arteriovenous malformations (AVM). (A) CT scan. (B) Angiography, lateral right carotid injection. (C) Intraoperative trans-sylvian exposure demonstrating the internal carotid artery and feeders to the medial aspect of the AVM by a very enlarged anterior temporal branch. (D) Postoperative right carotid arteriography demonstrating complete removal of the AVM.

the convexity. Lesions that are solely supplied by ACA feeders and do not reach the convexity are best approached through an interhemispheric approach. We prefer to position the patient in a lateral position with the ipsilateral hemisphere dependent to allow the brain to fall away from the falx. Lumbar drainage is occasionally used to facilitate brain relaxation. The craniotomy should extend across the midline. It is important to open the dura with a narrow flap based on the sinus to allow the brain to fall under and not against the dural edge. Every effort must be made at preserving the arterialized draining veins, which can be easily injured during brain retraction. Occasionally parasagittal AVMs are stuck by many small draining veins to the falx and sinus. It is, therefore, advisable to make a broad-based bone flap so that the lesion can be approached from a more anterior or posterior trajectory depending on the venous anatomy.

Parasagittal lesions with both ACA and MCA feeders and those that reach the convexity pose a technical problem. The position required to control the interhemispheric branches differs from that needed to control the MCA feeders along the convexity. Ideally, a parasagittal approach, with the head neutral or in a lateral position with the ipsilateral side down, is required to deal with the ACA feeders, while a lateral position with the ipsilateral side up is ideal for control of the MCA supply. One approach is to start with the head in a neutral position and control the interhemispheric branches first and then turn the head to a lateral position to deal with the convexity portion of the AVM. An alternative approach is to embolize the ACA feeders preoperatively and resect the AVM in the lateral position with the convexity uppermost in the field.

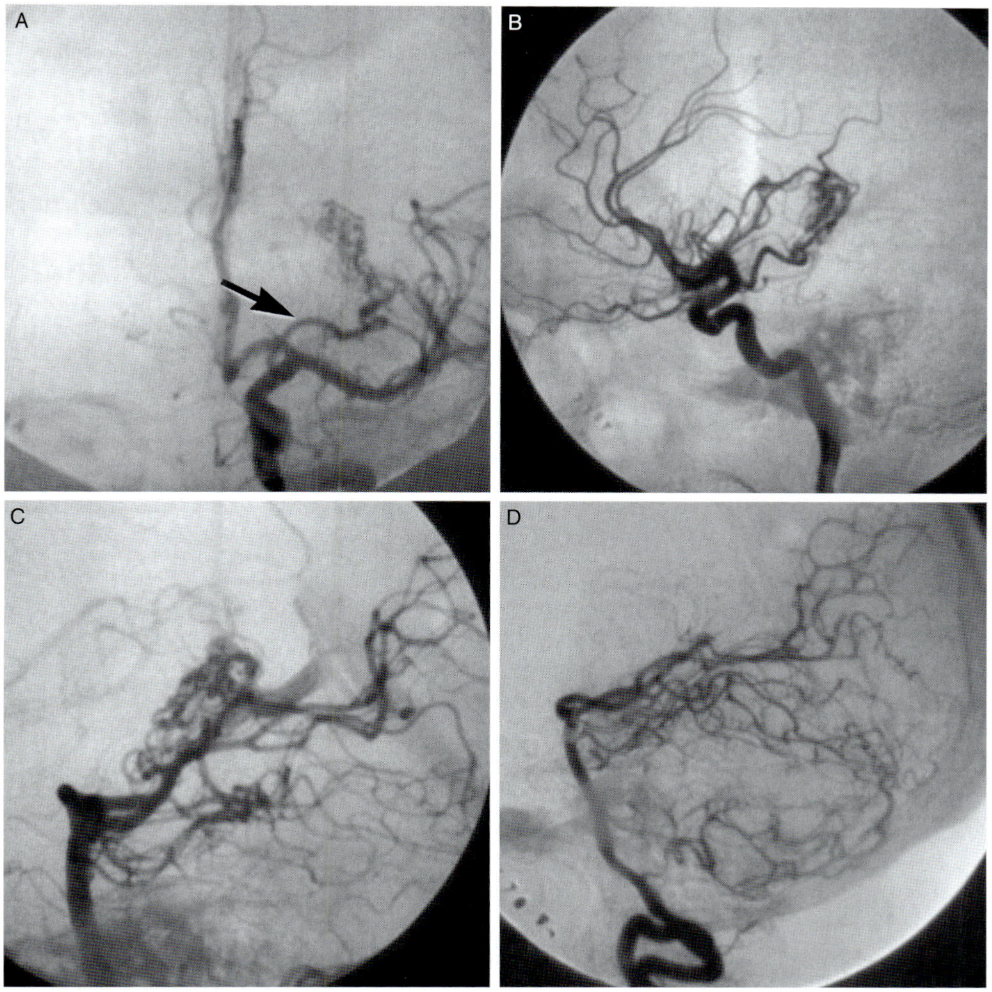

Fig. 11.4. Left posteromedial temporal arteriovenous malformations (AVM). (A) Left carotid injection demonstrating a large anterior choroidal feeder (arrow). (B) Lateral left carotid injection. (C) Lateral vertebral injection. (D) Postoperative vertebral injection demonstrating complete removal of the AVM.

Anterior corpus callosal locations

Anterior callosal malformations are usually fed by branches of the pericallosal and callosomarginal arteries and drain to the sagittal sinus as well as to the septal vein and deep venous system. These AVMs can extend laterally into the head of the caudate nucleus and acquire supply from the recurrent artery of Heubner and medial lenticulostriate arteries (Fig. 11.6). Evidence of lateral lenticulostriate supply, however, suggests involvement of the internal capsule and is an indicator of AVM inoperability. These lesions can also extend inferiorly below the genu to involve the basal frontal region and anterior aspect of the hypothalamus, where they receive additional supply from the anterior communicating complex perforators.

Anterior callosal AVMs are best approached through an anterior interhemispheric approach. The pericallosal and callosomarginal arteries feed the malformations by numerous small side-branches en passage through the lesion. As with sylvian AVMs, the main arterial trunks must be skeletonized and preserved. Malformations that involve the subcallosal region require a low frontal craniotomy and a subfrontal exposure to control feeders from the anterior communicating and early pericallosal arteries. An AVM that extends into the head of the caudate nucleus requires dissection through the ventricle and control of the medial lenticulostriate supply.

Splenial location

Splenial lesions are fed primarily by direct branches from the PCA, pericallosal branches of the PCA and ACA, and branches from the medial posterior choroidal artery. If the nidus extends laterally into the trigone, it can also obtain supply from the lateral posterior choroidal arteries (Fig. 11.7). Venous drainage is usually into the deep venous system. Because the majority of the blood supply comes from interhemispheric branches, these lesions are best approached through a posterior parasagittal approach. Splenial AVMs are frequently eccentric toward one hemisphere. We prefer to access these lesions in the lateral position placing the occipital lobe with the greater portion of the nidus down. The pericallosal feeders are controlled as they enter the malformations anteriorly whereas the PCA supply is accessed in the quadrigeminal cistern. As the AVM is dissected laterally toward the trigone, feeders from the medial posterior choroidal artery must be controlled. As with trigonal AVMs, this portion of the procedure requires some retraction of the

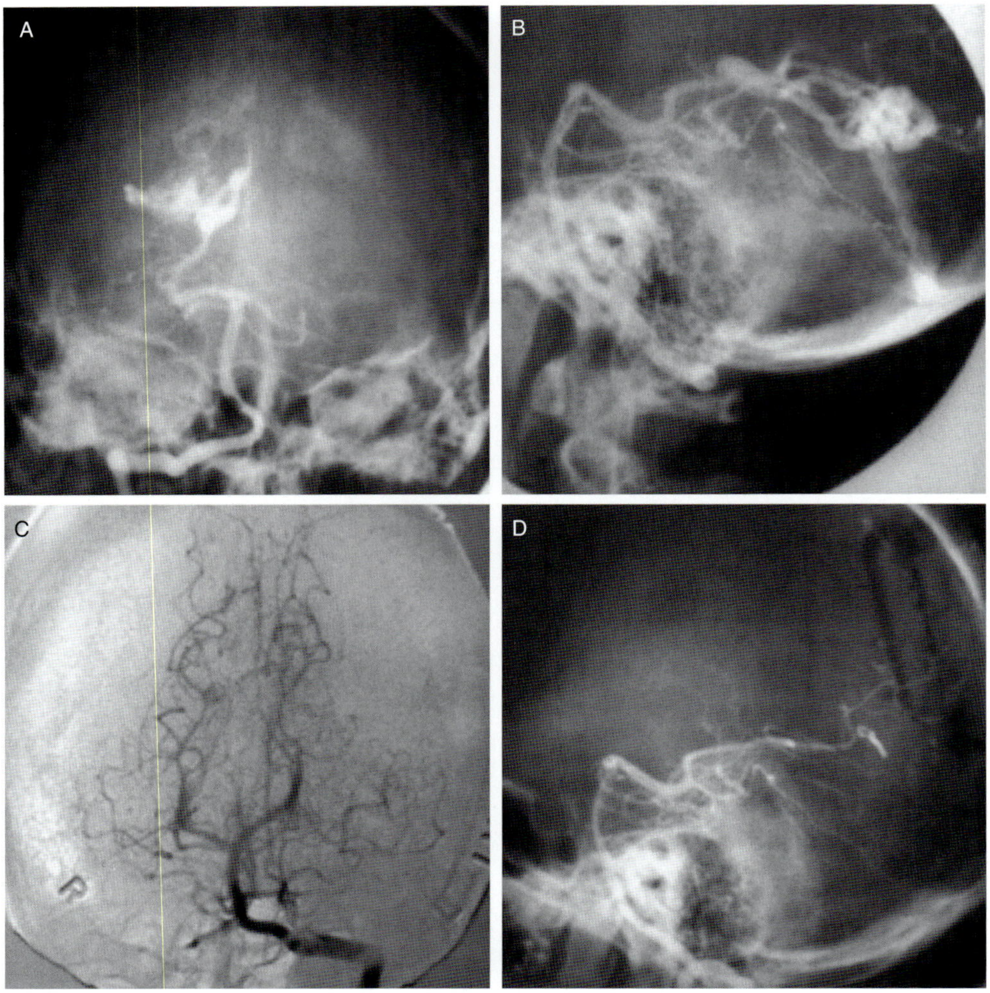

Fig. 11.5. Trigonal arteriovenous malformation (A) Anteroposterior vertebral injection. (B) Lateral vertebral injection. (C) Postoperative anteroposterior vertebral injection. (D) Postoperative lateral vertebral injection showing complete removal of the malformation through a posterior parietal bone flap.

occipital lobe and can be challenging because of the limited tangential working view. An alternative is accessing the AVM through a contralateral parafalcine approach by which a more direct view is possible. Another difficulty is that splenial AVMs may be intimately related to the deep venous system and care must be taken not to injure any of the important deep cerebral veins.

Intraventricular location

Intraventricular AVMs may be fed by deep perforating arteries and/or choroidal branches (Fig. 11.8). Venous drainage is usually into the deep venous system. Although it remains unproven, we believe that intraventricular AVMs may carry a higher rate of hemorrhage because of the lack of surrounding supportive parenchymal tissue and, therefore, should be considered for surgical resection, particularly in patients with a history of repeated bleeds. In general, the operability of these lesions is largely dependent on the source of arterial supply. Vascular lesions that are predominantly fed by perforating branches that traverse the basal ganglia and thalamus carry a significant risk of morbidity with surgical resection because of deep bleeding. Such lesions, if they are small enough, may be better managed with radiosurgery. If the majority of the blood supply arises from choroidal arteries, the AVM can be resected safely as the arterial feeders can be readily controlled at the various ependymal surfaces.

Intraventricular AVMs involving the head of caudate can be safely resected despite perforator supply from the recurrent artery of Heubner. Although control of deep arterial bleeding can be problematic during resection, damage to the anteromedial internal capsule is generally well tolerated. These lesions can be approached either through an anterior interhemispheric transcallosal approach or via a transfrontal trajectory if there is associated ventriculomegaly. Lesions involving the tela choroidea of the roof of the third ventricle can be reached via a transchoroidal approach by opening of the tenia fornices. Surgical approaches to trigonal AVMs have been discussed above.

Thalamus and basal ganglia

Surgical resection of thalamic and basal ganglial AVMs generally carries significant risk particularly if they are large and have predominant perforator supply. In general, these lesions are best managed conservatively or, if they are small enough, with

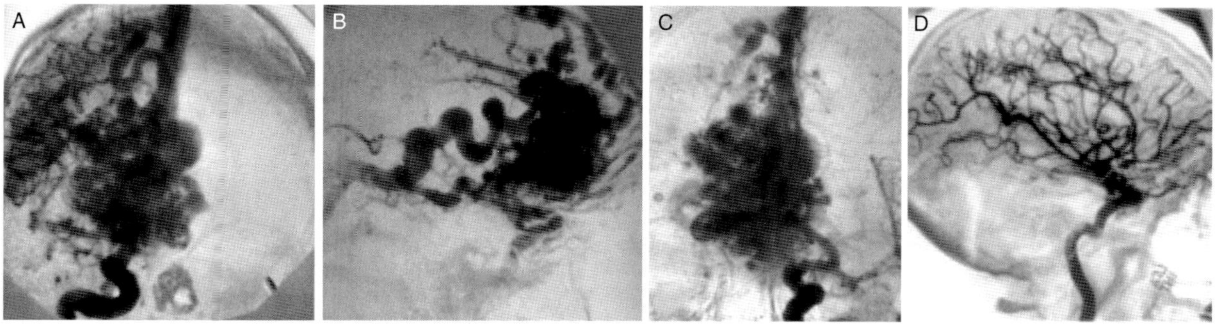

Fig. 11.6. Large anterior callosal arteriovenous malformation involving the caudate nucleus and anterior hypothalamus. (A) Anteroposterior right carotid injection. (B) Lateral right carotid injection showing a large septal draining vein. (C) Anteroposterior left carotid injection. (D) Postoperative lateral carotid arteriography showing complete removal of the malformations with preservation of both pericallosal arteries.

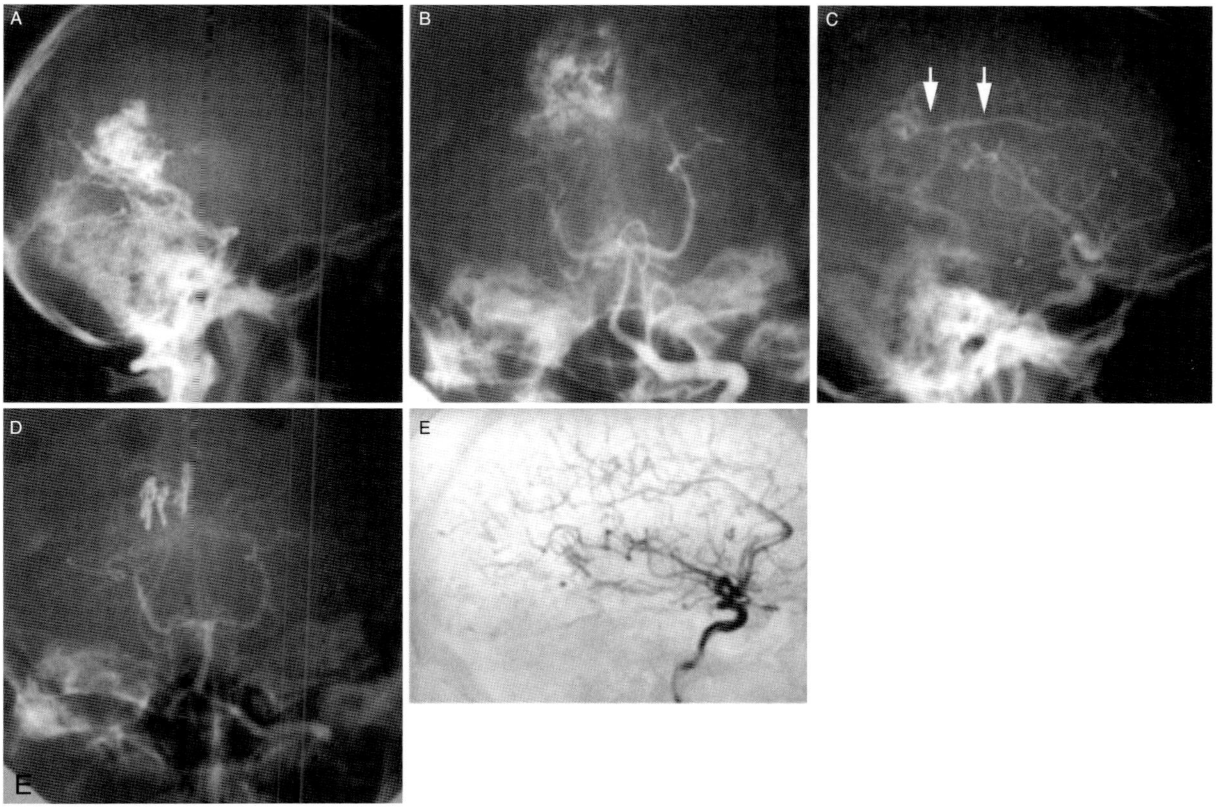

Fig. 11.7. Splenial arteriovenous malformation. (A) Lateral vertebral injection. (B) Anteroposterior vertebral injection. (C) Lateral carotid injection (arrows show a pericallosal feeder). (D) Postoperative anteroposterior vertebral injection showing complete removal of the malformation. (E) Postoperative lateral carotid injection.

stereotactic radiosurgery. Surgical resection may be considered for deep AVMs if the perforator supply can be safely occluded with endovascular therapy (Fig. 11.9) or for small to medium-sized AVMs in patients with a history of multiple hemorrhages and significant residual motor weakness following a sufficient time to allow for maximal functional recovery. Lesions located lateral to the internal capsule, involving the putamen and insula, may also be surgically resected with reasonable morbidity. Similarly, as discussed above, resection of AVMs involving the head of caudate nucleus or pulvinar of the thalamus can be performed with acceptable risk. An AVM involving the posterolateral inferior thalamus and lateral geniculate ganglia may also be amenable to surgical resection via a transtemporal approach in patients with pre-existing complete hemianopsia. Surgical resection of incompletely obliterated thalamic and basal ganglia AVMs following radiosurgery and/or embolization has also been reported [35].

Surgical outcomes

Microsurgical resection of Spetzler–Martin grades I, II, and most, although not all, grade III AVMs by experienced surgeons carries high cure rates and low complication rates, with immediate elimination of risk of hemorrhage [36–38]. Angiographic cure rate with microsurgery ranges from 94 to 100%. Microsurgery can achieve 100% angiographic obliteration for unruptured convexity AVMs <3 cm with superficial

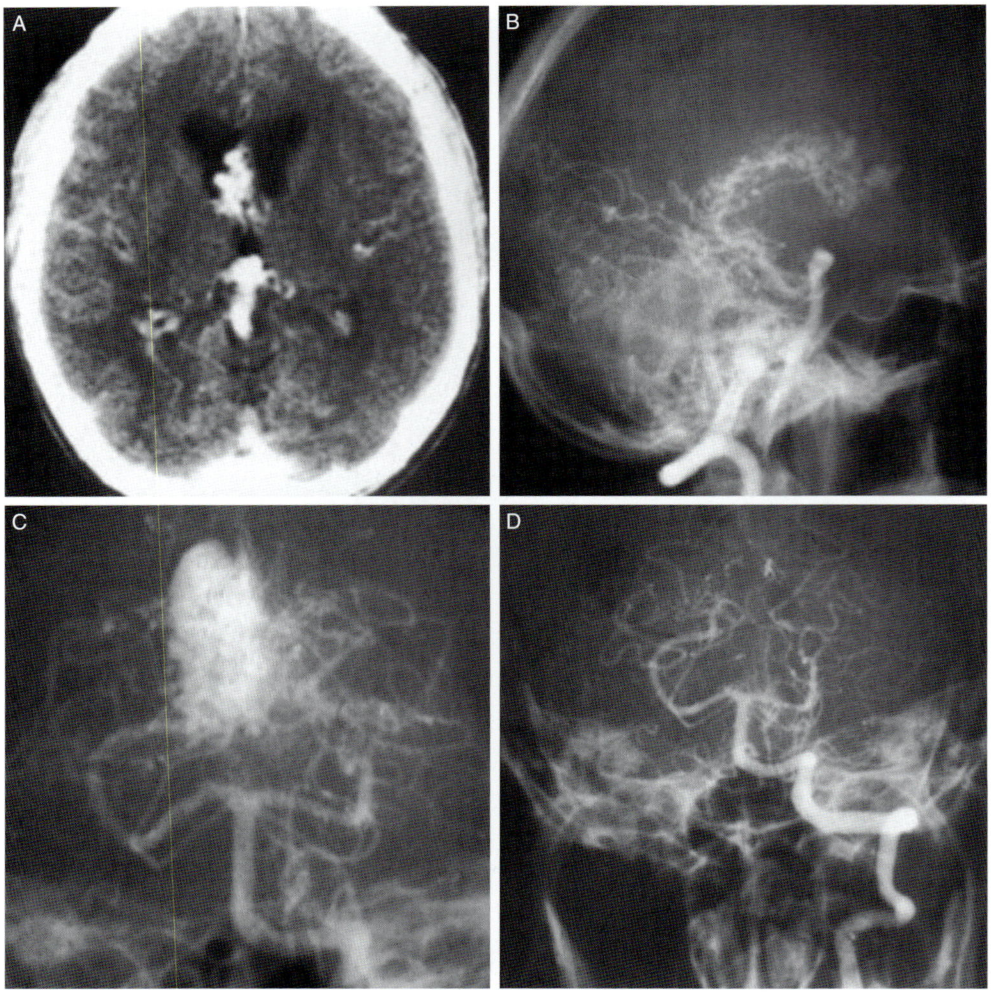

Fig. 11.8. Intraventricular arteriovenous malformation (AVM) involving the tela choroidea of the third ventricle. (A) CT demonstrated the AVM. (B) Lateral vertebral injection demonstrated the posteromedial choroidal supply to the AVM. (C) Anteroposterior vertebral injection. (D) Postoperative anteroposterior vertebral injection demonstrated complete removal of the AVM, which was accessed by a transcallosal transchoroidal approach.

venous drainage [39]. The combined surgical morbidity and mortality for AVMs of grades I–III is reported to be less than 10% in several large series [40–48]. Tables 11.2 and 11.3 summarize the microsurgical outcomes from some of the larger published case series for AVMs of Spetzler–Martin grades I–III and grades IV and V, respectively.

In a series of 311 patients with cerebral AVMs who underwent microsurgical resection alone before 1993, Heros *et al.* reported 89.9% of patients with grade I–III AVMs had a good outcome, 9.5% had significant disability, and 0.5% died during the early postoperative period [54]. However, only 60.7% of patients with grade IV and V AVMs had a good outcome, 37.5% having significant disability and 1.8% dying. In a follow-up study of 153 consecutive patients with AVMs of all grades, with a mean follow-up period of 3.8 years, we looked at the immediate morbidity and mortality rates and compared these with the late morbidity and mortality rates [36]. The overall immediate postoperative rate of serious morbidity was 24.2%; the serious morbidity at follow-up was 7.8%. The mortality rate at follow-up was 1.3%. There was no history of intracranial hemorrhage in any patient during the follow-up period. At follow-up, 97.8% of patients with grade I–III AVMs were in good or excellent condition; 1.1% experienced a poor outcome, and 1.1% died. In the group of patients with grade IV and V AVMs, 79.0% had good outcome, 17.7% had poor outcome, and 3.2% died.

As discussed above, grade III AVMs are a heterogeneous group, with subtypes possessing different surgical risks. Grade III AVMs that are 3 cm in size with superficial venous drainage in non-eloquent brain regions carry a low surgical risk similar to that of grade I or II AVMs. Grade III AVMs 3–6 cm in size with superficial drainage in eloquent brain regions have a surgical risk similar to that of grade IV or V AVMs. Grade III AVMs 3–6 cm in size with deep drainage in non-eloquent brain regions have intermediate risk [26].

Complete obliteration of AVMs leads to the best outcome in terms of seizure control. After surgical excision, 81% of patients with a history of seizures were seizure free, whereas seizure-free outcome after radiosurgery and embolization was at 43% and 50%, respectively [55]. Heros *et al.* [36] reported a seizure-free survival in 43.6% of patients with AVMs who had preoperative seizures.

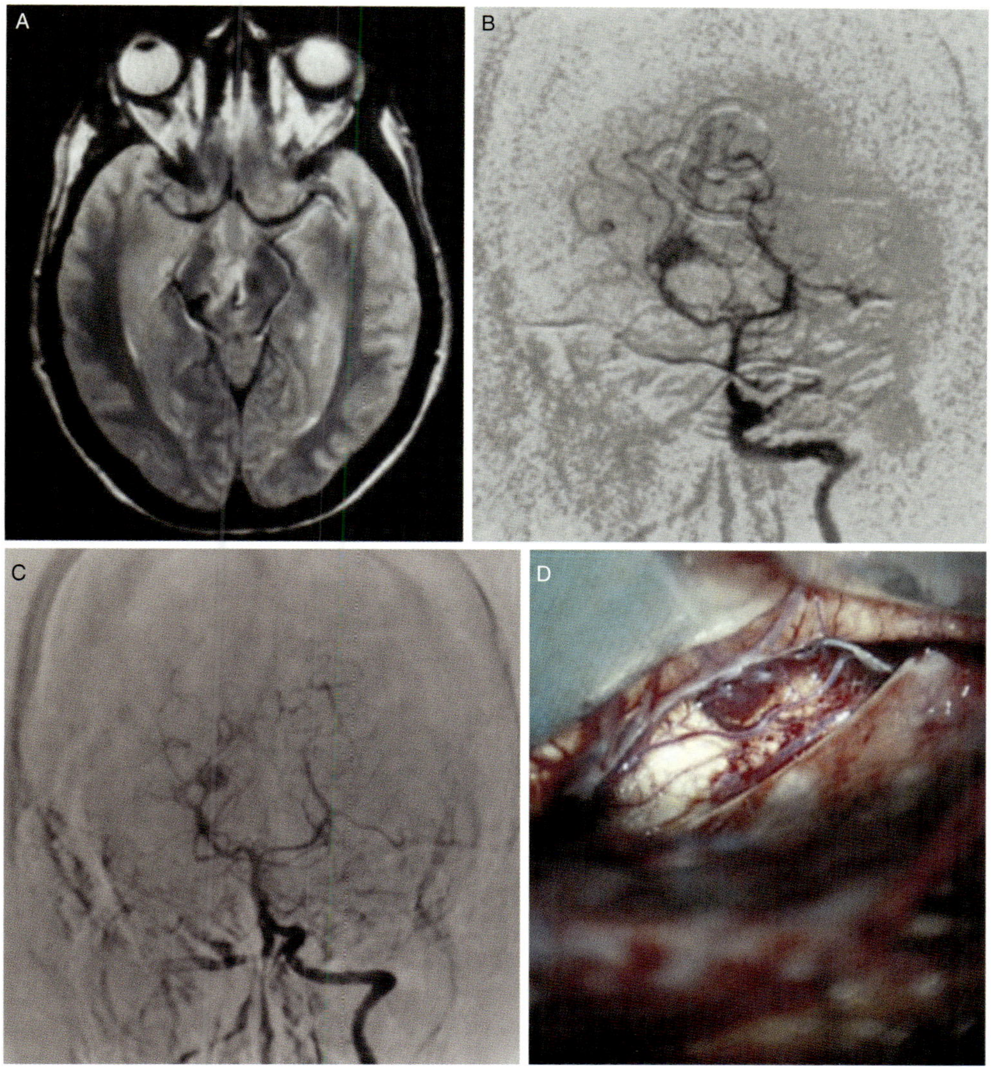

Fig. 11.9. Small inferolateral thalamic arteriovenous malformation. (A) Axial MRI. (B) Anteroposterior vertebral injection showed a large thalamic perforator. (C) Anteroposterior vertebral injection after successful embolization of the thalamic perforator. (D) Intraoperative photograph of the subtemporal approach to the malformation, which was successfully resected after embolization of the large single thalamic perforator.

Complications

Meticulous preoperative preparation, intraoperative technique and judgment, and postoperative precautions must be adhered to in order to minimize surgical morbidity and mortality. Surgical indications should be thoroughly analyzed, as many complications can be traced back to patients who underwent surgery inappropriately [56,57]. Many of the errors in judgment result from three-dimensional misinterpretation of eloquent anatomical relationships. This can be more easily avoided today with the utilization of modern anatomical and functional modalities to integrate anatomical, angiographic, hemodynamic, and functional data [58].

Intraoperative complications

Hemorrhage and intraparenchymal injury are two common complications encountered during AVM resection. Bleeding during surgery is either directly from the AVM during nidal dissection or secondarily from premature occlusion of major draining veins. Intraparenchymal injury can occur through several mechanisms. During nidal resection, caution must be exercised to remove a thin cortical rim without entering the AVM. However, a wide circumferential resection may lead to the destruction of functional parenchyma. Other mechanisms of injury include transecting arterial feeders too far from the nidus, excessive retraction, and bridging vein injury. Visual radiation injury is a specific concern during resection of temporal or occipital AVMs. Upon surgical planning, consideration must be given to the anatomical pathways of the geniculocalcarine fibers and Meyer's loop as they pass along the lateral ventricles. Additional considerations to avoid injury are cerebrospinal fluid release, thoughtful positioning, a wide craniotomy, and skull base approaches.

Postoperative complications

Hemorrhage

The most immediate and morbid postoperative complication is hemorrhage, either resulting from a residual nidus or

Table 11.2. Postoperative outcomes for grade I–III arteriovenous malformations

Study	No. patients	Morbidity and mortality rates
Pik and Morgan (2000) [44]	110	10.9% early morbidity; 2.7% late morbidity
Sisti *et al.* (1993) [47]	67 (small AVMs)	1.5% combined
Pikus *et al.* (1998) [45]	19	0%
Heros *et al.* (1990) [36]	91	1.1% late morbidity; 1.1% late mortality
Tokunaga *et al.* (2000) [48]	12	0% for grades I and II; 75% early morbidity, 50% late morbidity, and 0% mortality in grade III
Irie *et al.* (2000) [42]	27	0%
Hongo *et al.* (2000) [41]	20	4% mortality
Russell *et al.* (2002) [46]	35	8.6% morbidity; 0% mortality
Hartmann *et al.* (2000) [38]	95	5.3% morbidity; 0% mortality
Spetzler and Martin (1986) [23]	100	5% early morbidity
Lawton (2003) [25]	76 (grade III only)	3.9% morbidity; 3.9% mortality
Morgan *et al.* (2012) [49]	220 (grades I and II)	0.9% morbidity; 0.5% mortality; 9.5% adverse outcome for AVMs in eloquent cortex as opposed to 0.6% for AVMs in non-eloquent regions

AVM, arteriovenous malformation.

Table 11.3. Postoperative outcomes for grades IV and V arteriovenous malformations

Study	No. patients	Morbidity and mortality rates
Heros *et al.* (1990) [36]	62	17.7% late morbidity; 3.2% late mortality
Tokunaga *et al.* (2000) [48]	4	25% morbidity; 0% mortality
Irie *et al.* (2000) [42]	4	25% morbidity; 0% mortality
Hashimoto *et al.* (2000) [50]	3	75% morbidity; 0% mortality
Russell *et al.* (2002) [46]	9	22.2% morbidity; 11.1% mortality
Hartmann *et al.* (2000) [38]	29	6.9% morbidity; 0% mortality
Hamilton and Spetzler (1994) [40]	44	21.9% combined rate for grade IV; 16.7% combined rate for grade V
Hessler and Hejaza (1998) [51]	62	20.5% combined rate for grade IV; 30.4% combined rate for grade V
Nozaki *et al.* (2000) [52]	32	9% morbidity; 0% mortality
Jizong *et al.* (2000) [53]	50	26% early morbidity; 12% late morbidity; 0% mortality

inadequate hemostasis. Fortunately, the concern of inadvertent residual nidus has been resolved with intraoperative angiography.

Seizures

Of patients presenting with seizures, 55% have significant improvement, 35% remain unchanged, and 12% worsen. In addition, 15% of patients without a history of seizures develop first-time events postoperatively [36]. Because of this risk, we recommend a minimum of 6 months of antiepileptic treatment following the resection of a supratentorial AVM.

Normal perfusion pressure breakthrough

Normal perfusion pressure breakthrough refers to the theory that hemodynamic changes following AVM resection may lead to cerebral edema, hemorrhage, or both [59]. Angioarchitectural predictors include large caliber, long, high-flow feeding arteries that divert flow from surrounding parenchyma (steal phenomenon). Occurrence of normal perfusion pressure breakthrough can be avoided by selectively embolizing lesions with these high-risk characteristics.

Retrograde feeding artery thrombosis

Following AVM resection, angiographic feeding artery stasis is a common finding that can last up to 1 month [60]. Thrombosis of these arteries rarely occurs, being seen in 5 out of 76 patients (6.6%) reported by Miyasaka *et al.* [61]. The reported risk was highest in the elderly [62].

Retrograde venous thrombosis

Retrograde venous thrombosis can occur as a manifestation of venous stasis in large draining veins postoperatively.

Vasospasm

Vasospasm is an extraordinarily rare complication. In the series described by Yaşargil, postoperative vasospasm occurred in 2 out of 414 patients; in both there had been extensive A1 and M1 segment dissection during the procedures [63].

Conclusions

The management of patients harboring cerebral AVMs requires a thorough knowledge of the natural history as well as the efficacy and risks associated with the various treatment modalities. This chapter has discussed our general approach when faced with a patient harboring a cerebral AVM. Surgical approaches and technical nuances for the various supratentorial AVM locations were based on the experience of one author (RCH).

Decisions regarding the management of cerebral AVMs are complex and highly individualized. There is no fixed protocol to use to decide automatically for each patient. Each patient and each AVM is unique. The evaluation of an individual with a cerebral AVM begins with consideration of the various patient-related factors such as age, general health, clinical presentation and condition, occupation, and lifestyle. Similarly, AVM-related factors such as size, location, and presence of high-risk angiographic features, as well as the influence of these factors on the natural history and surgical risk, must be taken into account. Finally, the personal experience of the treating surgeon and interventionalist should be considered. In our opinion, the risk of intervention is best made by a neurosurgeon with experience in AVM surgery and preferably endovascular therapy and with at least a practical knowledge of the value and limits of radiosurgery. An alternative would be a multidisciplinary decision approach but, in our opinion, there has to be a "captain" of the team who is responsible for the final decision and its consequences. Information should be presented to the patient in an unambiguous manner with the best option being recommended. In general, patients with grade I and II AVMs should be offered surgical excision provided that they are relatively young and healthy. Radiosurgery may be a reasonable alternative in elderly patients with significant surgical comorbidities. Decisions regarding grade III AVMs are not straightforward; although many can be surgically resected with acceptable morbidity some are better left alone. The vast majority of grade IV and V lesions should be treated conservatively as surgical resection is associated with serious morbidity.

References

1. McCormick WF, Schochet SS. *Atlas of Cerebrovascular Disease*. Philadelphia, PA: Saunders, 1976.
2. Michelsen WJ. Natural history and pathophysiology of arteriovenous malformations. *Clin Neurosurg* 1979;**26**:307–13.
3. Ondra SL, Troupp H, George ED, *et al.* The natural history of symptomatic arteriovenous malformations of the brain: a 24-year follow-up assessment. *J Neurosurg* 1990;**73**:387–91.
4. Crawford PM, West CR, Chadwick DW, *et al.* Arteriovenous malformations of the brain: natural history in unoperated patients. *J Neurol Neurosurg Psychiatry* 1986;**49**:1–10.
5. Perret G, Nishioka H. Report on the cooperative study of intracranial aneurysms and subarachnoid hemorrhage. Section VI. Arteriovenous malformations. An analysis of 545 cases of cranio-cerebral arteriovenous malformations and fistulae reported to the cooperative study. *J Neurosurg* 1966;**25**:467–90.
6. Gross CR, Kase CS, Mohr JP, *et al.* Stroke in south Alabama: incidence and diagnostic features—a population based study. *Stroke* 1984;**15**:249–55.
7. Toffol GJ, Biller J, Adams HP, Jr. Nontraumatic intracerebral hemorrhage in young adults. *Arch Neurol* 1987;**44**:483–5.
8. Graf CJ, Perret GE, Torner JC. Bleeding from cerebral arteriovenous malformations as part of their natural history. *J Neurosurg* 1983;**58**:331–7.
9. Brown RD, Jr., Wiebers DO, Forbes G, *et al.* The natural history of unruptured intracranial arteriovenous malformations. *J Neurosurg* 1988;**68**:352–7.
10. Mast H, Young WL, Koennecke HC, *et al.* Risk of spontaneous haemorrhage after diagnosis of cerebral arteriovenous malformation. *Lancet* 1997;**350**:1065–8.
11. Halim AX, Johnston SC, Singh V, *et al.* Longitudinal risk of intracranial hemorrhage in patients with arteriovenous malformation of the brain within a defined population. *Stroke* 2004;**35**:1697–702.
12. Stapf C, Mast H, Sciacca RR, *et al.* Predictors of hemorrhage in patients with untreated brain arteriovenous malformation. *Neurology* 2006;**66**:1350–5.
13. Hernesniemi JA, Dashti R, Juvela S, *et al.* Natural history of brain arteriovenous malformations: a long-term follow-up study of risk of hemorrhage in 238 patients. *Neurosurgery* 2008;**63**:823–9.
14. Cunha e Sa MJ, Stein BM, Solomon RA, *et al.* The treatment of associated intracranial aneurysms and arteriovenous malformations. *J Neurosurg* 1992;**77**:853–9.
15. Marks MP, Lane B, Steinberg GK, *et al.* Hemorrhage in intracerebral arteriovenous malformations: angiographic determinants. *Radiology* 1990;**176**:807–13.
16. Redekop G, terBrugge K, Montanera W, *et al.* Arterial aneurysms associated with cerebral arteriovenous malformations: classification, incidence, and risk of hemorrhage. *J Neurosurg* 1998;**89**:539–46.
17. Thompson RC, Steinberg GK, Levy RP, *et al.* The management of patients with arteriovenous malformations and associated intracranial aneurysms. *Neurosurgery* 1998;**43**:202–11.
18. Turjman F, Massoud TF, Vinuela F, *et al.* Aneurysms related to cerebral arteriovenous malformations: superselective angiographic assessment in 58 patients. *AJNR Am J Neuroradiol* 1994;**15**:1601–5.
19. Kader A, Young WL, Pile-Spellman J, *et al.* The influence of hemodynamic and anatomical factors on hemorrhage from cerebral arteriovenous malformations. *Neurosurgery* 1994;**34**:801–7.
20. Miyasaka Y, Yada K, Ohwada T, *et al.* An analysis of the venous drainage system as a factor in hemorrhage from arteriovenous malformations. *J Neurosurg* 1992;**76**:239–43.
21. Turjman F, Massoud TF, Viñuela F, *et al.* Correlation of the angioarchitectural features of cerebral arteriovenous malformations with clinical presentation of hemorrhage. *Neurosurgery* 1995;**37**:856–60.
22. Cushing H, Bailey P. *Tumors Arising from the Blood-Vessels of the Brain; Angiomatous Malformations and Hemangioblastomas*. Springfield, IL: C. C. Thomas, 1928.
23. Spetzler RF, Martin NA. A proposed grading system for arteriovenous

malformations. *J Neurosurg* 1986;**65**:476–83.

24. Luessenhop AJ, Gennarelli TA. Anatomical grading of supratentorial arteriovenous malformations for determining operability. *Neurosurgery* 1977;**1**:30–5.
25. Lawton MT. Spetzler–Martin grade III arteriovenous malformations: surgical results and a modification of the grading scale. *Neurosurgery* 2003;**52**:740–8.
26. de Oliveira E, Tedeschi H, Raso J. Multidisciplinary approach to arteriovenous malformations. *Neurol Med Chir (Tokyo)* 1998;**38** (Suppl):177–85.
27. Spetzler RF, Hargraves RW, McCormick PW, *et al.* Relationship of perfusion pressure and size to risk of hemorrhage from arteriovenous malformations. *J Neurosurg* 1992;**76**:918–23.
28. Han PP, Ponce FA, Spetzler RF. Intention-to-treat analysis of Spetzler–Martin grades IV and V arteriovenous malformations: natural history and treatment paradigm. *J Neurosurg* 2003;**98**:3–7.
29. Fleetwood IG, Marcellus ML, Levy RP, *et al.* Deep arteriovenous malformations of the basal ganglia and thalamus: natural history. *J Neurosurg* 2003;**98**:747–50.
30. Nataf F, Meder JF, Roux FX, *et al.* Angioarchitecture associated with haemorrhage in cerebral arteriovenous malformations: a prognostic statistical model. *Neuroradiology* 1997;**39**:52–8.
31. Albert P, Salgado H, Polaina M, *et al.* A study on the venous drainage of 150 cerebral arteriovenous malformations as related to haemorrhagic risks and size of the lesion. *Acta Neurochir (Wien)* 1990;**103**:30–4.
32. Brown RD, Jr. Simple risk predictions for arteriovenous malformation hemorrhage. *Neurosurgery* 2000;**46**:1024.
33. Kondziolka D, McLaughlin MR, Kestle JR. Simple risk predictions for arteriovenous malformation hemorrhage. *Neurosurgery* 1995;**37**:851–5.
34. Jafar JJ, Rezai AR. Acute surgical management of intracranial arteriovenous malformations. *Neurosurgery* 1994;**34**:8–12.
35. Steinberg GK, Chang SD, Levy RP, *et al.* Surgical resection of large incompletely treated intracranial arteriovenous malformations following stereotactic radiosurgery. *J Neurosurg* 1996;**84**:920–8.
36. Heros RC, Korosue K, Diebold PM. Surgical excision of cerebral arteriovenous malformations: late results. *Neurosurgery* 1990;**26**:570–7.
37. Barrow DL. Controversies in neurosurgery: microsurgery versus radiosurgery for arteriovenous malformations: the case for microsurgery. *Clin Neurosurg* 2000;**46**:285–94.
38. Hartmann A, Stapf C, Hofmeister C, *et al.* Determinants of neurological outcome after surgery for brain arteriovenous malformation. *Stroke* 2000;**31**:2361–4.
39. Tew JM, Jr., Lewis AI. Honored guest presentation: management strategies for the treatment of intracranial arteriovenous malformations. *Clin Neurosurg* 2000;**46**:267–84.
40. Hamilton MG, Spetzler RF. The prospective application of a grading system for arteriovenous malformations. *Neurosurgery* 1994;**34**:2–6.
41. Hongo K, Koike G, Isobe M, *et al.* Surgical resection of cerebral arteriovenous malformation combined with pre-operative embolisation. *J Clin Neurosci* 2000;**7** (Suppl 1):88–91.
42. Irie K, Nagao S, Honma Y, *et al.* Treatment of arteriovenous malformation of the brain: preliminary experience. *J Clin Neurosci* 2000;**7**(Suppl 1):24–9.
43. Nussbaum ES, Heros RC, Camarata PJ. Surgical treatment of intracranial arteriovenous malformations with an analysis of cost-effectiveness. *Clin Neurosurg* 1995;**42**:348–69.
44. Pik JH, Morgan MK. Microsurgery for small arteriovenous malformations of the brain: results in 110 consecutive patients. *Neurosurgery* 2000;**47**:571–5.
45. Pikus HJ, Beach ML, Harbaugh RE. Microsurgical treatment of arteriovenous malformations: analysis and comparison with stereotactic radiosurgery. *J Neurosurg* 1998;**88**:641–6.
46. Russell SM, Woo HH, Joseffer SS, *et al.* Role of frameless stereotaxy in the surgical treatment of cerebral arteriovenous malformations: technique and outcomes in a controlled study of 44 consecutive patients. *Neurosurgery* 2002;**51**:1108–16.
47. Sisti MB, Kader A, Stein BM. Microsurgery for 67 intracranial arteriovenous malformations less than 3 cm in diameter. *J Neurosurg* 1993;**79**:653–60.
48. Tokunaga K, Kinugasa K, Meguro T, *et al.* Curative treatment of cerebral arteriovenous malformations by embolisation using cellulose acetate polymer followed by surgical resection. *J Clin Neurosci* 2000;**7** (Suppl 1):1–5.
49. Morgan MK, Patel NJ, Simons M, *et al.* Influence of the combination of patient age and deep venous drainage on brain arteriovenous malformation recurrence after surgery. *J Neurosurg* 2012;**117**:934–41.
50. Hashimoto H, Iida J, Hironaka Y, *et al.* Surgical management of cerebral arteriovenous malformations with intraoperative digital subtraction angiography. *J Clin Neurosci* 2000;**7** (Suppl 1):33–5.
51. Hessler W, Hejaza N. Complications of angioma surgery: personal experience in 191 patients with cerebral angiomas. *Neurol Med Chir (Tokyo)* 1998;**38**:238–44.
52. Nozaki K, Hashimoto N, Miyamoto S, *et al.* Resectability of Spetzler–Martin grade IV and V cerebral arteriovenous malformations. *J Clin Neurosci* 2000;**7** (Suppl 1):78–81.
53. Jizong Z, Shuo W, Jingsheng L, *et al.* Combination of intraoperative embolisation with surgical resection for treatment of giant cerebral arteriovenous malformations. *J Clin Neurosci* 2000;**7** (Suppl 1):54–9.
54. Heros RC, Morcos J, Korosue K. Arteriovenous malformations of the brain. Surgical management. *Clin Neurosurg* 1993;**40**:139–73.
55. Hoh BL, Chapman PH, Loeffler JS, *et al.* Results of multimodality treatment for 141 patients with brain arteriovenous malformations and seizures: factors associated with seizure incidence and seizure outcomes. *Neurosurgery* 2002;**51**:303–9.

56. Heros R, Korosue K. *Parenchymal Cerebral Arteriovenous Malformations. Brain Surgery: Complication Avoidance Management*. New York: Churchill Livingstone, 1993.

57. Heros RC. *Prevention and Management of Therapeutic Complications. Vascular Malformations of the Central Nervous System*. Philadelphia, PA: Lippincott Williams & Wilkins, 1999.

58. Latchaw RE, Hu X, Ugurbil K, *et al.* Functional magnetic resonance imaging as a management tool for cerebral arteriovenous malformations. *Neurosurgery* 1995;**37**:619–25.

59. Spetzler RF, Wilson CB, Weinstein P, *et al.* Normal perfusion pressure breakthrough theory. *Clin Neurosurg* 1978;**25**:651–72.

60. Meyer B, Urbach H, Schaller C, *et al.* Is stagnating flow in former feeding arteries an indication of cerebral hypoperfusion after resection of arteriovenous malformations? *J Neurosurg* 2001;**95**:36–43.

61. Miyasaka Y, Yada K, Ohwada T, *et al.* Retrograde thrombosis of feeding arteries after removal of arteriovenous malformations. *J Neurosurg* 1990;**72**:540–5.

62. Miyasaka Y, Kurata A, Tanaka R, *et al.* The significance of retrograde thrombosis following removal of arteriovenous malformations in elderly patients. *Surg Neurol* 1998;**49**:399–405.

63. Yaşargil MG. *Microneurosurgery*, Vol. IIIB: *AVM of the Brain, Clinical Considerations, General and Special Operative Techniques, Surgical Results, Nonoperated Cases, Cavernous and Venous Angiomas, Neuroanesthesia*. Stuttgart: Thieme, 1988.

Chapter 12

Surgical approaches and nuances for arteriovenous malformations in the posterior fossa

Najib E. El Tecle, Bernard R. Bendok, Tarek Y. El Ahmadieh, Samer G. Zammar, Byron Yip, Babu Welch, Jonathan White, Duke Samson, and H. Hunt Batjer

Introduction

Arteriovenous malformations (AVMs) of the brain are an important cause of hemorrhagic stroke particularly in the young. Posterior fossa AVMs carry a greater risk of hemorrhage than their supratentorial counterparts but also pose unique treatment challenges. Expanding awareness and increasing use of imaging studies have increased rates of posterior fossa AVM diagnosis and treatment. These intriguing AVMs account for 7–15% of brain AVMs. Studies suggest that their risk of morbidity and mortality is greater than that observed with supratentorial AVMs [1,2]. It is helpful to classify posterior fossa AVMs according to their anatomical location: hemispheric cerebellar AVMs, which constitute approximately 75% of all posterior fossa AVMs, and brainstem AVMs, which are less common but are associated with a worse prognosis in general. A number of factors make posterior fossa AVMs challenging to treat surgically, but success can be achieved with careful patient selection; judicious preoperative embolization; attention to details of positioning, technique, and anatomy; vigilant and attentive neuroanesthesia; and diligent postoperative care and rehabilitation. This chapter will present a global approach to the management of posterior fossa AVMs. The clinical presentation and natural history of these AVMs will be discussed followed by nuances in their management. Finally, in light of the surgical challenges of posterior fossa AVM resection, an overview of surgical techniques and approaches commonly used for the treatment of these lesions will be given.

History

Clingenstein's report of the first infratentorial AVM was published in 1908, almost half a century after the initial description of AVMs as a separate pathological entity by Luschka and Virchow [3,4]. In 1932, Olivercrona was the first to perform an excision of a posterior fossa AVM; however, outcomes of the surgical procedure were not documented [4]. Logue and Monckton reported the first posterior fossa AVM excision confirmed by postoperative angiography in 1954 [5]. These authors also described brainstem AVMs and judged them to be inoperable. In 1965, Mount performed the first surgical obliteration of a brainstem AVM but the patient had a poor neurological outcome [6]. In 1972, Green and Vaughan microsurgically removed a posterior fossa AVM, inaugurating the era of microsurgery for AVM treatment [7]. Since then, a significant knowledge base has been accumulated regarding patient selection, technique, and complication avoidance, which has led to improved outcomes [1,2,8,9].

Clinical presentation

Bleeding is the initial presentation in 50–92% of patients with posterior fossa AVMs. This rate is much higher than the reported rate of 50–61% for supratentorial AVMs [1,10]. Although this higher rate of bleeding as initial presentation has sometimes been linked to an increased propensity of supratentorial lesions to manifest via seizures or headaches, accumulating evidence suggests that this higher rate is related to a real higher risk of bleeding [11–13].

The second most common manifestation of posterior fossa AVMs is progressive neurological deficit, including those related to mass effect, ischemia, and hydrocephalus. Posterior fossa AVMs may also mimic diverse neurological conditions such as multiple sclerosis via a steal phenomenon [1,2]. Trigeminal neuralgia and hemifacial spasm may occur with posterior fossa AVMs involving the cerebellopontine angle [14].

Natural history

The known morbidity of posterior fossa AVMs and the absence of equipoise for most lesions have hindered prospective observational studies of these lesions. The few published multivariate analyses that have controlled for the location of AVMs, however, have shown that posterior fossa location is an independent predictor of future rupture [11–13]. The annual risk of hemorrhage for infratentorial AVMs was shown to be as high as 11.6% per year for the first five years after diagnosis and 6.7% per year overall [15], and the annual rate of rupture for non-ruptured posterior fossa AVMs can be as high as 8.4–9.4% per year [8]. Rehemorrhage is dependent on initial hemorrhagic presentation and the annual rate of rehemorrhage after initial bleeding can be as high as 34.3% [16,17].

Comprehensive Management of Arteriovenous Malformations of the Brain and Spine, ed. Robert F. Spetzler, Douglas S. Kondziolka, Randall T. Higashida, and M. Yashar S. Kalani. Published by Cambridge University Press.

While the evidence of an increased risk of rerupture after initial hemorrhage is overwhelming, data regarding other risk factors are not conclusive and originate from series reporting on both supratentorial and infratentorial lesions. Anatomical and hemodynamic features such as the presence of associated aneurysms have been among the investigated variables [18,19].

In terms of associated aneurysms, the presence of associated aneurysms was an independent predictor of poor outcome at follow-up for posterior fossa AVMs [20–22]. Further analysis of the effect of associated aneurysms was carried out in a series of 117 supratentorial and infratentorial AVMs with associated aneurysms [20–22]. Feeding artery aneurysms, as opposed to nidal and independent circle of Willis aneurysms, were found to be an independent predictor of increased risk of AVM hemorrhage.

Other factors such as involvement of perforating arteries, deep venous drainage, small nidus size, age and sex have been linked to rupture risk although with less statistical vigor [10].

Classification

While there is no formal classification system for posterior fossa AVMs, they are usually divided into brainstem AVMs and cerebellar AVMs. Autopsy studies suggest that 75–95% of posterior fossa AVMs are purely cerebellar, whereas the rest involve the brainstem [2,23]. Although many brainstem AVMs are deemed to be inoperable, cerebellar and cerebellopontine angle AVMs are often amenable to microsurgical intervention.

Decision making for unruptured asymptomatic arteriovenous malformations

While the elevated rupture risk of posterior fossa AVMs makes a compelling argument to treat asymptomatic lesions, the potential treatment morbidity must be carefully considered. Selecting appropriate patients for treatment and the most effective therapeutic strategy are the most important requisites for successful outcomes. Anatomical features, which may influence risk of treatment, should be carefully weighed against the risk of the disease. Patient age and comorbidities are additional important factors to consider. Alternative approaches for asymptomatic lesions are observation, radiosurgery, and embolization for cure or embolization of high-risk features, such as flow-related aneurysms.

Anatomical and hemodynamic nuances of posterior fossa AVMs may favor a specific management strategy. In general, radiosurgery for hemispheric cerebellar lesions is not indicated because of the acceptable morbidity associated with their resection and the potential morbidity of radiation necrosis in the tight confines of the posterior fossa. Endovascular surgery can be used to favorably modify the hemodynamics of an AVM and help to reduce the risk of bleeding, potentially enhancing surgical safety. These therapeutic options will be explored in further detail.

Preoperative care

The patient should undergo a thorough medical evaluation, including optimization of care for existing medical conditions. The anatomy and hemodynamics of the AVM should be studied in great detail. Thorough counseling of the patient should include a discussion of the potential for perioperative morbidity from both surgery and endovascular interventions. While functional imaging plays a lesser role in the posterior fossa, much of the hemodynamic information can be gained from angiographic evaluation of the lesion. In the posterior fossa, the differentiation between a pure dural arteriovenous fistula and fistulous AVM is crucial to the final management decision. Further, understanding the hemodynamics and associated aneurysms is crucial to making enlightened decisions on the advantages of preoperative embolization.

Preoperative embolization

Advances in microcatheters, microwires, embolic materials, and imaging have made endovascular techniques safer and more precise. The biggest advance, however, has been the evolving sophistication for patient selection and strategy creation, which have been refined through trial and error over several decades. Embolization strategies include complete angiographic occlusion for potential cure, preoperative embolization for flow reduction, preoperative embolization to secure difficult to access feeders, and preoperative embolization to secure a flow-related aneurysm or proximal aneurysm of the circle of Willis.

Embolization for potential cure

Despite increasing efficacy of nidal penetration with Onyx (Covidien, Dublin, Ireland) compared with other agents, cure rates for AVMs with embolization alone remain low (Fig. 12.1) [24]. Factors that predict the potential for achieving safe complete angiographic occlusion include smaller number of feeding arteries (usually one or two), small nidus (ideally ≤1 cm), and ease of access to the nidus. Questions remain regarding the potential for recanalization with embolization as a stand-alone approach [25]. Further evolution of embolic agents and better imaging of the embolysate cast are needed before this strategy can be used more widely [26,27].

Flow reduction for prevention of intraoperative and postoperative hemorrhage

The potential for intraprocedural hemorrhage can be significant for larger AVMs. Moreover, these AVMs can be associated with higher risk of postoperative hemorrhage, likely through the loss of autoregulation in the surrounding brain. Staged embolization may help to address both issues. The exact number of sessions, timing between sessions, and ultimate degree of embolization remain speculative. Advances in MRI may help to improve assessment of the impact of embolization on an AVM and the surrounding brain parenchyma [28]. Figure 12.2 describes a patient who presented with a history of several weeks of ataxia. Brain MRI demonstrated a large right

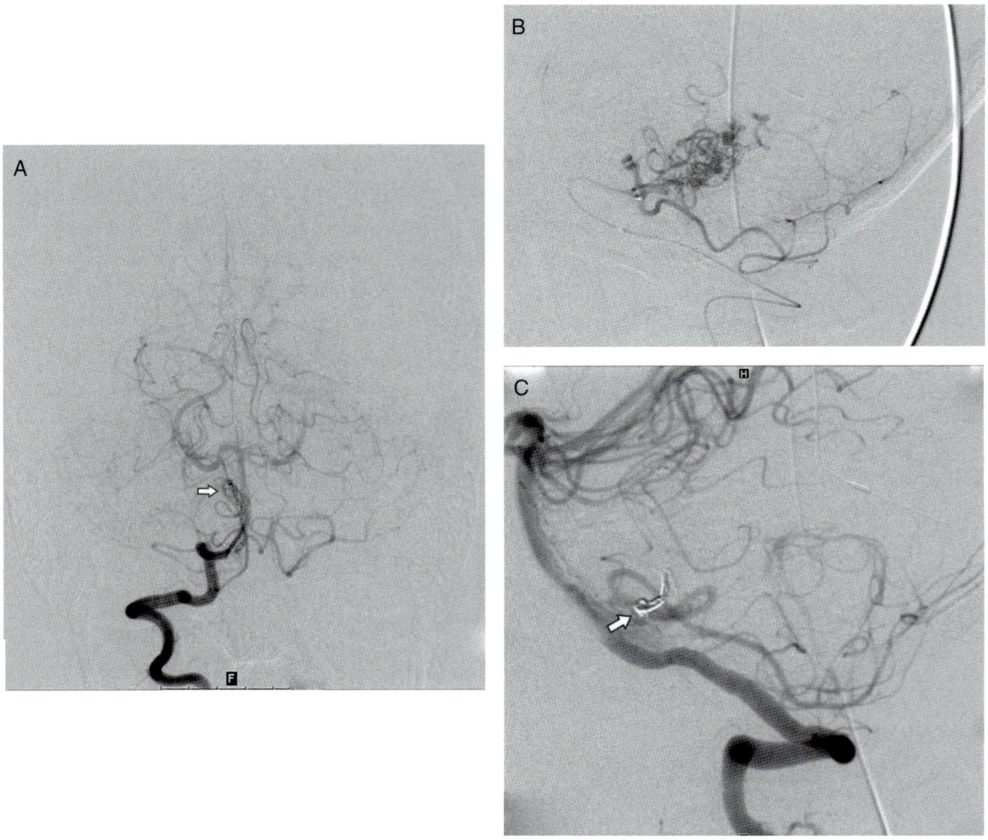

Fig. 12.1. A 32-year-old woman presented with a history of headache and occasional vertigo. MRI demonstrated a right cerebellar peduncle vascular lesion. (A) Anteroposterior digital subtraction angiography (DSA) identified a middle cerebellar peduncle arteriovenous malformation (AVM). (B) Lateral superselective DSA demonstrated the AVM arising from the anterior inferior cerebellar artery. The lesion was associated with a 3 mm nidal aneurysm at its superior posteromedial aspect. (C) Onyx embolization of the AVM was performed with an intention to secure the aneurysm and occlude the AVM. The Onyx cast is shown on lateral angiography.

cerebellar AVM. Embolization of the AVM was performed in a staged manner before proceeding to surgical resection.

Securing deep feeders

Deep feeders can increase surgical risk. They are often difficult to coagulate and securing them may require dissection through a deeper white matter plane than is considered ideal. Accessing and embolizing these feeders safely might help to enhance surgical safety. Unfortunately, such feeders are often too tortuous and/or too small for safe access.

Securing a high-risk aneurysm

Embolization can also be used to secure a feeding vessel aneurysm in order to enhance surgical safety. A prenidal aneurysm, which might be at increased risk of bleeding during surgery because of the sudden outflow obstruction associated with AVM resection, can be secured in order to prevent undesired perioperative bleeding (Fig. 12.3). This is particularly important if the aneurysm is not accessible surgically. Securing such aneurysms may also decrease bleeding after radiosurgery [29,30].

Occluding the source of hemorrhage

Using advanced three-dimensional angiography and CT angiography, the hemorrhage source from the AVM nidus or a proximal aneurysm can occasionally be identified. For prenidal aneurysms, surgical and endovascular options should be considered. If an intranidal aneurysm can be visualized with superselective catheterization, then occlusion of the nidal segment harboring the aneurysm may reduce the short-term rehemorrhage rate from the AVM [8,31,32].

Radiosurgery before surgery

Radiosurgery is a first-line option for select brainstem AVMs and a reasonable secondary option for cerebellar AVMs. While prior radiation typically makes most surgical procedures more complicated because of scarring, radiosurgery actually makes microsurgery easier for AVMs by thickening the walls of fragile nidal vessels and further defining the plane between the AVM and the surrounding white matter [33,34].

Acute management of ruptured posterior fossa arteriovenous malformations

Vigilant and timely intervention for patients with posterior fossa hemorrhage can be life saving and can result in gratifying patient outcomes. Patients with poor neurological examinations should undergo intubation and elevation of the head to reduce intracranial pressure. Both CT and CT

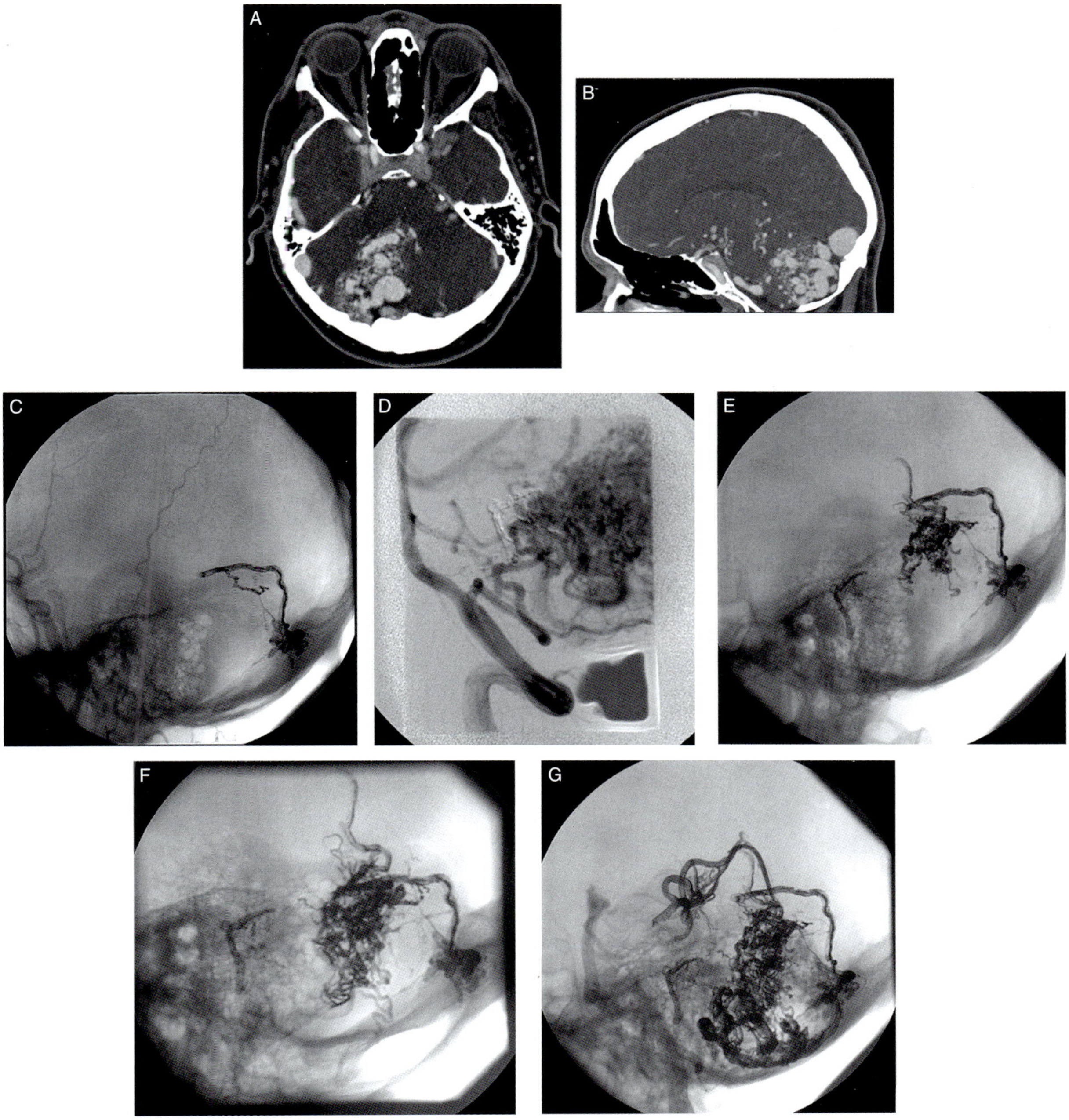

Fig. 12.2. A 51-year-old man presented with a history of several weeks of ataxia. (A,B) CT angiography demonstrated a large right cerebellar arteriovenous malformation (AVM) (A, axial view; B, sagittal view). (C–G) Embolization of the AVM was performed in a staged manner before proceeding to surgical resection: consecutive casts show stages 1–5 of the embolization.

angiography should be rapidly obtained for diagnosis and potential identification of a rupture source. The relationship of the hematoma to the AVM and the status of the fourth ventricle are all important for surgical decision making and planning. The presence of hydrocephalus and/or downward herniation is important to note. If the hematoma is >3 cm with a poor examination, immediate surgical intervention is indicated. The intervention can consist of ventriculostomy placement followed by immediate posterior fossa craniectomy and partial hematoma evacuation. The craniectomy may be complemented by a C1 laminectomy to help to assure complete decompression of the tonsils and allow access to thrombus in the fourth ventricle. A duraplasty at this time will allow for greater posterior fossa volume to accommodate the expected swelling in the ensuing days after an acute hemorrhage. It is advisable to open the ventriculostomy for drainage once the posterior fossa dura is opened to avoid upward herniation.

Special attention must be paid to the nidus and flow-related aneurysms. Surgical clipping of a flow-related aneurysm might be advisable if safely accessible. Unless the AVM is small and superficial, a common practice is to delay resection for a time when conditions are more optimal and the anatomy of the AVM has been better defined. A delay of 8 to 12 weeks is typical, but this may be tailored to the neurological condition of the patient. If it is not feasible to obtain an angiogram

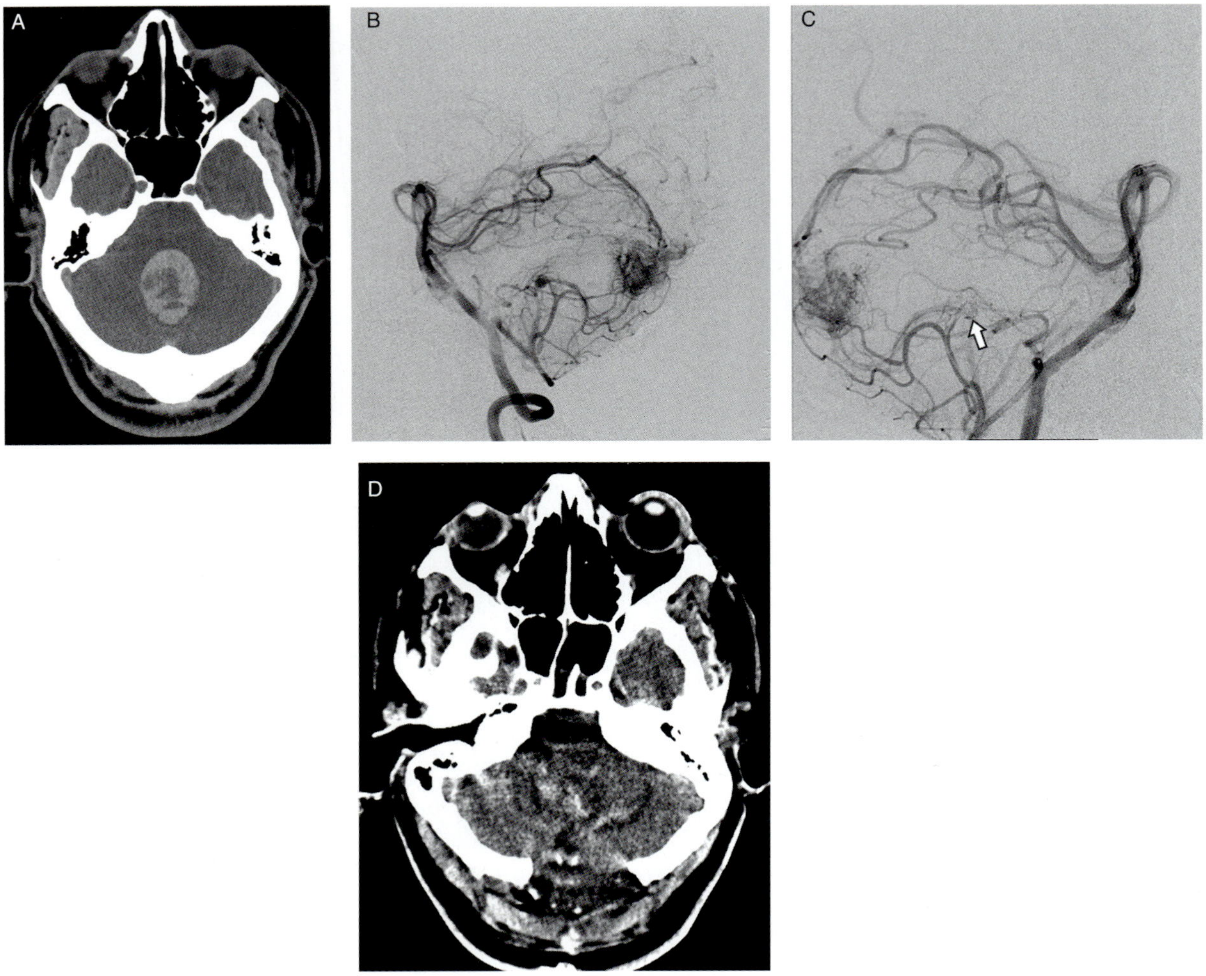

Fig. 12.3. A 51-year-old man collapsed at work and was found to have a significant posterior fossa hemorrhage from an arteriovenous malformation (AVM). (A,B) Posterior fossa hemorrhage shown with axial CT (A) and lateral angiography (B). After decompressive craniectomy and ventriculostomy placement, angiography revealed a flow-related aneurysm, which was the likely source of hemorrhage. (C) Lateral angiography demonstrated a flow-related aneurysm after it had been secured by coiling (arrow). (D) Axial CT after decompression of the cranial fossa. Three months later, the man underwent successful microsurgical resection.

before acute surgery because of impending or active herniation, then an angiogram should be obtained when the patient has been stabilized postoperatively. If a rupture site, such as a flow-related aneurysm, is found, occlusion of this site is warranted if it can be achieved safely by microsurgical or interventional means.

Microsurgical treatment

General principles

Preoperative preparation

Successful microsurgical treatment of posterior fossa AVMs requires careful preoperative preparation and planning. As stated above, surgery can be delayed after acute hemorrhage if the hematoma is small. Careful analysis of the anatomy and the angioarchitecture of the AVM are very important to develop an appropriate surgical strategy, which may or may not include preoperative embolization.

Relevant anatomy of the posterior fossa

Challenges of posterior fossa surgery result mainly from the small volume of the posterior fossa, and the neurovascular structures, which must be respected to achieve optimal and safe access.

Bony anatomy

The posterior fossa is delimited by the occipital bone posteriorly, which fuses laterally and anteriorly with the mastoid and the petrous bones. A midline occipital crest runs from the foramen magnum to the internal occipital protuberance and separates the cerebellar hemispheres. Grooves for the superior sagittal sinus run to the internal occipital protuberance and descend to the mastoid angle of the parietal bone to become continuous with the sigmoid sulcus. The porus acusticus is found on the posterior surface of the petrous bone. The jugular foramen extends laterally to the posterior aspect of the occipital condyle and the hypoglossal foramen is inferomedial to the jugular foramen and below the jugular tubercle.

Arterial anatomy

After the vertebral artery pierces the dura, it courses medially to enter the premedullary cistern where it passes between the hypoglossal nerve and the anterior root of the first cervical nerve and beneath the ligamentum denticulatum. It then gives rise to the ipsilateral posterior inferior cerebellar artery (PICA) and joins the contralateral vertebral artery at the pontomedullary junction to form the basilar artery. The left vertebral artery is usually dominant, with an average diameter of 3.2 mm compared with an average diameter for the right vertebral artery of 2.7 mm.

The basilar artery courses in the prepontine cistern in the sulcus basilaris, where it gives rise to the anterior inferior cerebellar arteries (AICAs), and in the interpeduncular cistern, where it divides into the posterior cerebellar arteries (PCA) and superior cerebellar arteries (SCA). The mean diameter of the basilar artery is 4.1 mm [35].

The PICA usually arises from the vertebral arteries but it can also arise from the basilar artery. It usually courses backward along the upper part of the medulla and passes between the origins of cranial nerves IX and X, supplying the medullary perforating arteries along the way. The PICA then passes over the inferior cerebellar peduncle to the undersurface of the cerebellum, where it divides into a medial branch that supplies the inferomedial surface of the cerebellar hemisphere and a lateral portion that supplies the undersurface of the cerebellum. The PICA also supplies the choroid plexus of the fourth ventricle.

The AICA arises in the prepontine cistern from the basilar artery. It is traversed by cranial nerve VI at 6–7 mm from the artery origin, defining the limit between the first segment and the second segment of the AICA. The second segment of the AICA courses laterally and posteriorly and comes in proximity to cranial nerve VII at the lateral portion of the flocculus. It supplies the anterior inferior quarter of the cerebellum and usually give rise to the labyrinthine artery.

The SCA courses laterally below cranial nerve III and winds around the cerebral peduncle in proximity to the trochlear nerve to reach the upper surface of the cerebellum, where it divides into its terminal branches. The SCA gives rise to multiple branches to the pineal body, the anterior medullary velum, the third ventricle, and the tela choroidea.

The PCA has two possible courses: a straight horizontal course or a looping cephalic course that goes under the medial temporal lobe. The PCA gives rise to a large number of arteries including the thalamoperforating branches and the peduncular perforating branches (also known as the central branches), the medial posterior and lateral posterior choroidal branches, the anterior and posterior temporal branches, the lateral medial occipital branches, and the splenial branches (known as the cortical branches of the PCA).

Venous anatomy

Posterior fossa veins can be divided into four groups: superficial veins, deep veins, veins of the brainstem, and bridging veins [36]. These groups exhibit diffuse and complex anastomotic patterns, making complications from small venous sacrifices in the posterior fossa unlikely.

Superficial veins drain the cortical surface of the cerebellum and can be divided into three groups based on the surface they drain: the tentorial surface is drained by the superior hemispheric and the superior vermian veins; the suboccipital surface is drained by the inferior hemispheric and inferior vermian veins; and the petrosal surface is drained by the anterior hemispheric veins.

Deep veins course in the cerebellomesencephalic, cerebellopontine, and cerebellomedullary fissures. This group also includes the vein of the superior cerebellar peduncle, which courses in the cerebellomesencephalic fissure; the vein of the inferior cerebellar peduncle, which courses in the cerebellomedullary fissure; and the vein of the middle cerebellar peduncle, which courses in the anterior part of the cerebellopontine fissure. In addition it includes the deep tonsilar veins.

Veins of the brainstem include longitudinally oriented and transverse veins, the latter coursing perpendicularly to the longitudinal veins. The longitudinally oriented veins coursing in the midline are the median anterior pontomesencephalic vein and the median anterior medullary veins. Longitudinally oriented veins coursing laterally include the lateral anterior medullary pontomesencephalic, the lateral anterior medullary veins, and the lateral mesencephalic veins. The horizontally running veins include the transverse pontine and transverse medullary veins. The peduncular veins usually empty into the petrosal sinus.

Bridging veins cross the subarachnoid and subdural spaces to reach venous sinuses in the dura. They organize into three groups: a superior group, which drains into the vein of Galen; an anterior group, which drains into the petrosal sinuses; and a posterior group, which drains into the sinuses converging into the torcula.

Anatomy of the cisterns and cranial nerves

Posterior fossa cisterns can be divided into unpaired cisterns, which include the interpeduncular cistern, the prepontine cistern, the premedullary cistern, the quadrigeminal cistern, the ambient cistern, and the cisterna magna, and paired cisterns, which include the cerebellopontine cisterns and the cerebellomedullary cistern [37].

The interpeduncular cistern extends between the cerebral peduncles and the leaves of Liliequist's membrane at the convergence of the supratentorial and infratentorial subarachnoid spaces. Liliequist's membrane gives rise to the diencephalic membrane and the mesencephalic membrane. The diencephalic membrane separates the interpeduncular cistern from the chiasmatic cistern. The mesencephalic membrane separates the interpeduncular cistern from the prepontine cistern. The basilar artery pierces the mesencephalic membrane. The oculomotor nerves course in the lateral wall of the interpeduncular cistern and form the pillars to which Liliequist's membrane attaches. The interpeduncular cistern also contains the posterior thalamoperforating arteries, the bifurcation of the basilar artery, and the origins of the posterior cerebral, superior cerebellar, and medial posterior choroidal arteries. It also contains the peduncular posterior communicating and median anterior pontomesencephalic veins.

The prepontine cistern extends between the anterior surface of the pons and the arachnoid membrane resting on the clivus. This cistern narrows inferiorly to reach the pontomedullary sulcus. The anterior pontine membrane laterally limits the prepontine cistern. The basilar artery usually courses in this cistern, where it gives rise to the anterior inferior cerebellar arteries that exit to the cerebellopontine cistern. This cistern also contains the transverse pontine veins and the vein of the pontomedullary sulcus.

The premedullary cistern extends between the anterior surface of the medulla and the arachnoid membrane covering the lower part of the clivus below the prepontine cistern, from which it is separated by the medial pontomedullary membrane. The rootlets of the hypoglossal nerves arise in the posterior wall of this cistern between the medullary pyramids and the inferior olives. The vertebral arteries enter this cistern through the foramen magnum. The major veins of this cistern are the traversing medullary veins, the median anterior medullary vein, and the vein of the pontomedullary sulcus.

The quadrigeminal cistern extends around the quadrigeminal plate, which constitutes the center of the anterior wall of the cistern. The roof of the cistern is formed by the lower surface of the splenium. The quadrigeminal cistern communicates with the posterior pericallosal cistern and opens inferiorly to the ambient cistern. Cranial nerve IV arises in this cistern. The PCA and SCA enter the lower two parts of the cistern. Usually, the PCA bifurcates into the calcarine and parieto-occipital branches within this cistern. The quadrigeminal cistern is also the site of convergence of the internal cerebral and basal veins. The internal cerebral veins enter the quadrigeminal cistern through the velum interpositum and the basal veins enter the quadrigeminal cistern through the ambient cistern. The cerebral veins and the basal veins join to form the vein of Galen, which then passes below the splenium to enter the straight sinus at the tentorial apex.

The ambient cistern refers to a thin extension of the quadrigeminal cistern that spreads laterally around the midbrain and connects it with the interpeduncular cistern. The term ambient cistern can also refer to the combination of these extensions with the quadrigeminal cistern. The ambient cistern has a supratentorial and infratentorial portion. The SCA and cranial nerve IV course in the infratentorial portion.

The cistern magna is dorsal to the medulla and cerebellar vermis and extends posteriorly to the arachnoid membrane lying on the inner surface of the occipital bone. The fourth ventricle opens to this cistern through the foramen of Magendie. The PICAs course posteriorly around the medulla to enter the cisterna magna. The major veins of the cistern are the inferior vermian vein, the median posterior medullary vein, and the vein of the cerebellomedullary fissure.

The cerebellopontine cistern extends between the anterolateral surface of the pons, the cerebellum, and the arachnoid membrane resting on the posterior surface of the petrous bone. In this cistern, the trigeminal nerve arises from the midpons and runs through the superolateral portion of the cistern and the abducens nerve arises at the level of the pontomedullary sulcus and ascends just lateral to the anterior pontine membrane. Cranial nerves VII and VIII arise in the lower part of the cerebellopontine cistern and are surrounded by the outer arachnoidal membrane as they enter the internal auditory canal. In terms of arterial structures, the SCA and the AICA course through this cistern. The veins in this cistern are the transverse pontine veins and the veins of the cerebellopontine fissure, pontomedullary sulcus, and middle cerebellar peduncle. They drain to the superior petrosal vein, which empties into the superior petrosal sinus.

The cerebellomedullary cistern is caudal to the junction of the medulla and pons and is separated from the cerebellopontine cistern by the lateral pontomedullary membrane and from the premedullary cistern by the trabeculae in front of cranial nerves IX, X, and XI, which arise and course though the cistern to reach the jugular foramen. The spinal portion of cranial nerve XI ascends from the posterior spinal cistern to reach the cerebellomedullary cistern. The lateral recess of the fourth ventricle opens to this cistern through the foramen of Luschka. The PICA runs in this cistern. The major veins are the vein of the pontomedullary sulcus and the lateral medullary vein.

Neuroanesthesia and principles of neuromonitoring

Successful neuroanesthesia has several elements including assisting with positioning to assure adequate ventilation, optimization of brain relaxation through pharmacological and physiological means, monitoring the physiological results of blood loss, monitoring for air emboli, and monitoring of relevant electrical potentials. Electrical potential monitoring is an essential part of the intraoperative team and can include motor and sensory evoked potentials, electroencephalography, brainstem auditory evoked potentials, and cranial nerve monitoring. When using the sitting position, precordial ultrasound and right central venous access should be used to diagnose and treat any possible air emboli. The exact strategy used depends on the specific characteristics of each patient and should be carefully discussed between the surgeon and neuroanesthesia team.

Close cooperation between the surgical and anesthesia teams is essential before and during the surgical procedure. The use of adenosine to produce cardiac pause and subsequent flow arrest is an important example of this collaboration. The use of this technique may help the surgeon to control deep feeders that are difficult to reach or resistant to coagulation.

General principles of surgical resection

Larger craniotomies than one would plan for a tumor or a cavernoma are usually advantageous in AVM surgery; they allow greater insight into the angioarchitecture of the AVM and the surrounding tissues and structures. The wider exposure is also advantageous should exuberant hemorrhage occur.

After opening the dura, the parenchyma is inspected in order to identify superficial feeding arteries and draining veins. Time should be taken to study the AVM anatomy and correlate it with angiographic and other radiographic data.

Image guidance may be advantageous in some cases and indocyanine green angiography can be useful to further understanding of the AVM hemodynamics in situ prior to proceeding with surgical resection. When the AVM does not present to the pial surface, a draining vein can be followed toward the nidus while paying attention not to compromise flow in that vein. Sharp dissection should be used to enter the subarachnoid space around the AVM and draining veins.

As typically performed in supratentorial AVMs, care should be taken to dissect the AVM margins with coagulation and division of arterial feeders on the periphery. It is essential not to compromise draining veins early in the operation. A spiral technique, as advocated by Yaşargil, should be used to progressively deepen all planes around the AVM. This avoids the hazards of working through a narrow channel that can easily and quickly well up with blood and obscure correct dissection planes. A gliotic plane is often present between the AVM and surrounding parenchyma. This can be a helpful plane to follow [38]. It is important to study and preserve en passage vessels so that ideally only branches supplying the AVM are divided while maintaining flow to normal brain tissue beyond the AVM. Preoperative superselective angiography can be helpful in understanding such vessels.

Ultimately, the AVM should be isolated on its venous pedicle. Deep small arterial feeders can be problematic as they tend to retract into white matter and present a source of bleeding. These vessels are difficult to coagulate and rupture easily when manipulated; AVM microclips are exceptionally helpful in tackling these petulant arteries. With efficient and careful application, hemostasis can be achieved by placing the clips on the small vessels prior to manipulation. After disconnection of all arterial feeders has been accomplished, it becomes safe to divide the large draining veins. Indocyanine green angiography and micro-Doppler can be used to monitor the resolution of venous arterialization throughout the procedure.

The surgical cavity should be inspected carefully for residual AVM. The surgeon should be suspicious of areas of the resection cavity that are not responsive to routine bipolar cautery. While this finding may be related to the relative loss of autoregulation of the surrounding tissue, the possibility of residual AVM or coagulopathy should also be considered. Repeated use of cotton tamponade in the cavity with meticulous bipolar cautery use between periods of tamponade is the best way to achieve hemostasis at this point. Coagulation profiles should also be checked at this stage as prolonged blood loss through the procedure can result in a coagulopathy that will work against the surgeon's efforts to keep the cavity dry [39]. Intraoperative or immediate postoperative angiography is required to assure complete AVM resection. Watertight dural closure is important. When feasible, harvesting pericranium can serve as an excellent adjunct for dural closure.

Surgical approaches to posterior fossa arteriovenous malformations

The need to access arterial feeders with minimal brain manipulation and preservation of draining veins until the end of resection should factor into choice of patient position and surgical approach. The common surgical approaches to posterior fossa AVMs are described according to the AVM location (Table 12.1 and Figs. 12.4 and 12.5) [40].

Table 12.1. Surgical approaches according to arteriovenous malformations location

Location	Surgical approach
Cerebellar	
Lower two-thirds of the vermis	Midline suboccipital
Paramedian hemisphere	Midline suboccipital
Tonsillar	Midline suboccipital
Cerebellopontine angle	Extended paramedian or retrosigmoid
Upper vermis and roof of the cerebellum	Supracerebellar infratentorial
Brainstem	
Anterior and anterolateral midbrain	Trans-sylvian
Interpeduncular cistern	Trans-sylvian
Lateral and posterolateral midbrain	Subtemporal
Tectum	Supracerebellar infratentorial or occipital transtentorial
Anterior and lateral pons	Transpetrosal approaches
Anterior and lateral medulla	Far lateral
Posterior medulla	Midline suboccipital with extension to the foramen magnum

Positioning

Proper positioning is critical for optimal surgical and anesthetic outcomes. While positioning is intended to provide direct access to the AVM and to minimize risk to surrounding tissues, attention to physiological consequences of positioning can help to prevent complications [41]. Positioning should be physically and physiologically safe for the anaesthetized patient and comfortable for the surgeon. It is important to realize that the longer duration of AVM surgeries may produce complications of positioning more often than shorter craniotomy procedures.

The main areas of concern related to neuroanesthesia from a positioning perspective include preventing increased intracranial pressure, avoiding prolonged pressure on pressure points, avoiding nerve stretching, and preventing thromboembolic complications. Prevention of increased intracranial pressure can be achieved by optimizing venous return. This is usually done by preventing kinking of the internal jugular veins by neutral neck position and by maintaining the heart below the level of the brain at all times during the surgery. The surgical and anesthesia teams should work together to secure the patient to the operative table so that table movement can enhance positioning but not endanger the patient.

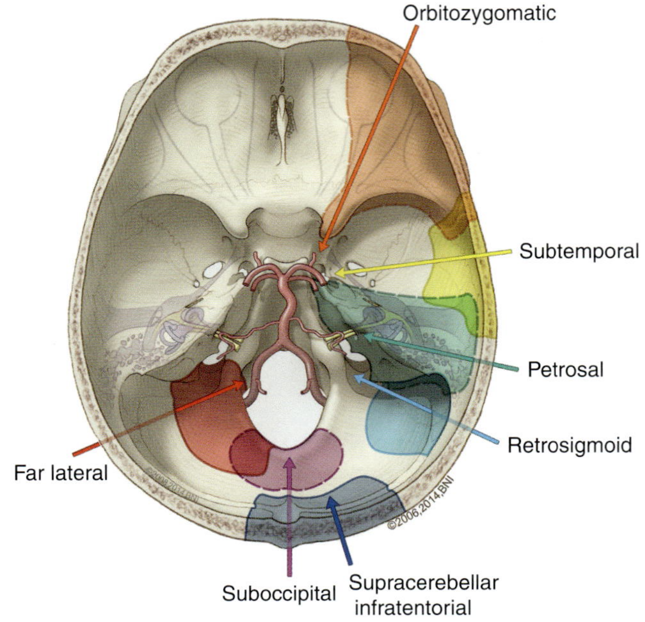

Fig. 12.4. Various skull base approaches to arteriovenous malformations in the posterior fossa depending on lesion location, eloquence of adjacent brain, patient habitus, and surgeon experience. The orbitozygomatic approach provides robust access to the anterior brainstem and basilar apex regions. Although the working distance is long compared with other posterior fossa approaches, the direct access afforded can be beneficial for lesions of the midbrain. Subtemporal and petrosal approaches can be used to provide more anterolateral views of the brainstem and cranial nerves. The subtemporal approach should be used judiciously, as it can place the vein of Labbé in danger during retraction. Petrosal approaches provide graded increased views of the lateral brainstem, particularly the midbrain and pons, but risk injury to cranial nerves VII and VIII. The retrosigmoid approach provides an alternative to petrosal approaches and allows for a posterolateral view of the brainstem without sacrifice of hearing. The far-lateral craniotomy, an extension of the retrosigmoid craniotomy, allows for visualization of the medulla, cervicomedullary junction, lower pons, and associated cranial nerves. The mobilization of the vertebral artery and partial condylectomy can provide a tangential view of the ventral brainstem. The suboccipital craniotomy exposes the medulla, cervicomedullary junction, and cerebellum. This approach is generally well tolerated and can be enlarged to address lesions along the dorsal brainstem. The midline and lateral supracerebellar infratentorial approaches can be used to address lesions in the midbrain and midbrain–pontine junction. (With permission from Barrow Neurological Institute.)

Positions used to access posterior fossa AVMs include the sitting position, the lateral park-bench position, the prone position, the Concorde position, and the supine position with head turned (with or without a shoulder roll depending on whether cerebellopontine angle access is needed).

The sitting position allows access to the supracerebellar region. Gravity allows the cerebellum to drop away from the tentorium. The sitting position can be complicated by air emboli formation, which can be minimized by careful attention to preserving sinus integrity and using a precordial Doppler to alert the surgical team if air is detected. Surgeon fatigue is a consideration in the sitting position and it is for this reason that many have replaced this positioning with the prone Concorde position (described below).

The park-bench position is optimal for lesions that involve the cerebellopontine angle (lateral cerebellar surface and lateral pons), which are accessed through a retrosigmoid craniotomy. The park-bench position can also be used to access hemispheric and even midline posterior fossa AVMs.

The prone neck flexed position is commonly used for access to the posterior fossa and the suboccipital region. In general, it is associated with a lower risk of air embolism compared with the sitting position [41]. This position is more difficult from the anesthesia perspective because of the challenges associated with ensuring adequate ventilation, maintaining hemodynamics, and securing intravenous lines and the tracheal tube. Further, injuries such as pressure ulcers, vascular compression, and brachial plexus or optic injuries have been reported, but these can be minimized with proper padding [41]. The Concorde position is a modification of the prone position that is best suited for surgical approaches to the occipital transtentorial and supracerebellar infratentorial areas. In this position, the head is flexed and the body is positioned in reverse Trendelenburg.

The supine position can be used when access to the anterior midbrain is needed through a pterional trans-sylvian approach. This position can also be used when anterior petrosectomy is needed (lateral position can be used when a posterior petrosectomy is needed). The supine position with head turned can also be used for a retrosigmoid approach.

Cerebellar lesions

Mid to lower vermian, tonsilar, and paramedian hemispheric lesions

Mid to lower vermian lesions, tonsilar lesions, and paramedian hemispheric lesions are usually accessed via the midline suboccipital approach in the sitting or prone position [42,43]. Depending on the extent of the lesion, this approach can be extended cranially to expose the torcula or caudally to expose the foramen magnum. Tonsilar lesions, for example, may require opening the foramen magnum; a C1 laminectomy can also be performed to enhance exposure if needed. For the midline suboccipital approach, the patient is usually maintained in the prone position with the neck flexed to ensure the interval between the foramen magnum and C1 is open. After a midline soft tissue incision tailored to the size of the lesion is performed, a craniotomy suited for the AVM size and location is completed to optimize exposure. Using a "reverse Trendelenburg" can optimize venous drainage. It is our preference to be seated during most microsurgical procedures so the head position should be optimized for this. After the craniotomy, the AVM is localized via direct inspection or with the help of stereotactic guidance and resected. Watertight closure of the dura is performed and the craniotomy and scalp are closed in standard fashion.

Cerebellopontine angle lesions

An AVM that primarily presents to the lateral cerebellar hemisphere can be accessed via a retrosigmoid (lateral suboccipital) craniotomy with the patient in either the park-bench or the supine position with the head flexed and turned toward the opposite shoulder.

A linear incision 2 cm behind the mastoid prominence can be tailored to meet the needs of the operation. The location of the

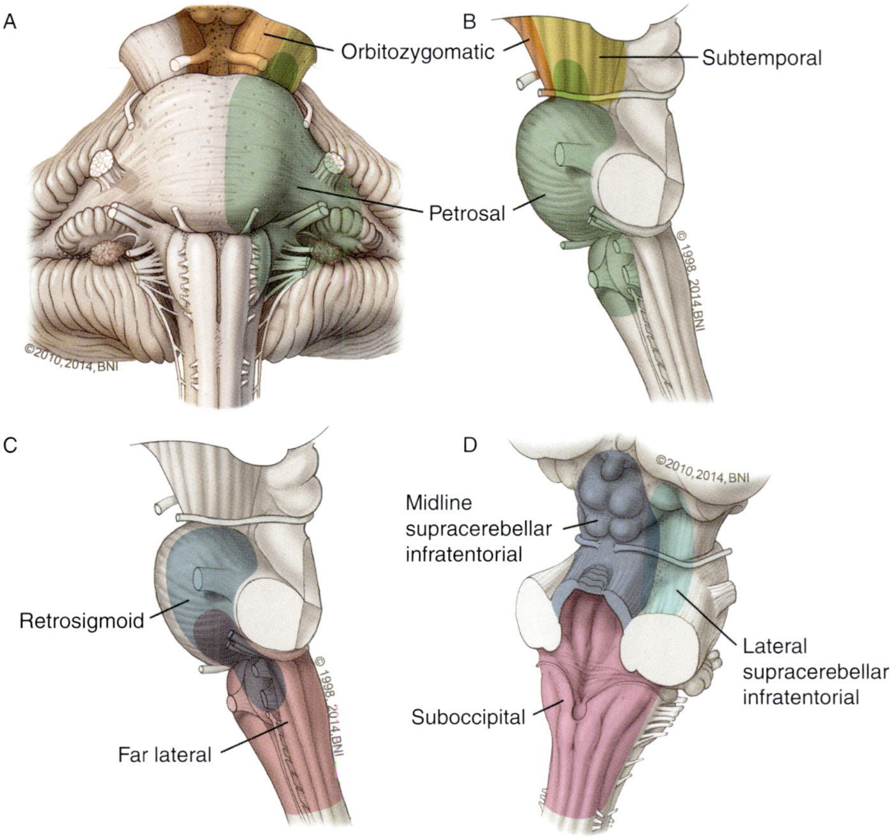

Fig. 12.5. Anatomical regions exposed by various skull base craniotomies for lesions in the posterior fossa and abutting the brainstem. (A,B) The brainstem showing exposure provided by the orbitozygomatic (to the ventral midbrain), subtemporal (lateral midbrain), and petrosal (lateral midbrain and pons) approaches (A, ventral view; B, lateral view). The orbitozygomatic, subtemporal, and petrosal approaches provide a mostly anterolateral view of these critical structures. Alternatively, posterior and posterolateral approaches can be used to access vascular malformations in the posterior fossa. (C,D) The brainstem demonstrate various domains exposed by posterior fossa skull base approaches. The retrosigmoid (providing access to the pons), far-lateral (providing access to the lower pons, medulla, and cervicomedullary junction), suboccipital (providing access to the dorsal pons, floor of fourth ventricle, medulla, and cervicomedullary junction), and supracerebellar infratentorial approaches (providing access to the dorsal midbrain) can be used to visualize and resect lesions in the posterior fossa (C, lateral view; D, dorsal view). (With permission from Barrow Neurological Institute.)

transverse–sigmoid junction and the mastoid tip are guiding points for surgical planning. The suboccipital bone is exposed to the foramen magnum or C1 as needed and the craniotomy can be extended to the transverse and sigmoid sinuses superiorly and laterally. Care should be taken to exenterate any exposed mastoid air cells. The dura is then opened in a triangular fashion with the base toward the sigmoid sinus. A second triangular flap can be based on the transverse sinus with the medial limb extending to the transverse–sigmoid junction. Success of the exposure depends on adequate cerebellar relaxation, which can be optimized by opening the cisterns. Care should be taken to gently expose and protect the cranial nerves to avoid postoperative neurological deficits.

Upper vermian and roof of the cerebellum lesions

A supracerebellar infratentorial approach is ideal for lesions involving the upper vermis or the roof of the cerebellum. A sitting or Concorde position can be used. It is important to expose the transverse sinuses, the torcula, and the dura overlying the superior cerebellar hemispheres. This requires that the craniotomy extends above and below the sinuses. We often prefer a two-piece craniotomy so the sinus can be carefully dissected off the bone under direct visualization. The dura is opened in a triangular fashion based on the transverse sinus–torcula junction. Bridging veins between the tentorium and superior surface of the cerebellum are then coagulated and divided while paying attention to avoid coagulation of any draining veins. Releasing cerebrospinal fluid optimizes this exposure.

Brainstem lesions

Midbrain

Anterior and anterolateral midbrain and interpeduncular cistern

The trans-sylvian approach can be used for AVMs involving the anterolateral midbrain and the interpeduncular cistern. A standard pterional craniotomy may be adequate but adjuncts such as a zygomatic osteotomy or orbitozygomatic osteotomy can widen the exposure and allow a more midline trajectory to the lesion. If a more lateral trajectory is needed, a frontotemporal craniotomy can be performed. Wide opening of the sylvian fissure is needed to allow adequate illumination in the depth and sufficient exposure to visualize relevant structures. Dissection of the fissure is gradually completed to expose the cerebral peduncles and the interpeduncular cistern. Although we do not commonly use retractors when the trans-sylvian approach is used for aneurysm clipping, frontal and temporal retractors can be used to facilitate access to deeper structures during AVM surgery. Preliminary work suggests that endoscopic approaches can be used to access anterior brainstem structures [44]. Combining endonasal and microsurgical techniques is needed for this approach to be viable. Risk of cerebrospinal fluid leak is one deterrent for this approach.

Lateral and posterolateral midbrain

The subtemporal approach gives limited but direct access to the lateral midbrain and pontomesencephalic region. The patient is positioned in the park-bench position or in the supine position with the head turned into a near horizontal angle. For heavier and larger patients, it is beneficial to suspend the bottom arm in a sling to allow the head to be tipped down. This allows the temporal lobe to migrate more easily off the middle fossa floor during exposure. Cerebrospinal fluid drainage via a lumbar drain is highly advantageous for this exposure. Enhancing this approach with a zygomatic osteotomy and a supralabyrinthine posterior petrosectomy may provide wider access. A linear or U-shaped incision can be used. The linear incision begins anterior to the ear at the level of the zygomatic root within 1 cm of the anterior tragus margin and extends cephalad for 10 cm. The U-shaped incision is more versatile and allows wider access. The anterior limb extends anteriorly to just in front of the ear and the posterior limb extends down to the mastoid tip when a partial petrosectomy is desired. Protection of the transverse and sigmoid sinuses should be kept in mind during the craniotomy. As in aneurysm surgery, through this approach the tentorium can be reflected back on itself and secured with a 4-0 nylon stitch just anterior to the junction of the fourth nerve and the tentorial edge. The dura is then opened and the temporal lobe retracted while paying attention not to injure the vein of Labbé and the inferior bridging veins. The AVM is then exposed and resected in standard fashion.

Tectum, superior cerebellar peduncles, and anterior vermis

The tectum, the superior cerebellar peduncles, and the anterior vermis can be accessed by the supracerebellar infratentorial approach or the occipital transtentorial approach. The supracerebellar infratentorial approach is usually used for AVMs of the tectal plate and the superior surface of the cerebellum, provided they do not extend above the incisura. The sitting or Concorde positions work well for AVMs extending above the incisura. The sitting position in particular allows gravity to assist in downward displacement of the cerebellum, which greatly facilitates exposure. In this position, the tentorium should ideally be parallel to the floor, which can be achieved by neck flexion. As noted above, the procedure is started with a midline vertical incision centered over the torcula and extending to the upper cervical spine. The craniotomy is then performed to expose the transverse sinuses and the torcula. The one flap can be taken in two pieces to minimize risk to the sinuses. The dural opening is made in triangular fashion based on the sinus–torcula junction. From this perspective, the anatomical landmarks are the P3 and P4 branches of the PCAs, the basal veins of Rosenthal, the vein of Galen, and the mesencephalon. Anterior cerebellar vermisectomy can be used if needed to expose the superior medullary velum and inferior mesencephalon.

The occipital transtentorial approach can be used to access AVMs of the superior cerebellar peduncle, the anterior cerebellar vermis, the superior medullary velum, and tectal plate of the mesencephalon. Occipital lobe relaxation can be optimized with lumbar or ventricular drainage. The patient is positioned in the prone position with the neck slightly flexed, or in the lateral position with the head turned toward the floor to optimize the surgical trajectory. An occipital craniotomy is performed to expose the torcula, distal superior sagittal sinus, and proximal ipsilateral transverse sinus. Extreme care should be taken not to injure the sinus. The dura is opened in a cruciate fashion and the tentorium is then divided 1 cm parallel to the straight sinus and retracted with sutures. Careful attention to preservation of the deep venous system is necessary to safely reach AVMs of the pineal region and the dorsal midbrain.

Pons

Exposure of the lateral pons

While a retrosigmoid craniotomy allows visualization of the lateral pontine surface, the exposure may not be adequate to achieve full control of an AVM in this location. The anterior transpetrosal approach consists of a subtemporal approach with anterior petrosectomy. It allows hearing preservation and is suited for anterior lesions. A U-shaped incision is made above the ear with the base of the incision along the superior temporal line. After exposing the zygomatic arch, it is cut in two points to free the temporal muscle, which is then retracted inferiorly. The petrous pyramid is exposed in the epidural space. The basal dura of the middle fossa is incised 2 cm inward toward the superior petrosal sinus and the incision is made adjacent to the sinus. Then an aperture in the posterior fossa dura is made below the superior petrosal sinus. The anterior inferior cerebellar artery and the petrosal vein serve as helpful landmarks in the cerebellopontine angle cistern. The translabyrinthine and transcochlear approaches offer the potential of a wider surgical view. However, both procedures sacrifice hearing and the latter places the facial nerve at significant risk. For these approaches, the patient is positioned supine with the head turned to the contralateral side. A C-shaped incision behind the ear exposes the mastoid tip and the underlying sigmoid sinus and transverse–sigmoid junction. Drilling begins with a standard mastoidectomy and skeletonization of the tegmen, the sigmoid sinus, and the posterior border of the external auditory canal. The drilling is continued to expose the dura of the middle fossa. During the dissection, the surgeon should identify the vertical segment of the facial nerve. This is followed by a labyrinthectomy that begins by opening the lateral and posterior semicircular canals. Eventually the sigmoid sinus can be traced toward the jugular bulb [45]. After identification of appropriate structures, the dura is opened and the AVM resected in a standard fashion. The retrolabyrinthine, presigmoid approach usually provides very small surgical view and is, therefore, rarely used for AVM resection.

Medulla

Anterior and lateral medulla

Access to the anterior and lateral cervicomedullary junction, medulla, and lower pons can be achieved using the far lateral approach. The patient is placed in a lateral or modified park-bench position with the operative side pointing up [42,43]. The patient's neck is flexed in the anteroposterior plane and rotated 45 degrees to the opposite shoulder, while at the same time flexed laterally 30 degrees down. To provide a better view of the cranial cervical junction, the superior shoulder can be retracted inferiorly with tape. During this retraction it is important to realize the potential for brachial plexus injury and respond accordingly. The patient's dependent arm can be suspended between the edge of the table and the Mayfield head holder; padding of the axilla is crucial. Two different scalp incisions can be performed to complete a far lateral approach. The first incision consists of an inverted hockey-stick incision going from the midline at C4 and curved anterolaterally to the mastoid tip. Detaching the musculature from the occiput is then performed, during which care should be taken to leave a cuff of muscle on the bone for reattachment at the time of closure. The soft tissue and musculature are then retracted inferolaterally to expose the craniocervical junction and the ipsilateral C1 and C2 laminae. The second incision is S-shaped and extends from the sigmoid–transverse junction to the level of C2. After performing the skin flap, subperiosteal dissection is performed to expose the ipsilateral C1 lamina. A C1 laminectomy is then performed while paying attention to the vertebral artery trajectory in the sulcus arteriosus.

After the subperiosteal dissection is performed, a lateral suboccipital craniotomy between the sigmoid sinus and the foramen magnum can be carried out. The medial foramen magnum and the posteromedial third of the occipital condyle are then removed. The dura is opened in a curvilinear fashion. The ipsilateral cerebellar hemisphere and tonsil can be retracted to expose the underlying anterolateral medulla and cervicomedullary junction. Landmarks that should be identified from this perspective include cranial nerves IX–XII, the vertebral artery, and the PICA. The AVM is then identified and resected using the technique described above. During closure, it is very important to be meticulous with dural approximation and exenteration of mastoid air cells.

Posterior medulla

Access to the posterior medulla can be achieved via a standard midline suboccipital craniotomy with extension to the foramen magnum. A C1 laminectomy can enhance visualization. Mobilizing and gently retracting one tonsil superiorly and laterally is usually sufficient to achieve adequate exposure.

Postoperative care

Postoperative care, consisting of neurological and hemodynamic monitoring, can be a major determinant of outcome in patients with AVMs. Following angiography after resection, it is customary to obtain a CT scan as a baseline. Patients should be carefully monitored in the intensive care unit and particular care is taken to address early signs of postoperative swelling, hemorrhage, and hydrocephalus. The potential for hyperperfusion breakthrough hemorrhage [46] should always be considered following the resection of any AVM. It is for this reason that relative hypotension should be instituted and closely monitored during the postoperative evaluation in the intensive care unit. Postoperative hyperemia may even require osmotic diuresis. Particular attention should be paid to coagulation status. A postoperative angiogram is essential to exclude residual AVM.

Surgical outcomes and complication management

Outcomes of posterior fossa AVM surgery have been improving over the past several decades [10]. This relates to accumulating experience with patient selection and advances in microsurgery, radiosurgery, and endovascular surgery, plus their thoughtful integration into practice [8].

In their classic 1986 series, Drake *et al.* reported on 66 posterior fossa AVMs of which 77% affected the cerebellum and 92% presented with hemorrhage. An obliteration rate of 92% was achieved, with 71% of patients achieving "excellent to good" outcomes [2]. In the same year, Batjer and Samson reported their series of 32 posterior fossa AVMs (17 vermian, 7 hemispheric, 4 brainstem, 2 tonsillar and 2 in the cerebellopontine angle) of which 23 (72%) presented with intracranial hemorrhage, and 15 (46%) were treated with the intention of primary resection. An obliteration rate of 100% was achieved in the treated group, with 80% of patients achieving "excellent to good" outcomes [47].

While these initial series described the outcomes of AVMs treated surgically, more recent studies have elaborated on the outcomes of AVMs treated with combined therapeutic modalities. In 2008, Kelly *et al.* reported on 76 patients with posterior fossa AVMs (36 cerebellar, 33 brainstem, and 7 involving both the cerebellum and brainstem) treated with radiosurgery (14), surgery (6), endovascular techniques (5), and multiple modalities (51). The mean follow up was 4.8 years. Of the 76 patients, 48 had high Spetzler–Martin grade (III–V). Of patients with high-grade AVMs, the obliteration rate was 52%, with 81% "excellent to good" outcomes despite 60% of the AVMs being in the brainstem [8]. Kelly *et al.* also assessed the effect of multimodal treatment on outcomes and found that multimodal treatment tripled the cure rate compared with radiosurgery alone; they concluded that brainstem AVMs are the only lesions that should be treated with radiosurgery alone [8].

In a single-center series over 15 years including 98 posterior fossa AVMs (46 cerebellar and 16 brainstem), 95 of the AVMs (97%) were symptomatic at presentation; 62 were treated and of those 18 had poor modified Rankin Scale (mRS) scores at presentation. The average follow up was 3.3 years. Of the 18 patients who had poor mRS scores at presentation, 12 (67%) improved to a good score at final visit. A multivariate analysis demonstrated correlation between the mRS score at presentation and mRS score at final visit. In the same series, the final clinical outcome was correlated with the presence of an associated aneurysm and the number of treatments needed to obliterate the AVM [20].

Optimizing surgical outcomes requires a proactive and vigilant approach to complication avoidance. The first step in complication avoidance begins with careful patient selection and is followed by creating a strategy that optimizes benefit and minimizes risk. Strategy development includes a decision regarding preoperative embolization. If the embolization is being carried out by a different surgeon, then a careful discussion regarding the goals of embolization should occur. Strategy formulation should also include issues related to positioning, neuroanesthesia, and neuromonitoring. Prior planning and discussion with the anesthesia team is worthwhile. Intraoperative complications can be minimized by careful positioning, optimization of the surgical corridor, brain relaxation, and careful attention to avoidance of venous injury during the craniotomy. During the procedure, the technical nuances regarding spiral technique, preservation of en passage vessels, and preserving venous outflow until arterial supply to the AVM has been disconnected will all contribute to a smoother operation. Careful management of deep feeders with AVM clips will avoid problematic deep bleeding. Careful hemostasis after AVM resection is paramount. Attentive postoperative care, as outlined above, will further ensure a desirable postoperative course. Edema, hemorrhage, and/or hydrocephalus should be suspected postoperatively if the patient does not have the expected results on examination. General complications of posterior fossa surgery, including cerebrospinal fluid leak and sinus thrombosis, should be kept in mind. If residual AVM is seen on postoperative angiography, consideration should be given to prompt re-exploration and resection.

Conclusions

The complex anatomy of the posterior fossa presents unique challenges for microsurgical management of AVMs within this compartment. However, the high morbidity and mortality associated with this subgroup of AVMs makes their treatment particularly rewarding. Assertive surgical, endovascular, and critical care interventions can salvage many patients who present with acute hemorrhage. With experience, thoughtful patient selection, and mastery of the issues outlined in this chapter, excellent outcomes can be achieved.

References

1. Batjer H, Samson D. Arteriovenous malformations of the posterior fossa. Clinical presentation, diagnostic evaluation, and surgical treatment. *J Neurosurg* 1986;**64**:849–56.
2. Drake CG, Friedman AH, Peerless SJ. Posterior fossa arteriovenous malformations. *J Neurosurg* 1986;**64**:1–10.
3. Bendok BR, El Tecle NE, El Ahmadieh TY, *et al.* Advances and innovations in brain arteriovenous malformations surgery. *Neurosurgery* 2014;**74**(Suppl 1):S60–73.
4. Yaşargil MG. *Microneurosurgery.* New York: Thieme, 1998.
5. Logue V, Monckton G. Posterior fossa angiomas; a clinical presentation of nine cases. *Brain* 1954;**77**:252–73.
6. Mount LA. Arteriovenous angioma derived from the anterior inferior cerebellar artery. Its diagnosis and treatment. *J Neurosurg* 1965;**22**:612–15.
7. Green JR, Vaughan RJ. Blood vessel tumors and hematomas of the posterior fossa in adolescence. *Angiology* 1972;**23**:474–87.
8. Kelly ME, Guzman R, Sinclair J, *et al.* Multimodality treatment of posterior fossa arteriovenous malformations. *J Neurosurg* 2008;**108**:1152–61.
9. Samson DS, Batjer HH. Posterior fossa arteriovenous malformations. In Carter LP, Spetzler RF, eds. *Neurovascular Surgery*. New York: McGraw Hill, 1995, pp. 1005–15.
10. Arnaout OM, Gross BA, Eddleman CS, *et al.* Posterior fossa arteriovenous malformations. *Neurosurg Focus* 2009;**26**:E12.
11. Khaw AV, Mohr JP, Sciacca RR, *et al.* Association of infratentorial brain arteriovenous malformations with hemorrhage at initial presentation. *Stroke* 2004;**35**:660–3.
12. Ondra SL, Troupp H, George ED, *et al.* The natural history of symptomatic arteriovenous malformations of the brain: a 24-year follow-up assessment. *J Neurosurg* 1990;**73**:387–91.
13. Wilkins RH. Natural history of intracranial vascular malformations: a review. *Neurosurgery* 1985;**16**:421–30.
14. Garcia-Pastor C, Lopez-Gonzalez F, Revuelta R, *et al.* Trigeminal neuralgia secondary to arteriovenous malformations of the posterior fossa. *Surg Neurol* 2006;**66**:207–11.
15. Hernesniemi JA, Dashti R, Juvela S, *et al.* Natural history of brain arteriovenous malformations: a long-term follow-up study of risk of hemorrhage in 238 patients. *Neurosurgery* 2008;**63**:823–9.
16. da Costa L, Wallace MC, terBrugge KG, *et al.* The natural history and predictive features of hemorrhage from brain arteriovenous malformations. *Stroke* 2009;**40**:100–5.
17. Stapf C, Mast H, Sciacca RR, *et al.* Predictors of hemorrhage in patients with untreated brain arteriovenous malformations. *Neurology* 2006;**66**:1350–5.
18. Duong DH, Young WL, Vang MC, *et al.* Feeding artery pressure and venous drainage pattern are primary determinants of hemorrhage from cerebral arteriovenous malformations. *Stroke* 1998;**29**:1167–76.
19. Hademenos GJ, Massoud TF. Risk of intracranial arteriovenous malformations rupture due to venous drainage impairment. A theoretical analysis. *Stroke* 1996;**27**:1072–83.
20. da Costa L, Thines L, Dehdashti AR, *et al.* Management and clinical outcome of posterior fossa arteriovenous malformations: report on a single-centre 15-year experience. *J Neurol Neurosurg Psychiatry* 2009;**80**:376–9.
21. Stapf C, Mohr JP, Pile-Spellman J, *et al.* Concurrent arterial aneurysms in brain arteriovenous malformations with haemorrhagic presentation. *J Neurol Neurosurg Psychiatry* 2002;**73**:294–8.
22. Thompson RC, Steinberg GK, Levy RP, *et al.* The management of patients with arteriovenous malformations and associated intracranial aneurysms. *Neurosurgery* 1998;**43**:202–11.
23. George B, Celis-Lopez M, Kato T, *et al.* Arteriovenous malformations of the posterior fossa. *Acta Neurochir (Wien)* 1992;**116**:119–27.
24. Katsaridis V, Papagiannaki C, Aimar E. Embolization of brain arteriovenous malformations for cure: because we could and because we should. *AJNR Am J Neuroradiol* 2009;**30**:e67.

25. Natarajan SK, Ghodke B, Britz GW, *et al.* Multimodality treatment of brain arteriovenous malformations with microsurgery after embolization with Onyx: single-center experience and technical nuances. *Neurosurgery* 2008;**62**:1213–25.
26. Panagiotopoulos V, Gizewski E, Asgari S, *et al.* Embolization of intracranial arteriovenous malformations with ethylene–vinyl alcohol copolymer (Onyx). *AJNR Am J Neuroradiol* 2009;**30**:99–106.
27. Pierot L, Januel AC, Herbreteau D, *et al.* Endovascular treatment of brain arteriovenous malformations using Onyx: preliminary results of a prospective multicenter study. *Interv Neuroradiol* 2005;**11**:159–64.
28. Thakrar D, Popescu A, Gupta S, *et al.* Complex 3D blood flow pathways in two cases of aorta to right heart fistulae: a 4D flow MRI study. *Magn Reson Imaging* 2013;**31**:1453–5.
29. El Ahmadieh TY, El Tecle NE, Stadler JA, III, *et al.* Taming the beast: treating associated aneurysms to reduce risk of hemorrhage after radiosurgery for arteriovenous malformations. *Neurosurgery* 2013;**72**:N15–17.
30. Kano H, Kondziolka D, Flickinger JC, *et al.* Aneurysms increase the risk of rebleeding after stereotactic radiosurgery for hemorrhagic arteriovenous malformations. *Stroke* 2012;**43**:2586–91.
31. Dashti SR, Spalding AC, Yao TL. Multimodality treatment of a ruptured grade IV posterior fossa arteriovenous malformations in a patient pregnant with twins: case report. *J Neurointerv Surg* 2012;**4**:e21.
32. Mpotsaris A, Loehr C, Harati A, *et al.* Interdisciplinary clinical management of high grade arteriovenous malformations and ruptured flow-related aneurysms in the posterior fossa. *Interv Neuroradiol* 2010;**16**:400–8.
33. Sanchez-Mejia RO, McDermott MW, Tan J, *et al.* Radiosurgery facilitates resection of brain arteriovenous malformations and reduces surgical morbidity. *Neurosurgery* 2009;**64**:231–8.
34. Zaidi HA, Abla AA, Nakaji P, *et al.* Prospective evaluation of preoperative stereotactic radiosurgery followed by delayed resection of a high grade arteriovenous malformations. *J Clin Neurosci* 2014;**21**:1077–80.
35. Shrontz C, Dujovny M, Ausman JI, *et al.* Surgical anatomy of the arteries of the posterior fossa. *J Neurosurg* 1986;**65**:540–4.
36. Matsushima T, Rhoton AL, Jr., de Oliveira E, *et al.* Microsurgical anatomy of the veins of the posterior fossa. *J Neurosurg* 1983;**59**:63–105.
37. Matsuno H, Rhoton AL, Jr., Peace D. Microsurgical anatomy of the posterior fossa cisterns. *Neurosurgery* 1988;**23**:58–80.
38. Steinberg GK, Chang SD, Levy RP, *et al.* Surgical resection of large incompletely treated intracranial arteriovenous malformations following stereotactic radiosurgery. *J Neurosurg* 1996;**84**:920–8.
39. Zacharia BE, Bruce S, Appelboom G, *et al.* Occlusive hyperemia versus normal perfusion pressure breakthrough after treatment of crania arteriovenous malformations. *Neurosurg Clin N Am* 2012;**23**:147–51.
40. Sinclair J, Kelly ME, Steinberg GK. Surgical management of posterior fossa arteriovenous malformations. *Neurosurgery* 2006;**58**:ons201.
41. Rozet I, Vavilala MS. Risks and benefits of patient positioning during neurosurgical care. *Anesthesiol Clin* 2007;**25**:631–53.
42. Porter RW, Detwiler PW, Spetzler RF, *et al.* Cavernous malformations of the brainstem: experience with 100 patients. *J Neurosurg* 1999;**90**:50–8.
43. Stein BM, Solomon RA. Surgical approaches to posterior fossa arteriovenous malformations. *Clin Neurosurg* 1991;**37**:353–71.
44. Kassam AB, Thomas AJ, Zimmer LA, *et al.* Expanded endonasal approach: a fully endoscopic completely transnasal resection of a skull base arteriovenous malformations. *Childs Nerv Syst* 2007;**23**:491–8.
45. Nickele CM, Akture E, Gubbels SP, *et al.* A stepwise illustration of the translabyrinthine approach to a large cystic vestibular schwannoma. *Neurosurg Focus* 2012;**33**:E11.
46. Tamano Y, Ujiie H, Hori T. [Postoperative hemorrhage due to normal pressure hyperperfusion breakthrough after a trapping of VA–PICA dissecting aneurysm]. *No Shinkei Geka* 2000;**28**:257–62.
47. Batjer H, Samson D. Arteriovenous malformations of the posterior fossa: clinical presentation, diagnostic evaluation and surgical treatment. *Neurosurg Rev* 1986;**9**:287–96.

Chapter 13

Surgical management of cerebral dural arteriovenous fistulae

Ramsey Ashour and Jacques Morcos

Introduction

A cerebral dural arteriovenous fistula (DAVF) is an abnormal arteriovenous shunt, supplied primarily by dural feeding arteries, in which the fistulous connection occurs within the dural leaflets that surround the brain. Venous drainage then occurs via an adjacent dural venous sinus, cortical vein, or both. Pathologically increased blood flow through these venous pathways may remain clinically silent or may manifest in a variety of ways, including pulsatile tinnitus, bruit, headache, cranial nerve palsy, orbital venous congestion, seizures, cognitive decline, focal neurological deficit, cerebral venous hypertension, or intracranial hemorrhage. Importantly, DAVFs with retrograde cortical venous drainage often behave in a "malignant" fashion, with high associated rates of intracranial hemorrhage, neurological deficits, and death.

While endovascular approaches have emerged as the primary treatment for most DAVFs, certain fistula types are still best dealt with via open surgery as the first-line strategy. Furthermore, surgery has been used to successfully treat DAVFs after previous partial, incomplete, or failed endovascular treatment. Finally, surgery can be used adjunctively in a combined approach to provide direct access for embolization of DAVFs that are inaccessible by a purely endovascular route. This chapter will briefly review historical and clinical features of cerebral DAVFs and then describe the principles of their treatment through open surgical techniques.

History

Pre-angiography era

Although the first detailed clinicopathological descriptions of intracranial vascular malformations did not begin to appear until the late nineteenth century, Travers [1] likely carried out the first successful surgical treatment of a DAVF in 1809, when he curatively ligated the cervical carotid artery of a woman with spontaneous "pulsating exophthalmos," which was presumably secondary to a dural carotid–cavernous fistula (CCF). In 1873, Rizzoli reported both the clinical course and autopsy analysis of a child with a scalp/peritorcular fistula, and this was considered by Yaşargil to be the first clinicopathological description of a dural vascular malformations [2]. In 1924, Locke [3] collected all previously reported cases in the literature of pulsating exophthalmos and reported that a dural CCF was found in 16 of 30 spontaneous (non-traumatic) cases with autopsy data available. Notably, Locke also reported that cervical carotid ligation performed in 293 patients with pulsating exophthalmos between 1809 and 1923 resulted in 27 (9%) deaths.

Post-angiography era

Sachs [4] is widely credited with the first angiographic description of a DAVF in 1931. Subsequently, physicians armed with angiographic visualization and clinicopathological correlation began to characterize the various types of dural vascular lesion [5–10], although most attempts at treatment remained limited to feeding artery ligation. Over the course of the mid 20th century, many individuals recognized the limitations of feeding artery ligation alone, with its high associated morbidity and lesion recurrence rates. Novel treatments began to emerge primarily in the realm of both traumatic and dural CCFs, including combined cervical and intracranial internal carotid artery ligation [11,12], cavernous internal carotid artery embolization using a plug of muscle [13,14], and even direct cavernous sinus surgery with sinus packing and/or fistula ligation [15].

In 1972, Debrun and Chartres [5] provided an important angiographic and clinical description of non-CCF dural arteriovenous "malformations" in the post-angiography era, which had received much less attention in the literature than CCFs. In 26 treated patients with DAVFs collected from the literature up to that time, a successful outcome was achieved in 14 (54%) patients; 11 of these were treated by fistula excision, and 3 were treated by afferent vessel ligation. Of the remaining 12 patients, there were six recurrences (all external carotid artery ligations), two deaths, and four were lost to follow-up.

In 1974, Hugosson and Bergstrom [16] described four patients with transverse–sigmoid DAVFs treated surgically by circumferentially cutting the dural attachments to, and thus isolating, the involved sinuses. In view of the unique

Comprehensive Management of Arteriovenous Malformations of the Brain and Spine, ed. Robert F. Spetzler, Douglas S. Kondziolka, Randall T. Higashida, and M. Yashar S. Kalani. Published by Cambridge University Press.

pathoanatomy of DAVFs, surgical skeletonization of the sinus represented a promising step forward in the treatment of these lesions. In 1983, Sundt and Piepgras [17] reported their experience in 27 patients with transverse–sigmoid DAVFs using a more aggressive surgical approach that entailed complete resection of the lesion along with ligation and packing of the involved sinuses. Although 23 patients experienced excellent/good outcomes, two experienced poor outcomes (one related to venous infarction) and two patients died of excessive blood loss (one exsanguinated on the table). Consequently, although DAVFs had become amenable to curative surgical treatment, they remained formidable lesions even in the best hands.

The seminal contributions of Serbinenko [18] and Debrun *et al.* [19], both using detachable balloons to elegantly embolize CCFs, decisively shifted the momentum toward endovascular techniques as the primary approach toward traumatic CCFs in particular. Transvenous endovascular approaches to the cavernous sinus were later pioneered by Debrun and allowed successful treatment of dural CCFs as well. In the 1990s, the introduction of detachable coils, among other factors, resulted in a highly accelerated period of neuroendovascular technological advances, which facilitated treatment not just for cerebral aneurysms but also for several types of cerebrovascular lesions, including DAVFs. Indeed, improvements in catheter design, novel embolic agents, and enhanced angiographic imaging capabilities have combined over the past several years to allow most DAVFs to be safely and successfully treated endovascularly. Nevertheless, surgery remains the primary approach for certain DAVF types and is also an important second option in failed endovascular treatment.

Clinical features

Epidemiology

Dural arteriovenous fistulae account for approximately 10–15% of all cerebrovascular malformations [20]. The majority of affected patients are between 40 and 60 years of age [21]. Considering all DAVF locations, women are slightly more often affected than men [21]; however, dural CCFs have a particularly strong female preponderance [22].

Pathophysiology

While congenital DAVFs may rarely occur in children and are typically more complex than adult DAVFs, the majority of adult DAVFs are considered to be acquired idiopathic lesions. Consequently, while the term "malformations" has been used in the past, this term implies a congenital lesion and, therefore, the term "fistula" is now preferred to reflect the contemporary view that these are typically acquired lesions. Notably, while DAVFs can rarely recruit or "parasitize" pial arterial feeders, they are distinguished from cerebral arteriovenous malformations (AVMs) in that DAVFs are extrapial dural-based lesions that lack a true parenchymal nidus.

There exists a well-recognized association between DAVFs and dural venous sinus thrombosis, and multiple animal studies have demonstrated that surgically induced venous hypertension leads to increased angiogenic activity and to the development of de novo DAVFs [23–25]. Nevertheless, the exact pathogenesis of DAVFs and their relationship to venous sinus thrombosis are not fully established. One theory is that spontaneous venous sinus occlusion is the initiating event, and the resulting venous hypertension "awakens" pre-existing embryonic dural arteriovenous channels [26]. Another possibility is that venous hypertension/thrombosis may induce local angiogenesis and promote the de novo formation of an arteriovenous shunt [27]. Yet another possibility is that the DAVF may arise first [6] and then the fistula itself promotes venous sinus thrombosis/hypertension, which is a common clinical observation in lesions followed over time. However, many patients with DAVFs do not develop sinus thrombosis, and most patients with sinus thrombosis do not develop DAVFs. Finally, a subset of "secondary" DAVFs are known to occur after head trauma [28], infection, or iatrogenically after surgery/embolization [29].

Signs and symptoms

The signs and symptoms are predictably related to an abnormal pattern of arterialized venous drainage. Intracerebral hemorrhage secondary to venous hypertension occurs frequently in lesions exhibiting cortical venous drainage; this is both the most common cause of death and the strongest indication for treatment in patients with DAVFs. Non-hemorrhagic focal neurological deficits may result from venous hypertension, mass effect in venous ectasias, or, rarely, from hypoperfusion secondary to arterial steal. Global cognitive decline and seizures are also well-recognized sequelae of venous hypertension in patients with DAVFs. Pathological turbulent flow, which may occur within the transverse, sigmoid, or petrosal sinuses, results in pulsatile tinnitus, the most common symptom reported by patients harboring a DAVF [30]. Headaches may also occur secondary to stretching of the dura and/or venous hypertension itself. Cranial nerve palsies may result from arterialization of the petrosal sinuses (superior or inferior) and/or from arterialization of the cavernous sinuses. Orbital congestive signs/symptoms are typically associated with CCFs but may also be caused by non-CCF DAVFs that arterialize the cavernous sinus, and include proptosis, chemosis, ocular bruit, restrictive ophthalmoparesis, glaucoma, neovascular retinopathy, and vision loss [31].

Classification

Numerous DAVF classification systems have been proposed (Table 13.1) [6, 32–37]. Importantly, in 1978, Djindjian and Merland [32] presented the first DAVF classification scheme to emphasize the concept that the presence of cortical venous drainage is associated with an aggressive clinical course. In 1995, Borden *et al.* [35] and Cognard *et al.* [34] presented classification systems based on angiographic features. These have emerged as the two most commonly used contemporary DAVF grading schemes. While each of these classification systems has its particular strengths and weaknesses, cortical venous drainage is the defining angiographic feature that

Table 13.1. Classification schemes for dural arteriovenous fistulae

Classification	Type	Drainage	Retrograde sinus flow?	CVD
Aminoff (1973) [6]	Anteroinferior	Basal sinuses (cavernous, petrosal, sphenoparietal)	±	±
	Posterosuperior	Dural sinuses (superior sagittal, transverse, sigmoid)	±	±
Djindjian and Merland (1978) [32]	I	Into sinus or meningeal vein	No	No
	II	Into sinus with CVD or retrograde flow into another sinus	Yes	Yes
	III	Direct CVD	No	Yes
	IV	Directly into dural venous lake	No	Yes
Lalwani *et al.* (1993) [33]	1	Antegrade sinus flow only; no retrograde sinus flow or CVD	No	No
	2	Antegrade and retrograde sinus flow with or without CVD	Yes	±
	3	No antegrade sinus flow; only retrograde sinus flow with CVD	Yes	Yes
	4	CVD only; no antegrade or retrograde sinus flow	No	Yes
Cognard *et al.* (1995) [34]	I	Into sinus with antegrade flow	No	No
	IIa	Into sinus with retrograde flow	Yes	No
	IIb	Into sinus with CVD	No	Yes
	IIa+b	Into sinus with retrograde flow and CVD	Yes	Yes
	III	Direct CVD	No	Yes
	IV	Direct CVD with venous ectasia	No	Yes
	V	Spinal venous drainage	No	Yes
Borden *et al.* (1995) [35]	I	Into sinus or meningeal vein	±	No
	II	Into sinus with CVD	±	Yes
	III	Direct CVD	No	Yes
Zipfel *et al.* (2009) [36]	1	Same as Borden I	±	No
	2+aCVD	Borden II with asymptomatic CVD	±	Yes
	2+sCVD	Borden II with symptomatic CVD	±	Yes
	3+aCVD	Borden III with asymptomatic CVD	No	Yes
	3+sCVD	Borden III with symptomatic CVD	No	Yes
Barrow *et al.* (1985) [37] (CCFs *only*)	A	Direct CCF; rent in the cavernous ICA	±	±
	B	Dural CCF; fed by ICA branches only	±	±
	C	Dural CCF; fed by ECA branches only	±	±
	D	Dural CCF; fed by ICA and ECA branches	±	±

CCF, dural carotid–cavernous fistula; CVD, cortical venous drainage; ECA, external carotid artery; ICA, internal carotid artery.

distinguishes those DAVFs with high potential for future morbidity and mortality if left untreated.

Natural history

The concept that DAVFs can be categorized as "benign" or "malignant" based on the absence or presence, respectively, of cortical venous drainage was validated by the natural history data reported by the University of Toronto Brain Vascular Malformations Study Group. Specifically, in lesions without cortical venous drainage followed over a mean period of 33 months, 98% of lesions remained benign and 2% developed new cortical venous drainage and interval aggressive behavior [38]. By comparison, in lesions with cortical venous drainage followed over a mean period of 4.3 years, the annual rates of hemorrhage, non-hemorrhagic neurological deficit, and death were 8.1%, 6.9%, and 10.4%, respectively [39]. The location of the DAVF is another important consideration that relates to the clinical presentation of a given lesion. In a meta-analysis of 377 patients, clinical behavior was evaluated in the context of DAVF location and this identified three particularly aggressive DAVF locations (aggressive:benign ratio): tentorial incisura (31:1), sylvian/middle fossa (2.5:1), and orbital/falx/anterior fossa (2.1:1) [40]. Cortical venous drainage and variceal venous distension were identified as the most important angiographic risk factors associated with aggressive DAVF behavior [40].

In summary, the prevailing view that emerged in the latter half of the 20th century is that lesions without cortical venous drainage tend to remain benign but require angiographic follow-up if clinical changes occur, whereas lesions with cortical venous drainage tend to behave aggressively and almost always require treatment. However, two contemporary studies have led some to reconsider this notion. In 2008, Soderman *et al.* [41] retrospectively reviewed 85 patients with DAVFs with cortical venous drainage evaluated at their institution over a 30-year period and found that the risk of future hemorrhage was 7.4% per year in those who presented initially with intracranial hemorrhage versus 1.5% per year in those who did not present with hemorrhage. Similarly in 2009, Strom *et al.* [42] retrospectively reviewed 28 patients with DAVFs with cortical venous drainage (some untreated or only partially treated) and found that the risk of future hemorrhage was 7.6% per year in those who presented initially with either hemorrhage or a neurological deficit (median follow-up of 9.7 months) versus 1.4% per year in those who did not present with hemorrhage/neurological deficits (median follow-up of 31.4 months). On the basis of these data, Zipfel *et al.* [36] have recently proposed a modified DAVF classification scheme that closely mirrors the Borden classification but distinguishes asymptomatic versus symptomatic cortical venous drainage based on the mode of clinical presentation (i.e., with or without hemorrhage/neurological deficit).

While the association between cortical venous drainage and aggressive clinical behavior has received much attention, it is also important to recognize that significant orbital venous congestion, which is typically seen in dural CCFs, threatens vision and so should also be considered a malignant feature of these unique lesions even in the absence of cortical venous drainage.

Diagnosis

The clinical presentation of DAVFs overlaps with a variety of other conditions, and imaging studies play an important role in clarifying the diagnosis. However, if the possibility of a DAVF is not suspected (e.g., a patient with pulsatile tinnitus presumed to have a vestibular problem), the appropriate imaging may not be obtained, causing a delay in diagnosis. Importantly, a DAVF is the most frequent cause of objective pulsatile tinnitus in a patient with a normal otoscopic examination [30]. Pulsatile tinnitus that resolves with manual compression of the ipsilateral occipital artery is virtually pathognomonic for the presence of a DAVF, particularly if the lesion involves the transverse/sigmoid sinuses. In such patients, the occipital artery is often enlarged, and a bruit can be auscultated. However, pulsatile tinnitus that resolves with compression of the ipsilateral internal jugular vein is pathognomonic for jugular venous hum [43], which can be treated if disabling but typically poses no potential for future neurological morbidity.

Imaging

Non-contrast brain CT is best used to screen for intracerebral hemorrhage but often will not disclose the presence of a DAVF in a patient presenting with a neurological complaint. Dilated tortuous vessels, which correspond to enlarged arterial feeders or ectatic cortical veins, are better visualized by contrast CT angiography. Similarly, MRI/MR angiography may reveal dilated pial vessels, prominent early venous sinus filling, venous sinus enlargement or occlusion, and white matter edema related to venous hypertension. Formal diagnostic cerebral angiography will clarify an uncertain diagnosis and is required to fully evaluate all DAVFs in order to plan and execute treatment. Six-vessel angiography should be performed to identify arterial supply, venous drainage pattern, vascular steal and global hemispheric flow, and potential transarterial and transvenous endovascular access options. Some DAVFs may appear quite complex angiographically, receiving arterial supply from the internal carotid, external carotid, and vertebrobasilar circulations. While the various angiographic runs performed from each of these different circulations may appear drastically different during the early arterial phase, often a "final common pathway" emerges during the late arterial phase, as the venous drainage appears the same regardless of which arterial feeder is injected. Careful study of these different runs side by side through the venous phase is necessary to determine the location of the fistulous point upon which the arterial feeders from each territory ultimately converge into the final common venous outflow of the lesion.

Surgical management

Treatment indications

Intracranial hemorrhage is the strongest and most urgent indication for treatment of a DAVF. Indeed, after an initial DAVF hemorrhage, the chance of experiencing a second hemorrhage is as high as 35% within the first two weeks [44]. A DAVF with cortical venous drainage carries a yearly event rate (hemorrhage or non-hemorrhagic neurological deficit) of 15% and a yearly mortality rate of 10.4%; therefore, most of these high-risk lesions should also be treated [39]. Conversely, the majority of DAVFs without cortical venous drainage do not require treatment; however, any clinical changes must be correlated with angiography to investigate for lesion progression, which is rare (~2%) [38]. A DAVF without cortical venous drainage may be considered for palliative treatment in the setting of an intolerable bruit, headaches, orbital venous congestion, or symptoms of venous hypertension related to retrograde dural venous sinus flow; however, caution must be exercised because partial treatment in such patients may lead to the unintended consequence of converting a benign lesion into an aggressive one.

Treatment options and principles

Surgical options for the treatment of DAVFs include the following techniques:

- radical fistula excision
- sinus skeletonization
- disconnection of cortical venous drainage
- ligation of the fistulous point and/or outflow vein
- sinus packing
- coagulation of arterial feeders to the lesion.

Radical DAVF excision including the involved sinus, as described by Sundt and Piepgras, has proven in the past to be an effective, yet potentially dangerous, surgical option, with significant risks of massive intraoperative blood loss as well as postoperative venous infarction [17]. Furthermore, the experience of Sundt and Piepgras was limited to transverse–sigmoid DAVFs; radical excision of deeper lesions, such as tentorial DAVFs, requires more extensive surgical approaches and entails greater operative risk.

Sinus skeletonization, as described by Hugosson and Bergstrom [16], achieves DAVF arterial deafferentation by circumferentially cutting the dural attachments alongside the involved sinus and is useful for lesions in which the involved sinus must be preserved and a discrete fistulous point is difficult to localize and ligate directly. However, complete DAVF arterial deafferentation may not always be possible, and because the venous outflow remains patent, it is not uncommon for lesions treated by this technique to persist or recur as new arterial feeders are recruited to supply the shunt. This is supported by good evidence that the fistulization occurs within the layers of the sinus wall [45].

Since the mid 1990s, it has been recognized and emphasized by many that interruption of the venous drainage, either surgically or endovascularly, is effective for achieving complete DAVF obliteration [46–48]. Unlike cerebral AVMs, in which early occlusion of the venous outflow in the face of persistent arterial inflow carries a high risk of potentially disastrous intracerebral hemorrhage, occlusion of the venous outflow of a DAVF is safe because these lesions do not harbor an intraparenchymal nidus; rather, the fistulous connection is contained within the dural leaflets. However, while the risk of arterial hemorrhage after DAVF venous outflow occlusion is low, the risk of venous infarction/hypertension is potentially significant if the venous drainage of normal adjacent brain is also sacrificed simultaneously. Therefore, a careful and thoughtful review of the pretreatment angiograms, including the late venous phase, is necessary to fully evaluate not only the pathological DAVF venous outflow but also the venous drainage of surrounding normal brain. For example, a DAVF that is seen to cause retrograde flow through the transverse sinus during systole does not necessarily preclude drainage of normal brain via the vein of Labbé into the non-arterialized portion of this sinus during diastole.

In general, when surgery is utilized for DAVFs that drain directly into cortical veins (without an intervening sinus), surgical interruption of the venous outflow is the treatment of choice and can often be achieved by directly clipping the vein as close as possible to its exit from the dura. From an endovascular standpoint, transvenous approaches are often required to achieve complete obliteration of a DAVF; however, lesions with direct cortical venous drainage are quite difficult to approach transvenously because of the lack of an intervening sinus. Furthermore, a transarterial approach is unlikely to be curative unless embolic material can be injected across the point of the arteriovenous shunt to cast the venous outflow, which is difficult to achieve precisely compared with surgical clipping under direct vision.

For DAVFs that drain into an intervening sinus and then into cortical veins, sinus excision with disconnection of the cortical venous drainage continues to be an option when surgery is required. Unlike DAVFs that drain directly into cortical veins, where simple interruption of the cortical venous drainage directly obliterates the fistula at the point of arteriovenous shunting, simple interruption of the cortical venous drainage alone is controversial for lesions that drain first into a sinus, as this strategy leaves the fistula open and results in a potential for recruitment of pre-existing venous channels to reconstitute and maintain a new fistula. In one study, 23 patients with Borden type II DAVFs who previously underwent failed endovascular treatments were subsequently successfully treated by selective surgical disconnection of the cortical venous drainage only [49]. In other words, the sinus component of the fistula itself was not excised or packed, and essentially all of the DAVFs were converted from Borden type II to type I lesions. No episode of intracranial hemorrhage or worsening neurological deficit was seen over a mean follow-up period of 4.9 years, indicating that this treatment strategy is effective while avoiding the increased surgical risks associated with radical sinus excision.

Techniques by location

Transverse–sigmoid locations

Transverse–sigmoid DAVFs are typically supplied by transosseous branches of the occipital artery but may also be fed by branches of the posterior auricular, ascending pharyngeal, middle meningeal, posterior meningeal, and tentorial arteries. Venous drainage occurs initially through the ipsilateral transverse–sigmoid sinuses; however, sinus occlusion may result in retrograde flow to the contralateral sinuses or into temporal, occipital, or cerebellar cortical veins.

Several surgical positions and skin incisions could be entertained, but we generally prefer the very versatile lateral decubitus position and the C-shaped retroauricular incision (similar to our approach to acoustic neuromas). The major arterial supply via the occipital artery is encountered and ligated during the exposure. Significant hemorrhage may occur during the craniotomy from transosseous feeders, from diploic veins, or from enlarged dural feeding arteries if

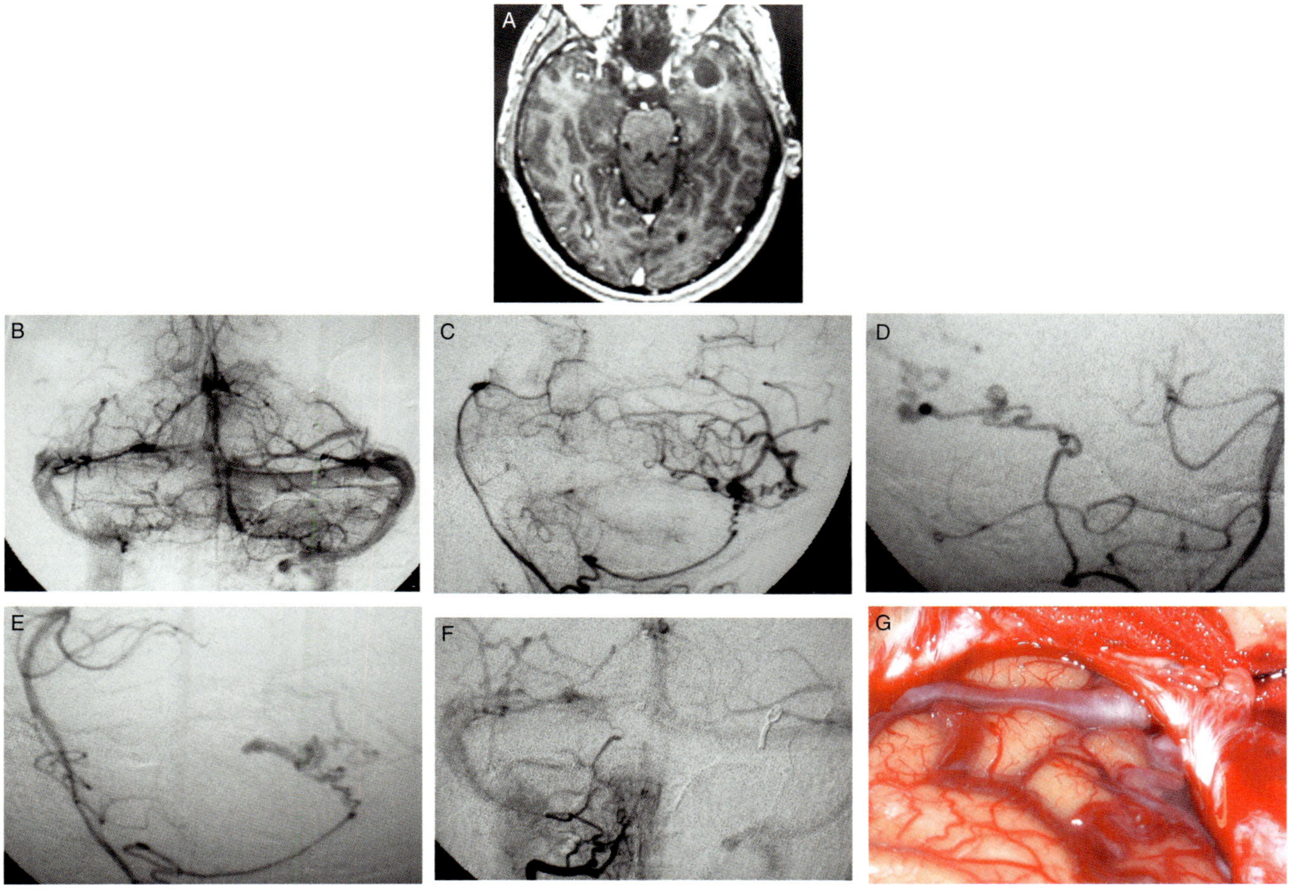

Fig. 13.1. A 45-year-old man with a history of a clipped unruptured left middle cerebral artery aneurysm who developed right-sided headaches. (A) MRI of the brain with gadolinium revealed a clip artifact on the left, and evidence of congested veins in the right occipitoparietal area. (B–D) Cerebral angiography with right vertebral artery (VA) injections demonstrated a right transverse sinus dural arteriovenous fistula with a patent sinus but retrograde cortical venous drainage. Right VA injection, demonstrated arterialization of the right transverse sinus wall via the posterior meningeal artery and two distinct arterialized cortical veins draining supratentorially (B, anteroposterior view; C, lateral view; D, oblique view). (E) Left VA injection revealed supply from the left posterior meningeal artery as well. (F) An anteroposterior venous phase view demonstrated well-patent transverse sinuses bilaterally. (G) At surgery, through a right occipital craniotomy, the two arterialized occipital veins were well visualized and clipped (not shown).

a dural laceration occurs. The widest craniotomy to expose the entire region needs to be partly infratentorial retrosigmoid, partly infratentorial presigmoid, and partly supratentorial in order to expose the respective dural surfaces. Therefore a combined bone flap straddling the transverse sinus with additional drilling of the "retrolabyrinthine" portion of the temporal bone is ideal. As many burr holes as necessary can be placed to make the craniotomy safe, and the use of diamond drill bits is extremely valuable to deal with particularly bloody portions of the bone resection.

After exposing the transverse sinus, the dura is coagulated above and below and then cut parallel to the sinus. Arterialized cortical veins emanating from the sinus should then be identified, coagulated, and divided or clipped as close as possible to the sinus in order to achieve disconnection of the fistula's cortical venous drainage. If necessary, the transverse sinus can be sacrificed proximally, and the tentorium cut anterior to the sinus to interrupt any tentorial supply to the fistula. The dural cuts above, below, and anterior to the transverse sinus can be carried distally beyond the transverse–sigmoid junction, and subsequently the sinus can be sacrificed or packed distally if not required for normal drainage, as determined by preoperative angiographic review. Bone wax is helpful for control of arterial feeders emanating from the petrous bone and should also be used to obliterate exposed mastoid air cells.

Depending on the extent of the arterialization, a fourth layer of dura may need to be divided – the presigmoid dura. When all the dural cuts have been completed, the remaining dural edges will have undoubtedly been coagulated as well, leading to a substantial dural defect. A duraplasty, ideally using autologous pericranium, is used to prevent a leak of cerebrospinal fluid. Intraoperative angiography and/or indocyanine green videography can be utilized to document complete skeletonization.

This general technique may need to be adapted to particular variations. Two such instances are important. A non-arterialized vein of Labbé complex requires complete preservation of its drainage pathway. The presence of a non-arterialized tentorial venous sinus also requires preservation through a tailoring of the tentorial durotomy.

Figures 13.1 and 13.2 demonstrate two different variations in the surgical treatment of transverse–sigmoid DAVFs.

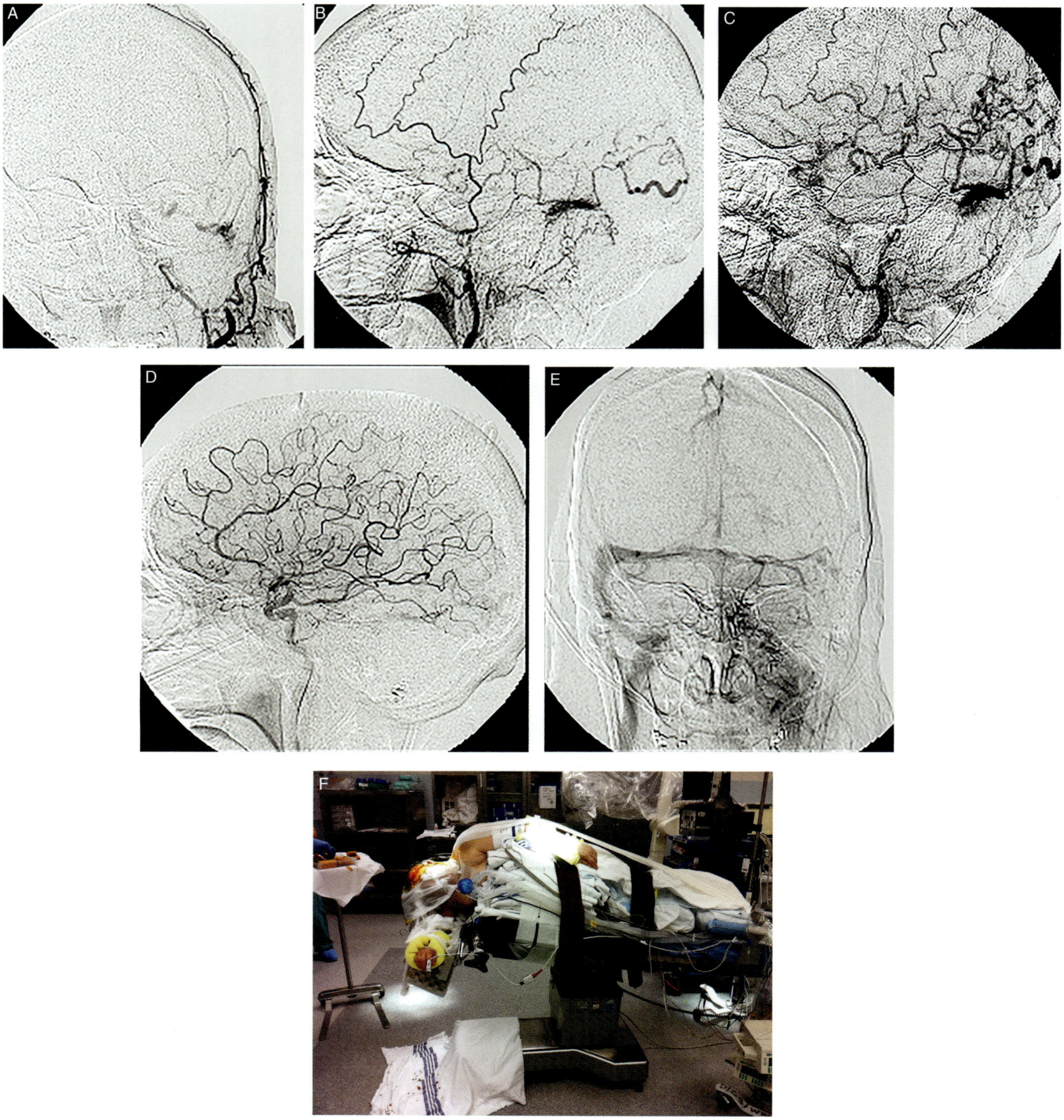

Fig. 13.2. A 60-year-old man had presented to an outside institution with dizziness, ataxia, and a bruit. The diagnosis of a left transverse–sigmoid dural arteriovenous fistula Borden type III was made. Partial transarterial embolization was carried out and the man was referred for further treatment. (A–C) A selective left external carotid artery (ECA) injection demonstrated an isolated segment of the left transverse–sigmoid junction, with arterialization via transosseous supply from the left occipital artery, and retrograde venous drainage through cortical veins of the temporo-occipital region, including the vein of Labbé. A cast of old Onyx can be seen in the left middle meningeal artery, best seen in (C). (D) Selective left internal carotid artery (ICA) injection showed a modest contribution from the tentorial branch from the cavernous ICA. (E) An anteroposterior view of the venous phase demonstrated the occluded left and patent right transverse sinuses. (F–J) For surgery, the plan was a combined left supratentorial and infratentorial exposure of the transverse–sigmoid junction for "triple" dural division and skeletonization/excision of the isolated transverse sinus, as well as clip ligation of the arterialized cortical veins. The patient was positioned in the three-quarter prone position, left side up (F). Following the craniotomy, the dura was opened above and below the left transverse sinus (G). A large arterialized occipital vein was well visualized (H). The vein was clipped, in addition to clipping the more lateral arterialized vein of Labbé (I). After ligating the medial part of the transverse sinus with a 2-0 silk tie, a tentorial incision was started in order to interrupt the ICA contribution to the fistula (J). (K) A tentorial venous (non-arterialized) sinus was encountered and, in an effort to preserve it, the plan changed to intraoperative embolization of the transverse–sigmoid sinus. A small opening was made at the transverse–sigmoid junction, and the delivery catheter of a tissue sealant (Evicel) was placed intraluminally and the tissue sealant delivered manually under pressure, immediately obliterating the arterial bleeding. The patient suffered no complications. (L) MRI on postoperative day 2 revealed no evidence of venous infarction. The evidence of chronic venous hypertension was still seen at this early stage. (M,N) Angiography of the left common carotid artery on postoperative day 5 revealed no residual fistula (M, lateral view; N, anteroposterior view). (O–Q) Repeat angiography at 4 months showed a cure (lateral views: O, selective left ECA; P, left vertebral artery; Q, selective left ICA).

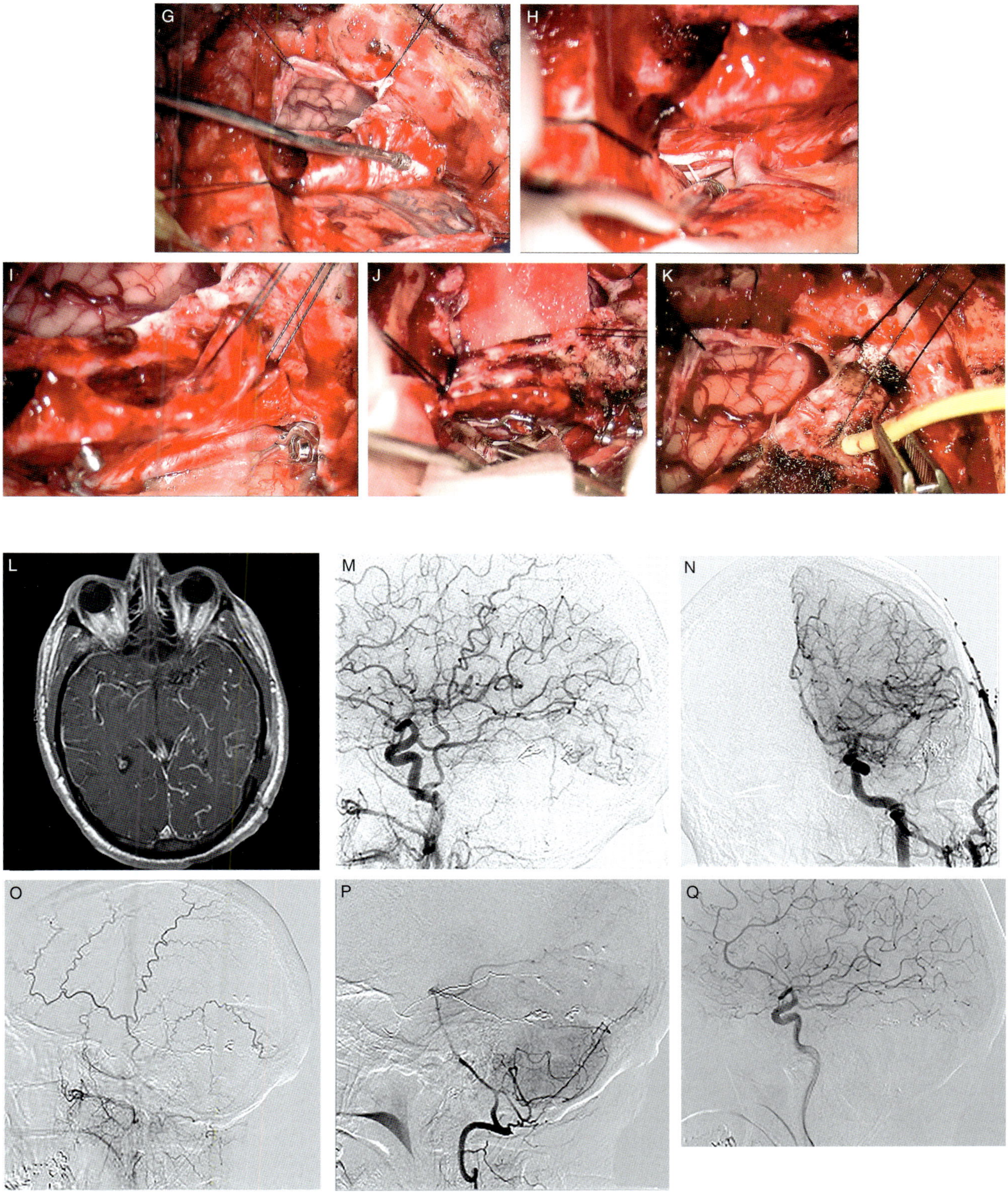

Fig. 13.2. (cont.)

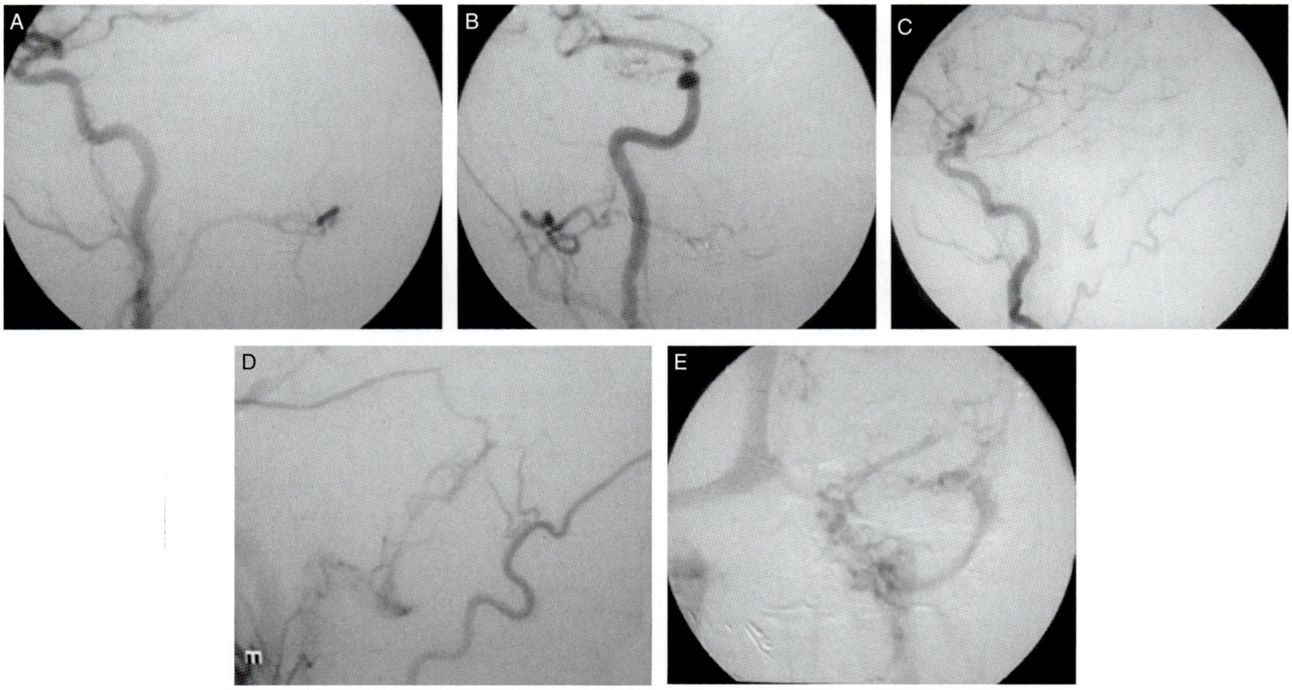

Fig. 13.3. A 55-year-old woman was treated for a dissecting right distal posterior inferior cerebellar artery (PICA) aneurysm. She had undergone a right occipital artery–PICA bypass and trapping of the aneurysm without sequelae. The surgery was performed through a right hockey-stick incision and the right suboccipital craniotomy had crossed the midline. She was doing well and was scheduled for her routine (and last) angiography at 4 years postoperatively. (A,B) The right common carotid artery (CCA) injection showed a patent occipital–PICA anastomosis (A, lateral view; B, anteroposterior view). There was no visualized aneurysm on vertebral artery injection (not shown). (C) However, the left CCA injection showed an unexpected subtle early opacification of the left sigmoid sinus. (D,E) Selective left external carotid artery injection confirmed a small dural arteriovenous fistula Borden type I of the left sigmoid sinus with contribution from transosseous–meningeal branches of the left occipital artery as well as from the left middle meningeal artery (D) with no retrograde venous flow and moderate venous prominence (E). In view of the benign nature of these lesions, its low Borden grade, and lack of symptoms, it was left untreated, with no sequelae over the last 10 years.

Figure 13.3 shows a patient with incidental benign postoperative development of a DAVF.

Anterior fossa/ethmoidal locations

Anterior fossa DAVFs are typically supplied by the ophthalmic artery via the anterior and/or posterior ethmoidal arteries. The anterior division of the middle meningeal artery and transcranial scalp feeders may also supply DAVFs in this region. Cortical venous drainage is a constant feature of anterior fossa DAVFs, which often occur through dilated varicose frontal and olfactory veins and account for the characteristic aggressive clinical behavior of these lesions. Endovascular treatment by a transarterial approach is limited by the fact that the ethmoidal branches of the ophthalmic artery are difficult to catheterize and dangerous to embolize because of the risk of central retinal artery occlusion and subsequent visual compromise. Furthermore, transvenous access to anterior fossa DAVFs is severely limited both by their anterior location and their propensity to drain directly into cortical veins. However, an open surgical approach via a unilateral or bilateral frontal craniotomy provides direct access to the lesion and allows for coagulation and division of its arterialized cortical venous drainage on either or both sides of the falx (with/without falx resection), resulting in high cure rates with minimal surgical morbidity. Figure 13.4 shows a typical example of an ethmoidal/anterior fossa DAVF.

Parasagittal locations

Parasagittal DAVFs are typically fed by bilateral middle meningeal, posterior meningeal, and/or transosseous occipital artery branches, and may drain into the superior sagittal sinus, cortical veins, or both. Global intracranial hypertension may result from sinus occlusion or from retrograde arterialization of a patent sinus from the high flow through the shunt. In the presence of discrete cortical venous drainage, a craniotomy over the site of the fistula allows for curative surgical disconnection of the venous outflow; however, preoperative transarterial embolization may be used to prevent significant blood loss from the scalp and dura during the exposure. Given the important role of the superior sagittal sinus in the venous drainage of normal brain, particular care must be taken to preserve it during sinus skeletonization, which becomes necessary when the lesion is diffuse. Curative endovascular treatment for parasagittal DAVFs has traditionally been difficult to achieve from either a transarterial or transvenous route because of difficulties of access; however, the use of the liquid embolic agent Onyx (Covidien ev3 Neurovascular, Irvine, CA, USA),

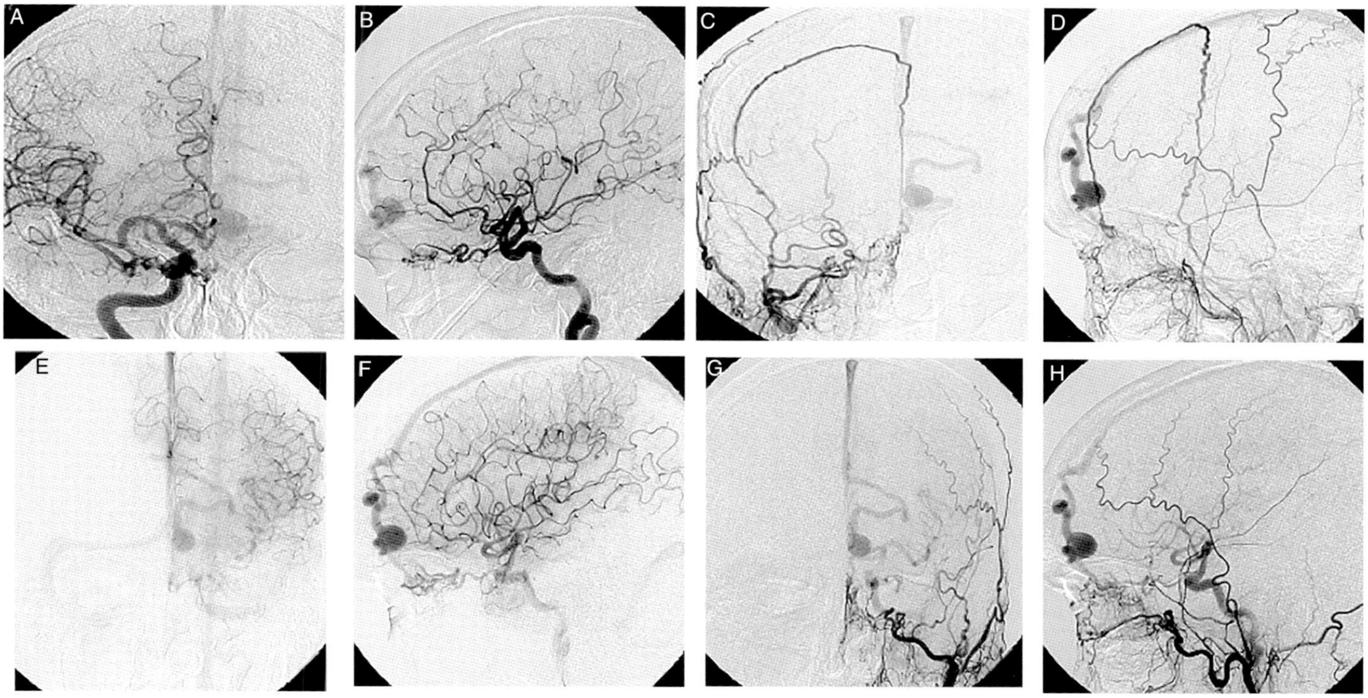

Fig. 13.4. A 43-year-old man presented with a mild subarachnoid hemorrhage. Angiography revealed a classic ethmoidal anterior fossa dural arteriovenous fistula with a large variceal draining vein. The fistula point and the single draining vein were just to the left of midline next to crista galli, but the arterial supply converged from multiple directions. (A–D) From the right side, supply was from ethmoidal arteries off the ophthalmic artery of the right internal carotid artery (A,B) and the falcine branch of the frontal branch of the middle meningeal artery (C,D). (E–H) From the left side, supply was from the ethmoidal arteries off the ophthalmic artery of the left internal carotid artery (E,F) and the internal maxillary artery (G,H). (I) A bifrontal craniotomy, avoiding the frontal sinus, was fashioned with a larger exposure on the left side. After unilateral dural opening, a worm-like, arterialized, red cortical venous complex was seen, reminiscent of the appearance of the "angioma racemosa venosa" of the spinal dural fistula type I. (J–L) With the identical strategy, all that was needed was a clip division of the single vein immediately downstream from the fistula point (J,K), and the arterialized veins turned blue immediately (L). (M,N) Postoperative angiography demonstrated the clip and the disappearance of the fistula.

which can be injected from the arterial side across the fistula to cast the venous outflow with better control than with older embolic agents, may represent a new frontier in the management of such lesions. Its limitations are the danger of inadvertently casting and occluding the superior sagittal sinus itself, or incompletely obliterating the lesion.

The surgical position is supine with various degrees of head flexion/elevation. A midline sagittal straight incision is ideal. It avoids skin flaps that may necrose, particularly if aggressive preoperative embolization was utilized, and it places the surgeon exactly where the exposure is needed – the midline. A bilateral parasagittal craniotomy is almost always needed to expose both sides and carefully select and divide the "red" bridging veins from the "blue" ones. An autologous pericranial duraplasty ends up often being necessary for closure. Figure 13.5 shows an extensive example.

Tentorial locations

Tentorial DAVFs are supplied by dural branches of the external carotid, internal carotid, and vertebral arteries and may involve the tentorial incisura, straight sinus, and posterior falx. Enlargement of the tentorial branch of the meningohypophyseal trunk (artery of Bernasconi and Cassinari) is often noted on angiography; less commonly, abnormal enlargement of the dural branch of the posterior cerebral artery (artery of Davidoff and Schecter) or the petrosquamosal branch of the middle meningeal artery may also be visualized. Venous drainage typically occurs through the deep venous system via the basal vein of Rosenthal, mesencephalic veins, and the vein of Galen. Cortical venous drainage is almost universally present in tentorial DAVFs and may occur above or below the tentorium, including into spinal perimedullary veins. Endovascular access is often difficult to achieve within the relatively small and tortuous dural branches that often supply tentorial DAVFs; furthermore, transarterial embolization into or transvenous embolization through the deep venous system is technically challenging and dangerous. Given the tendency of these lesions to be the most aggressive, open surgery is ideal. Disconnecting the cortical venous drainage and coagulating tentorial arterial feeders is effective and often can be achieved with low risk.

This is the location par excellence, among all DAVFs, where a thoughtful strategy is needed because multiple corridors are potentially available. The choice of the approach is guided by two principles:

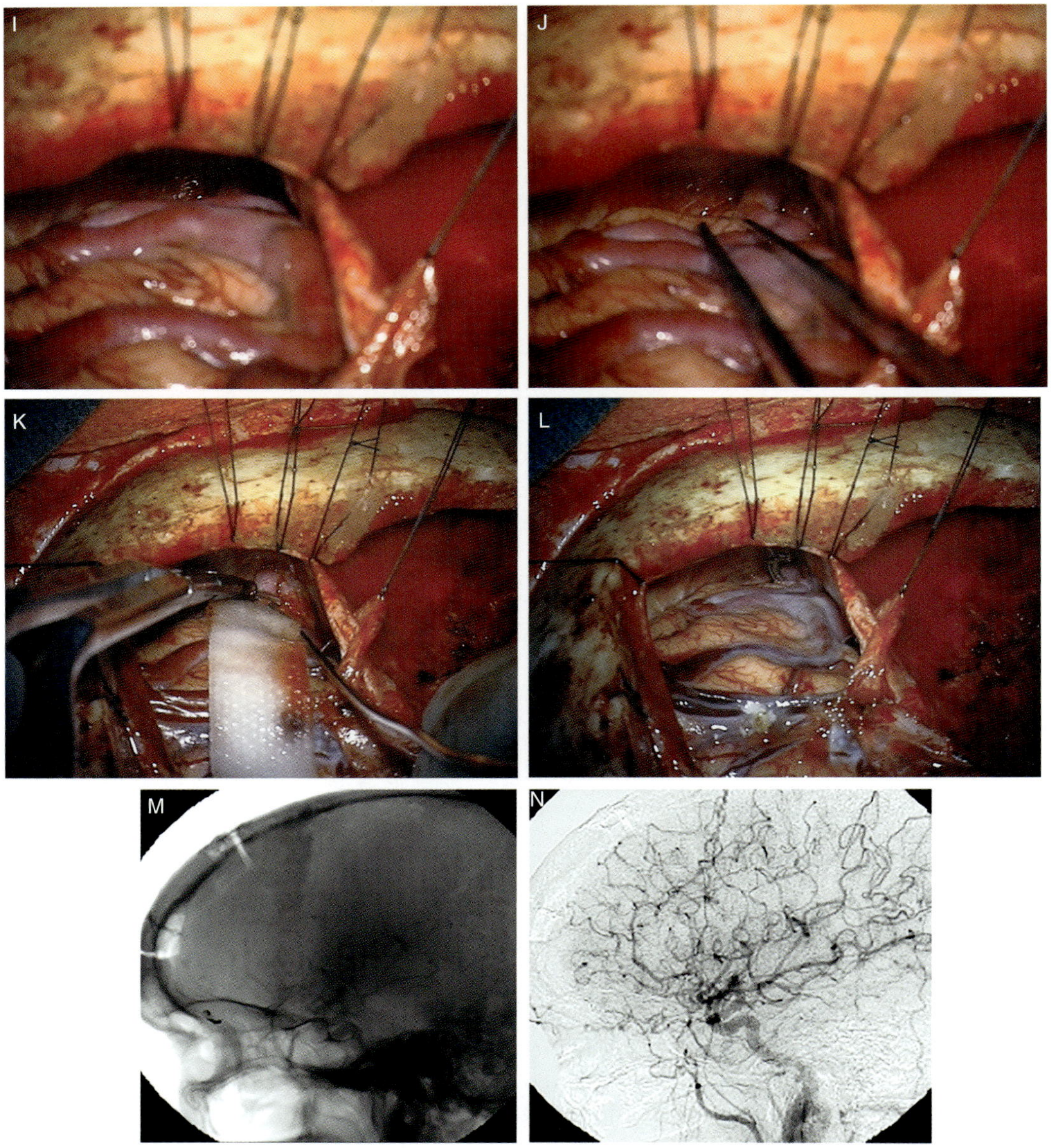

Fig. 13.4. (cont.)

Location of the exact fistulous point, and therefore that of the nascent arterialized vein. To the inexperienced, this may not be straightforward, since it is easy to become lost in the multiple worm-like formations of vessels from multiple injections that are not easily classifiable at first glance as arteries or veins. Through careful analysis of independent arterial injections (via the vertebral and internal and external carotid artery routes) and, most importantly, after superposition of these different angiographic runs (digitally or mentally), the surgeon needs to discover the "final common venous pathway:" the vascular angiographic configuration that is identical in all runs carried out at the same angulation. It is where treatment should be directed for cure.

Relative location of nearby non-arterialized veins. Once the fistulous point is defined, there will undoubtedly exist more than one surgical approach to it. The best approach should merge simplicity with avoidance of normal veins that may act as obstacles.

The commonly used approaches are supracerebellar–infratentorial, paraoccipital–posterior interhemispheric, subtemporal, retrosigmoid, and infraoccipital–supratentorial. The first two approaches are the most versatile.

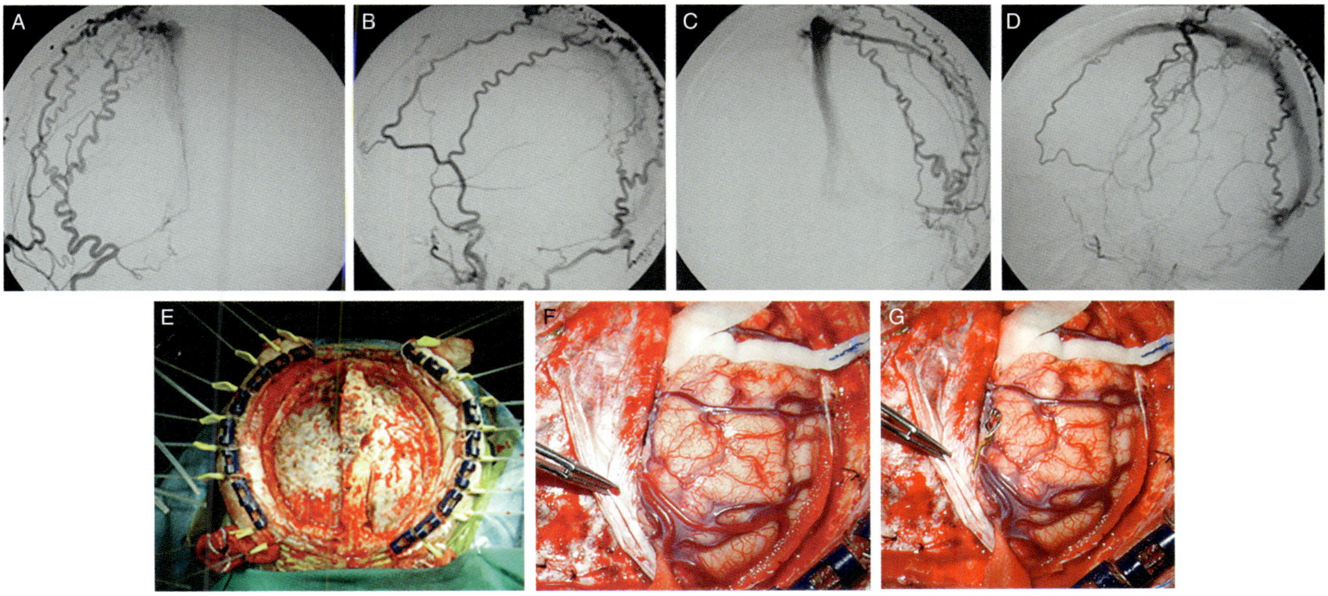

Fig. 13.5. A 38-year-old woman was referred with an extensive superior sagittal sinus dural arteriovenous fistula. (A–D) Selective bilateral external carotid artery injections revealed extensive enlargement of superficial temporal arterial supply right (A,B) and left (C,D), with some contribution from both middle meningeal arteries. Retrograde cortical venous drainage via bridging veins was particularly appreciated in (C) and (D). An extensive extracranial subgaleal venous channel network, communicating via emissary veins with the superior sagittal sinus, was particularly impressive (B,D). (E–G) A partial transarterial preoperative embolization was carried out to limit blood loss during the craniotomy. Through a midline sagittal incision, a bilateral, primarily biparietal, craniotomy was made, sparing a midline bony bridge to avoid injury to and/or excessive dural bleeding from the superior sagittal sinus (E). The dura was opened on both sides and all arterialized bridging veins were clip ligated, turning immediately from red to blue (F,G).

The supracerebellar–infratentorial approach is a workhorse to many infratentorial but also supratentorial lesions. Its advantages are simplicity, applicability to bilateral lesions, and relative absence of critical structures along the way. Its drawbacks are the limited visualization and control of the falx and supra-Galenic structures. A very steep (semivertical) tentorial orientation renders this approach less favorable. We favor placing the patient in the prone Concorde position rather than the semi-sitting position in order to avoid anesthetic drawbacks and have not regretted this strategy. However, proper brain relaxation and cerebrospinal fluid diversion are critical. No self-retaining retraction is needed, just gravity, to mobilize the cerebellum. The incision can be midline or paramedian, based on the particular patient. The bone flap crosses above the transverse sinus to allow upward mobilization/retraction of that sinus to improve visualization. The fistulous point is identified and divided. If necessary, a tentorial window can be created to extend the view superiorly and/or coagulate arterial dural feeders.

The paraoccipital–posterior interhemispheric approach would be preferred in the presence of a very steep tentorium and when the fistulous point involves the falx more than the tentorium. It is also best suited for midline/near midline lesions, since the occipital cortex is likely to suffer from excessive lateral mobilization. We prefer to place the patient in the "lateral decubitus, ipsilateral side down" position, with the back and head elevated 30 degrees. A lumbar drain is often very useful since there is no reliable cerebrospinal fluid cistern during the approach. We favor the hockey-stick incision, one limb of which is midline. It is not generally necessary to expose the transverse sinus unless the fistula is just anterior to it. It is also important to expose the superior sagittal sinus to mobilize it contralaterally. The dura is opened in an obliquely set T-configuration, creating two dural triangles, one based on the superior sagittal sinus and one on the transverse sinus. Gravity and cerebrospinal fluid drainage will allow the occipital lobe to "fall down" and, again, no self-retaining retraction is necessary. As required, various extents of the falx and tentorium can be excised and the fistula divided, with special attention to preservation of the Galenic system.

The other listed approaches are commonly known and will not be described individually. Figure 13.6 and 13.7 illustrate and contrast the decision-making process and the surgical techniques utilized in two different types of tentorial DAVFs.

Torcular locations

Torcular DAVFs are particularly challenging lesions to treat because of the proximity and convergence of multiple important venous sinuses at this site. These fistulae may present in adults as an acquired lesion with signs and symptoms of intracranial venous hypertension, but they more typically present as a complex congenital malformations in young children, with high-output cardiac failure, dilated scalp veins, macrocephaly, seizures, and in older

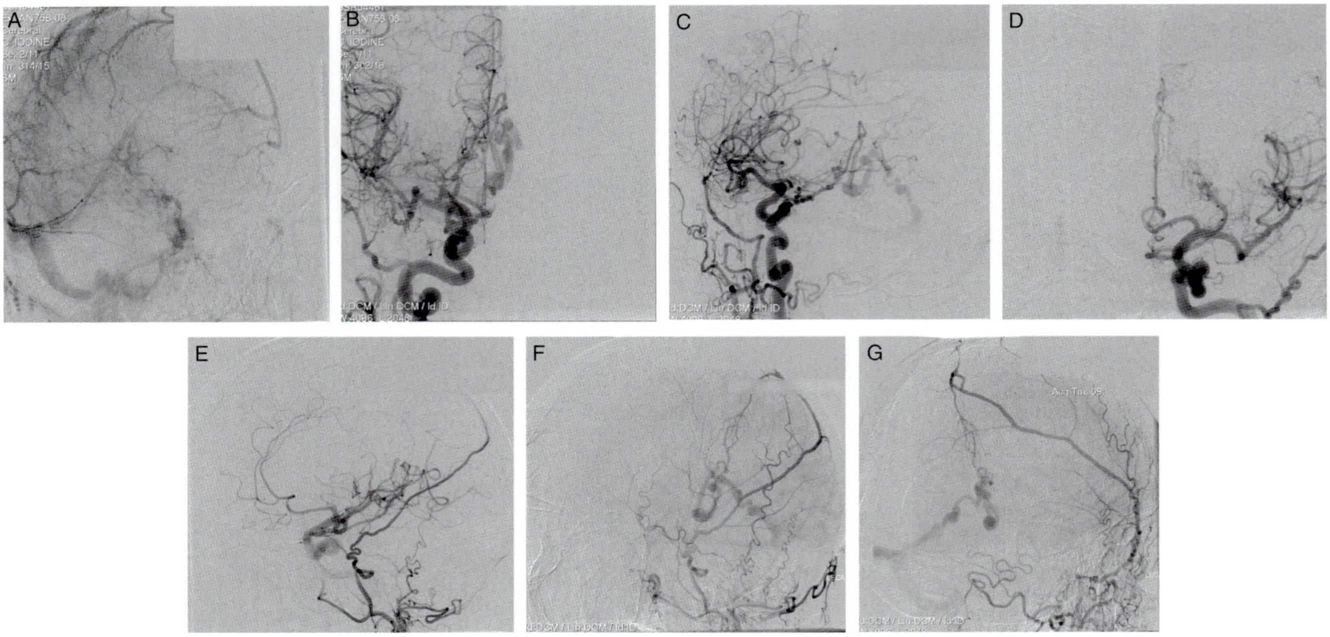

Fig. 13.6. A 64-year-old woman presented to an outside facility with a subacute history of headaches, dizziness, and imbalance as well as a relatively acute deterioration of mental status. Obstructive hydrocephalus at the level of the aqueduct was diagnosed (CT and MRI scans not available). The etiology was confirmed to be a falco-tentorial dural fistula with varicose venous dilatation directly compressing the aqueduct. An urgent endoscopic third ventriculostomy was carried out, dramatically relieving her symptoms, and the patient was referred to our institution for further treatment of the dural arteriovenous fistula (DAVF). The DAVF is best described as a falco-tentorial lesion with a single arterialized precentral cerebellar vein coursing in the subarachnoid space, parallel and caudal to the straight sinus and eventually draining into the peritorcular area. (A) The straight sinus and the inferior sagittal sinus were clearly patent and non-arterialized. (B–G) The feeders were from three main sources: artery of Bernasconi and Cassinari off the right internal carotid artery (ICA) (B,C) and to a lesser extent off the left ICA (D,E), and a large posterior falcine branch off a hypertrophic left parietal middle meningeal branch, with a "rete mirabile-like" neovascular configuration in the falx (F,G). As in most DAVFs, note that all arterial inputs converged to a single point from which the same venous outline emerged with every injection. The right and left vertebral artery injections did not contribute to the fistula (not shown). Two surgical approaches were entertained: infratentorial supracerebellar and posterior parieto-occipital interhemispheric transtentorial. Both approaches have advantages and disadvantages. The former is simple and does not involve manipulation of a potentially hyperemic tentorium/falx, but it has the limitation in this case of encountering the arterialized vein very posteriorly first rather than near its emergence from the fistula point. The latter is slightly more complex in its involvement of parieto-occipital mobilization, necessitates at least partial tentorial section, but has the advantage of providing a more comprehensive exposure of the fistulous area, both infra- and supratentorially, division of some of the arterial input, and allowing the obliteration of potential small venous channels not clearly involved at present but which may provide alternative arterialization in the future. We chose the latter approach. (H–M) The patient was positioned three-quarter prone, with the head and trunk elevated and the right side down to allow the right hemisphere to "fall away" from the falx (H). Following a right parieto-occipital craniotomy that crossed the midline to allow falx and superior sagittal sinus mobilization, an interhemispheric dissection posterior to the last parietal bridging vein was carried out. No self-retaining retraction was needed. A partial section of the right tentorial leaf was done, exposing the quadrigeminal cistern and the peri-Galenic venous complex (I). Following dissection of a thickened arachnoid, the arterialized precentral cerebellar vein was seen, immediately posterior to a "blue" uninvolved vein of Galen (J). A segment of arterialized vein was skeletonized and mobilized (K). An aneurysm clip was placed across it (L). Further dissection was made closer to the fistula point, and an incision through the falx was made just above and parallel to the inferior sagittal sinus to explore briefly the left side, not to miss small, arterialized venous branches. One such branch was encountered off the precentral cerebellar vein, and so a second clip was placed at a higher point across both (M). (N–R) Angiography at postoperative day 1 revealed complete obliteration of the DAVF (N, right ICA; O, left vertebral artery; P, left common carotid artery; Q, left external carotid artery; R, venous phase).

children, with hydrocephalus and developmental delay [50,51]. Torcular DAVFs often receive supply from bilateral middle meningeal arteries and may also be fed by the occipital, posterior meningeal, posterior inferior cerebellar, and anterior inferior cerebellar arteries. The transverse–sigmoid sinuses and jugular veins may become enlarged, stenosed, or occluded depending on the unique hemodynamics of the lesion and the stage at which it is diagnosed. Retrograde arterialization of the superior sagittal sinus, beginning at the torcula, accounts for the tendency of these lesions to present with signs and symptoms of intracranial venous hypertension. For treatment planning, in addition to noting the lesion's arterial supply and the venous drainage pattern of normal brain as well as the fistula, it is important to specifically recognize whether there is complete communication at the torcula between the superior sagittal sinus and the bilateral transverse sinuses or whether one of these components is "isolated" from the sinus confluence.

Torcular DAVFs are typically treated by embolization, either in a single session or in a staged fashion; however, if complete fistula obliteration is attempted, there is a high risk of inadvertent sinus occlusion, regardless of whether a transarterial or a transvenous endovascular approach is utilized. To this end, some have attempted to use balloons to protect the sinus during embolization or covered stents within the sinus to further reduce arteriovenous shunting after partial embolization [52]. Surgery is most often used adjunctively to achieve direct

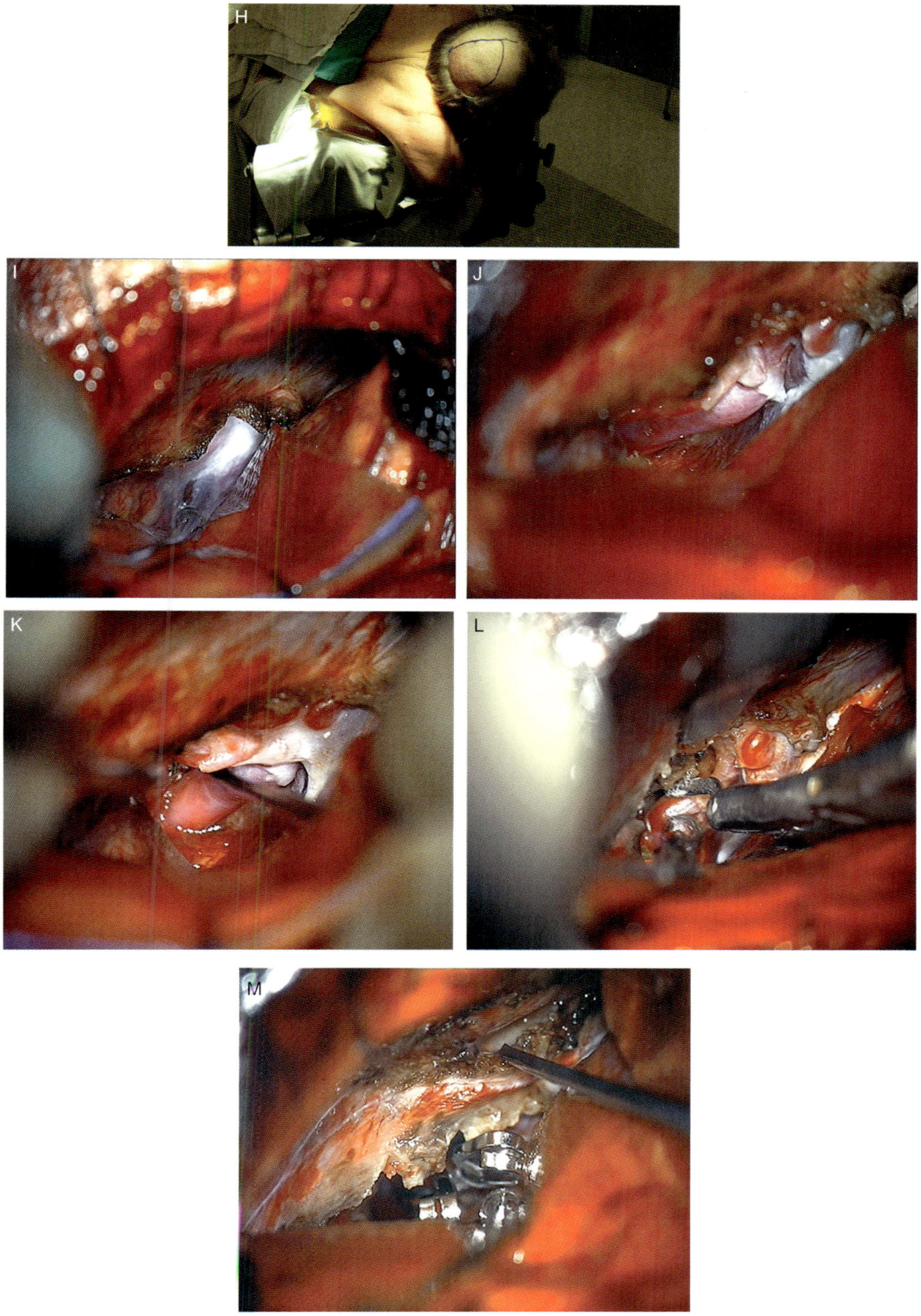

Fig. 13.6. (cont.)

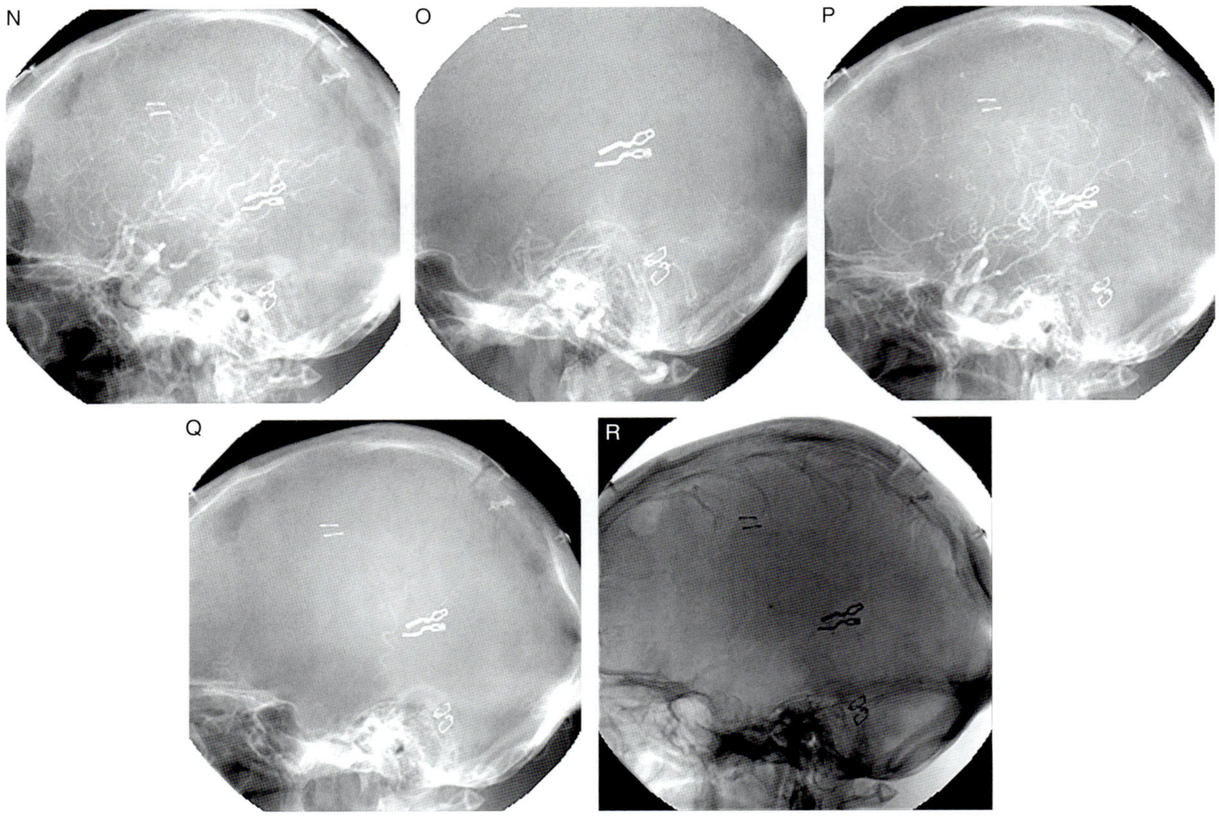

Fig. 13.6. (cont.)

operative exposure for embolization in the setting of difficult transfemoral/transjugular endovascular access, as occurs when the sinuses and jugular veins progress to become occluded [53,54]. In select patients, surgical packing of an isolated diseased sinus segment may be performed [55]; other surgical options include sinus skeletonization or even resection [56], which can be performed by making dural cuts and coagulating arterial feeders parallel to the transverse, superior sagittal, straight, and occipital sinuses up to their convergence at the torcula. These techniques are generally reserved for patients for whom endovascular approaches are not feasible or have failed.

Petrous locations

Petrous DAVFs are located along the petrous ridge and are typically supplied by the same arterial distribution that is seen to supply tentorial DAVFs; in addition, vertebral artery muscular branches, ascending pharyngeal artery neuromeningeal branches, and the dorsal meningeal branch of the meningohypophyseal trunk may contribute significantly to petrous DAVFs. Unlike true tentorial DAVFs, however, petrous DAVF venous drainage tends to occur through either the superior or the inferior petrosal sinuses rather than through the Galenic system. Because of the normal petrosal sinus connections to the posterior cavernous sinuses, both superior petrosal sinus DAVFs and inferior petrosal sinus DAVFs tend to arterialize the cavernous sinus, which often results in orbital venous congestive signs/symptoms. Pulsatile tinnitus may result from increased flow through the jugular bulb. Furthermore, the relatively small caliber of the petrosal sinuses makes them prone to thrombosis in the setting of a DAVF, which promotes cortical venous drainage and increases the likelihood of aggressive clinical behavior.

Multiple surgical corridors may be utilized to access petrous DAVFs for disconnection of cortical venous drainage, including retrosigmoid, subtemporal, anterior petrosal, posterior petrosal, and far lateral approaches. However, the ubiquitous and simple retrosigmoid approach remains the best approach for this location. All that is required in most instances is an exposure of the arterialized superior (or less commonly, inferior) petrosal vein and placement of an aneurysm clip on it. Figure 13.8 shows a classical example of the findings and surgical treatment of a petrous DAVF.

Carotid–cavernous locations

Endovascular techniques have evolved and emerged as the primary treatment method for CCFs. This is in part because there are many venous avenues to the cavernous sinus, and in part because operating on a highly arterialized

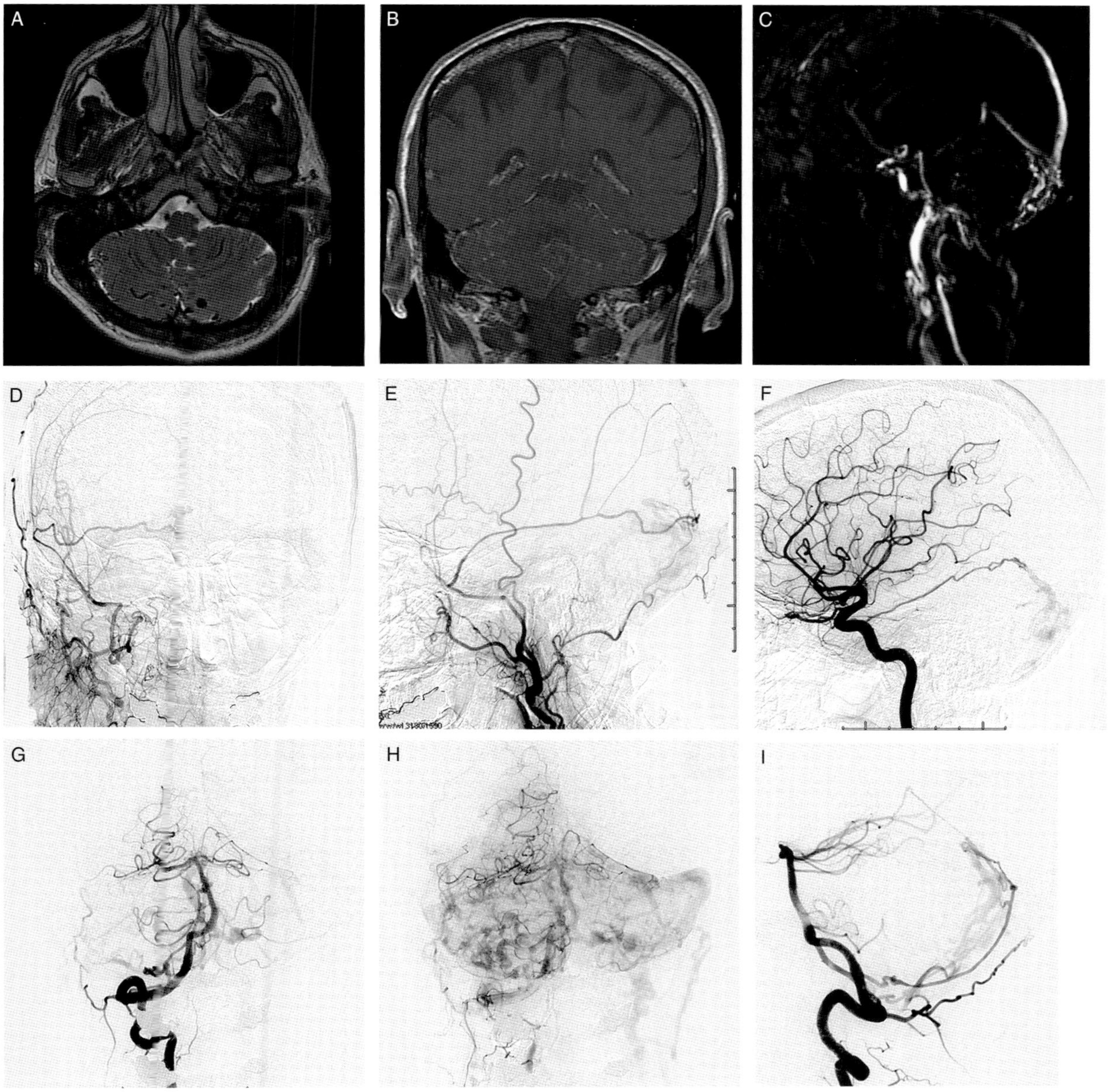

Fig. 13.7. A 69-year-old man presented with a 1-week history of acute left cranial nerve VI palsy and no other neurological symptoms or signs. He was diagnosed with a dural arteriovenous fistula (DAVF) at another institution through MRI/MR angiography and subsequent angiography. They attempted a curative embolization of his fistula but the treatment was partial. He was then referred for further care. (A–C) The MRI/MR angiography revealed large venous flow voids in the posterior fossa. (D–M) Angiography showed that there were two distinct fistulous points. The main one was midline, about 1.5 cm anterior to the torcula, in the tentorium. Blood supply originated from the right middle meningeal artery (D,E), the tentorial branch of the right internal carotid artery (ICA) (F), the posterior meningeal branches of the right vertebral artery (VA) (G–I), the left VA (J,K), and the left middle meningeal artery (L,M). (N) Additionally, the left middle meningeal artery supplied a separate small DAVF of the superior border of the left transverse sinus that drained slowly and retrogradely into the left vein of Labbé. (O,P) A three-dimensional angiographic reconstruction of the right VA injection clearly demonstrated the main fistula, as well as its single superior vermian-draining vein that led to pancerebellar venous engorgement. (Q–S) A selective right posterior meningeal injection during embolization (Q) showed significant decrease in flow (R,S). (T) Interestingly, the left transverse sinus fistula became more prominent/visible after the partial embolization of the tentorial fistula. (U–Z) The patient underwent a midline suboccipital craniotomy that straddled the torcula. The arterialized superior vermian vein and branches were clearly seen (U), with change to normal blue color after simple clip placement (V). Additionally, the supratentorial dura was opened and a small, currently non-arterialized, occipital vein was test-clipped (W) and then divided to reduce the risk of recurrence. (X) Postoperative angiography at day 3 revealed cure of the tentorial DAVF. At the same time, the second fistula was occluded with *N*-butyl cyanoacrylate embolization via the left middle meningeal artery, the cast reaching the vein of Labbé (Y,Z). (AA–FF) At follow-up at 5 months, both fistulae remain cured.

cavernous sinus, while feasible, is a high-risk, high-complexity endeavor. The endovascular bag of tricks includes catheter access via the inferior or superior petrosal sinuses (including "blind burrowing" through them even if non-opacified), the angular vein into superior or inferior ophthalmic veins, and the intercavernous sinus via the contralateral cavernous sinus. Even if catheter access is not possible by any route, direct transorbital percutaneous

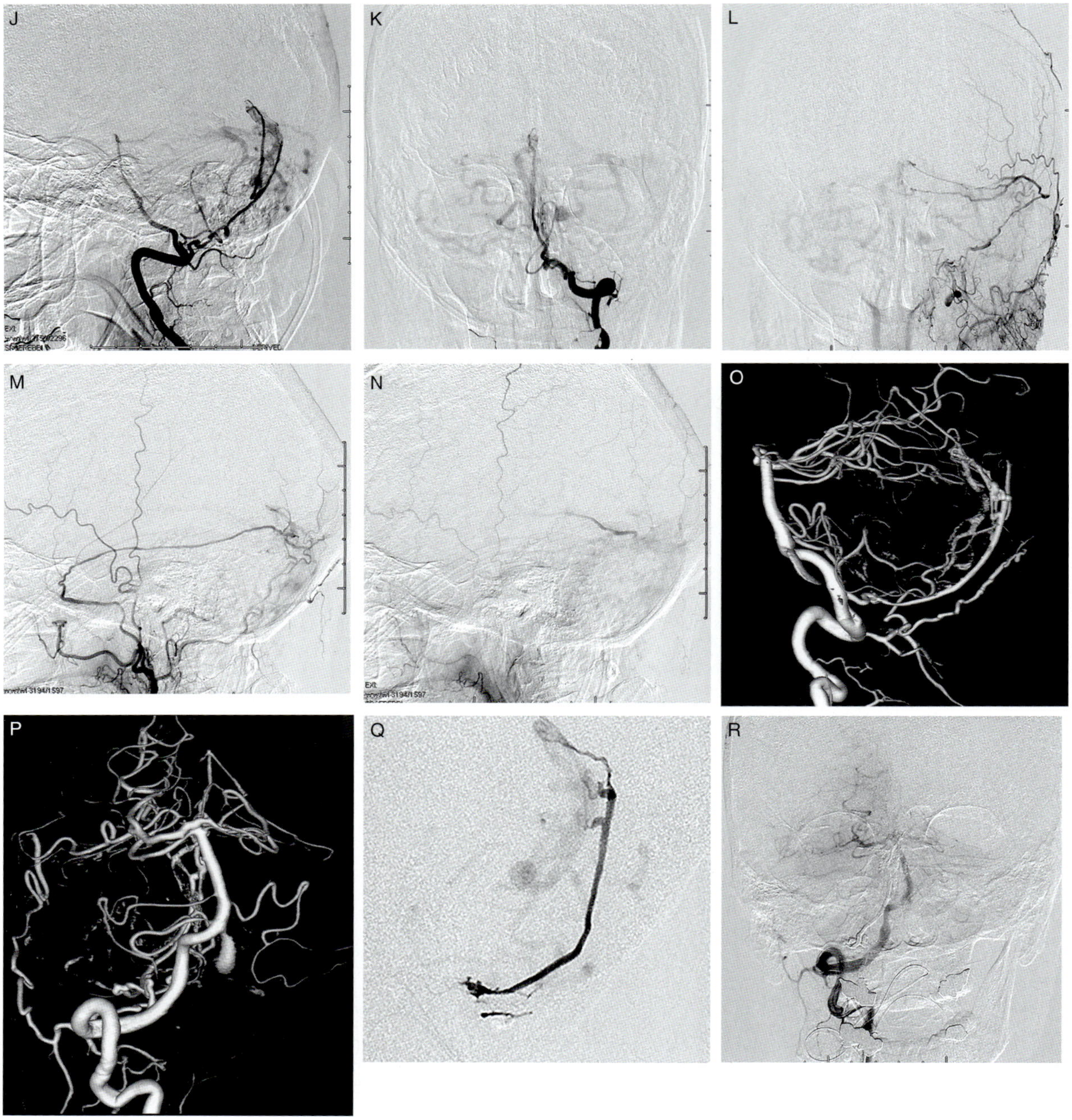

Fig. 13.7. (cont.)

fluoroscopic or three-dimensional CT-guided puncture of the anterior cavernous sinus is possible [57,58]. An alternative technique is an open surgical access to an arterialized superior ophthalmic vein via the eyelid, which we have preferred performing under microscopic magnification and have achieved excellent results [59].

In spite of these advancements, there remains a small group of patients where a craniotomy is still necessary. These patients fall in one of two groups:

- failed endovascular management: catheter access proved impossible, superior ophthalmic vein is not enlarged enough, multiple previous endovascular treatments have resulted in recurrences
- fistula located within leaflets of the lateral wall of the cavernous sinus.

The latter group is to be distinguished from the true "intracavernous" fistula, because its drainage pattern often involves the sphenoparietal sinus and then retrogradely the sylvian veins. If the superior petrosal sinus is excluded from the drainage pattern, endovascular access may become impossible, and a craniotomy to disconnect cortical venous drainage coming off the lateral cavernous sinus wall becomes the most effective means of cure.

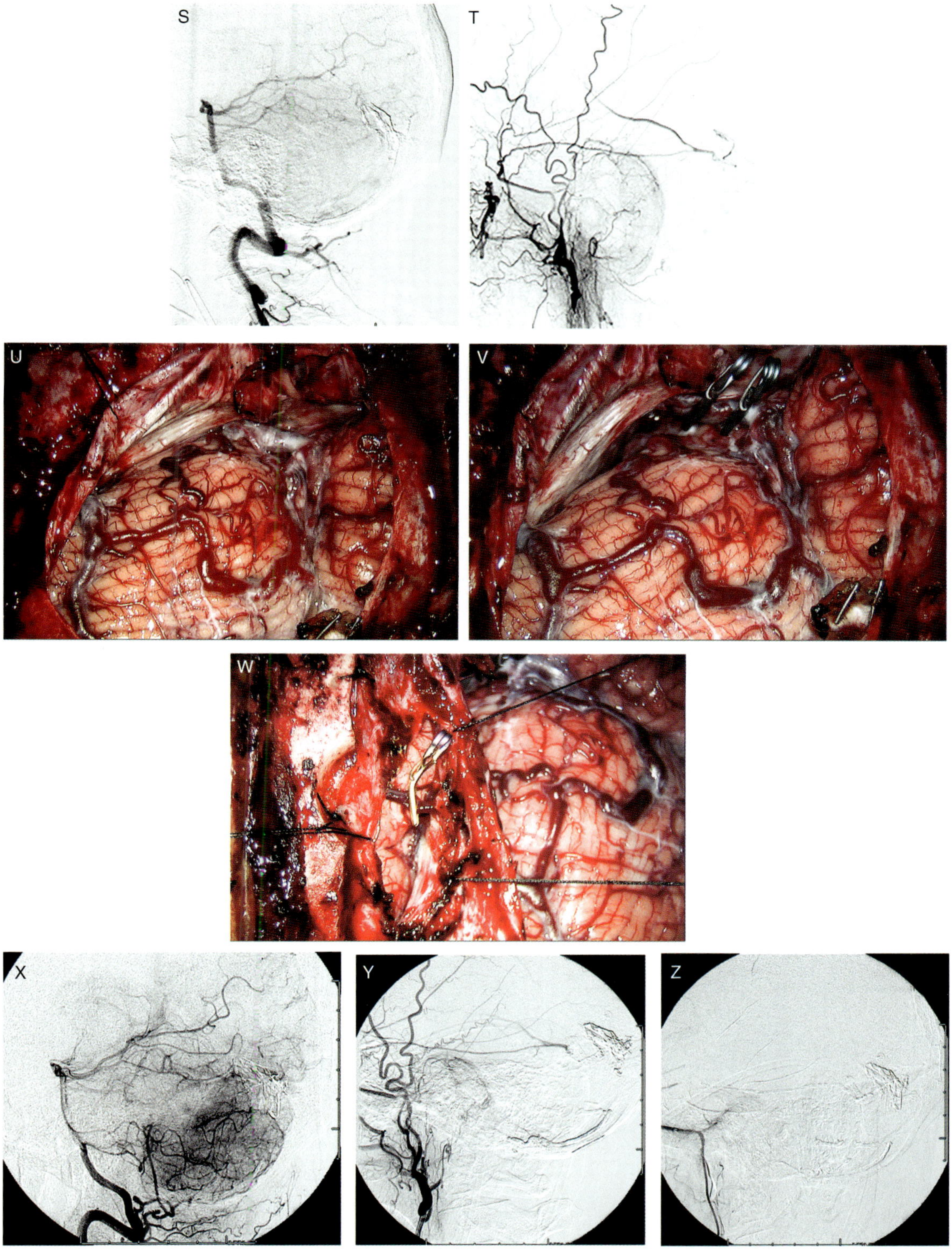

Fig. 13.7. (cont.)

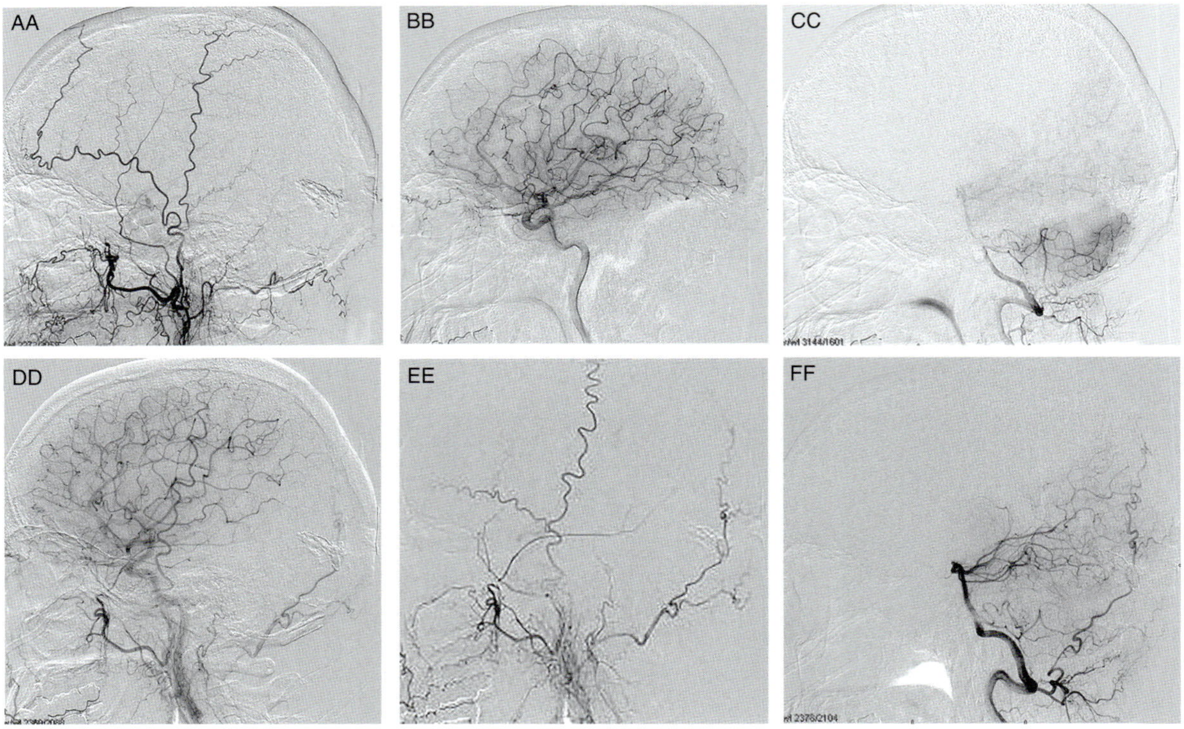

Fig. 13.7. (cont.)

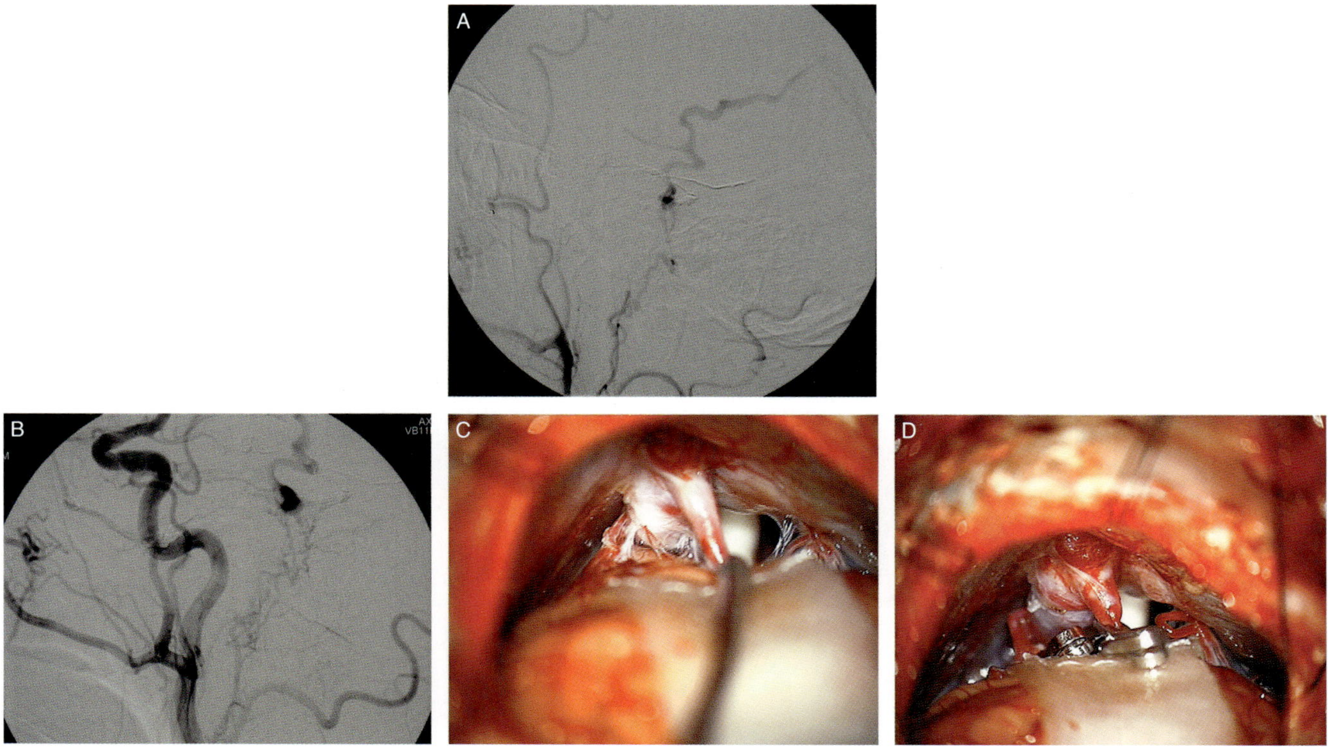

Fig. 13.8. A 50-year-old man presented with an acute headache and a mild subarachnoid hemorrhage on CT (not shown). (A,B) Selective right external carotid artery angiography demonstrated a right petrosal dural arteriovenous fistula supplied by ascending pharyngeal arterial branches and draining into the superior petrosal vein. (C,D) Through a simple right retrosigmoid approach, the petrous–tentorial junction was approached and the two arterialized branches of the superior petrosal vein were clipped. Postoperative angiography (not shown) showed a cure.

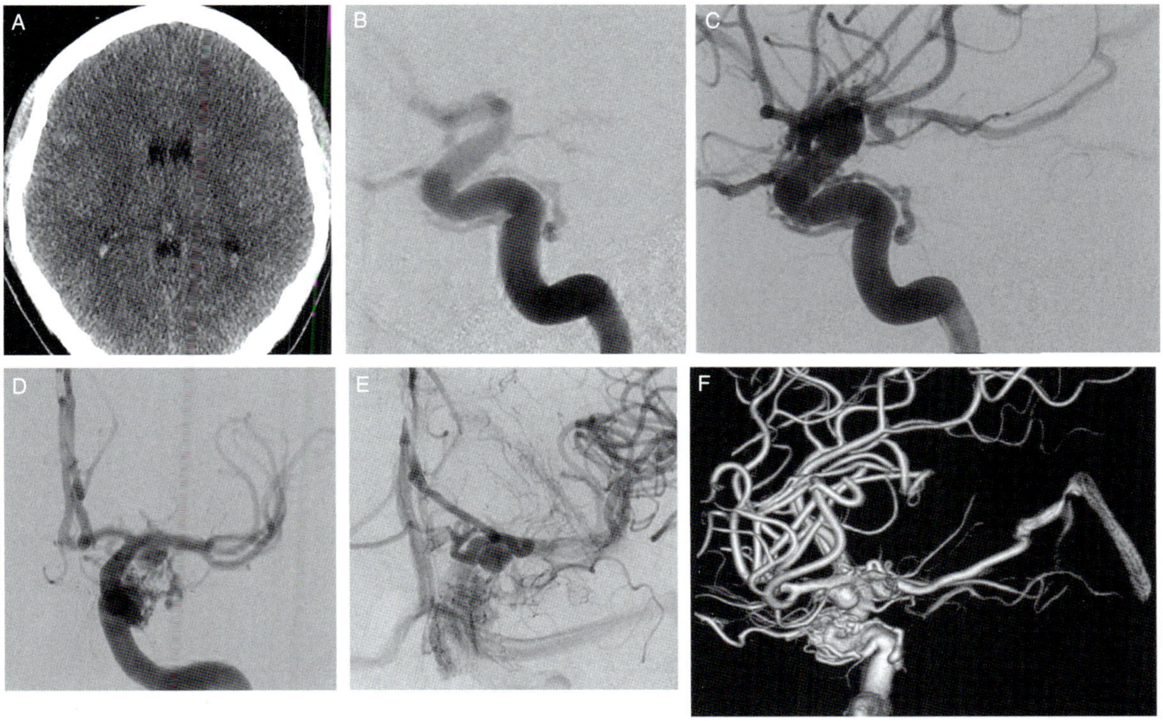

Fig. 13.9. A 44-year-old woman presented to an outside institution with a subarachnoid hemorrhage. (A) CT on day 1 showed diffuse sulcal blood on both sides. (B–E) Selective left internal carotid artery (ICA) angiography demonstrated a classical dural arteriovenous fistula confined to the lateral wall of the cavernous sinus (not holocavernous), fed by direct cavernous ICA branches and draining through the left vein of Rosenthal into the Galenic system. A subarachnoid venous varix could clearly be seen (B,C, lateral views; D,E, anteroposterior views). (F) The three-dimensional reconstruction depicts all the significant findings. The patient refused treatment and was lost to follow-up.

The standard contemporary surgical approach to the cavernous sinus, as pioneered by Dolenc [60], consists of a combined extradural/intradural frontotemporal exposure with anterior clinoidectomy, unroofing of the optic nerve, superior orbital fissure, foramen ovale, and foramen rotundum. This complete access is, of course, most appropriate for tumor surgery and rarely necessary to treat a DAVF of the cavernous sinus. Bony exposure therefore needs to be tailored with emphasis on simplicity. The surgical goal is usually one of two:

- craniotomy to provide access to an isolated arterialized "lake" that drains retrogradely into cortical veins, by open puncture and embolization intraoperatively (usually with Onyx, and biplane fluoroscopy), or immediately postoperatively in the angiographic suite using a fixated catheter access tunneled through the craniotomy [61]
- craniotomy to achieve cure intraoperatively by disconnecting arterialized cortical veins; this needs to be as thorough as possible to avoid incomplete treatment and future recurrences through alternative recruited venous pathways: the cavernous sinus is a notorious region for this biological behavior and in the absence of a discrete, easily localizable fistulous point, the cavernous sinus may need to be accessed and packed via multiple windows [62].

Figures 13.9 and 13.10 demonstrate two lateral wall cavernous sinus DAVFs almost exclusively treatable surgically. Figure 13.11 shows a classic CCF where drainage is anterior into a large superior ophthalmic vein requiring open cannulation for access.

Sphenoparietal locations

Sphenoparietal sinus DAVFs may be regarded by some as a subtype of cavernous sinus DAVFs, but, as alluded to earlier, there is value in considering them distinct. They are typically fed by the middle meningeal artery, and may occur after head trauma [63]. Venous drainage may occur medially into the cavernous sinus resulting in orbital venous congestion, in which case they can be treated endovascularly as outlined for the CCFs. However, lateral drainage results in cortical venous drainage, typically into the superficial middle cerebral/sylvian veins. In those patients with cortical venous reflux requiring intervention, a frontotemporal craniotomy allows for extradural interruption of the meningeal supply (perhaps not crucial, but helpful), followed by intradural ligation of the enlarged draining sylvian vein at its connection to the sphenoparietal sinus along the sphenoid ridge. Figures 13.12 and 13.13 illustrate a spectrum of complexity in the treatment of two such patients.

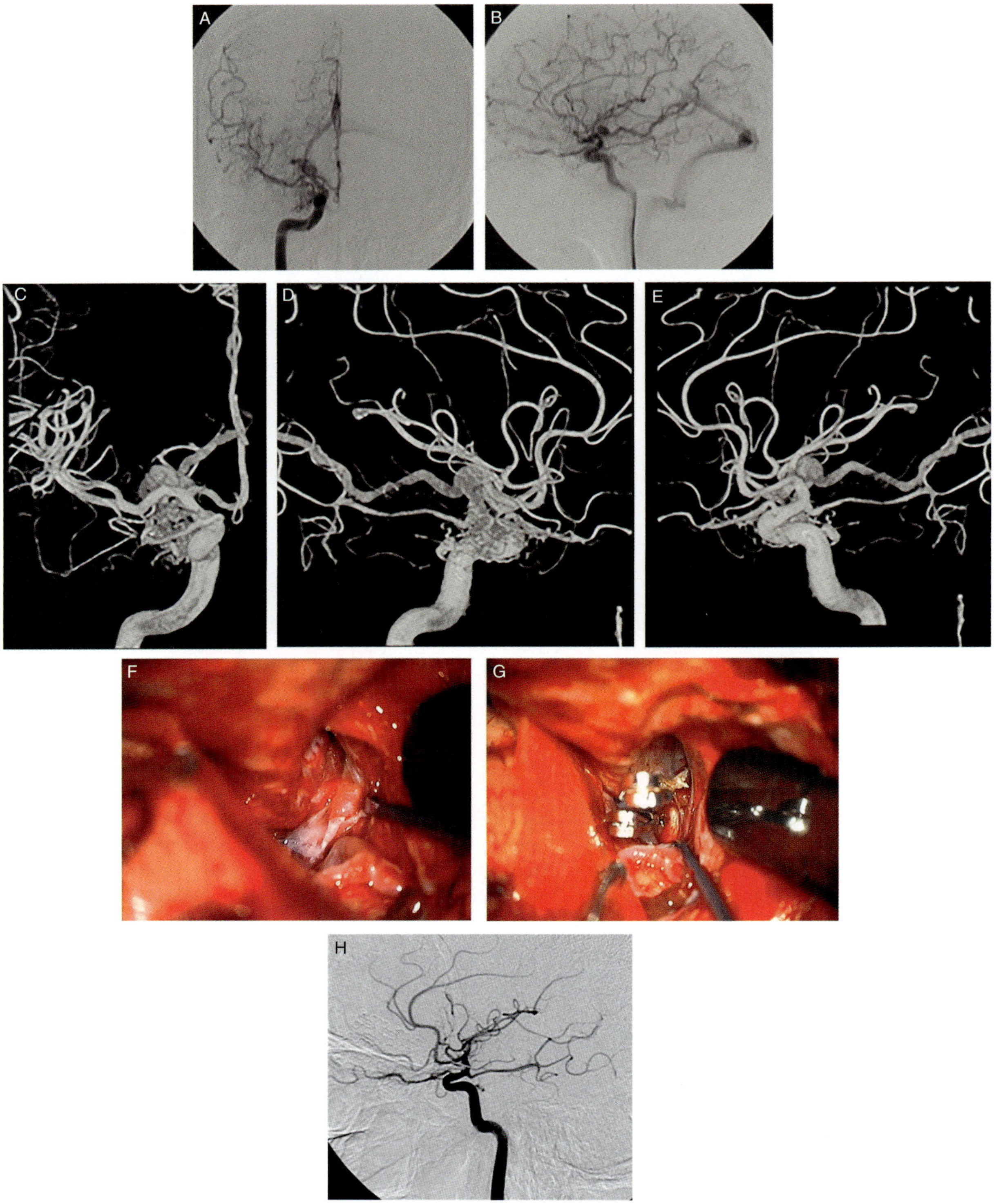

Fig. 13.10. A 48-year-old man presented having had intermittent diplopia for several months. After a brain MRI (not shown) and angiography, a diagnosis of a right lateral cavernous sinus wall dural arteriovenous fistula was made. This situation was nearly identical to the patient in Fig. 13.9, with the same arterial and venous flows. (A, B) Angiography with selective right internal carotid artery injection. (C–E) Three-dimensional reconstruction. (F,G) Through a right trans-sylvian approach, the obvious arterialized single vein emerging from the lateral wall of the cavernous sinus and draining into the vein of Rosenthal was visualized, clipped, and then could be seen to collapse. There clearly was no need to enter the cavernous sinus proper in this type of fistula. (H) Postoperative lateral carotid angiography demonstrated occlusion of the fistula.

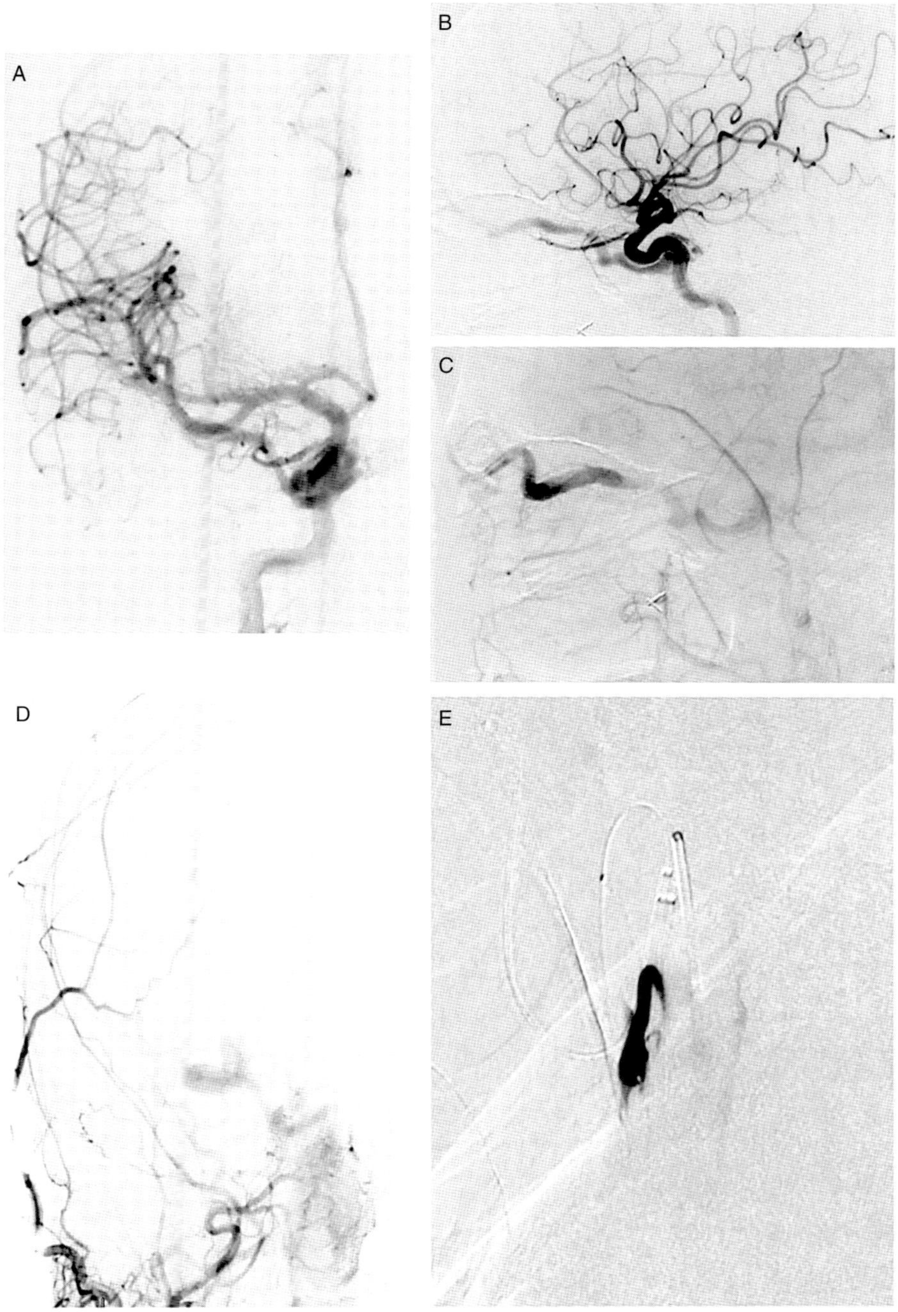

Fig. 13.11. A 62-year-old woman presented with unilateral right-sided pulsatile exophthalmos, rapid decline in visual acuity, and injected sclera. A right carotid–cavernous fistula (CCF) exclusively draining into the superior ophthalmic vein (SOV) was diagnosed. (A–C) Selective right internal carotid artery injection demonstrating the enlarged right SOV draining forward toward the angular vein. (D) Selective right external carotid artery injection demonstrated contribution from internal maxillary artery. (E) Multiple endovascular transfemoral attempts at accessing the cavernous sinus failed, including "blind" catheterization of the superior and inferior petrosal sinus, as well as through the angular vein. (F) The patient was taken to the operating room to access the right SOV directly through a superior eyelid skin crease approach under microscope magnification. The large, worm-like SOV was quickly identified above the tarsal plate, medially and within the superficial part of the orbital fat. (G) The direction of arterialized blood flow was confirmed through the "milking" test, the arrow indicating the direction of the catheter insertion (counterflow, from anterior to posterior). (H) The 10-cm (4-inch) puncture set used. (I) The cannula was inserted and absorbable sutures secured it to the vein. (J) The skin incision was closed subcuticularly. The patient was transported to the angiography suite, under general anesthesia, with an arterial pressurized heparinized system dripping into the SOV access. (K) An SOV venogram confirmed good catheter placement. (L,M) Onyx was used to obliterate the CCF. The access cannula was removed without difficulty (not shown).

Foramen magnum locations

Foramen magnum DAVFs are typically supplied by vertebral artery muscular branches, occipital artery branches, ascending pharyngeal neuromeningeal branches, and the dorsal meningeal branch of the meningohypophyseal trunk. Venous drainage through the marginal sinus may then communicate with:

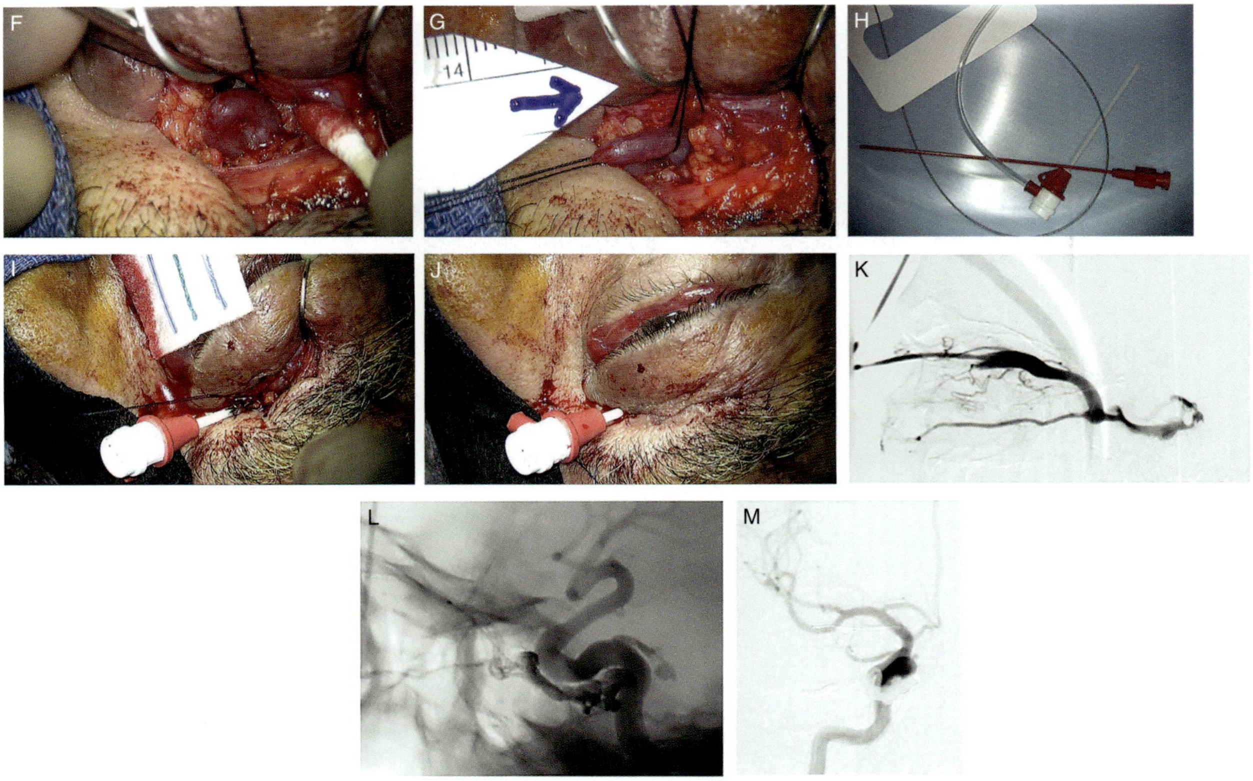

Fig. 13.11. (cont.)

- the sigmoid sinus/jugular bulb, resulting in tinnitus
- the inferior petrosal sinus and subsequently the cavernous sinus, resulting in orbital venous congestion
- the spinal perimedullary veins, resulting in myelopathy/quadriparesis; this latter type often presents a diagnostic challenge, as one rarely considers a cranial pathology as a cause of spinal symptomatology.

Midline, paramedian, or far lateral suboccipital approaches, along with upper cervical laminectomy, are characteristically utilized to access foramen magnum DAVFs. The rich venous arterialization can render the approach difficult because of excessive bleeding, particularly from the suboccipital venous plexus. Again, the goal should be to perform as targeted a craniotomy as possible to reach and divide the venous end of the fistulous point.

Outcomes

Favorable outcomes have been reported after surgery for "high-risk" DAVFs (i.e., with cortical venous drainage); however, most series include highly selected patients harboring a variety of fistula types/locations and treated with a combination of varied endovascular and surgical approaches. Collice *et al.* [64] reported no mortality or permanent morbidity in 34 patients with high-risk DAVFs treated surgically; all lesions were completely obliterated with no clinical or radiographic evidence of recurrence at mean follow-up of 33 months. In 23 DAVFs with cortical venous drainage treated surgically over a 14-year period, Liu *et al.* [65] achieved complete obliteration in all patients without complications and no recurrences or repeat hemorrhages over a mean follow-up period of 45 months. Wachter *et al.* [66] reported that in 41 patients with high-risk DAVFs treated surgically, complete lesion obliteration was achieved in 97.6% and permanent surgical morbidity was seen in 7.1%. No clinical or radiographic recurrences were noted over a mean follow-up period of 4.2 years, and the one lesion with known residual fistula after treatment remained angiographically and clinically stable as well. Kakarla *et al.* [55] reported that in 53 patients with high-risk DAVFs treated surgically, 49 (92%) had good/excellent clinical outcomes, 3 (6%) died, and complete lesion obliteration was achieved in 48 (91%). Tirakotai *et al.* [67] achieved complete surgical obliteration of four deep DAVFs draining into the jugular bulb, and the only complication was a partial hypoglossal nerve palsy. In a meta-analysis of 248 patients with DAVFs, Lucas *et al.* [68] compared treatment success rates for surgical, endovascular, and combined therapies by lesion location. For transverse–sigmoid DAVFs, the success rate for combined therapy (68%) was greater than that for either embolization (41%) or surgery (33%) alone. For tentorial DAVFs, the success rate for combined therapy (89%) was greater than that for either surgery (78%) or embolization (31%) alone. For anterior fossa DAVFs, 238 (96%) were

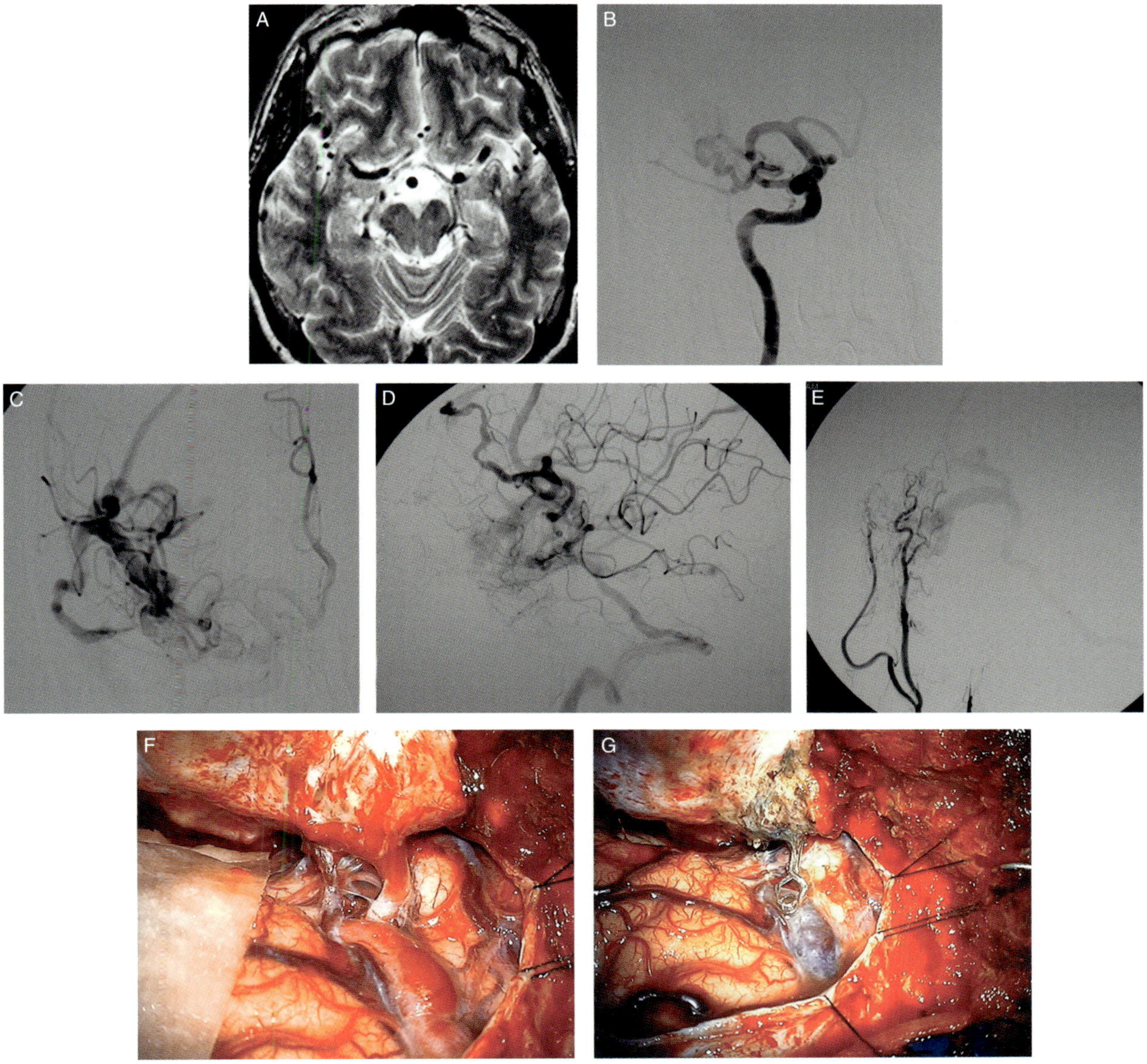

Fig. 13.12. A 60-year-old man presented with headaches and a bruit. (A) Brain MRI showed flow voids in and around the right sylvian fissure. (B–D) Angiography confirmed a dural arteriovenous fistula that was best classified as a sphenoparietal sinus fistula. There was input from middle cerebral artery branches (B) and drainage into the superficial sylvian vein and from there on to the vein of Labbé posteriorly and superior sagittal sinus superiorly (C,D). (E) Additionally there was recruitment from branches of the internal maxillary artery, but the venous outflow was identical to the one seen with right internal carotid artery injection, making the localization of the fistula point clearer. (F,G) In view of a single accessible draining vein, a right craniotomy was performed. A red bridging vein emerged from the sphenoparietal sinus and drained retrogradely into a large red superficial sylvian vein (F). Simple clip division of the fistulous point eliminated arterial input to the vein, and bipolar coagulation of the dura around the sphenoparietal sinus was added to guarantee complete dural disconnection (G).

treated surgically, with a successful outcome in all surgical patients. In summary, contemporary surgical series suggest that excellent technical outcomes can be achieved with reasonably low morbidity and mortality rates in well-selected patients harboring high-risk DAVFs.

Conclusions

High-risk DAVFs often require treatment. Endovascular techniques have emerged as the primary approach to many DAVFs; however, open surgical approaches continue to play an important role as the primary option in selected patients and also as a secondary option in patients where endovascular attempts have failed. In order to determine the best course of treatment for a given patient, the unique clinical and angiographic features of the patient should be closely evaluated as the risks of surgery are weighed against those of endovascular embolization, while taking into account the likelihood of completely obliterating the fistula. Over time, many have come to recognize that radical DAVF excision is rarely necessary, and that simple disconnection of the lesion's cortical venous drainage is often curative and safe in appropriately selected patients.

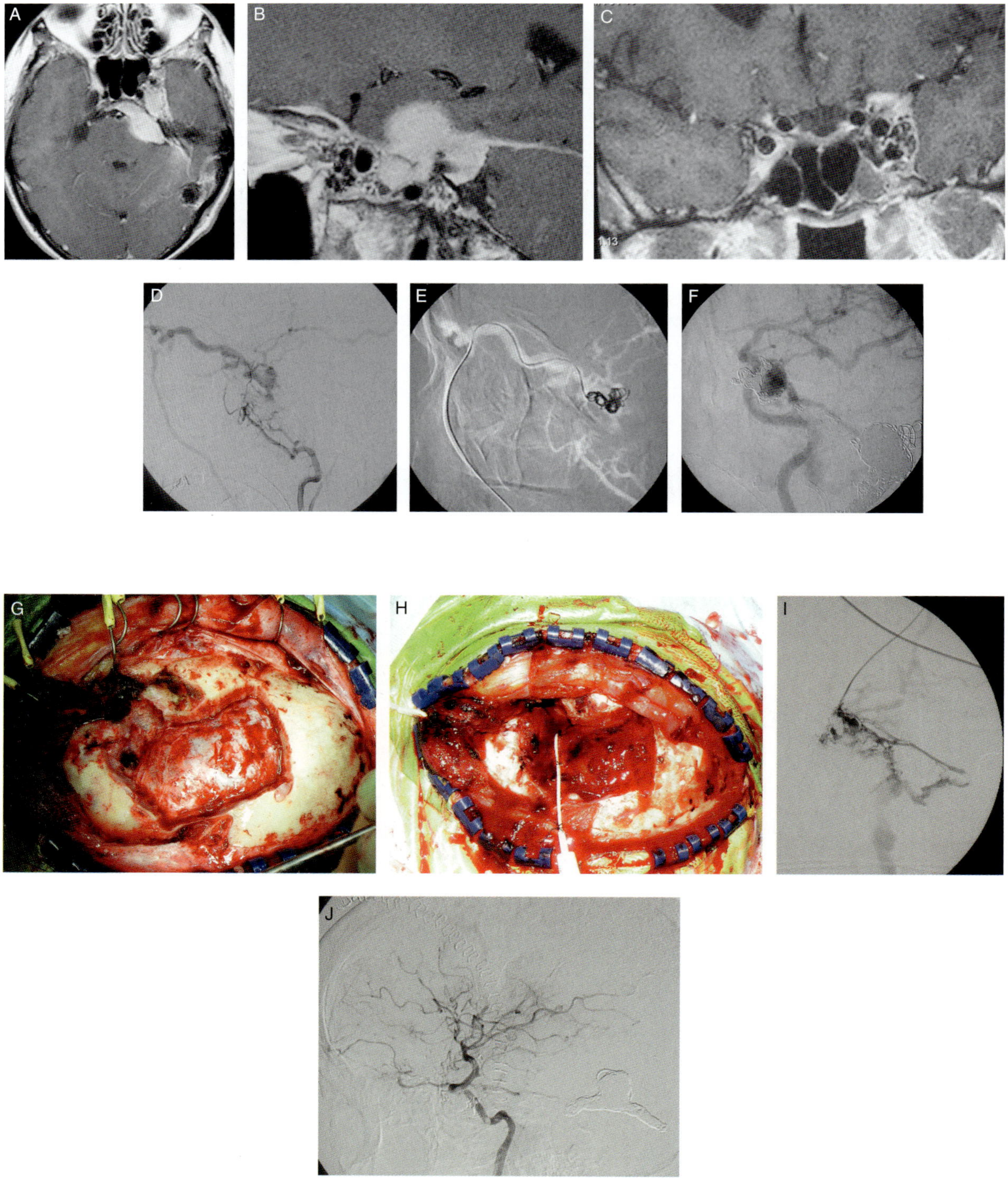

Fig. 13.13. A 46-year-old woman had been diagnosed with a large left petroclival meningioma as well as multifocal multicentric dural arteriovenous fistulae (DAVFs) affecting the left cavernous sinus, the left transverse–sigmoid junction, and the posterior fossa. She had been treated over a few years with multiple sessions of embolizations but with a tendency for recurrence in an aggressive pattern. (A–C) MRI demonstrated the meningioma intermixed with a left cavernous sinus DAVF. (D,E) Angiography demonstrated retrograde drainage into the superior ophthalmic vein and the cortical veins. On the last session, it was partially embolized via the angular vein. (F) However, this essentially isolated the cavernous sinus, which now drained arterialized blood only into cortical veins. (G,H) A left frontotemporal craniotomy was carried out and, under microscopic magnification, an extradural pretemporal approach was used to expose the arterialized sphenoparietal sinus, which was cannulated. (I) The access was used to obtain a venogram of the fistula and inject *N*-butyl cyanoacrylate (this was prior to the advent of Onyx) and obliterate the fistula. (J) Angiography on postoperative day 1 confirmed the obliteration of the fistula.

References

1. Travers B. A case of aneurism by anastomosis in the orbit, cured by the ligature of the common carotid artery. *Med Chir Trans* 1811;**2**:1–420.
2. Perrini P, Nannini T, Di LN. Francesco Rizzoli (1809–1880) and the elusive case of Giulia: the description of an "arteriovenous aneurysm passing through the wall of the skull." *Acta Neurochir (Wien)* 2007;**149**:191–6.
3. Locke CE. Intracranial arteriovenous aneurism or pulsating exophthalmos. *Ann Surg* 1924;**80**:272–85.
4. Sachs E. *The Diagnosis and Treatment of Brain Tumors*. St. Louis, MO: Mosby, 1931.
5. Debrun G, Chartres A. Infra and supratentorial arteriovenous malformations, a general review. About 2 cases of spontaneous supratentorial arteriovenous malformation of the dura. *Neuroradiology* 1972;**3**:184–92.
6. Aminoff MJ. Vascular anomalies in the intracranial dura mater. *Brain* 1973;**96**:601–12.
7. Newton TH, Weidner W, Greitz T. Dural arteriovenous malformation in the posterior fossa. *Radiology* 1968;**90**:27–35.
8. Newton TH, Hoyt WF. Spontaneous arteriovenous fistula between dural branches of the internal maxillary artery and the posterior cavernous sinus. *Radiology* 1968;**91**:1147–50.
9. Fincher EF. Arteriovenous fistula between the middle meningeal artery and the greater petrosal sinus; case report. *Ann Surg* 1951;**133**:886–8.
10. Olivecrona H, Ladenheim J. *Congenital Arteriovenous Aneurysms of the Carotid and Vertebral Arterial Systems*. Berlin: Springer, 1957.
11. Hamby WB. Carotid–cavernous fistula: report of 32 surgically treated cases and suggestions for definitive operation. *J Neurosurg* 1964;**21**:859–66.
12. Dandy WE. The treatment of carotid cavernous arteriovenous aneurysms. *Ann Surg* 1935;**102**:916–26.
13. Hamby WB. Carotid–cavernous fistula (pulsating exophthalmos). *GP* 1968;**37**:92–4.
14. Brooks B. The treatment of traumatic arteriovenous fistula. *South Med J* 1930;**23**:100–6.
15. Parkinson D. Carotid cavernous fistula: direct repair with preservation of the carotid artery. *J Neurosurg* 1973;**38**:99–106.
16. Hugosson R, Bergstrom K. Surgical treatment of dural arteriovenous malformation in the region of the sigmoid sinus. *J Neurol Neurosurg Psychiatry* 1974;**37**:97–101.
17. Sundt TM, Jr., Piepgras DG. The surgical approach to arteriovenous malformations of the lateral and sigmoid dural sinuses. *J Neurosurg* 1983;**59**:32–9.
18. Serbinenko FA. Balloon catheterization and occlusion of major cerebral vessels. *J Neurosurg* 1974;**41**:125–45.
19. Debrun G, Lacour P, Caron JP, *et al.* Detachable balloon and calibrated-leak balloon techniques in the treatment of cerebral vascular lesions. *J Neurosurg* 1978;**49**:635–49.
20. Newton TH, Cronqvist S. Involvement of dural arteries in intracranial arteriovenous malformations. *Radiology* 1969;**93**:1071–8.
21. Satomi J, van Dijk JM, terBrugge KG, *et al.* Benign cranial dural arteriovenous fistulas: outcome of conservative management based on the natural history of the lesion. *J Neurosurg* 2002;**97**:767–70.
22. Friedman A. Etiologic factors in intracranial dural arteriovenous malformations. In Awad IA, Barrow DL, eds. *Dural Arteriovenous Malformations*. Park Ridge, IL: American Association of Neurological Surgeons, 1993, pp. 35–47.
23. Terada T, Higashida RT, Halbach VV, *et al.* Development of acquired arteriovenous fistulas in rats due to venous hypertension. *J Neurosurg* 1994;**80**:884–9.
24. Herman JM, Spetzler RF, Bederson JB, *et al.* Genesis of a dural arteriovenous malformation in a rat model. *J Neurosurg* 1995;**83**:539–45.
25. Lawton MT, Jacobowitz R, Spetzler RF. Redefined role of angiogenesis in the pathogenesis of dural arteriovenous malformations. *J Neurosurg* 1997;**87**:267–74.
26. Graeb DA, Dolman CL. Radiological and pathological aspects of dural arteriovenous fistulas. Case report. *J Neurosurg* 1986;**64**:962–7.
27. Houser OW, Campbell JK, Campbell RJ, *et al.* Arteriovenous malformation affecting the transverse dural venous sinus: an acquired lesion. *Mayo Clin Proc* 1979;**54**:651–61.
28. Debrun G, Lacour P, Vinuela F, *et al.* Treatment of 54 traumatic carotid–cavernous fistulas. *J Neurosurg* 1981;**55**:678–92.
29. Pigott TJ, Holland IM, Punt JA. Carotico–cavernous fistula after trans-sphenoidal hypophysectomy. *Br J Neurosurg* 1989;**3**:613–16.
30. Sila CA, Furlan AJ, Little JR. Pulsatile tinnitus. *Stroke* 1987;**18**:252–6.
31. Miller NR. Diagnosis and management of dural carotid–cavernous sinus fistulas. *Neurosurg Focus* 2007;**23**:E13.
32. Djindjian R, Merland J. *Super-selective Arteriography of the External Carotid Artery*. Berlin: Springer, 1978.
33. Lalwani AK, Dowd CF, Halbach VV. Grading venous restrictive disease in patients with dural arteriovenous fistulas of the transverse/sigmoid sinus. *J Neurosurg* 1993;**79**:11–15.
34. Cognard C, Gobin YP, Pierot L, *et al.* Cerebral dural arteriovenous fistulas: clinical and angiographic correlation with a revised classification of venous drainage. *Radiology* 1995;**194**:671–80.
35. Borden JA, Wu JK, Shucart WA. A proposed classification for spinal and cranial dural arteriovenous fistulous malformations and implications for treatment. *J Neurosurg* 1995;**82**:166–79.
36. Zipfel GJ, Shah MN, Refai D, *et al.* Cranial dural arteriovenous fistulas: modification of angiographic classification scales based on new natural history data. *Neurosurg Focus* 2009;**26**:E14.
37. Barrow DL, Spector RH, Braun IF, *et al.* Classification and treatment of spontaneous carotid–cavernous sinus fistulas. *J Neurosurg* 1985;**62**:248–56.
38. Davies MA, Saleh J, terBrugge K, *et al.* The natural history and management of intracranial dural arteriovenous fistulae. Part 1: benign lesions. *Interv Neuroradiol* 1997;**3**:295–302.
39. van Dijk JM, terBrugge KG, Willinsky RA, *et al.* Clinical course of cranial dural arteriovenous fistulas with long-term persistent cortical venous reflux. *Stroke* 2002;**33**:1233–6.

40. Awad IA, Little JR, Akarawi WP, *et al.* Intracranial dural arteriovenous malformations: factors predisposing to an aggressive neurological course. *J Neurosurg* 1990;**72**:839–50.

41. Soderman M, Pavic L, Edner G, *et al.* Natural history of dural arteriovenous shunts. *Stroke* 2008;**39**:1735–9.

42. Strom RG, Botros JA, Refai D, *et al.* Cranial dural arteriovenous fistulae: asymptomatic cortical venous drainage portends less aggressive clinical course. *Neurosurgery* 2009;**64**:241–7.

43. Chandler JR. Diagnosis and cure of venous hum tinnitus. *Laryngoscope* 1983;**93**:892–5.

44. Duffau H, Lopes M, Janosevic V, *et al.* Early rebleeding from intracranial dural arteriovenous fistulas: report of 20 cases and review of the literature. *J Neurosurg* 1999;**90**:78–84.

45. Mullan S. Reflections upon the nature and management of intracranial and intraspinal vascular malformations and fistulae. *J Neurosurg* 1994;**80**:606–16.

46. Collice M, D'Aliberti G, Talamonti G, *et al.* Surgical interruption of leptomeningeal drainage as treatment for intracranial dural arteriovenous fistulas without dural sinus drainage. *J Neurosurg* 1996;**84**:810–17.

47. Thompson BG, Doppman JL, Oldfield EH. Treatment of cranial dural arteriovenous fistulae by interruption of leptomeningeal venous drainage. *J Neurosurg* 1994;**80**:617–23.

48. van Dijk JM, terBrugge KG, Willinsky RA, *et al.* Selective disconnection of cortical venous reflux as treatment for cranial dural arteriovenous fistulas. *J Neurosurg* 2004;**101**:31–5.

49. da Costa LB, terBrugge K, Farb R, *et al.* Surgical disconnection of cortical venous reflux as a treatment for Borden type II dural arteriovenous fistulae. *Acta Neurochir (Wien)* 2007;**149**:1103–8.

50. Komiyama M, Nishikawa M, Kitano S, *et al.* Transumbilical embolization of a congenital dural arteriovenous fistula at the torcular herophili in a neonate. Case report. *J Neurosurg* 1999;**90**:964–9.

51. Herman TE, Siegel MJ. Congenital dural arteriovenous fistula at torcula Herophili. Endovascular embolization. *J Perinatol* 2007;**27**:730–1.

52. Spiotta AM, Sivapatham T, Hussain MS, *et al.* Combined surgical and endovascular approach to a complex dural arteriovenous fistula involving the superior sagittal sinus and torcula. *J Stroke Cerebrovasc Dis* 2012;**21**:283–8.

53. Liu JK, Choudhry OJ, Barnwell SL, *et al.* Single stage transcranial exposure of large dural venous sinuses for surgically assisted direct transvenous embolization of high-grade dural arteriovenous fistulas: technical note. *Acta Neurochir (Wien)* 2012;**154**:1855–9.

54. Houdart E, Saint-Maurice JP, Chapot R, *et al.* Transcranial approach for venous embolization of dural arteriovenous fistulas. *J Neurosurg* 2002;**97**:280–6.

55. Kakarla UK, Deshmukh VR, Zabramski JM, *et al.* Surgical treatment of high-risk intracranial dural arteriovenous fistulae: clinical outcomes and avoidance of complications. *Neurosurgery* 2007;**61**:447–57.

56. Fiumara E, Tumbiolo S, Bellomonte ML, *et al.* Resection of the transverse sinuses and confluence of sinuses for treatment of multiple dural arteriovenous fistulas. Case report. *J Neurosurg* 2004;**100**:348–52.

57. Elhammady MS, Peterson EC, ziz-Sultan MA. Onyx embolization of a carotid cavernous fistula via direct transorbital puncture. *J Neurosurg* 2011;**114**:129–32.

58. White JB, Layton KF, Evans AJ, *et al.* Transorbital puncture for the treatment of cavernous sinus dural arteriovenous fistulas. *AJNR Am J Neuroradiol* 2007;**28**:1415–17.

59. Wolfe SQ, Cumberbatch NM, Aziz-Sultan MA, *et al.* Operative approach via the superior ophthalmic vein for the endovascular treatment of carotid cavernous fistulas that fail traditional endovascular access. *Neurosurgery* 2010;**66**:293–9.

60. Dolenc V. Direct microsurgical repair of intracavernous vascular lesions. *J Neurosurg* 1983;**58**:824–31.

61. Mullan S. Treatment of carotid–cavernous fistulas by cavernous sinus occlusion. *J Neurosurg* 1979;**50**:131–44.

62. Day JD, Fukushima T. Direct microsurgery of dural arteriovenous malformations type carotid–cavernous sinus fistulas: indications, technique, and results. *Neurosurgery* 1997;**41**:1119–24.

63. Smith JE, Epps J, Press HC, Jr., *et al.* Traumatic arteriovenous fistula between the middle meningeal artery and the sphenoparietal sinus: a case report and review of the world literature. *J Natl Med Assoc* 1981;**73**:274–8.

64. Collice M, D'Aliberti G, Arena O, *et al.* Surgical treatment of intracranial dural arteriovenous fistulae: role of venous drainage. *Neurosurgery* 2000;**47**:56–66.

65. Liu JK, Dogan A, Ellegala DB, *et al.* The role of surgery for high-grade intracranial dural arteriovenous fistulas: importance of obliteration of venous outflow. *J Neurosurg* 2009;**110**:913–20.

66. Wachter D, Hans F, Psychogios MN, *et al.* Microsurgery can cure most intracranial dural arteriovenous fistulae of the sinus and non-sinus type. *Neurosurg Rev* 2011;**34**:337–45.

67. Tirakotai W, Benes L, Kappus C, *et al.* Surgical management of dural arteriovenous fistulas with transosseous arterial feeders involving the jugular bulb. *Neurosurg Rev* 2007;**30**:40–8.

68. Lucas CP, Zabramski JM, Spetzler RF, *et al.* Treatment for intracranial dural arteriovenous malformations: a meta-analysis from the English language literature. *Neurosurgery* 1997;**40**:1119–30.

Chapter 14

Surgery of spinal arteriovenous malformations and fistulae

M. Yashar S. Kalani, George A. C. Mendes, Maziyar A. Kalani, and Robert F. Spetzler

Introduction

The first reports of a spinal vascular malformations were by Hebold [1] and Gaupp [2] in the 1880s. These were followed by the first successful surgical treatment of a spinal malformations (a fistula) by Krause in 1911 [3] and the first major series by Wyburn-Mason in 1943 [4]. With the introduction and widespread use of spinal angiography, these lesions have become more frequently identified and treated. Aminoff and Logue are credited with the first systematic review of the presentation and natural history of spinal malformations, which they reported in 1974 [5]. They proposed that abnormal shunting and the resultant venous congestion were responsible for the decreased intramedullary blood flow and the symptoms noted in most patients. This mechanistic observation was further refined to the current theory of venous congestion as the etiology behind these lesions. Indeed, the treatment strategies for spinal vascular malformations are based on this mechanistic understanding of venous congestion inciting neurological decline.

Spinal arteriovenous fistulae (AVFs) and spinal arteriovenous malformations (AVMs) have distinct characteristics with respect to incidence, sex predominance, age at onset of symptoms, etiology, pathophysiology, location along the spinal axis, clinical presentation, and natural history [6]. The current therapies for these lesions, including endovascular and microsurgical treatments, depend on disconnecting the shunt and decreasing venous congestion. This chapter focuses on the microsurgical treatment of spinal AVFs and AVMs. In many cases, treatment of spinal vascular malformations requires a multidisciplinary approach with surgeons, interventionalists, and radiation therapists working side by side to provide optimal holistic care for the patient.

Incidence and prevalence of spinal vascular malformations

Spinal vascular malformations account for 3–4% of all intradural spinal cord lesions [6]; the three main types are AVFs, AVMs, and cavernous malformations (see Classification, below). Spinal AVFs are by far the most common, constituting 70% of all spinal vascular malformations and affecting 5–10 people per million annually [7]. These lesions are most frequently identified in men (with an 80% male predominance) between 50 and 60 years of age [8]. Given their late presentation, they are thought to be acquired lesions. Spinal AVMs, including all the various subtypes, are much less common than spinal AVFs and account for approximately 20% of spinal vascular malformations [7]. These lesions are frequently observed in younger patients (most younger than 30 years) and are occasionally associated with inherited disorders such as Klippel–Trénaunay–Weber syndrome [9–12], hereditary hemorrhagic telangiectasia [13], familial cutaneous hemangiomas [14], familial cerebral cavernous malformations [15], and pulmonary AVMs [16].

Etiology

Spinal AVFs do not have a clear etiology or associations with other diseases; however, they are more common in men and are considered acquired lesions because of their presentation in adulthood. In contrast, spinal AVMs are considered congenital lesions and are usually seen in children or young adults. There is no sex predominance in young adults, but a male predominance is noted in children. Occasionally, spinal AVMs may present in association with other vascular malformations. Some authors have postulated that spinal AVMs are caused by disturbances occurring early in embryogenesis during the development of spinal cord vasculature [6,17].

Metameric vascular malformations encompass a group of lesions that extend beyond the spinal cord and affect bone, paraspinal muscles, and skin related to a segmental dermatome. The full spectrum is seen in Cobb syndrome, which affects all of the involved dermatome. In other congenital, non-hereditary syndromes, such as Klippel–Trénaunay–Weber syndrome and Parkes–Weber syndrome, the full dermatome is not involved. In these patients, the vascular malformations typically affect the lower extremities and have three remarkable clinical features: cutaneous capillary malformations, varicose veins, and limb hypertrophy, frequently associated with lymphatic abnormalities [18,19].

Comprehensive Management of Arteriovenous Malformations of the Brain and Spine, ed. Robert F. Spetzler, Douglas S. Kondziolka, Randall T. Higashida, and M. Yashar S. Kalani. Published by Cambridge University Press.

Pathophysiology

Myelopathy is a predominant presentation of spinal vascular malformations. The three pathophysiological mechanisms that are thought to contribute to its development are venous hypertension, arterial steal phenomenon, and subarachnoid hemorrhage. Pathological and clinical studies have demonstrated the prominent role of venous hypertension in the pathophysiology of spinal AVFs. The blood supply of spinal AVFs usually arises from a radicular artery, which shunts into a radicular vein within the dural sleeve of a nerve root thereby increasing pressure in the coronal venous plexus and radial veins [6,20]. Venous hypertension reduces the arteriovenous gradient and tissue perfusion; consequently, the spinal cord is affected by progressive hypoxia [20,21]. Berenstein *et al.* postulated that increased venous pressure causes progressive intramedullary vasodilatation, which may result in loss of vessel autoregulation in affected areas [21].

Angiographic findings of slow drainage through dilated medullary veins support the theory that venous hypertension is the main cause of the pathophysiology of spinal AVFs. In some fistulae, the arterialization of the coronal venous plexus may reach the anterior and posterior surface of the spinal cord. The increased pressure may extend into the spinal cord veins, mostly those located in the posterolateral white matter and the corticospinal tract but, subsequently, those in the gray matter [21].

The vascular steal mechanism is unlikely to contribute to the pathophysiology of spinal AVFs. Since the fistula and spinal cord have distinct blood supplies, the fistula would have to steal enough blood to reduce the intra-aortic pressure and divert normal spinal cord blood. This is unlikely in a low-flow spinal fistula [6].

Spinal AVMs are intradural lesions usually located along the surface of the spinal cord or intramedullary, or both. They are supplied by the anterior spinal artery, the pial network, radicular arteries, perforators, or a combination of these feeders [22]. Spinal AVMs are typically high-flow malformations; therefore, vascular steal is the primary mechanism involved in spinal cord ischemia. Usually, these high-flow shunts are associated with multiple feeders, supplied by medullary arteries, which can divert blood directly from the spinal cord parenchyma into the malformations. Arterial and venous aneurysms are associated with high-flow spinal AVMs and significantly increase the risk of spinal cord hemorrhage [6].

The rupture of spinal AVFs or AVMs can result in subarachnoid hemorrhage and, consequently, in compression of the spinal cord and nerve roots. The released blood (and its breakdown products) can cause irritation of the spinal cord nervous tissue and vasculature. Subarachnoid hemorrhage is discussed further in the next section.

Clinical presentation

The clinical presentation and natural history of the lesions are distinct between spinal AVFs and AVMs [23,24]. The most common presenting symptoms for both groups are motor weakness, sensory impairment, sphincter disturbances, and pain, but spinal hemorrhage is remarkably more common in spinal AVMs (Table 14.1) [6].

Table 14.1. Initial signs and symptoms in the series of Jellema *et al.*

Signs and symptoms	Initial (No. [%])	At time of diagnosis (No. [%])
Walking disturbances	27 (34)	50 (63)
Sensory disturbances	19 (24)	55 (69)
Paresthesiae	17 (21)	27 (34)
Paraparesis	13 (16)	62 (78)
Low back pain	11 (14)	21 (26)
Pain in legs	10 (13)	20 (25)
Weakness of one leg	7 (9)	–
Cramps	4 (5)	–
Micturition problems	3 (4)	64 (80)
Anal sphincter disturbances	–	31 (39)
Erectile dysfunction	–	20 (25)

Source: from Jellema *et al.* [24], with permission from BMJ Publishing Group Ltd.

Spinal AVFs are commonly seen in the lower thoracic and lumbar spine [6], and clinical presentation ranges from non-specific symptoms to severe motor deficits. The usual presenting symptoms are weakness, sensory disturbances, and micturition problems; of these, motor symptoms are clearly the most common and the group that best responds to treatment [23,24]. Back or radicular pain in isolation is an infrequent presentation. Subarachnoid hemorrhage is extremely rare in spinal AVFs [25]. There is a robust male predominance (more than 80% of patients in most series) and late presentation (median age, 60 years) [23,24,26]. The diagnosis is typically delayed because of the rarity of the disease and the non-specificity of the symptoms: a median interval of 15 months has been reported between onset of symptoms and diagnosis [20].

Patients with spinal AVFs usually report a progressive worsening of symptoms with the Valsalva maneuver, physical exercise, and postural modifications. The increased intra-abdominal and intrathoracic pressure from these maneuvers can lead to increased vena caval pressure, which causes higher intraspinal venous pressure [22]. Pregnancy is also correlated with worsening of symptoms through the higher intra-abdominal pressure, augmented intravascular volume, hormonal changes, and increased venous pressure associated with delivery.

Spinal AVMs, by comparison, most commonly affect the upper thoracic and cervical spine. The most common presenting symptom is sudden-onset back pain, usually correlated to the level of the lesion along the spinal axis and associated nerve root. Patients with spinal AVMs are much younger than patients with spinal AVFs (patients generally present in their twenties; range, 15–40 years) [22]. There appears to be a male predominance in children [18], and no sex predominance in adults [22]. The hemorrhagic presentation occurs in a half of patients, which may be either subarachnoid hemorrhage or hematomyelia [22]. Patients with spinal AVFs complain of exacerbation of myelopathic symptoms with exertion. Conversely, exacerbation of symptoms after physical activity is less likely to occur in patients with spinal AVMs [6, 27].

Pregnancy is also correlated with worsening of symptoms with spinal AVMs, for the same reasons as for spinal AVFs.

Natural history

Spinal AVFs and AVMs are associated with a malignant course. Half of all patients will become severely disabled within three years after the onset of motor symptoms [28]. Usually, the progressive myelopathy is caused by venous hypertension [28] and the sudden neurological deficit or worsening of previous symptoms is caused by hemorrhage from the lesions. Less commonly, an acute deterioration is associated with thrombosis of the draining vein of the malformations. Even with modern imaging methods, late detection is noted in most modern series and the time to diagnosis from the onset of symptoms ranges from 12 to 22 months [29]. It is well demonstrated that without treatment the symptoms will escalate to severe neurological impairment leading to disability [28].

Classification

Although spinal vascular malformations were known pathological entities, it was not until the turn of the 20th century that Krause reported the first case of spinal AVM treated with surgery [3]. Subsequently, Elsberg published a successful treatment of an extradural spinal AVM [30]. Later, in 1926, Foix and Alajouanine identified a syndrome linked to an acute thrombosis of the pathological vessels [31]. In 1943, Wyburn-Mason published the first major series of spinal AVMs and proposed a classification system based on the histological criteria observed in 110 patients [4]. This divided the spinal AVMs into two main categories: arteriovenous angiomas and venous angiomas. In 1977, Kendall and Logue [32], using angiographic criteria, were the first to distinguish the spinal AVMs as dural and intradural types based on the location of the nidus. Since then, several classification schemes, mostly based on morphological data, have been proposed that aim to facilitate better understanding and management of spinal AVMs and AVFs [18,33,34].

Borden and colleagues [33] proposed a classification scheme in which they unified cranial and spinal dural AVFs in groups based on the site of venous drainage. This system divides the dural AVFs into three types: type I fistulae are considered to have a benign course, drain directly into dural venous sinuses or meningeal veins intracranially, or into the Batson epidural venous plexus in the spine; types II and III are associated with an aggressive course and have a higher risk of intracranial hemorrhage, venous hypertension, and neurological deficits. Type II fistulae drain into venous sinuses and have a retrograde flow into subarachnoid veins or epidural venous plexus and perimedullary veins. Type III fistulae drain into subarachnoid veins. Moreover, the system recognizes two different grades of complexity: type A has a single feeding artery, and type B has multiple feeding arteries and is considered a complex dural AVF with multifocal arteriovenous shunts [20].

Rodesch and colleagues [18] reviewed the charts and radiological files of 155 patients with spinal cord arteriovenous shunts and elaborated a classification system based on anatomical, biological, and genetic features. They divided the spinal shunts into three groups. The first group, genetic hereditary lesions, includes single shunts linked to disorders such as hereditary hemorrhagic telangiectasias (usually these syndromes are associated with single spinal AVMs in children). The second group, genetic hereditary lesions, has two subgroups: metameric and non-metameric. Lesions in the metameric subgroup have multiple shunts in different myelomeres of the cord and intradural nerve roots and are linked to disorders such as Cobb syndrome (which the authors named spinal arteriovenous metameric syndrome). In the non-metameric subgroup, shunts are usually associated with lower extremity vascular malformations in syndromes such as Klippel–Trénaunay–Weber syndrome and Parkes–Weber syndrome. The third group includes AVF and AVM shunts that are located in the intradural space and found in patients without associated genetic syndromes.

In 2006, Kim and Spetzler [34] introduced a new grading system based on anatomical and pathophysiological factors (see also Surgical management, below). They divided spinal vascular malformations into five groups: extradural AVFs, intradural AVFs (subclassified into dorsal and ventral), extradural–intradural AVMs, intramedullary AVMs, and a newly proposed group of conus medullaris AVMs.

Evaluation of spinal arteriovenous malformations and fistulae

The evaluation of spinal AVFs and AVMs requires spinal angiography. Although MRI and MR angiography have improved in resolution and can now delineate the source of many shunts, they have not replaced spinal angiography as the gold standard imaging modality for the study of spinal vascular malformations.

In spinal AVFs and AVMs, spinal angiography demonstrates a tangle of vessels at the level of the spinal cord parenchyma. These lesions may have a single or multiple arterial feeders arising from the anterior or posterior spinal arteries. The extradural–intradural AVMs (also called metameric or juvenile AVMs) are complex lesions associated with multiple arterial feeders in which the nidus usually involves spinal cord, spinal canal, nerve roots, bone, muscles, and skin. Angiography in conus medullaris AVMs shows a direct arteriovenous shunt with arterial feeders arising from the

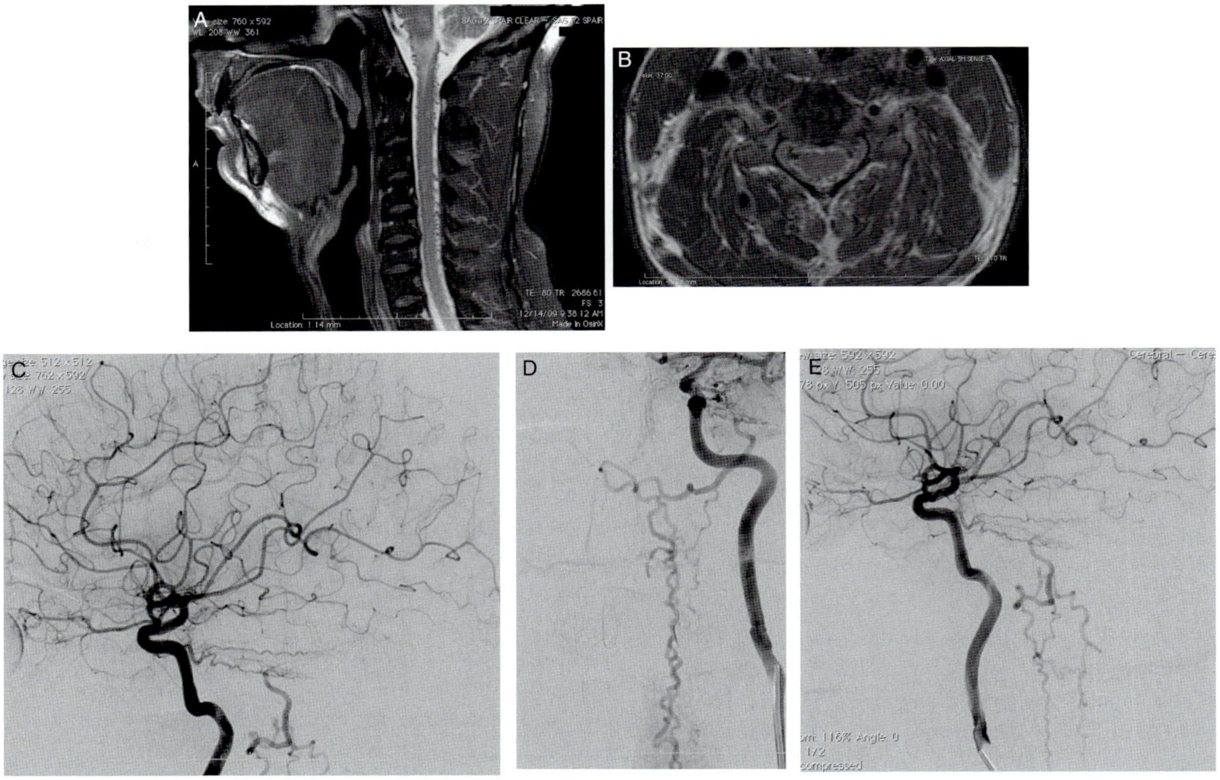

Fig. 14.1. A 58-year-old man presented with progressive myelopathy. (A,B) MRI demonstrating flow voids in the subarachnoid space and central spinal cord, with hyperintensity on T_2-weighted images (A, sagittal view; B, axial view). Spinal angiography was unremarkable (not shown). (C–E) Cerebral angiography through left internal carotid injection demonstrated a tentorial dural fistula supplied by the tentorial artery of Bernasconi and Cassinari. The intradural arteriovenous fistula was associated with reflux to the perimedullary veins.

anterior or posterior spinal arteries and associated with engorged veins [34].

After delineation of the lesion, the neighboring vessels should be studied to identify potential feeders and to evaluate the effect of the lesion on the spinal cord. Anteroposterior angiography should be performed to identify feeding vessels and their origin from the anterior or posterior spinal artery (if any). Mass effect can distort the midline structures on frontal projection angiography and in this situation, the lateral projection angiography may help to delineate angioarchitecture. Three-dimensional angiography may help to define the relationship between the vascular malformations, bony structures, and the spinal cord. During the selective injection, contrast reflux into the lesion helps to identify the contributing feeders immediately above and below and is critical for planning endovascular treatment. Postprocedural complications are rare; most are related to ischemic events caused by incidental air or clot emboli [22,26].

Intracranial dural AVFs can also present with symptoms of myelopathy, associated with spinal MRI findings of dilated, tortuous, and arterialized coronal venous plexus, but an unremarkable appearance on spinal angiography. In these patients, selective internal carotid angiography is indispensable for identifying tentorial or posterior fossa dural fistulae supplied by intracranial branches that may drain into the perimedullary plexus (Fig. 14.1).

Arterial phase

Berenstein *et al.* [22] have described some features of the angioarchitecture that may help to localize the level of vascular malformations, such as arterial anastomosis in axial and longitudinal planes and intrinsic or extrinsic spinal cord arteries supply. These parameters may help to differentiate intramedullary from extramedullary lesions. The caliber of the feeders may also help to differentiate direct from indirect shunts. Usually, larger branches going into the fistula suggest a direct fistula, whereas smaller feeders with anastomoses to normal neighboring vessels suggest an indirect fistula [22].

Aneurysms

Aneurysms associated with spinal AVMs are more frequently seen in high-flow lesions, which are mostly at the cervical level and in patients with a history of spinal hemorrhage. Aneurysms located on the radicular arteries are associated with multiple bleeds. Spinal angiography may exhibit an irregular dilatation proximal to the AVM. An AVM-associated aneurysm may be flow-related or dysplastic when associated with congenital disorders such as Klippel–Trénaunay–Weber syndrome. Similar to flow-related aneurysms in the brain, aneurysms associated with spinal vascular malformations tend to regress after occlusion of the shunt [22]. Unlike brain AVMs, spinal AVMs do not frequently demonstrate dilatation of the draining vein on angiography [22].

Nidus

In contrast to the nidus of a brain AVM, delineating the nidus of a spinal vascular malformations is difficult because of the numerous anastomoses in the spinal vasculature, including axial, transmedullary, arterio–arterial, venovenous, and complex intrinsic and complex extrinsic longitudinal anastomoses [22]. Certain parameters in the arterial phase help to define the flow type of the lesions. Fistulae supplied by the anterior spinal artery are usually high flow, except those located in the filum terminale, and are considered macro-AVFs, whereas the micro-AVFs are associated with slow and moderate flow. Dorsal AVFs are micro-AVFs and, if located off from the midline, can be mistaken for dural AVFs because of the location and clinical presentation of venous congestion [22].

The filum terminale arteriovenous shunts are usually micro-AVFs, exclusively supplied by the anterior spinal artery. However, fistulae located at the nerve roots and conus medullaris frequently encompass radicular, pial, and anterior spinal artery supply [22].

Venous phase

Venous pouches, ectasias, and kinking are frequently seen in spinal AVMs and result in mechanical compression of the cord inside the spinal canal. While the radicular veins are usually patent in spinal AVMs, in spinal AVFs, thrombosis of the radicular veins contributes to the pathophysiology of the disease. Congestion of the radicular veins is commonly demonstrated in spinal angiography and may result in brachial nerve deficits [22].

Surgical management

Preoperative planning is essential for understanding the location and anatomy of the malformations and the surgical strategy necessary to treat it. The management of spinal vascular malformations requires a multidisciplinary team consisting of neurovascular surgeons, interventionalists, and radiation therapists. This chapter will focus on the surgical nuances associated with the treatment of these rare and complex lesions. Later chapters will discuss the role of endovascular and radiation therapies as primary treatments and as adjuncts to surgery.

General principles

All patients must have a thorough preoperative evaluation, including neurological, radiographic, and angiographic evaluations. The decision to treat vascular malformations of the spine should be made after discussion between the various members of the team and with the patient or caregivers. Endovascular embolization should be considered as a stand-alone procedure or as an adjunct to microsurgical resection for spinal vascular malformations, when appropriate [35]. At Barrow Neurological Institute, all patients undergo intraoperative monitoring of cortical somatosensory evoked potentials and motor evoked potentials. These techniques monitor spinal cord function throughout the intervention and help to guide the extent of resection, particularly for large AVMs. We maintain the mean arterial pressure between 60 and 80 mmHg throughout the procedure to prevent hypotension and cord hypoperfusion, which may place the cord at risk for injury, particularly if vascular spasm occurs during dissection.

Patients are usually placed in the prone position, although anterior approaches have been used in rare situations [36]. The patient is positioned prone on a Wilson frame or chest rolls, and the appropriate level is verified by radiography. In certain patients, we recommend placement of radiopaque fiducial markers intraoperatively under fluoroscopic guidance to help in identifying the level of interest. Subperiosteal dissection is performed through a midline approach to expose the posterior elements overlying the level of pathology. A laminectomy is performed using the Midas Rex high-speed drill with the pediatric craniotomy footplate (Medtronic; Minneapolis, MI, USA). The lamina and spinous processes are removed as one piece and preserved to repair the laminotomy at the end of the procedure. Microsurgical technique is used to perform the operations. Pathology-specific considerations are discussed below.

Intradural dorsal arteriovenous fistulae

The goal of the surgical treatment of intradural dorsal AVFs is to relieve venous hypertension by disconnecting the fistula and the arterialized draining vein. Before opening the dura, care must be taken to evaluate for the presence of a nidus within the dura mater. This fistulous point is usually located on the lateral aspect of the spinal dura adjacent to the nerve root entry. The dura is opened under microscopic visualization and anchored using 4-0 nylon sutures. Next, the arachnoid is opened and anchored with small hemoclips, and the arterialized vein is identified, which will lead to the fistulous point (Fig. 14.2). We now routinely use indocyanine green (ICG) videoangiography to identify the arterialized vein [10,37,38]. The vessel is dissected free using sharp dissection, ensuring that the vessels are not avulsed from the radial veins of the spinal cord, which could cause venous congestion if the vessels are damaged. The efferent vein is identified, coagulated with bipolar cautery, and cut. The inner dural surface at the fistulous point is carefully inspected for other possible feeding vessels. Once the fistulous point is identified and disconnected, the dorsal spinal cord veins should be less engorged. We routinely perform ICG videoangiography after disconnection to confirm interruption of the fistula.

Watertight closure of the dura is achieved using 6-0 nylon sutures reinforced with fibrin glue. The lamina is repaired with laminectomy plates and attached to the lateral elements. In our experience, replacement of the lamina helps to decrease the incidence of kyphotic deformity. The superficial wound is closed in the usual fashion.

Intradural ventral arteriovenous fistulae

The surgical approach to intradural ventral AVFs is complicated by their ventral position and intimate association with the anterior spinal artery. The goal of surgery for intradural ventral AVFs, similar to that of intradural dorsal AVFs, is to disconnect

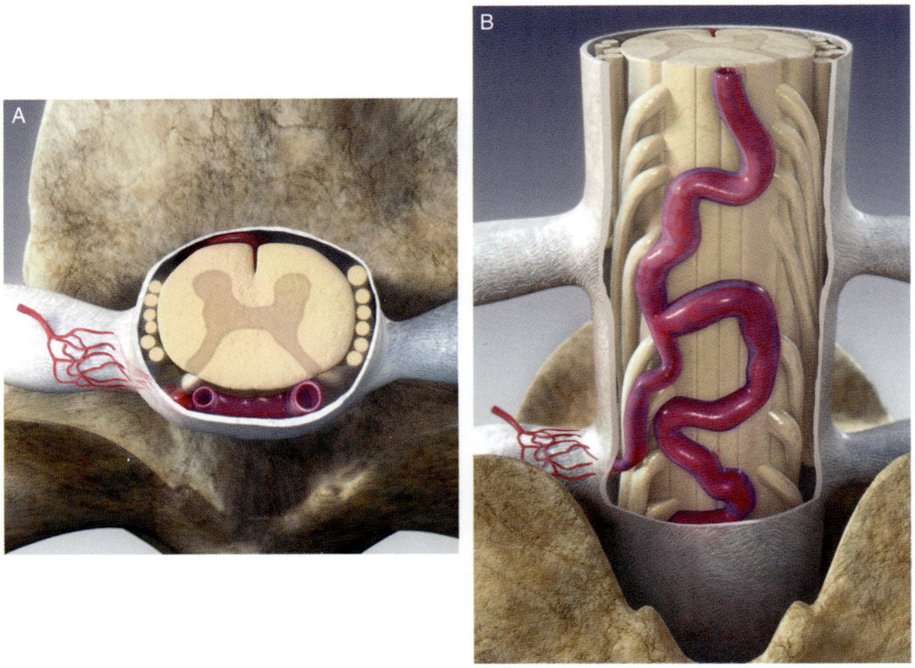

Fig. 14.2. Intradural dorsal arteriovenous fistula. (A) Axial view of an abnormal radicular feeding artery along the nerve root on the right. The glomerular network of branches coalesces at the site of the fistula along the dural root sleeve. (B) Posterior view demonstrates the dilatation of the coronal venous plexus. Arterialization of these veins and venous outflow obstruction (not shown) produces venous hypertension. Focal disruption of the point of the fistula by endovascular or microsurgical methods will obliterate the lesion and decrease the venous congestion. (Used with permission from Barrow Neurological Institute.)

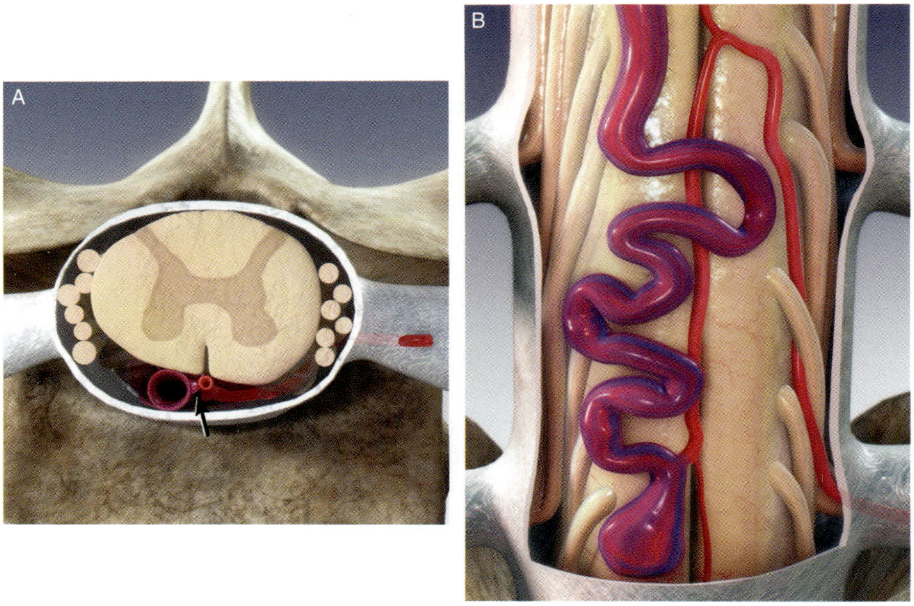

Fig. 14.3. Intradural ventral arteriovenous fistula. (A) Axial view of a midline lesion derived from a fistulous connection (arrow) between the anterior spinal artery and the coronal venous plexus. (B) Anterior view demonstrates a type A fistula along the anteroinferior aspect of the spinal cord. Proximal and distal to this lesion, the course of the anterior spinal artery is normal. (Used with permission from Barrow Neurological Institute.)

the arteriovenous fistulous point. The other vessels in proximity to the fistulous point are usually normal and should be preserved. Intradural ventral AVFs are subclassified as types A, B, and C (Fig. 14.3) [34,39]. Type A lesions are small and have a single feeder. Type B lesions are intermediate in size and have a major feeder from the anterior spinal artery. Type C lesions are giant lesions with dilated venous varices and multiple feeding pedicles, usually from the anterior spinal artery. Surgery is indicated for type A and B lesions but is excessively risky for type C lesions.

Intradural ventral AVFs may be approached via anterior, posterior, or posterolateral approaches. If the perimedullary fistula is located along the dorsal or dorsolateral aspects of the spinal cord, a standard posterior or posterolateral approach can be used. An anteriorly located lesion requires an anterior or anterolateral approach. Once the approach has been performed, the dura is opened and secured in the usual fashion. The fistula is identified on the anterior surface of the spinal cord. The point of fistulous connection can be confirmed using ICG videoangiography. An area of venous ectasia is often present at the fistulous point and can aid in its visual identification. The junction between the anterior spinal artery and the feeding vessels is identified and disconnected using a small clip. We do not

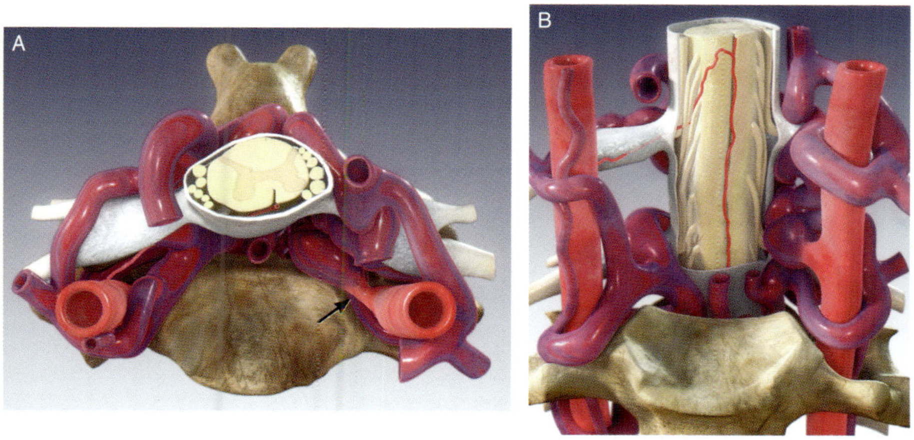

Fig. 14.4. Extradural arteriovenous fistula. (A) Axial view along a perforating branch of the left vertebral artery (arrow). (B) Posterior view showing engorgement of epidural veins. This congestion can produce a mass effect on adjacent nerve roots and spinal cord. (Used with permission from Barrow Neurological Institute.)

advocate the use of electrocautery at this location because the current may spread to the anterior spinal artery. Once the fistula is disconnected, the dura is closed in the usual watertight fashion and the wound is closed. If an extensive anterior approach has been used, the vertebral column may need to be reconstructed. In patients with type B or C fistulae, the decision to perform microsurgical intervention depends on the location, size, and number of vessel feeders. The location and relation of the feeders to the anterior spinal artery may also influence the decision to intervene with an endovascular or open microsurgical approach.

Extradural arteriovenous fistulae

Extradural AVFs, also known as epidural fistulae, represent an abnormal communication between an extradural branch of a radicular artery and an epidural venous plexus (Fig. 14.4). These lesions can be treated using both endovascular and microsurgical techniques. Depending on the location of these lesions, an anterior or posterior approach may be used. Upon exposure of the dura, the fistulous connection is identified and disconnected using a small clip or via electrocautery-assisted ligation. Considerations for the approach and closure of intradural AVFs are applicable to these lesions as well.

Intramedullary arteriovenous malformations

Resection of intramedullary AVMs is more challenging than that of AVFs. These high-flow lesions have thin walls; therefore, they tend to rupture and are difficult to coagulate and control. Although surgical resection remains the gold standard for treating intramedullary AVMs [40,41], embolization alone [42] or in combination with surgery [10,36,43] has provided acceptable results. Preoperative spinal angiography must be used to identify the relationship of the AVM to the anterior spinal artery. If it is not possible to identify this relationship, embolization of the vessels should be avoided to minimize the risk of neurological injury.

The positioning, incision, and approach used for intramedullary AVMs are similar to those used for AVFs, but an anterior approach may be used in certain patients [36,40,44,45]. Intraoperatively, there is little extradural evidence of the vascular malformations, although enlarged vessels may be noted (Figs. 14.5 and 14.6). Once the dura is opened, the surface of the spinal cord is examined and the relationship of vessels to the AVM is noted. We routinely perform intraoperative ICG videoangiography to evaluate the contribution of feeding vessels and the relationship of en passage vessels to the nidus [37,38]. In contrast to the surgical strategy for AVFs, the strategy for intramedullary AVMs does not include obliteration of feeding vessels at their dural entry because they may have feeders joining the anterior spinal artery. In AVMs of the lower thoracic spine, the artery of Adamkiewicz (great anterior radiculomedullary artery) should be identified early and preserved. Next, the AVM nidus is devascularized and resected using a microsurgical technique. We prefer circumferential dissection of the AVM at a pial surface. Intraparenchymal components of AVMs can be resected by one of four classic myelotomies: midline dorsal, dorsal root entry zone, lateral, and anterior midline. If the nidus is completely intraparenchymal without an exophytic component, we prefer a midline myelotomy. If there is significant posterior column dysfunction, the myelotomy may also be placed off midline toward the side of greatest neurological dysfunction. Dorsal nerve rootlets may be sacrificed in certain patients to improve exposure. We routinely section the dentate ligaments to further augment anterolateral exposure and spinal cord mobilization as necessary. We prefer to shrink large venous varices early in the procedure to provide additional room for dissection. Under high magnification and with thorough irrigation, the nidus is coagulated and resected. Inflow arterial vessels are skeletonized and obliterated prior to sacrifice of the draining pedicles. In our practice, we routinely use multiple runs of ICG videoangiography at various points during the resection to identify residual pedicles. Embolic material casts from endovascular embolization can further assist in identification of feeding arteries.

We do not advocate chasing vascular loops of the malformations that may dive into the spinal cord parenchyma; we believe that it is better to truncate vessels embedded in the parenchyma at the pial surface rather than to seek deeper

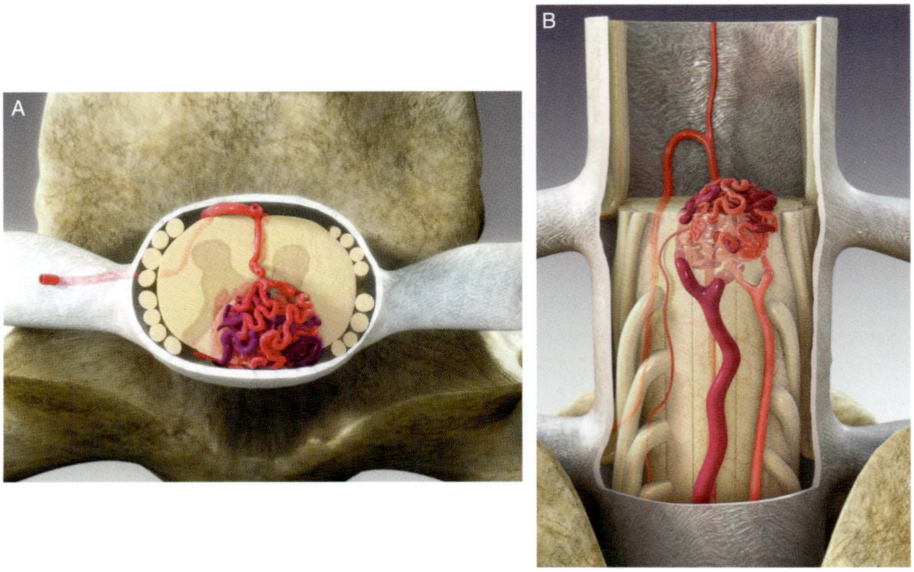

Fig. 14.5. Compact intramedullary arteriovenous malformations (AVM). (A) Axial view of a compact nidus. An arterial feeder from the anterior spinal artery can be identified. (B) Posterior view of the same lesion demonstrates additional feeding branches from the posterior spinal artery. Portions of the AVM are evident along the surface of the spinal cord while deeper loops of vessel may be present. (Used with permission from Barrow Neurological Institute.)

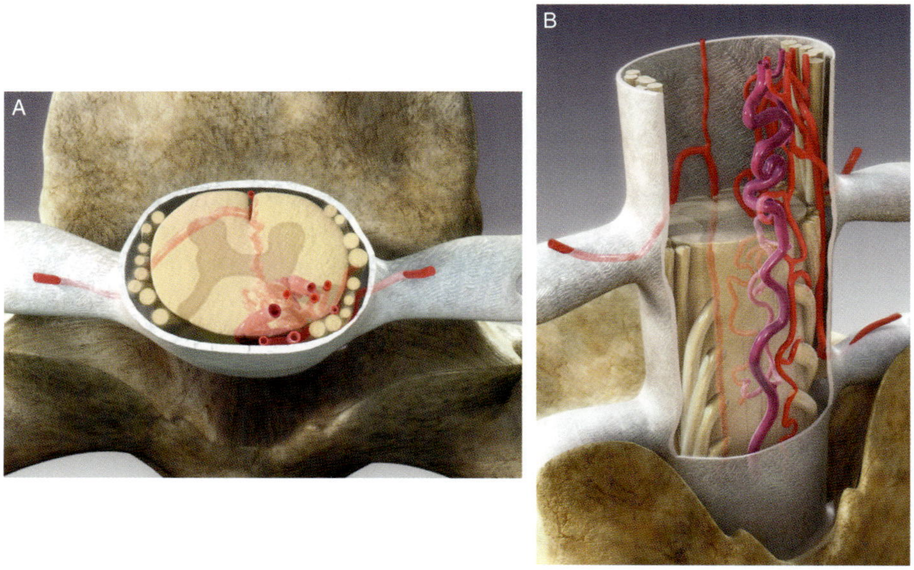

Fig. 14.6. Diffuse intramedullary arteriovenous malformations (AVM). (A) Axial view of a diffuse lesion with areas of intervening neural tissue between the intraparenchymal loops of the AVM. Portions of the AVM also course along the pial surface and subarachnoid space. (B) Oblique posterior view of the loops of the AVM coursing in and out of the spinal cord. This view accentuates the diffuse character of these lesions, with normal neural tissue present between loops of the AVM. (Used with permission from Barrow Neurological Institute.)

loops, which may cause neurologically devastating injury [10,36,43] (Fig. 14.7). Partial resection is performed in some patients and depends on which component of the AVM is causing the patient's symptoms, on the thoroughness of embolization, and on the flow dynamics of the AVM. It is prudent to leave completely embolized components of the AVM if resection would require additional pial dissection or results in changes in spinal monitoring. Specifically, in cases of large superficial AVMs with diving vessel loops that penetrate the spinal cord, we do not advocate following the diving vessels because the risk of causing neurological injury outweighs the benefit of complete resection (Fig. 14.8) [36]. In our hands, this technique has allowed for the resection of complex AVMs with minimal morbidity and often with improvement of premorbid deficits. In stark contrast to cranial AVMs, in which partial resection does not alter the natural history, so far, we have not encountered significant bleeding, spinal infarction, or neurological deterioration associated with partial resection of intramedullary AVMs. Care must be taken to work within the plane of gliotic tissue immediately surrounding the AVM and to prevent violation of adjacent, normal spinal cord tissue. Once resection is complete and hemostasis is obtained, the dura is closed, the myelotomy is repaired, and the wound is closed in the usual fashion.

Extradural–intradural arteriovenous malformations

Extradural–intradural AVMs are challenging lesions that involve neural structures, bone, and soft tissue along the affected spinal level and are usually impossible to resect completely, although a few cases have been reported (Fig. 14.9)

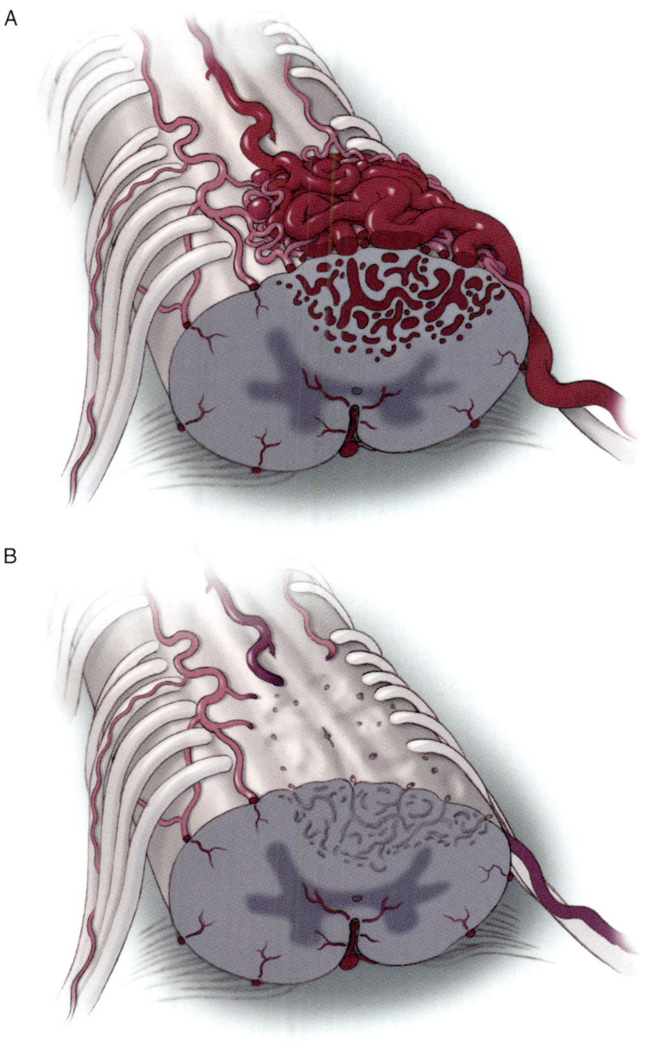

Fig. 14.7. Resection technique used for a glomus spinal arteriovenous malformations (AVM). (A) The AVM nidus extends through the spinal parenchyma into the extrapial space on the dorsal surface of the cord. (B) The extrapial portion of the AVM nidus has been resected, leaving the parenchymal portion of the nidus, including diving loops of vessels. Despite subtotal nidal resection, the glomus spinal AVM has been essentially devascularized and obliterated. (Used with permission from Barrow Neurological Institute.)

[44,46,47]. The surgical strategy for these lesions is to disconnect the large feeding vascular pedicles (thereby minimizing vascular steal and venous hypertension) and to decompress the mass effect along the nerve roots and spinal cord. These lesions usually contain multiple large feeders; therefore, surgery may result in significant bleeding. We recommend multiple stages of aggressive embolization of these lesions. The treatment goal is to decrease congestion caused by venous hypertension.

After routine exposure of extradural–intradural AVMs, we recommend identifying and disconnecting the easily accessible feeding pedicles. We do not recommend en bloc resection for these lesions because the procedure may result in significant bleeding and will likely harm residual neurological function. Considerable involvement of multiple structures makes these entities extremely difficult to treat. Although cures have been reported, the primary goal of treatment is usually palliative.

Conus medullaris arteriovenous malformations

Conus medullaris lesions typically exhibit multiple feeders from the anterior spinal artery and posterior spinal artery with direct arteriovenous shunts and large dilated veins (Fig. 14.10) [43]. These AVMs are treated with a combined endovascular and microsurgical approach. Angiography is used to identify the anterior and posterior spinal arteries and to embolize the feeders from these vessels. The venous vasculature associated with conus medullaris AVMs is vastly dilated, and surgical decompression and resection through a posterior approach can relieve neurological symptoms (Fig. 14.11). In our experience, aggressive combined treatment can result in good outcomes [43].

The surgical approach to conus medullaris lesions involves a posterior approach, and the positioning and exposure are similar to those used for other spinal AVMs. In our experience, many of these lesions have a glomus-type nidus with intramedullary and extramedullary components at the level of the conus [43]. The resection technique for the nidal component is similar to that used for intramedullary AVMs. The nidus may be associated with functional nerve roots at the conus, which can complicate resection. We do not recommend routine sacrifice of functional nerve roots to obtain complete resection. If venous aneurysms are identified, they should be obliterated and shrunken using electrocautery. The dura and wound are closed in the standard fashion.

Postoperative angiographic evaluation

Angiography must be used after resection to confirm the obliteration of the lesion. Initially, frequent radiographic and clinical follow-up should be performed; if recurrence does not occur, the interval can be lengthened. We recommend follow-up imaging at 1, 3, 5, and 10 years after treatment. In our experience, some patients develop tethering of the spinal cord after treatment; therefore, a return of symptoms should include evaluation for possible tethering of spinal elements. Any new neurological symptoms should be thoroughly investigated with MRI and catheter angiography as soon as possible.

Outcomes

Spinal vascular malformations are rare, and most reports in the literature are case reports or small case series (Table 14.2) [6,10,26,28,36,40,43,48–54]. The obliteration of the shunt and the associated vascular congestion improves symptoms and can be achieved through either microsurgical or endovascular methods. In most published series, both methods have resulted in acceptable outcomes.

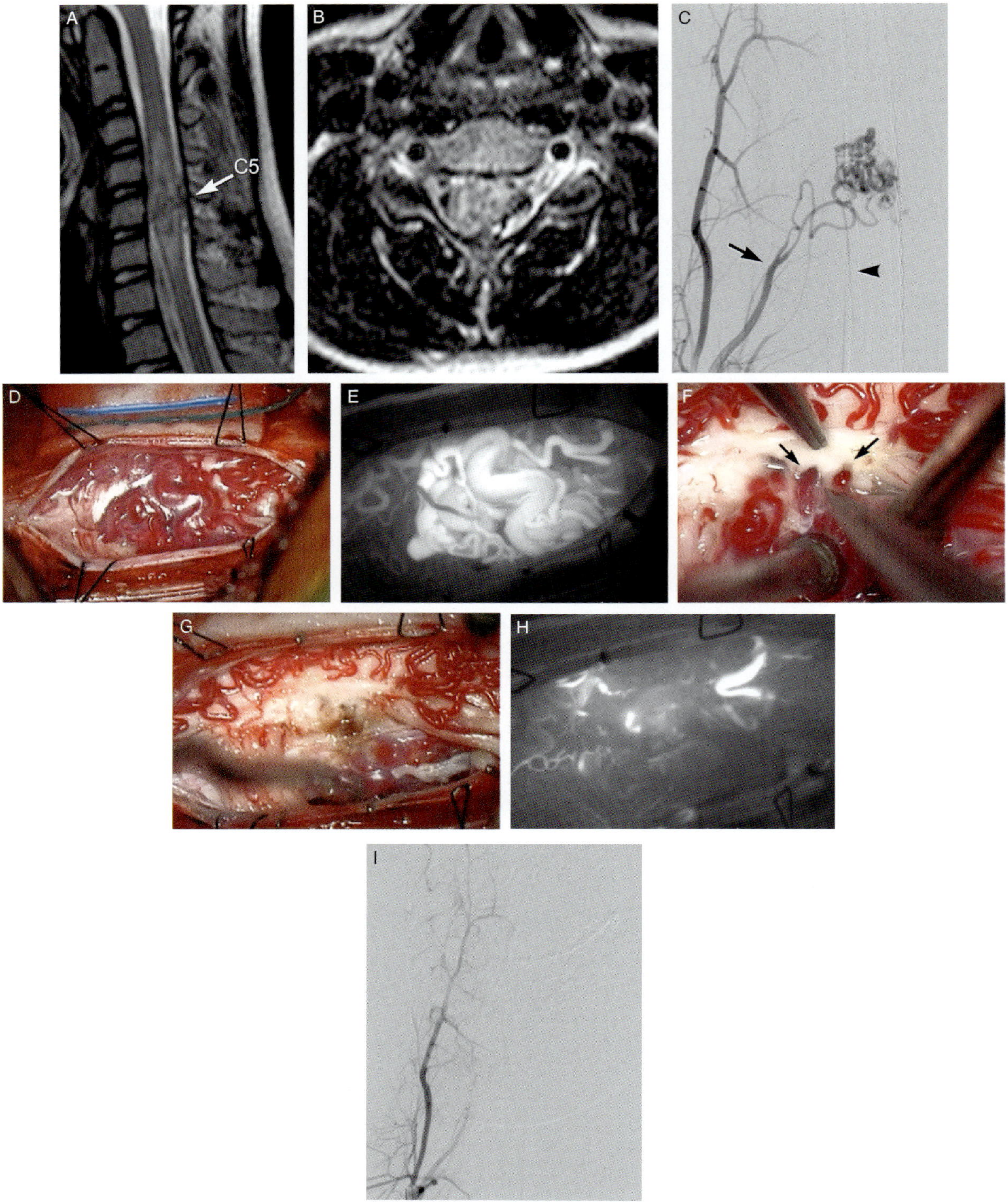

Fig. 14.8. A 12-year-old boy presented with progressive bilateral upper-extremity paresis and paresthesiae. (A,B) MRI shows characteristic flow voids and extensive edema consistent with the intramedullary C5 spinal arteriovenous malformations (AVM, arrow) (A, sagittal view; B, axial view). (C) Preoperative anteroposterior angiography demonstrates feeders from a right thyrocervical feeder (arrow). Given the contribution of this arterial pedicle to the anterior spinal artery (arrowhead), embolization was not performed. (D) Intraoperative photograph acquired after C4–C6 laminoplasties were performed, illustrating an extensive extrapial AVM nidus involving the posterolateral surface of the spinal cord. (E) Indocyanine green videoangiography demonstrated early filling of the extrapial AVM nidus. (F) The pial resection technique was used to devascularize the extrapial AVM nidus. Sharp dissection was used to expose vascular pedicles that traverse the spinal cord parenchyma (arrows) prior to coagulation and division. (G) The extrapial portion of the AVM nidus was resected along the posterolateral margin of the spinal cord. (H) Indocyanine green videoangiography confirmed resection of the extrapial AVM nidus. (I) Postoperative anteroposterior angiography of the right thyrocervical artery verified complete obliteration of the AVM despite the subtotal nidal resection achieved using the pial resection technique. (A–C, I reprinted from Velat *et al.*, 2012 [36], with permission from the American Association of Neurological Surgeons; D–H used with permission from Barrow Neurological Institute.)

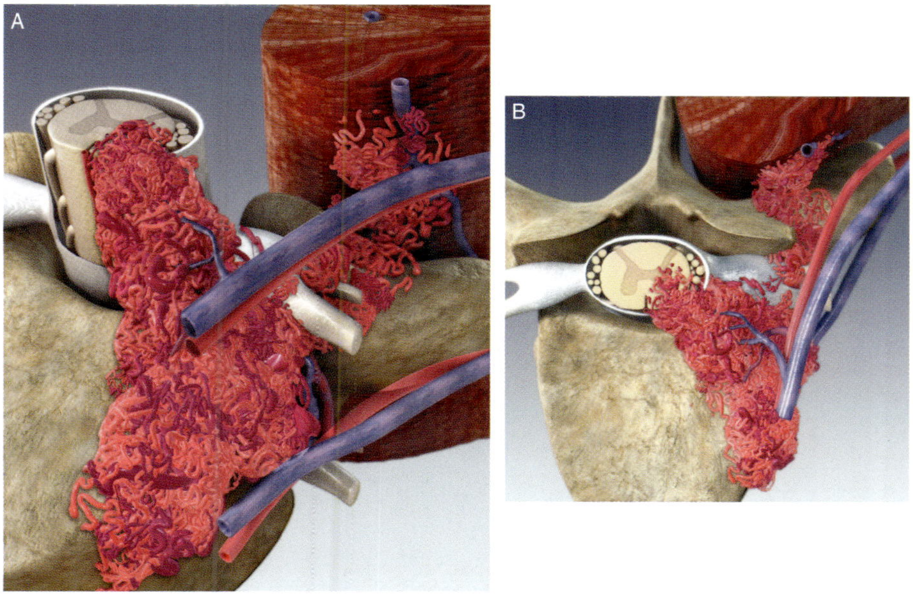

Fig. 14.9. Extradural–intradural arteriovenous malformations. (A,B) Anterolateral oblique (A) and axial (B) illustrations of this complex pathology. These lesions can encompass soft tissues, bone, spinal canal, spinal cord, and spinal nerve roots along an entire spinal level. (Used with permission from Barrow Neurological Institute.)

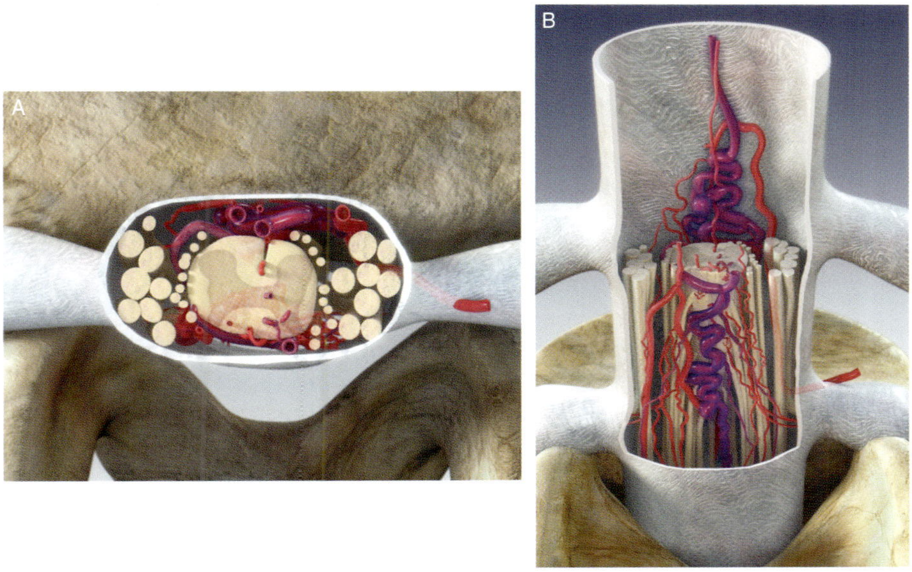

Fig. 14.10. Conus medullaris arteriovenous malformations (AVM). (A) Axial view of feeding arteries and draining veins from both the anterior and posterior aspects of the spinal cord. Note the proximity of the AVM to branches of the cauda equina. (B) Posterior view recapitulates the complexity of the angioarchitecture of these lesions. Conus medullaris AVMs can consist of regions of direct arteriovenous shunts and regions of true AVM nidus. (Used with permission from Barrow Neurological Institute.)

Logue reported the first large series (24 patients) of treatment of spinal AVFs by directly clipping the feeding artery and removing the related dura; 15 patients (62.5%) showed improvement in motor symptoms [50]. Subsequently, Symon and colleagues showed improvement in motor symptoms in 32 of 46 patients (69%) [55]. More recently, obliteration rates as high as 100% with improvement in 91% of patients treated with surgery, have been reported [54]. The results of the endovascular treatment of spinal AVFs are variable, with successful obliteration rates between 30 and 90%. Recanalization has been reported more frequently after endovascular procedures than after surgery and has reached up to 19% in some series [23].

Spinal AVMs are much rarer than spinal AVFs, and, consequently, there is a paucity of data on treatment outcomes. In 41 patients who underwent surgical treatment, complete exclusion of the spinal AVM was reported for 30 (73%), with improvement of symptoms in 20 (48%) of patients and worsening of symptoms in 8 (19.5%) [56]. Rosenblum and colleagues reported improvement of motor symptoms in 73% of patients in their series [6], and Anson and Spetzler reported improvement in motor function after surgery in 17 of 24 patients (71%) and stabilization of symptoms in 6 of the 24 (25%) [51]. Mourier and colleagues reported improvements in 10 of a series of 20 patients (50%) [57,58]. In 2012, we reported our results from a series of 20 patients with intramedullary spinal AVMs, which achieved an obliteration rate of 75% [36]. Of note, 70% of patients were functionally independent at long-term follow-up.

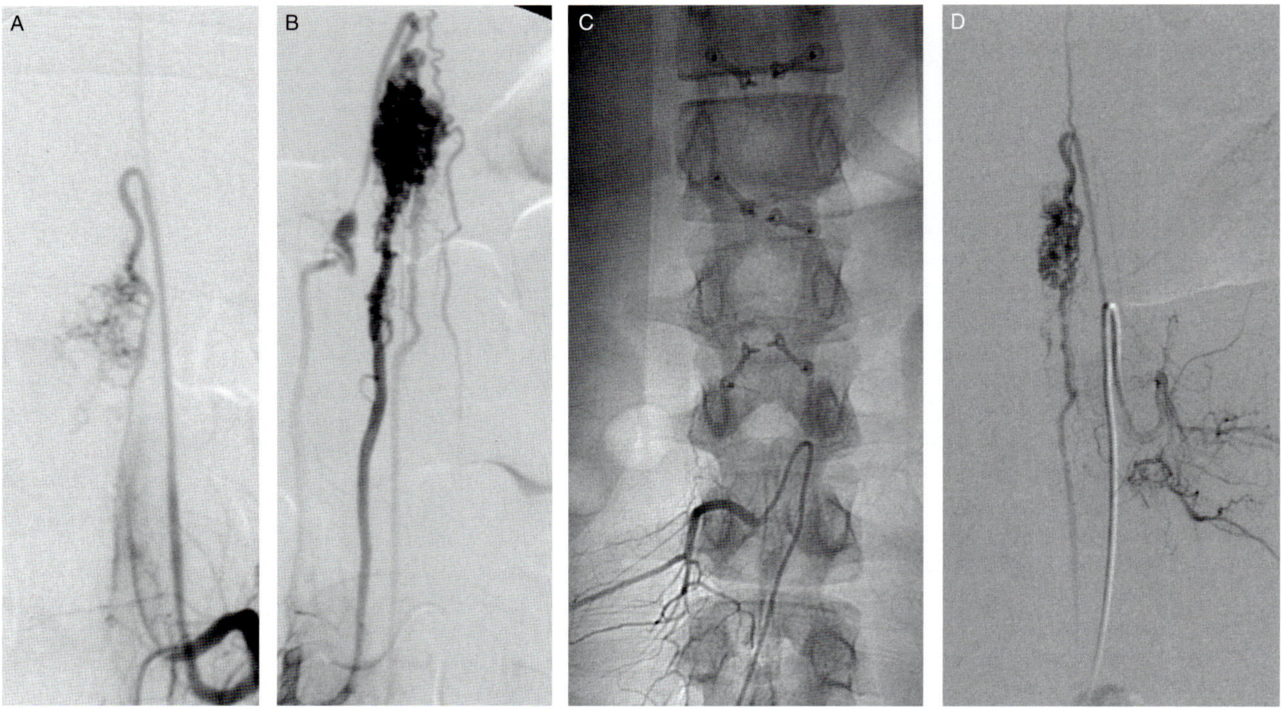

Fig. 14.11. Partial treatment of a conus medullaris arteriovenous malformations (AVM). (A,B) Spinal angiography before treatment demonstrated arterial supply to the lesion from the left L1 (A) and right L3 (B) radicular arteries. The right L3 feeder was embolized with *N*-butyl cyanoacrylate. Intraoperatively, after most of the AVM nidus was resected, a portion of nidus supplied by the left L1 radicular artery was invested within the conus medullaris. This portion of the nidus was not completely resected. (C,D) Post-treatment angiography showed obliteration of feeders from the right L3 radicular artery (C) and expected residual supply from the left L1 feeder (D). (Used with permission from Barrow Neurological Institute.)

Wilson *et al.* have reported their results from combined endovascular and microsurgical treatment of 16 conus medullaris AVMs, in which they achieved complete angiographic obliteration in 88% [43]. At last follow-up (mean, 70 months), 43% of patients had improved neurologically, 43% were stable, and 14% had declined relative to their pretreatment examination. All patients who were ambulatory before treatment remained ambulatory at follow-up, and 75% of patients who were non-ambulatory before treatment became ambulatory.

In 2012, we published a series of nine children with spinal AMVs who underwent combined microsurgical and endovascular treatment; the children achieved a mean improvement of at least 1 point on the World Health Organization/Zubrod score, with one recurrence [10].

Factors influencing outcomes

Clinical outcomes for patients with spinal AVMs and AVFs are correlated with the clinical presentation at the time of surgery: patients who present with minimal neurological impairment are more likely to experience better outcomes than those presenting in a neurologically devastated condition. However, patients who present with severe neurological impairment tend to stabilize neurologically and may improve after surgery. In patients undergoing intensive rehabilitation, control of micturition and independent ambulation are the abilities that are most likely to improve. In contrast to motor deficits, sensory deficits and sphincter disturbances are less responsive to treatment. After successful surgical or endovascular treatment, almost all patients will improve an average of 1 to 2 points on the Aminoff–Logue scale. Motor improvements are the most widely reported, and at least 70% of patients exhibit them to some degree [23]. In published reports, sensory symptoms improved in 12–43% of patients but declined in 14–22%. Sphincter disturbances usually do not improve, with one series reporting improvements in a modest 15% of patients [23]. The correlation between patient age and clinical outcome is well established, with younger patients exhibiting better outcomes [59].

Onset of symptoms

The time between the onset of symptoms and treatment is not associated with operative outcomes in most series [23]. In most patients with spinal AVFs, neurological symptoms present progressively, whereas in patients with spinal AVMs, an acute presentation is more common. Cenzato and colleagues reported that a gradual onset of symptoms was linked to greater neurological recovery than an acute presentation [28].

Length and intensity of symptoms

Most authors agree that no correlation exists between the duration of symptoms and postoperative outcomes. In a

Table 14.2. Surgical series on management of spinal vascular malformations

Study	No. patients	Adjuvant embolization	Type[a]	Mean follow-up (years)	Good or independent outcome (%)	Perioperative complication rate (%)	Perioperative obliteration rate (%) (imaging modality)
Cogen and Stein (1983) [48]	6	No	N/A	5	83	N/A	N/A
Yaşargil *et al.* (1984) [49]	41	No	II	2.9	80.1 (48.4 improved; 31.7 stable)	N/A	60
Logue (1979) [50]	24	No	N/A	5	87.5	12.5	N/A
Rosenblum *et al.* (1987) [6]	14	Yes	II	N/A	73	N/A	N/A
Anson and Spetzler (1995) [51]	24	No	I	N/A	71 improved; 25 stable	N/A	N/A
van Dijk *et al.* (2002) [26]	35	Yes	I	2.7	N/A	3	N/A
Velat *et al.* (2012) [36]	20	Yes	II	3.8	70	5	75 (angio)
Wilson *et al.* (2012) [43]	16	Yes	V	5.9	85	8.3	88 (angio)
Connolly *et al.* (1998) [40]	15	Yes	II	8.9	67	7	93 (angio)
Zozulya *et al.* (2006) [52]	30	Yes	II	N/A	87	N/A	100 (N/A)
Boström *et al.* (2009) [53]	12	Yes	II	3.9	80	8	83 (8 patients angio, 2 patients MRI)
Ropper *et al.* (2012) [54]	11	No	I	0.4 (4.7 months)	100	0	100 (angio)
Cenzato *et al.* (2012) [28]	55	No	I	3	80	0	100 (angio)
Kalani *et al.* (2012) [10]	9	Yes	II, V	2.4	77.8	12.5	88.9 (angio)

N/A, not available; angio, angiography.
[a]Types: Ia, intradural dorsal arteriovenous fistula; II, intramedullary arteriovenous malformation; V, conus arteriovenous malformation.

retrospective chart review of 65 patients, Cenzato and colleagues found no statistical correlation between the duration of pretreatment clinical symptoms and post-treatment improvement [28].

Location of the shunt

Spinal AVMs may be seen with equal probability at any level, whereas spinal AVFs are more commonly seen at the middle and lower thoracic and upper lumbar spine levels. Cenzato and colleagues reported a significant association between dural AVFs located in the lower thoracic spine and better motor outcomes. They postulated that the rich vasculature in this region decreased the degree of ischemia and lessened the likelihood of ischemic injury to the spinal cord [28].

Conclusions

Effective treatment of spinal AVFs and AVMs depends on reducing congestion caused by shunting through the aberrant arteriovenous connection. Despite their complex angioarchitecture, spinal vascular malformations are amenable to combined therapy consisting of endovascular embolization and microsurgical resection. Even with varied clinical presentations, patients tend to improve after treatment. Residual AVM in the spine does not appear to have the same natural history as its cranial counterpart. In the case of spinal AVFs and simple AVMs, complete obliteration should be the goal; however, with complex glomus AVMs, partial devascularization and resection of exophytic components without resection of the deeper components appears to lead to satisfactory clinical outcomes. Patients with these lesions require long-term follow-up. Given the high incidence of spinal AVMs with other inherited disorders of the vasculature, workup for syndromes including Klippel–Trénaunay–Weber syndrome, familial cavernous malformations, and hereditary hemorrhagic telangiectasia is recommended.

References

1. Hebold O. Aneurysms der Kleisnten Rucken Marksgefass. *Arch Psychiatr Nervnkr* 1885;**16**:813.
2. Gaupp J. Hamorrhoiden der Pia Mater Spinalis im Gebiet des Lendenmarks. *Beitr Pathol* 1888;516–18.
3. Krause F. *Chirurgie des Gehirns und Rückenmarks*. Berlin: Urban & Schwarzenberg, 1911.
4. Wyburn-Mason R. *The Vascular Abnormalities and Tumours of the Spinal Cord and its Membranes*. London: Klimptom, 1943.
5. Aminoff MJ, Logue V. The prognosis of patients with spinal vascular malformations. *Brain* 1974;**97**: 211–18.
6. Rosenblum B, Oldfield EH, Doppman JL, *et al.* Spinal arteriovenous malformations: a comparison of dural arteriovenous fistulas and intradural AVMs in 81 patients. *J Neurosurg* 1987;**67**:795–802.
7. da Costa L, Dehdashti AR, terBrugge KG. Spinal cord vascular shunts: spinal cord vascular malformations and dural arteriovenous fistulas. *Neurosurg Focus* 2009;**26**:E6.
8. Steinmetz MP, Chow MM, Krishnaney AA, *et al.* Outcome after the treatment of spinal dural arteriovenous fistulae: a contemporary single-institution series and meta-analysis. *Neurosurgery* 2004;**55**:77–87.
9. Alexander MJ, Grossi PM, Spetzler RF, *et al.* Extradural thoracic arteriovenous malformation in a patient with Klippel–Trénaunay–Weber syndrome: case report. *Neurosurgery* 2002;**51**:1275–8.
10. Kalani MY, Ahmed AS, Martirosyan NL, *et al.* Surgical and endovascular treatment of pediatric spinal arteriovenous malformations. *World Neurosurg* 2012;**78**:348–54.
11. Iizuka Y, Suzuki M, Komura S, *et al.* Conus medullaris spinal arteriovenous malformation in a patient with Klippel–Trénaunay–Weber syndrome. A case report and review of the literature. *Interv Neuroradiol* 2008;**14**:185–90.
12. Rohany M, Shaibani A, Arafat O, *et al.* Spinal arteriovenous malformations associated with Klippel–Trénaunay–Weber syndrome: a literature search and report of two cases. *AJNR Am J Neuroradiol* 2007;**28**:584–9.
13. Poisson A, Vasdev A, Brunelle F, *et al.* Acute paraplegia due to spinal arteriovenous fistula in two patients with hereditary hemorrhagic telangiectasia. *Eur J Pediatr* 2009;**168**:135–9.
14. Kaplan P, Hollenberg RD, Fraser FC. A spinal arteriovenous malformation with hereditary cutaneous hemangiomas. *Am J Dis Child* 1976;**130**:1329–31.
15. Hu MH, Wu CT, Lin KL, *et al.* Intramedullary spinal arteriovenous malformation in a boy of familial cerebral cavernous hemangioma. *Childs Nerv Syst* 2008;**24**:393–6.
16. Rosenow J, Rawanduzy A, Weitzner I, Jr., *et al.* Type IV spinal arteriovenous malformations in association with familial pulmonary vascular malformation: case report. *Neurosurgery* 2000;**46**:1240–4.
17. Muralidharan R, Saladino A, Lanzino G, *et al.* The clinical and radiological presentation of spinal dural arteriovenous fistula. *Spine (Phila Pa 1976)* 2011;**36**:E1641–7.
18. Rodesch G, Hurth M, Alvarez H, *et al.* Classification of spinal cord arteriovenous shunts: proposal for a reappraisal – the Bicêtre experience with 155 consecutive patients treated between 1981 and 1999. *Neurosurgery* 2002;**51**:374–9.
19. Kim DJ, Willinsky R, Geibprasert S, *et al.* Angiographic characteristics and treatment of cervical spinal dural arteriovenous shunts. *AJNR Am J Neuroradiol* 2010;**31**:1512–15.
20. Eskandar EN, Borges LF, Budzik RF, Jr., *et al.* Spinal dural arteriovenous fistulas: experience with endovascular and surgical therapy. *J Neurosurg* 2002;**96**:162–7.
21. Berenstein A, Lasjaunias P, terBrugge KG, Lasjaunias PL. Spinal dural arteriovenous fistulae. In Berenstein A, Lasjaunias P, terBrugge KG, eds. *Surgical Neuroangiography:* Vol. 2. *Clinical and Endovascular Treatment Aspects in Adults*. New York: Springer, 2004, pp. 847–72.
22. Berenstein A, Lasjaunias P, terBrugge KG, Lasjaunias PL. Spinal arteriovenous malformations. In Berenstein A, Lasjaunias P, terBrugge KG, eds. *Surgical Neuroangiography:* Vol. 2. *Clinical and Endovascular Treatment Aspects in Adults*. New York: Springer, 2004, pp. 738–847.
23. Fugate JE, Lanzino G, Rabinstein AA. Clinical presentation and prognostic factors of spinal dural arteriovenous fistulas: an overview. *Neurosurg Focus* 2012;**32**:E17.
24. Jellema K, Canta LR, Tijssen CC, *et al.* Spinal dural arteriovenous fistulas: clinical features in 80 patients. *J Neurol Neurosurg Psychiatry* 2003;**74**:1438–40.
25. Sato K, terBrugge KG, Krings T. Asymptomatic spinal dural arteriovenous fistulas: pathomechanical considerations. *J Neurosurg Spine* 2012;**16**:441–6.
26. van Dijk JM, terBrugge KG, Willinsky RA, *et al.* Multidisciplinary management of spinal dural arteriovenous fistulas: clinical

presentation and long-term follow-up in 49 patients. *Stroke* 2002;**33**:1578–83.

27. Raynor RB, Weiner R. Transthoracic approach to an intramedullary vascular malformation of the thoracic spinal cord. *Neurosurgery* 1982;**10**:631–4.
28. Cenzato M, Debernardi A, Stefini R, *et al.* Spinal dural arteriovenous fistulas: outcome and prognostic factors. *Neurosurg Focus* 2012;**32**:E11.
29. Mull M, Nijenhuis RJ, Backes WH, *et al.* Value and limitations of contrast-enhanced MR angiography in spinal arteriovenous malformations and dural arteriovenous fistulas. *AJNR Am J Neuroradiol* 2007;**28**:1249–58.
30. Elsberg C. *Treatment of Surgical Diseases of Spinal Cord and its Membranes*. Philadelphia, PA: Saunders, 1916.
31. Foix C, Alajouanine T. La myélite nécrotique subaique: myélite central angéiphypertrophique a évolution progressive: paraplégie amyotrophique lentement ascendante, d'abord spasmodique, puis flasque, s'accompagnant de dissociation, albumino-cytologique. *Rev Neurol* 1926;**2**:1–42.
32. Kendall BE, Logue V. Spinal epidural angiomatous malformations draining into intrathecal veins. *Neuroradiology* 1977;**13**:181–9.
33. Borden JA, Wu JK, Shucart WA. A proposed classification for spinal and cranial dural arteriovenous fistulous malformations and implications for treatment. *J Neurosurg* 1995;**82**:166–79.
34. Kim LJ, Spetzler RF. Classification and surgical management of spinal arteriovenous lesions: arteriovenous fistulae and arteriovenous malformations. *Neurosurgery* 2006;**59**: S195–201.
35. Ducruet AF, Crowley RW, McDougall CG, *et al.* Endovascular management of spinal arteriovenous malformations. *J Neurointerv Surg* 2012.
36. Velat GJ, Chang SW, Abla AA, *et al.* Microsurgical management of glomus spinal arteriovenous malformations: pial resection technique – clinical article. *J Neurosurg Spine* 2012;**16**:523–31.
37. Killory BD, Nakaji P, Maughan PH, *et al.* Evaluation of angiographically occult spinal dural arteriovenous fistulae with surgical microscope-integrated intraoperative near-infrared indocyanine green angiography: report of 3 cases. *Neurosurgery* 2011;**68**:781–7.
38. Oh JK, Shin HC, Kim TY, *et al.* Intraoperative indocyanine green video-angiography: spinal dural arteriovenous fistula. *Spine (Phila Pa 1976)* 2011;**36**: E1578–80.
39. Anson JA, Spetzler RF. Classification of spinal arteriovenous malformations and implications for treatment. *BNI Quarterly* 1992;**8**:2–8.
40. Connolly ES, Jr., Zubay GP, McCormick PC, *et al.* The posterior approach to a series of glomus type II intramedullary spinal cord arteriovenous malformations. *Neurosurgery* 1998;**42**:774–85.
41. Spetzler RF, Detwiler PW, Riina HA, *et al.* Modified classification of spinal cord vascular lesions. *J Neurosurg* 2002;**96**:145–56.
42. Ausman JI, Gold LH, Tadavarthy SM, *et al.* Intraparenchymal embolization for obliteration of an intramedullary AVM of the spinal cord. *J Neurosurg* 1977;**47**:119–25.
43. Wilson DA, Abla AA, Uschold TD, *et al.* Multimodality treatment of conus medullaris arteriovenous malformations: 2 decades of experience with combined endovascular and microsurgical treatments. *Neurosurgery* 2012;**71**:100–8.
44. Martin NA, Khanna RK, Batzdorf U. Posterolateral cervical or thoracic approach with spinal cord rotation for vascular malformations or tumors of the ventrolateral spinal cord. *J Neurosurg* 1995;**83**:254–61.
45. Williams FC, Zabramski JM, Spetzler RF, *et al.* Anterolateral transthoracic transvertebral resection of an intramedullary spinal arteriovenous malformation. Case report. *J Neurosurg* 1991;**74**:1004–8.
46. Spetzler RF, Zabramski JM, Flom RA. Management of juvenile spinal AVMs by embolization and operative excision. Case report. *J Neurosurg* 1989;**70**:628–32.
47. Touho H, Karasawa J, Shishido H, *et al.* Successful excision of a juvenile-type spinal arteriovenous malformation following intraoperative embolization. Case report. *J Neurosurg* 1991;**75**:647–51.
48. Cogen P, Stein BM. Spinal cord arteriovenous malformations with significant intramedullary components. *J Neurosurg* 1983;**59**:471–8.
49. Yaşargil MG, Symon L, Teddy PJ. Arteriovenous malformations of the spinal cord. *Adv Tech Stand Neurosurg* 1984;**11**:61–102.
50. Logue V. Angiomas of the spinal cord: review of the pathogenesis, clinical features, and results of surgery. *J Neurol Neurosurg Psychiatry* 1979;**42**:1–11.
51. Anson JA, Spetzler RF. Spinal arteriovenous malformations: surgical treatment. In Carter LP, Spetzler RF, Hamilton MG, eds. *Neurovascular Surgery*. New York: McGraw-Hill, 1995, pp. 1197–212.
52. Zozulya YP, Slin'ko EI, Al-Qashqish II. Spinal arteriovenous malformations: new classification and surgical treatment. *Neurosurg Focus* 2006;**20**:E7.
53. Boström A, Krings T, Hans FJ, *et al.* Spinal glomus-type arteriovenous malformations: microsurgical treatment in 20 cases. *J Neurosurg Spine* 2009;**10**:423–9.
54. Ropper AE, Gross BA, Du R. Surgical treatment of type I spinal dural arteriovenous fistulas. *Neurosurg Focus* 2012;**32**:E3.
55. Symon L, Kuyama H, Kendall B. Dural arteriovenous malformations of the spine. Clinical features and surgical results in 55 cases. *J Neurosurg* 1984;**60**:238–47.
56. Yaşargil MG, DeLong WB, Guarnaschelli JJ. Complete microsurgical excision of cervical extramedullary and intramedullary vascular malformations. *Surg Neurol* 1975;**4**:211–24.

57. Mourier KL, Gelbert F, Rey A, *et al.* Spinal dural arteriovenous malformations with perimedullary drainage. Indications and results of surgery in 30 cases. *Acta Neurochir (Wein)* 1989;**100**:136–41.

58. Mourier KL, Gobin YP, George B, *et al.* Intradural perimedullary arteriovenous fistulae: results of surgical and endovascular treatment in a series of 35 cases. *Neurosurgery* 1993;**32**:885–91.

59. Nagata S, Morioka T, Natori Y, *et al.* Factors that affect the surgical outcomes of spinal dural arteriovenous fistulas. *Surg Neurol* 2006;**65**:563–8.

Chapter 15

Surgery of basal ganglia, thalamic, and brainstem arteriovenous malformations

Matthew B. Potts, Seunggu J. Han, and Michael T. Lawton

Introduction

Surgical management of arteriovenous malformations (AVMs) of the basal ganglia, thalamus, and brainstem poses significant challenges that distinguish these lesions from more superficial AVMs. While convexity or cerebellar AVMs are approached with simple craniotomies that widely expose the nidus for safe, perpendicular dissection of margins, the deep location of basal ganglia, thalamic, and brainstem AVMs requires more elaborate surgical approaches. Such approaches provide limited exposure that often requires more tangential dissection of the AVM margins. In addition, the location of these deep AVMs within eloquent tissue and their supply by critical perforators adds to the surgical challenges. Consequently, neurosurgeons often favor stereotactic radiosurgery or observation over surgical resection for these lesions. However, AVMs of the basal ganglia, thalamus, and brainstem have more aggressive natural histories than other AVMs and, therefore, warrant intervention. Annual hemorrhage rates have been reported to be as high as 10–34% [1–3], with associated hemiparesis rates up to 85% [1] and mortality rates as high as 63% [4]. These lesions also have increased risks associated with radiosurgical management because the basal ganglia, thalamus, and brainstem are exquisitely sensitive to radiation side-effects and hemorrhage during the latency period [5–10]. Finally, radiosurgical obliteration rates with deep-seated AVMs are lower than in other locations [6,11]. For these reasons, experienced neurosurgeons have challenged the belief that AVMs of the basal ganglia, thalamus, and brainstem are inoperable [12]. As discussed here, with careful patient selection and a firm understanding of the relevant anatomy, microsurgical resection of basal ganglia, thalamic, and brainstem AVMs can be a safe and definitive treatment.

Relevant anatomy

Basal ganglia and thalamic arteriovenous malformations

The basal ganglia and thalamus originate from the deep core of the cerebrum where the telencephalon and diencephalon fuse during embryological development. This complex region has been variably described as the insular block, central area, and central core, among other names. Surgically, it is most informative to divide this region into the basal ganglia, thalamus, and insula.

An AVM of the basal ganglia lies deep to the insular cortex and extends into the caudate nucleus, putamen, globus pallidus, and/or the anterior limb of the internal capsule. It also sits lateral to the posterior limb of the internal capsule and deep to the M2 segments of the middle cerebral artery (MCA). Conversely, thalamic AVMs lie in the thalamus medial to the posterior limb of the internal capsule.

The vascular supply to basal ganglia and thalamic AVMs also distinguishes these two lesions. Basal ganglia AVMs are supplied by the anterior choroidal artery and/or MCA branches, including large branches from the M2 segment, small insular perforators, and lenticulostriate arteries from the M1 segment. In contrast, thalamic AVMs are supplied from below by thalamoperforating arteries from the posterior communicating artery and the P1 segment of the posterior cerebral artery (PCA), the posterior choroidal arteries (lateral more often than medial), and the anterior choroidal artery. Feeding arteries to basal ganglia and thalamic AVMs are often en passage arteries that continue on to supply normal brain in distal territories. In addition, the distal perforators feeding these deep AVMs are often small in caliber. For these reasons, preoperative embolization is both difficult and risky and is performed less often than with more superficial AVMs [12,13].

Venous drainage of basal ganglia and thalamic AVMs is most often deep, draining medially into thalamostriate and internal cerebral veins or inferiorly to the basal veins of Rosenthal. Superficial drainage is much less common and is through lateral subependymal veins and sylvian veins. In our experience, we have only seen deep drainage in thalamic AVMs, but have seen superficial drainage in approximately 20% of basal ganglia AVMs. When present, arterialized sylvian veins are good landmarks to basal ganglia AVMs during a trans-sylvian–transinsular approach. Similarly, arterialized ventricular veins are good landmarks for thalamic and basal ganglia AVMs during transcallosal-transventricular approaches.

Comprehensive Management of Arteriovenous Malformations of the Brain and Spine, ed. Robert F. Spetzler, Douglas S. Kondziolka, Randall T. Higashida, and M. Yashar S. Kalani. Published by Cambridge University Press. © Cambridge University Press 2015.

Brainstem arteriovenous malformations

The brainstem arises from two of the primary neural vesicles: the mesencephalon, which gives rise to the midbrain, and the rhombencephalon, which ultimately gives rise to the cerebellum, pons, and medulla. The three structures comprising the brainstem – midbrain, pons, and medulla – contain the nuclei for all cranial nerves except I, II, and XI, as well as all motor, sensory, and autonomic pathways traveling between the cerebrum, spinal cord, and cerebellum. It is, therefore, not surprising that both microsurgical and radiosurgical treatments of brainstem AVMs carry such high risks. In our experience, brainstem AVMs are most commonly found in six general locations: anterior and posterior midbrain, anterior and lateral pons, and anterior and lateral medulla. These regions are associated with different cranial nerves, vascular supply, and venous drainage.

Anterior midbrain AVMs are intimately associated with the oculomotor nerves and cerebral peduncles. They lie amongst the thalamoperforators from the basilar bifurcation and the P1 segment of the PCA and are fed from these branches. Venous drainage is through anterior mesencephalic veins and the basal vein of Rosenthal. In this location, AVMs are rare but also affect highly eloquent areas. Conversely, posterior midbrain AVMs are associated with the quadrigeminal plate, trochlear nerves, and the Galenic venous complex. They are fed by branches from the superior cerebellar artery and sometimes PCA branches as well. Arterial supply is typically bilateral. Venous drainage is directly into the vein of Galen.

Anterior pontine AVMs lie on the anterior surface of the pons between the basilar trunk and the trigeminal root entry zone. The arterial supply is from the anterior inferior cerebellar artery and enlarged branches off the basilar trunk. The superior cerebellar artery will sometimes also contribute inferiorly directed branches to the nidus. Interestingly, these AVMs can also receive supply from dural arteries, specifically branches from the meningohypophyseal trunk that travel along Meckel's cave and the trigeminal nerve to reach the AVM nidus. These AVMs are intimately associated with the pons and the trigeminal nerve. Their medial location makes them difficult to visualize around the trigeminal nerve and they often infiltrate the nerve itself, without a clear plane of separation. Venous drainage can be medial through anterior pontine veins or laterally to the petrosal vein and superior petrosal sinus. In contrast, lateral pontine AVMs lie on the lateral surface of the pons between the trigeminal root and the cerebellopontine angle. There is variability in the extent of pial invasion, with some lying in the pia and others penetrating deeply into the cerebellar peduncles. This portion of the brachium pontis is tolerant of surgical transgression, unlike the body of the pons. Lateral pontine AVMs have arterial supply and venous drainage similar to anterior pontine AVMs.

Within the medulla, we have found that lateral medullary AVMs are the most common. The AVMs reside on the medullary surface lateral to the hypoglossal nerve rootlets and preolivary sulcus. They are mainly fed by small branches from the ipsilateral vertebral artery but also receive supply from the posterior inferior cerebellar artery. Venous drainage is typically through lateral or anterior medullary veins. They tend to be small in size and respectful of pia. Anterior medullary AVMs are rare and lie anterior to the hypoglossal rootlets. They are typically fed bilaterally from vertebral artery and posterior inferior cerebellar artery feeders and drain into anterior medullary veins.

Approaches

General considerations

Appropriate approach selection is critical to the successful microsurgical management of deep AVMs. In general, we favor generous craniotomies that maximize a given exposure. The working corridors for deep AVMs are often very narrow at their deepest extent so it is important to have room to maneuver more superficially. Patient positioning is also an important component of the surgical approaches used for deep AVMs. When possible, we position patients so that gravity can be used to retract the dependent hemisphere without the need for retractors. [14]. Finally, the presence of intraparenchymal hemorrhage surrounding a ruptured AVM should be used to the surgeon's advantage. Hematomas or encephalomalacia often provide a direct path to an AVM nidus through what would have otherwise been eloquent tissue.

Basal ganglia and thalamus

Three main approaches can be used to access AVMs of the basal ganglia and thalamus: trans-sylvian, transcallosal, and transcortical. Most AVMs of the basal ganglia and rare anteriorly located thalamic AVMs can be accessed through a trans-sylvian–transinsular approach. Two distinct variants of this approach exist: anterior and posterior. Both approaches require wide splitting of the sylvian fissure to expose the insular cortex, but they differ in the direction of the sylvian fissure split. With the anterior trans-sylvian–transinsular approach, the dissection parallels the sphenoid portion of the sylvian cistern and is directed at the sphenoidal (M1) and insular (M2) segments of the MCA. Final exposure accesses the limen insulae and short gyri. With the posterior trans-sylvian–transinsular approach, the sylvian dissection parallels the opercular cleft and is directed along the opercular (M3) segments of the MCA (Fig. 15.1). Final exposure separates the opercular surfaces of the frontal, parietal, and temporal lobes and accesses the circular sulcus and long gyri of the insula. Both approaches preserve frontal, parietal, and temporal cortex around the sylvian fissure but access the lesion by crossing insular cortex, working through the candelabra of MCA vessels.

Both trans-sylvian–transinsular approaches use a pterional craniotomy for access to the sylvian fissure. With the anterior approach, the head is positioned as it would be for an MCA aneurysm – it is rotated 15–20 degrees away from the side of the lesion and extended 20 degrees. This position aligns the plane of the proximal sylvian fissure vertically, allowing the frontal and temporal lobes to fall naturally to either side as the fissure is split. This eliminates the need for retractors during the sylvian

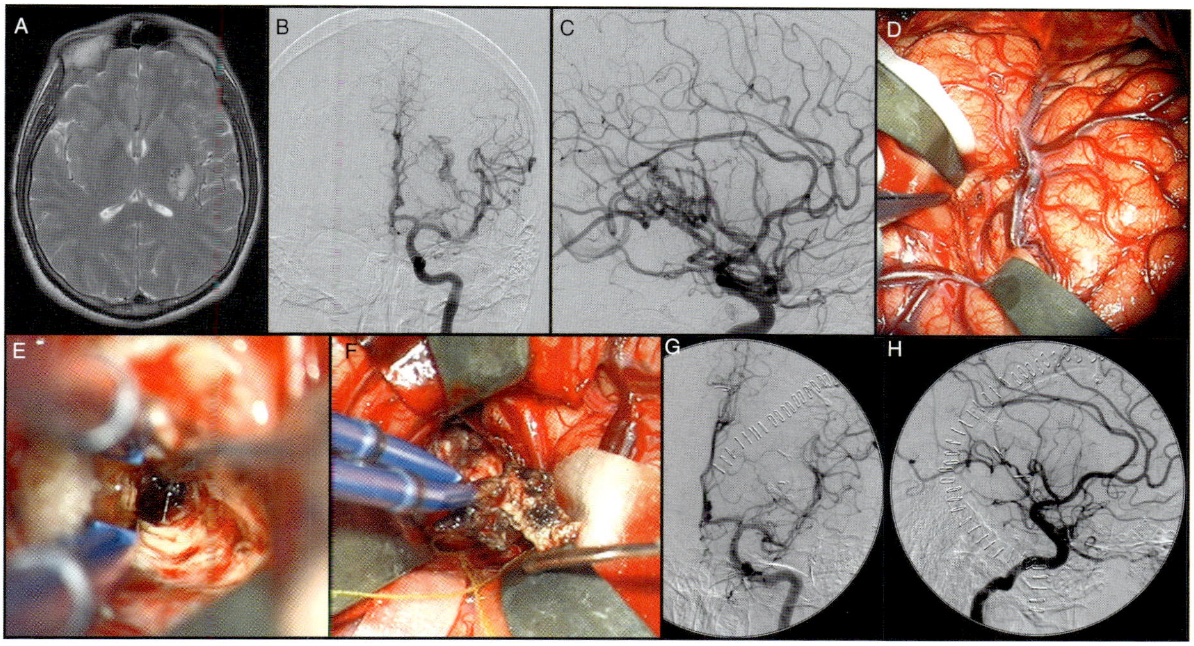

Fig. 15.1. Case example of the posterior trans-sylvian approach. This 26-year-old patient presented with right hemisensory loss resulting from hemorrhage from a small arteriovenous malformation (AVM) in the left putamen behind the posterior limb of the internal capsule. (A) Axial T_2-weighted MRI of the lesion. (B,C). Digital subtraction angiography with left internal carotid artery injection revealed a modified Spetzler–Martin grade III, supplementary grade II AVM (B, anteroposterior view; C, lateral view). (D) The AVM was exposed through a posterior trans-sylvian–transinsular approach. Splitting the left distal sylvian fissure opened the opercular cleft, preserved overlying sylvian veins, and exposed insular M2 segments. (E) Transinsular dissection through the long gyrus led to the hematoma associated with the nidus. (F) The AVM was dissected circumferentially and removed completely. The posterior trans-sylvian–transinsular approach preserved language cortex and the patient awoke with no language deficit, but did have a mild hemiparesis related to dissection near the internal capsule. (G,H) Postoperative angiography confirmed complete AVM resection (left internal carotid artery injection; G, anteroposterior view; H, lateral view).

fissure dissection. With the posterior approach, the head is positioned nearly laterally to align the plane of the opercular cleft vertically, again allowing the frontal and temporal lobes to separate naturally to either side. A standard pterional skin incision is used with the anterior approach whereas a "question mark" incision is used for the posterior approach to allow a more posterior exposure of the angular gyrus. Similarly, a standard pterional craniotomy is used with the anterior approach while additional parietal and posterior temporal bone is incorporated into the craniotomy used with the posterior trans-sylvian–transinsular approach.

Another variant of the trans-sylvian approach that can be used for inferomedially located basal ganglia AVMs (i.e., globus pallidus) is the supracarotid–infrafrontal approach [15]. This approach exploits the supracarotid triangle between the A1 segment of the anterior cerebral artery and the M1 segment of the MCA to pass medial and inferior to the insula through the medial orbital gyrus of the frontal lobe. The trajectory of this approach is directed superiorly and, therefore, requires an orbitozygomatic craniotomy to increase the upward viewing angle.

Transcallosal approaches are most often employed for thalamic AVMs or superolateral basal ganglia AVMs (i.e., head of caudate). The transcallosal approaches expose the midline, dissect the interhemispheric fissure, traverse the corpus callosum, and extend transventricularly to reach medial targets through the ependyma [16,17]. These approaches do not typically access any cortical tissue but only a portion of corpus callosum. Variations include anterior, posterior, ipsilateral, contralateral, and transchoroidal fissure. The anterior–ipsilateral transcallosal approach offers a direct view of the floor of the lateral ventricle and superior thalamus, whereas the anterior–contralateral transcallosal creates a steeper viewing angle across to the lateral wall of the ventricle and caudate nucleus. The transcallosal–transchoroidal approach deepens the exposure by opening the taenia fornicis of the choroid plexus, following the thalamostriate and internal cerebral veins into the roof of the third ventricle, and widening the foramen of Monro to gain access into the third ventricle (Fig. 15.2). This approach exposes the lateral wall of the third ventricle and medial thalamus. The posterior transcallosal approach crosses the splenium for a more posterior view of the superior thalamus. It also provides access to arterial feeders and draining veins around the Galenic complex that are inaccessible from anterior transcallosal approaches.

All of the transcallosal variations require a craniotomy that crosses the midline to expose the superior sagittal sinus. For the anterior approaches, the patient is positioned supine with the head turned laterally 90 degrees away from the lesion with the sagittal midline plane parallel to the floor. The neck is then flexed upwards about 45 degrees. This position allows gravity to retract the dependent hemisphere down away from the falx, opening up the interhemispheric fissure. The scalp incision is C-shaped, beginning at the widow's peak and coursing posteriorly and slightly across midline (to the side of the lesion) before arcing back across midline and anteriorly. The incision should

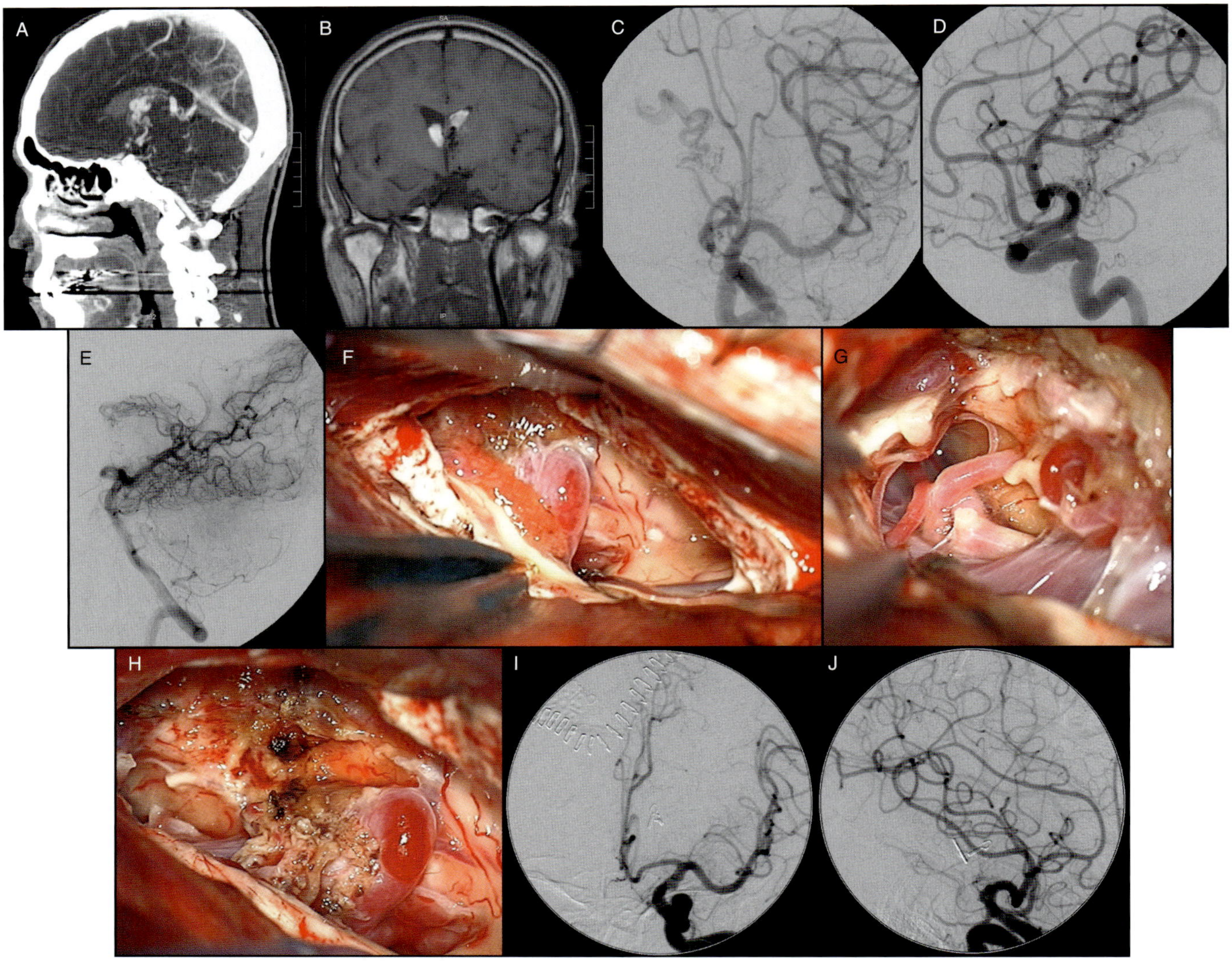

Fig. 15.2. Case example of the transcallosal–transchoroidal approach. This 45-year-old man presented with intraventricular hemorrhage from a left medial thalamic arteriovenous malformations (AVM). (A) Sagittal CT angiography. (B) Coronal T_1-weighted MRI. He was treated radiosurgically and had persistent AVM 5 years later. (C–E) Digital subtraction angiography showed that the AVM was supplied by anterior thalamoperforators from the internal carotid artery (ICA) terminus (left ICA injection; C, anterior oblique view; D, lateral view), and from the medial posterior choroidal artery (left vertebral artery injection; E, lateral view). His modified Spetzler–Martin grade was III, supplementary grade III. (F) The contralateral transcallosal approach exposed the left foramen of Monro (head turned to the right, right hemisphere down, and left-sided AVM up). (G) By opening the choroidal fissure between the fornix and choroid plexus, the foramen was enlarged, the velum interpositum was entered, and an arterialized internal cerebral vein was followed posteriorly to feeders from the posterior choroidal artery. (H) The AVM was dissected out of the thalamus and removed completely. (I,J) Postoperative angiography confirmed complete resection (left ICA injection; I, anteroposterior view; J, lateral view).

accommodate a craniotomy flap that is two-thirds anterior and one-third posterior to the coronal suture. The craniotomy crosses the superior sagittal sinus to allow dura to be retracted medially to the edge of the superior sagittal sinus and maximize access to the interhemispheric fissure without overhanging bone. Conversely, the posterior transcallosal approach requires a torcular craniotomy that exposes the junction of the superior sagittal sinus and transverse sinuses [18]. The patient is positioned in a lateral position with the head turned away from the lesion, the head flexed on the neck, and the neck extended on the shoulders. Care should be taken to avoid undue compression of cerebral venous outflow, which could increase venous pressures and therefore risk of intraoperative bleeding or AVM rupture. An upside-down U-shaped skin incision is made, starting below the superior nuchal line slightly across the midline on the side contralateral to the lesion, extending upward to the occiput, then going across and then down just behind the ear on the side ipsilateral to the lesion. While the craniotomy is centered over the ipsilateral occipital lobe, it traverses both the superior sagittal sinus and bilateral transverse sinuses to expose the entire torcula. The dura is opened over the ipsilateral occipital lobe and typically flapped in two pieces: one towards the superior sagittal sinus and one towards the ipsilateral transverse sinus.

A variation of the contralateral transcallosal approach is the contralateral transcingulate approach [19]. While this approach is typically used for lesions within the cingulate gyrus and deep white matter of the frontal lobe, it can also be used for superiorly located caudate AVMs. The patient is positioned supine with the head turned laterally 90 degrees as with a contralateral–

transcallosal approach. The head, however, is angled upward even more (60 degrees) to achieve a steeper crossing trajectory to the contralateral cingulated gyrus.

The final group of approaches that can be used for AVMs of the basal ganglia and thalamus are the transcortical approaches (Fig. 15.3). In the presence of a sizable hematoma or encephalomalacia connecting the cortical surface with an AVM, transcortical approaches (transfrontal, transtemporal, or transparietal) can be used instead of subarachnoid or transventricular routes. In short, the surgeon should exploit direct, non-anatomical corridors to deep AVMs when such paths already exist and otherwise select anatomical corridors through subarachnoid spaces (sylvian or interhemispheric fissures) and ventricles that will minimize brain transgression.

Brainstem

Microsurgical resection of brainstem AVMs requires a distinct set of surgical approaches to those for AVMs of the basal ganglia and thalamus. These skull-base approaches often require a far reach to the target lesion, and the close proximity of critical cranial nerves and vessels often allows for only a very narrow operative corridor. Bony removal is, therefore, often critical to maximizing view and minimizing retraction on brain and surrounding structures. For these reasons, appropriate

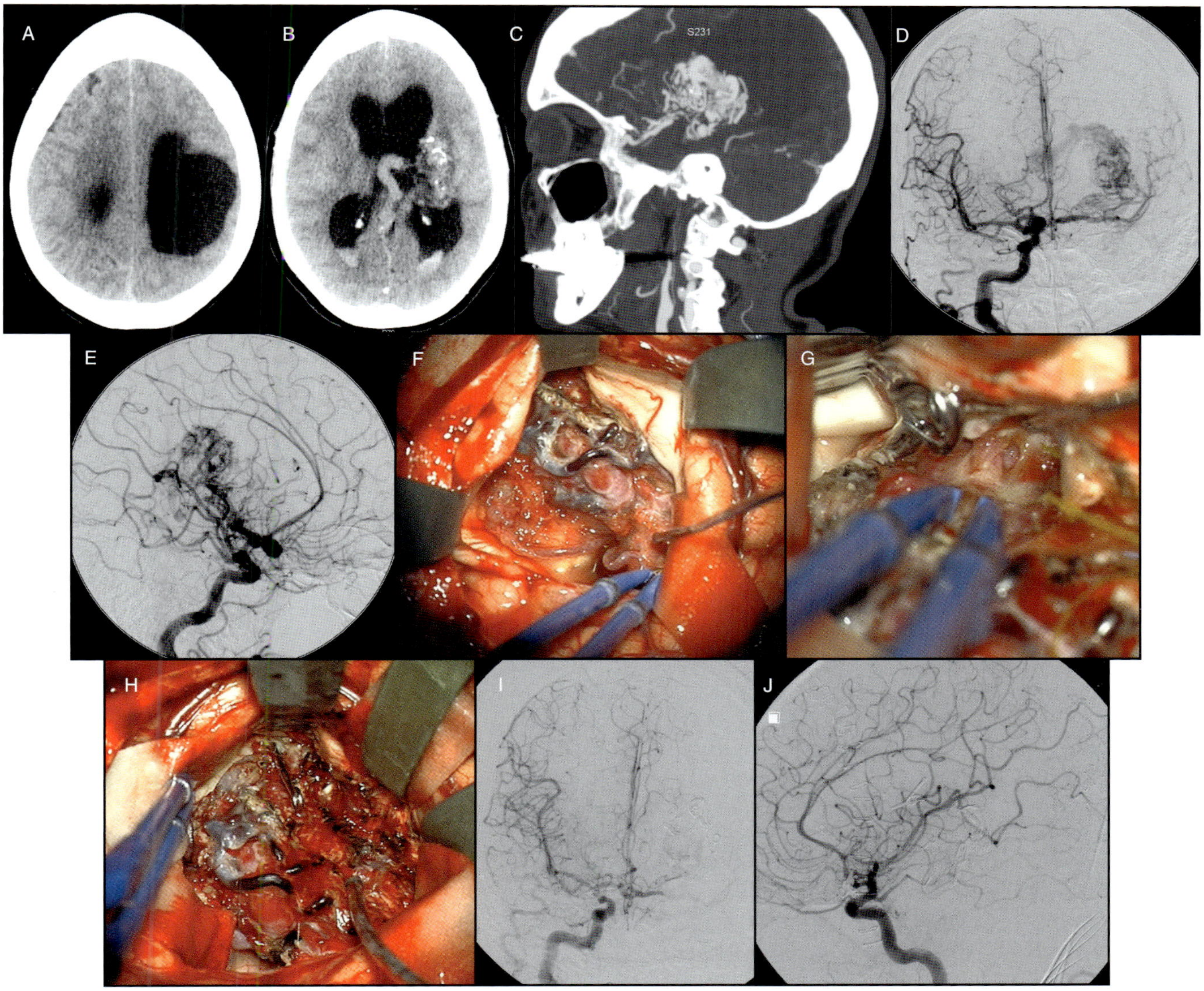

Fig. 15.3. Case example of the transcortical approach. This 57-year-old woman had a history of hemorrhage in childhood from a left thalamic arteriovenous malformation (AVM) that left her hemiparetic (Spetzler–Martin grade IV, supplementary grade III). The AVM was not treated. She presented decades later with headache and altered mental status. (A,B) Axial CT showed intraventricular hemorrhage. (C) Sagittal CT angiography (and the axial CT) demonstrated encephalomalacia extending from the cortical surface to the thalamic nidus. (D,E) Angiography showed an occluded left internal carotid artery (ICA), cross-filling from the right ICA, an anterior communicating artery aneurysm, and AVM supply from medial and lateral lenticulostriate arteries (left ICA injection; D, anteroposterior view; E, lateral view), and the posterior choroidal arteries (not shown). (F) The AVM was exposed through a transparietal approach with minimal cortical transgression. (G) Lenticulostriate feeding arteries were occluded along the anterior AVM margin and posterior choroidal arteries were occluded along the lateral and inferior margins. (H) The AVM was circumscribed but not resected. (I,J) Postoperative angiography demonstrated some residual AVM filling (left ICA injection; I, anteroposterior view; J, lateral view). Her anterior communicating artery aneurysm was clipped. She improved neurologically, and the residual AVM was treated radiosurgically.

approach selection is necessary for the safe resection of brainstem AVMs.

The orbitozygomatic–pterional craniotomy is used for anterior midbrain lesions, providing an anterolateral view of the midbrain. Compared with a standard pterional craniotomy, addition of orbital and zygomatic osteotomies provides a more superior-looking viewing angle. It is also important to drill the temporal bone down to the floor of the middle fossa in order to maximally mobilize the temporal lobe. A wide sylvian fissure split, ligation of sylvian veins entering the sphenoparietal sinus, and release of any bridging veins on the underside of the temporal lobe allow the temporal lobe to be retracted laterally and the frontal lobe to be retracted medially to create a wide view into the carotid and basal cisterns. Cerebrospinal fluid can be released from the third ventricle by opening the lamina terminalis, facilitating subsequent arachnoid dissection. Medially located lesions can be accessed through the carotid–optic or carotid–oculomotor triangles, although they may be concealed by the basilar artery. More lateral lesions can be accessed by opening the tentorial incisura and dissecting lateral to the oculomotor nerve to expose the distal S1 segment of the superior cerebellar artery [20] and P2 segment of PCA, between which can be found the cerebral peduncle.

Dorsal mesencephalic, pontomesencephalic, and superior pontine AVMs can be approached from a supracerebellar–infratentorial approach, either midline for midline lesions or laterally for more lateral lesions. We prefer to perform this approach with the patient in the sitting position to allow for gravity-retraction of the cerebellum, although a prone position may be more comfortable for the neurosurgeon. If a sitting position is selected, preoperative workup should include transthoracic echocardiography with agitated saline ("bubble") contrast to exclude the presence of a right-to-left cardiac or pulmonary shunt, which could allow a venous air embolism to enter the arterial circulation. For a midline approach, a torcular craniotomy is made to allow maximal retraction of the posterior fossa dura up to the transverse sinuses. Bridging veins between the superior cerebellar surface and tentorium should be coagulated and divided to prevent avulsion. The arachnoid of the quadrigeminal cistern is opened to reveal the Galenic complex, superior and inferior colliculi, and the pineal gland. For more lateral posterior mesencephalic, pontomesencephalic, and superior pontine lesions, a paramedian supracerebellar–infratentorial approach can be used [21]. The patient is positioned either seated or prone with the head turned toward the side of the lesion and a paramedian craniotomy over the ipsilateral occiput is made. Again, the transverse sinus must be exposed to maximize dural retraction. Finally, for lesions involving the lateral-most aspects of the midbrain and upper pons, the extreme lateral supracerebellar–infratentorial approach can be used [21]. This approach requires a retrosigmoid craniotomy with exposure of the distal transverse sinus and provides a view of the dorsal midbrain and upper pons from the lateral aspects of the ipsilateral colliculi posteriorly to the back of the cerebral peduncle and trigeminal nerve root anteriorly. The patient is positioned laterally or in a park-bench position. Alternative approaches to the dorsal midbrain and upper pons include the occipital transtentorial approach and transpetrosal approaches: the former risks retraction injury to the occipital lobes while the latter requires extensive drilling and only supplies a very narrow exposure. In addition, a subtemporal approach can be taken to the lateral and posterolateral aspects of the midbrain, although this again requires significant retraction of the temporal lobe for adequate exposure.

The retrosigmoid or extended retrosigmoid [22] approaches are best for lateral lesions of the pons (Fig. 15.4). The patient is placed in the lateral or park-bench position and a postauricular C-shaped incision is made, arcing from the mastoid tip to just above the ear. While a standard retrosigmoid craniotomy exposes the posterior edge of the sigmoid sinus, the extended retrosigmoid craniotomy involves a partial mastoidectomy from the asterion down to the mastoid tip that exposes the entire sigmoid sinus. In addition, the transverse–sigmoid junction is exposed superiorly while the jugular bulb is exposed inferiorly. This allows the posterior fossa dura to be retracted forward as far as possible, maximizing the view of the cerebellopontine angle down the posterior petrous face. An additional dural flap can be made superiorly along the transverse sinus. Cerebrospinal fluid should be released from the cisterna magna followed by dissection of the cerebellopontine angle arachnoid and identification of the lower cranial nerves. The extended retrosigmoid approach is also used for anterior pontine AVMs, requiring a deeper reach medial to the trigeminal, facial, and vestibulocochlear nerves.

Medullary AVMs are best approached through a far lateral craniotomy for anterolateral and lateral lesions or a midline suboccipital approach for dorsal lesions. For the far lateral craniotomy (Fig. 15.5), the patient is placed in a lateral or park-bench position with the head flexed, rotated away from the side of the lesion, and then tilted laterally away from the lesion. The skin incision can be varied depending on the location and size of the lesion. The largest involves a midline incision from C2 up to the inion, which then passes laterally and down along the mastoid to the mastoid tip. This incision is described as the hockey-stick incision. Other variants include the "lazy S" and paramedian incisions. The ipsilateral C1 arch should be removed from the midline to the sulcus arteriosus with care taken to mobilize the vertebral artery and surrounding venous plexus laterally. The craniotomy extends from midline laterally and opens the foramen magnum. The ipsilateral occipital condyle is then drilled down to expand the view of the lateral medulla. The extent of condylar drilling depends on the location of the AVM, with more extensive removal required to see further anteriorly. The dura is flapped laterally with a C-shaped opening beginning over the ipsilateral cerebellar hemisphere and arcing to the midline and then laterally over the exposed cervical region. Once the arachnoid is opened, this exposure reveals the ipsilateral posterior inferior cerebellar artery and lower cranial nerves.

Surgical adjuncts

As discussed above, microsurgical resection of basal ganglia, thalamic, and brainstem AVMs poses inherent risks to the

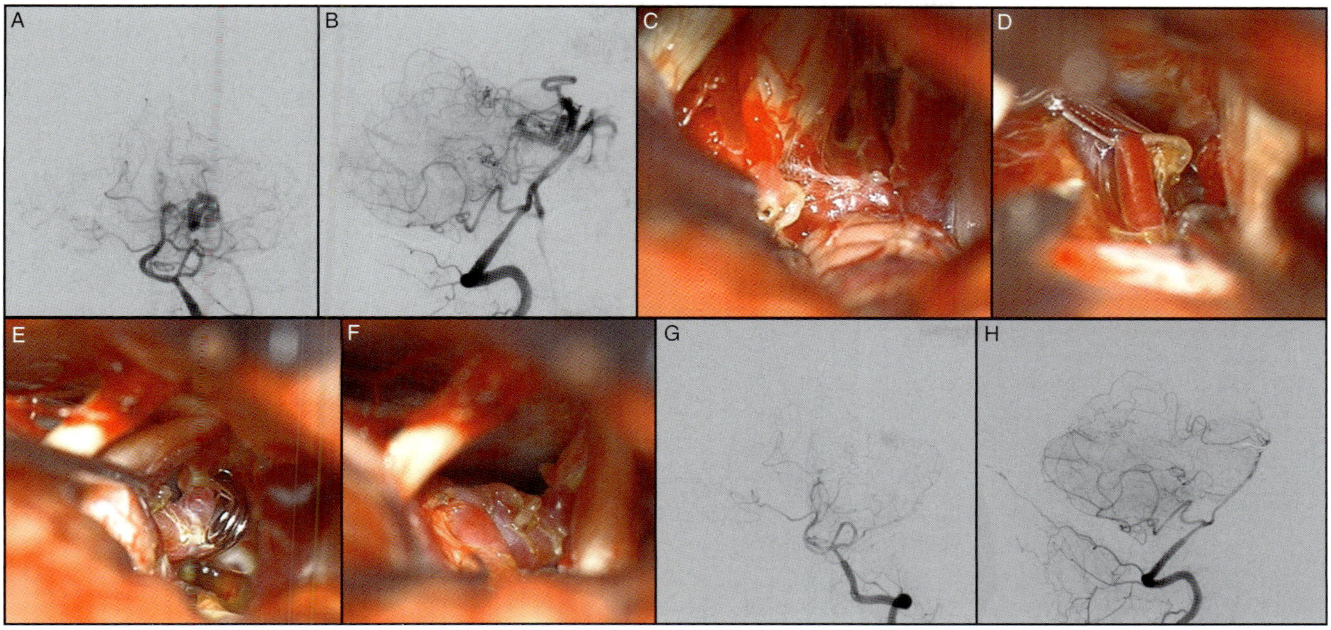

Fig. 15.4. Case example of the extended retrosigmoid approach for a pontine arteriovenous malformations (AVM). This 59-year-old man presented with subarachnoid hemorrhage from this Spetzler–Martin grade II, supplementary grade IV AVM. (A,B) Digital subtraction angiography showed supply by the left superior cerebellar artery (SCA), a duplicate left SCA, and the left anterior inferior cerebellar artery (AICA) (left vertebral artery injections; A, anteroposterior view; B, lateral view). A ruptured SCA feeding artery aneurysm was treated endovascularly. (C) The AVM was then exposed surgically through an extended retrosigmoid approach, which skeletonized the sigmoid sinus to maximize access to the cerebellopontine angle. (D,E). Feeding artery branches from the SCA (D) and AICA (E) were clip-ligated. (F) Having been devascularized, the AVM nidus was left in situ. (G,H) Postoperative angiography showed complete obliteration (left vertebral artery injections; G, anteroposterior view; H, lateral view).

cerebral vasculature, deep nuclei, and subcortical pathways. Surgical adjuncts, such as neuronavigation, neuromonitoring, and intraoperative imaging can be used during microsurgical resection to maximize the chance of complete resection while minimizing surgical morbidity.

Preoperative embolization

Preoperative embolization of AVM feeding arteries has been shown to significantly reduce AVM volume in certain situations [23]; however, its use for AVMs of the basal ganglia, thalamus, and brainstem is more controversial [12]. The arteries feeding such deep-seated AVMs are often small in caliber, en passage, or give off critical perforators to eloquent territory, making them difficult to catheterize for preoperative embolization. In addition, deep venous drainage and location within eloquent brain are associated with neurological complications after embolization [24]. For these reasons, embolization may be more dangerous for basal ganglia, thalamic, and brainstem AVMs than for more superficial lesions. Intra-arterial sodium amytal testing may be useful in predicting morbidity from embolization of AVM feeding arteries [25,26].

Neuronavigation

Neuronavigation based on preoperative MRI or CT is often used for surgical resection of cerebral tumors and cavernous malformations. Its use for AVM surgery is more limited but has been successfully demonstrated [27,28]. Neuronavigation based on preoperative digital subtraction angiography performed during preoperative embolization procedures has also been described [29]. In general, we have found neuronavigation to be most helpful for deep AVMs of the basal ganglia and thalamus, where it can help to determine the correct transinsular, transcallosal, or transcortical trajectory. Often, arterial feeders or draining veins may lead the surgeon directly to the AVM nidus without the need for neuronavigation. In the brainstem, anatomical landmarks are typically sufficient to localize an AVM.

Neuromonitoring

While direct visualization of critical structures is an important component of any cerebrovascular surgery, visualization alone cannot always detect irritation and impending damage to such structures. Small perforators and en passage vessels are at risk for occlusion during AVM surgery, while deep nuclei, tracts, and cranial nerves may be damaged during resection. Neurophysiological monitoring methods are, therefore, used to assess various cerebral functions during AVM surgery. These monitoring techniques can detect changes in cerebral and cranial nerve function caused by either ischemia or direct damage. Somatosensory evoked potentials monitor the somatosensory pathways, including the nuclei cuneatus and gracilis, medial lemniscus, and thalamocortical projections, while motor evoked potentials monitor the integrity of the corticospinal tracts, all of which may be damaged during resection of basal ganglia, thalamic, or brainstem AVMs. Brainstem auditory evoked potentials monitor the auditory pathways, which include several nuclei with synapses sensitive to pontine ischemia [30]. In addition, electromyography and direct stimulation can be used to detect and monitor motor nuclei and nerves [31]. In general, no neuromonitoring method alone can assess all

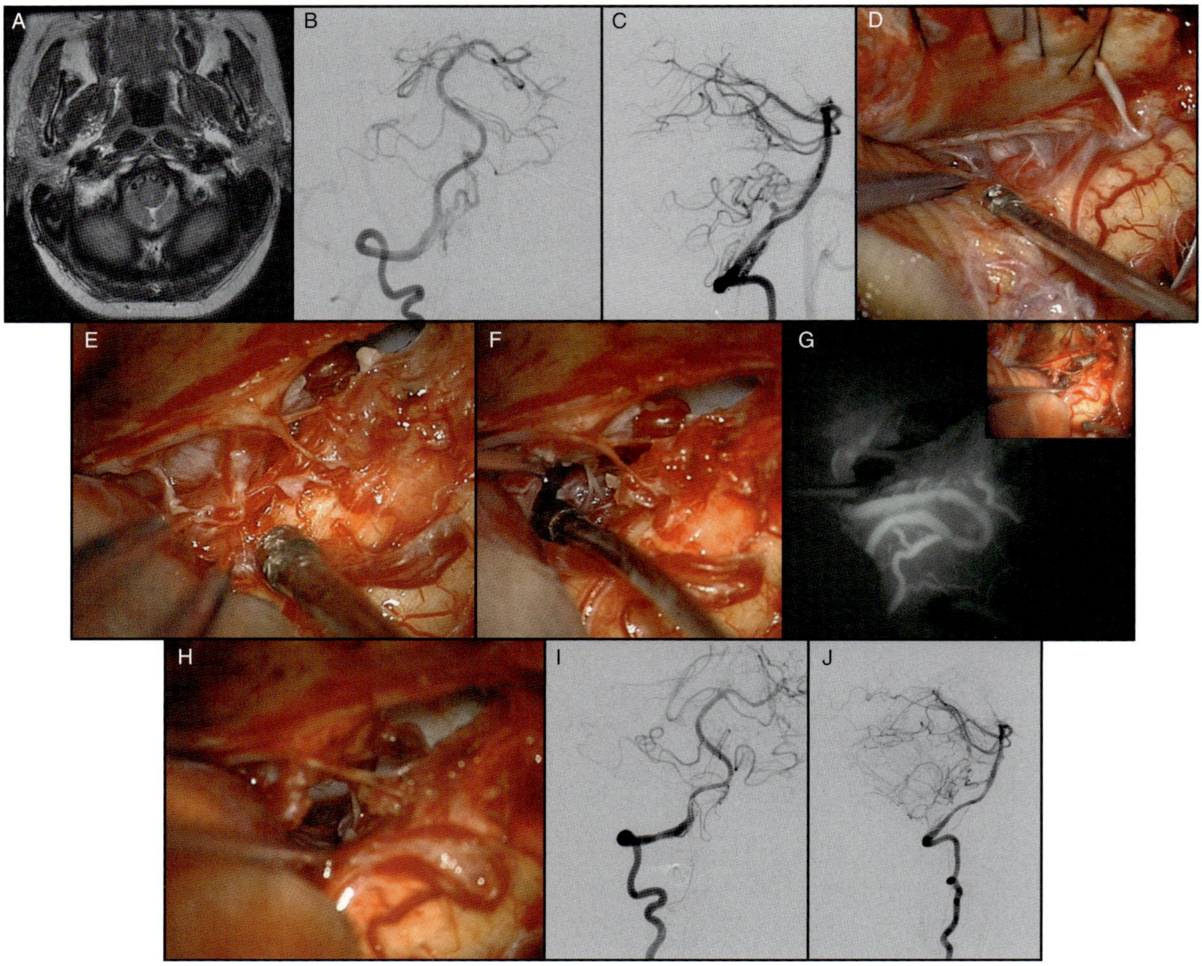

Fig. 15.5. Case example of the far lateral approach for a medullary arteriovenous malformation (AVM). This 55-year old woman presented with subarachnoid hemorrhage. (A) Axial T_2-weighted MRI showed increased vascularity along the anterolateral surface of the medulla. (B,C) Digital subtraction angiography revealed this to be Spetzler–Martin grade III, supplementary grade III AVM supplied by anterior medullary branches of the right posterior inferior cerebellar artery and anterior spinal artery (right vertebral artery injections; B, anteroposterior view; C, lateral view). (D) This AVM was approached through a right far lateral craniotomy, which requires drilling of the occipital condyle to obtain wide lateral exposure of the medulla. (E,F) Careful subarachnoid dissection between lower cranial nerves revealed the AVM and the arterial feeders were ligated. (G) Intraoperative indocyanine green videoangiography confirmed no further shunting into the draining vein, which was then coagulated. (H) The AVM nidus was left in situ. (I,J) Postoperative angiography showed complete obliteration (left vertebral artery injections; I, anteroposterior view; J, lateral view).

brain functions. We typically monitor both somatosensory and motor evoked potentials during surgery for basal ganglia and thalamic AVMs, while somatosensory, motor, and brainstem auditory evoked potentials are used for brainstem AVMs.

Intraoperative imaging

Digital subtraction angiography is the gold standard for diagnosing cerebral AVMs and may also be performed postoperatively to evaluate the success of microsurgical resection. Intraoperatively, however, the extent of AVM resection is typically assessed with visual inspection, which in rare cases can fail to detect residual AVM. Combined operative/angiography suites, so-called "hybrid" operating rooms, allow for the use of intraoperative digital subtraction angiography and immediate confirmation of AVM obliteration. In a retrospective study of over 1000 craniotomies for vascular lesions, including 101 AVM surgeries, intraoperative angiography revealed residual AVM nidus in nearly 9% of patients with AVMs [32]. This allowed the surgeons to further explore and resect the residual AVM during the same operation, preventing the need for a second surgery in all but two of these patients.

While intraoperative digital subtraction angiography may provide a definitive assessment of AVM obliteration, it requires specialized facilities and significantly lengthens the surgery time. Indocyanine green (ICG) videoangiography is another intraoperative imaging technique that can be performed easily and rapidly in any operating room with the addition of a surgical microscope with near-infrared video integration. The fluorescent dye ICG is non-toxic with a peak spectral absorption of 800 nm and emission of 835 nm. For angiographic evaluation, the anesthesiologist administers an intravenous bolus of 25 mg in 5 mL of normal saline. Under illumination from the microscope's near-infrared light source, flow of ICG through the exposed cerebral vessels can be visualized in real-time through the surgical microscope. Indocyanine green videoangiography can be used to identify AVM feeding arteries and draining veins as well as the nidus. In addition, it can be used after resection to confirm absence of the AVM nidus and absence of flow through the draining veins [33]. This technique, however, has a significant limitation in that only exposed vessels can be visualized and its results must be interpreted accordingly. Overall, intraoperative ICG angiography is a safe and rapid alternative to intraoperative digital subtraction angiography but is best used for assessment of blood flow through superficial vessels [34].

Results

While several modern series have retrospectively described the results of microsurgical management of basal ganglia, thalamic, and brainstem AVMs, these series are all relatively small. For the purposes of this chapter, the focus is on those series that report 15 or more surgically treated patients for a given deep AVM subtype. While basal ganglia and thalamic AVMs are distinct entities, they are routinely grouped together in the literature. Therefore, surgical results for these two subtypes will be discussed as a group, noting important differences when indicated.

Basal ganglia and thalamic arteriovenous malformations

Table 15.1 summarizes the larger reports of basal ganglia and thalamic AVMs treated with microsurgery since the late 1980s [4,35–40]. It is important to note that the largest of these series only reported 39 patients [38], indicating how rarely such lesions are treated surgically. Overall, complete obliteration rates were achieved in 71–100% of patients. While it is difficult to make an accurate generalization about outcomes given differences in outcome reporting, the majority of patients were reported to have favorable outcomes, with only four deaths attributable to AVM surgery and 12 instances of worsened neurological status among 140 patients. These studies used variations of the trans-sylvian, transcallosal, and transcortical approaches as described above. Interestingly, U *et al.* described changing their preferred approach to basal ganglia and thalamic AVMs abutting the ventricles from a trans-sylvian approach to a transfrontal transventricular approach in order to have access to the ventricular system in case of hemorrhage [37].

The most common reported postoperative deficits were memory disturbances and visual deficits. Solomon and Stein reported the use of a posterior interhemispheric transcallosal transventricular approach to AVMs of the thalamus and caudate in 22 patients, which required sectioning of the ipsilateral fornix; transient postoperative memory deficits were identified in 11 of the patients, homonymous hemianopsia in 6, permanent hemisensory loss in 2, and Perinaud syndrome in 1 [35]. Despite these permanent deficits, all patients in this series were able to return to their presurgical occupation. Sasaki *et al.* similarly described several patients with postoperative visual field cuts presumably related to damage to the optic radiations during transtemporal and transparietal approaches [4]. In addition, they report several patients with postoperative speech deficits, two of which occurred after interhemispheric transventricular approaches and three after transtemporal transventricular approaches. All but one were transient. Interestingly, motor and sensory deficits were less common and usually transient. It is unclear if this is a feature of the use of intraoperative neuromonitoring or the surgeons' ability to avoid motor and sensory pathways.

Several of these studies have reported the use of staged surgical resections [35,37,39]. Subsequent resections were most often used for residual AVM; however, Solomon and Stein reported the use of planned staged resections in two patients: one with a large AVM that required both an anterior and posterior transcallosal approach and a second patient who underwent a subfrontal approach to occlude AVM feeding arteries followed by a posterior interhemispheric approach to remove the nidus [35].

Brainstem arteriovenous malformations

Table 15.2 describes the results of larger published series of brainstem AVMs treated with surgical resection. Results among these series vary, both in terms of extent of resection and neurological outcomes. The early series emphasized the technical difficulties of these operations, with Drake *et al.* [41] commenting that these lesions are "treacherous to treat." The most important theme that arises from these series is that unacceptable surgical morbidity and mortality may be associated with brainstem AVMs within the parenchyma of the brainstem while those that abut or involve the pial surface or extend into the subarachnoid space are more amenable to surgical resection. Yaşargil [42] noted this in his series of 14 midbrain AVMs while Drake *et al.* [41] were only able to successfully resect two extrapial midbrain AVMs among a series of 15 brainstem AVMs. Lawton *et al.* [39] reported excellent results of eight patients with brainstem AVMs treated surgically. Complete resection was achieved in all but one, with only one patient having worsened neurological function postoperatively. These authors noted that a lesion must project to a subarachnoid space in order to be considered surgically accessible, emphasizing the importance of proper patient selection.

Conclusions

Treatment of deep-seated AVMs of the basal ganglia, thalamus, and brainstem is challenging regardless of the treatment modality. The technical difficulties of surgical resection and poor outcomes reported in the early literature led many neurosurgeons to avoid surgical resection as a treatment option, favoring instead radiosurgery, embolization, or simply observation. As discussed above, a firm understanding of the surgical approaches and principles, and use of surgical adjuncts such as preoperative embolization and intraoperative neuromonitoring and angiography, can lead to safe operations for deep-seated AVMs. Most importantly, proper patient selection is critical, with a preference for lesions that reach the subarachnoid space, ventricles, hematoma cavities, or other non-eloquent tissue (Fig. 15.6). If these principles are adhered to, surgical resection can be a safe treatment option in a multidisciplinary approach to AVMs of the basal ganglia, thalamus, and brainstem.

Table 15.1. Summary of published large series reporting microsurgical management of basal ganglia and thalamic arteriovenous malformations

Study	No. patients	Hemorrhagic presentation	Preoperative functional status	Preoperative embolization	Surgical approaches	Complete resection	Long-term functional outcomes
U *et al.* (1992) [37]	16	8	2 normal, 11 hemiparetic, 1 comatose, 2 other deficits	6	Trans-sylvian in 3; then transfrontal–transventricular in remaining 13	12 (75%)	10 good/excellent, 3 fair, 2 poor, 1 death (4 worsened)
Shi and Chen (1987) [36]	16	16	2 normal, 14 hemiplegic + other deficits	No mention	Trans-sylvian	13 (81%) (2 treated with feeding artery ligation only)	12 excellent, 1 permanent deficit, 1 postoperative death, 2 late deaths (unclear if related)
Solomon and Stein (1987) [35]	22	21	All independent, 3 mild hemiparesis, 8 other mild deficits	No mention	Interhemispheric–transcallosal, 5 patients with 2 stages	18 (82%)	All returned to previous occupation, 6 visual deficit, 2 hemisensory loss, 1 sterile ventriculitis, 1 extraocular movement deficit, no deaths
Tew *et al.* (1995) [38]	39	Not specified for AVMs[a]	Not specified for AVMs[a]	No mention	Transcallosal, transcortical–transventricular, trans-sylvian	38 (97%)	26 improved, 7 unchanged, 5 worsened, 1 death
Lawton *et al.* (1995) [39]	14	13	6 normal, 5 hemi/paraplegic, 2 other deficits, 1 comatose	7	Transcortical, transcallosal, occipital–transtentorial	10[b] (71%)	6 improved, 7 unchanged, 1 worse, no deaths
de Oliveira *et al.* (1997) [40]	18	16	11 deficits, 7 symptomatic with normal neurological examination	2	Various trans-sylvian, transcortical, transcallosal approaches	15 (83%)	17 improving/unchanged, 1 death
Sasaki *et al.* (1998) [4]	15	15	8 weakness, 7 no weakness	1	Transcortical, interhemispheric, and trans-sylvian	15 (100%)	10 working, 4 living independently, 1 bedridden, no deaths

[a] This report describes a series of 65 patients with deep-seated vascular malformations. Pretreatment hemorrhage occurred in 91%.
[b] This includes patients treated with multimodal therapies.

Table 15.2. Summary of published large series reporting microsurgical management of brainstem arteriovenous malformations

Study	No. patients	Hemorrhagic presentation	Preoperative functional status	Preoperative embolization	Surgical approaches	Complete resection	Long-term functional outcomes
Nozaki *et al.* (2006) [3]	20	19	6 with hemiparesis, 2 with tetraplegia, 12 cranial nerve deficits	6 preoperatively	No mention	Complete in 14	Glasgow Outcome Scale Score 1–2 for 2, 3 for 4, 4 for 6, 5 for 8
Solomon and Stein (1986) [43]	9	11	6 cranial nerve deficits, 1 with hemiparesis, 2 with ataxia	No mention	Suboccipital lateral or sitting	Complete in 8	5 unchanged, 2 with new cranial nerve deficit

Table 15.2. (cont.)

Study	No. patients	Hemorrhagic presentation	Preoperative functional status	Preoperative embolization	Surgical approaches	Complete resection	Long-term functional outcomes
Yaşargil (1998) [42]	Midbrain 6, pontine 4	Midbrain 6, pontine 3	Midbrain with deficits 3, pontine with deficits 3	No mention	Dorsal midbrain: sitting, paramedian infratentorial Dorsolateral midbrain: paramedian supracerebellar Upper ventral pontine: subtemporal–transtentorial Sulcus pontomedullaris: sitting, midline approach	Midbrain complete in 5/6 Pontine complete in 4	Midbrain good in 5, 1 death Pontine: 2 unchanged/ improved, 2 worse
Lawton *et al.* (1995) [39]	8	6	4 comatose, 3 with hemiparesis, 1 with paraplegia	None	Midline suboccipital, infratentorial–supracebellar, or far lateral	Complete in all	5 improved, 2 unchanged, 1 worse

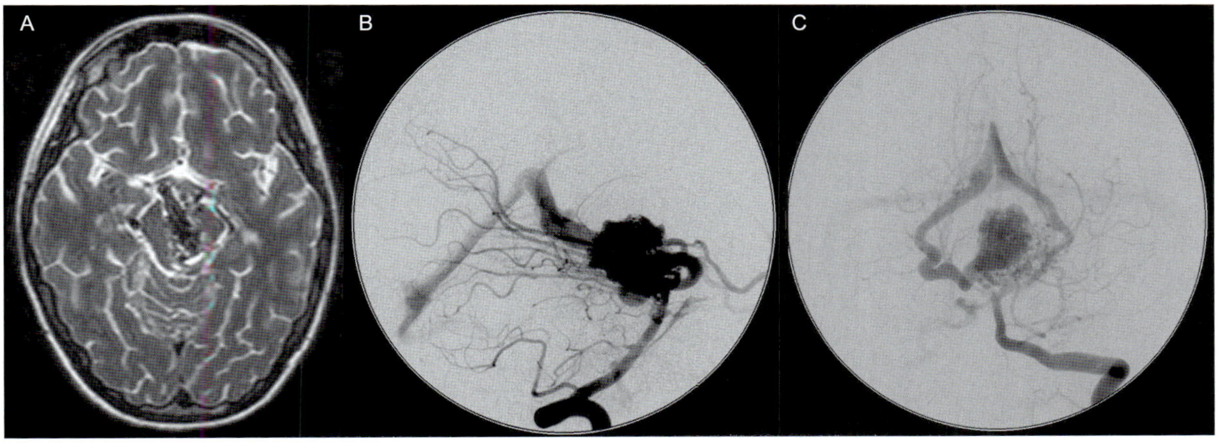

Fig. 15.6. Case example of an inoperable midbrain arteriovenous malformation (AVM) in a 14-year-old girl who presented with subarachnoid hemorrhage. (A) Increased vascularity within the midbrain on axial T_2-weighted MRI. (B,C) Digital subtraction angiography revealed a Spetzler–Martin grade III, supplementary grade I AVM (left vertebral artery injections; B, anteroposterior view; C, lateral view). Given the AVM location within the midbrain parenchyma, it was decided that the morbidity of surgical resection was unacceptable and the patient underwent stereotactic radiosurgery with a dramatic reduction in the size of her AVM. At last follow-up, she had a small remnant and salvage stereotactic radiosurgery was recommended.

References

1. Fleetwood IG, Marcellus ML, Levy RP, *et al.* Deep arteriovenous malformations of the basal ganglia and thalamus: natural history. *J Neurosurg* 2003;**98**:747–50.
2. Stapf C, Mohr JP, Pile-Spellman J, *et al.* Epidemiology and natural history of arteriovenous malformations. *Neurosurg Focus* 2001;**11**:E1.
3. Nozaki K, Hashimoto N, Kikuta K, *et al.* Surgical applications to arteriovenous malformations involving the brainstem. *Neurosurgery* 2006;**58**(Suppl):ons8.
4. Sasaki T, Kurita H, Saito I, *et al.* Arteriovenous malformations in the basal ganglia and thalamus: management and results in 101 cases. *J Neurosurg* 1998;**88**:285–92.
5. Pollock BE, Gorman DA, Brown PD. Radiosurgery for arteriovenous malformations of the basal ganglia, thalamus, and brainstem. *J Neurosurg* 2004;**100**:210–14.
6. Kiran NA, Kale SS, Kasliwal MK, *et al.* Gamma knife radiosurgery for arteriovenous malformations of basal ganglia, thalamus and brainstem – a retrospective study comparing the results with that for AVMs at other intracranial locations. *Acta Neurochir (Wein)* 2009;**151**:1575–82.
7. Kano H, Kondziolka D, Flickinger JC, *et al.* Stereotactic radiosurgery for arteriovenous malformations. Part 4: management of basal ganglia and thalamus arteriovenous malformations. *J Neurosurg* 2012;**116**:33–43.

8. Kano H, Kondziolka D, Flickinger JC, *et al.* Stereotactic radiosurgery for arteriovenous malformations. Part 5: management of brainstem arteriovenous malformations. *J Neurosurg* 2012;**116**:44–53.
9. Kurita H, Kawamoto S, Sasaki T, *et al.* Results of radiosurgery for brain stem arteriovenous malformations. *J Neurol Neurosurg Psychiatry* 2000;**68**:563–70.
10. Flickinger JC, Lunsford LD, Kondziolka D, *et al.* Radiosurgery and brain tolerance: an analysis of neurodiagnostic imaging changes after gamma knife radiosurgery for arteriovenous malformations. *Int J Radiat Oncol Biol Phys* 1992;**23**:19–26.
11. Koga T, Shin M, Terahara A, *et al.* Outcomes of radiosurgery for brainstem arteriovenous malformations. *Neurosurgery* 2011;**69**:45–51.
12. Gross BA, Duckworth EA, Getch CC, *et al.* Challenging traditional beliefs: microsurgery for arteriovenous malformations of the basal ganglia and thalamus. *Neurosurgery* 2008;**63**:393–410.
13. Morgan MK, Zurin AA, Harrington T, *et al.* Changing role for preoperative embolisation in the management of arteriovenous malformations of the brain. *J Clin Neurosci* 2000;**7**:527–30.
14. Spetzler RF, Sanai N. The quiet revolution: retractorless surgery for complex vascular and skull base lesions. *J Neurosurg* 2012;**116**:291–300.
15. Waldron JS, Lawton MT. The supracarotid-infrafrontal approach: surgical technique and clinical application to cavernous malformations in the anteroinferior basal ganglia. *Neurosurgery* 2009;**64**:ons86–95.
16. Shucart WA, Stein BM. Transcallosal approach to the anterior ventricular system. *Neurosurgery* 1978;**3**:339–43.
17. Lawton MT, Golfinos JG, Spetzler RF. The contralateral transcallosal approach: experience with 32 patients. *Neurosurgery* 1996;**39**:729–34.
18. Chi JH, Lawton MT. Posterior interhemispheric approach: surgical technique, application to vascular lesions, and benefits of gravity retraction. *Neurosurgery* 2006;**59**: ons41–9.
19. Davies J, Tawk RG, Lawton MT. The contralateral transcingulate approach: operative technique and results with vascular lesions. *Neurosurgery* 2012;**71**:4–13.
20. Rodriguez-Hernandez A, Rhoton AL, Jr., Lawton MT. Segmental anatomy of cerebellar arteries: a proposed nomenclature. Laboratory investigation. *J Neurosurg* 2011;**115**:387–97.
21. de Oliveira JG, Lekovic GP, Safavi-Abbasi S, *et al.* Supracerebellar infratentorial approach to cavernous malformations of the brainstem: surgical variants and clinical experience with 45 patients. *Neurosurgery* 2010;**66**:389–99.
22. Quinones-Hinojosa A, Chang EF, Lawton MT. The extended retrosigmoid approach: an alternative to radical cranial base approaches for posterior fossa lesions. *Neurosurgery* 2006;**58**: ons14.
23. Loh Y, Duckwiler GR. A prospective, multicenter, randomized trial of the Onyx liquid embolic system and *N*-butyl cyanoacrylate embolization of cerebral arteriovenous malformations. *J Neurosurg* 2010;**113**:733–41.
24. Hartmann A, Stapf C, Hofmeister C, *et al.* Determinants of neurological outcome after surgery for brain arteriovenous malformation. *Stroke* 2000;**31**:2361–4.
25. Purdy PD, Batjer HH, Samson D, *et al.* Intraarterial sodium amytal administration to guide preoperative embolization of cerebral arteriovenous malformations. *J Neurosurg Anesthesiol* 1991;**3**:103–6.
26. Rauch RA, Vinuela F, Dion J, *et al.* Preembolization functional evaluation in brain arteriovenous malformations: the ability of superselective Amytal test to predict neurologic dysfunction before embolization. *AJNR Am J Neuroradiol* 1992;**13**:309–14.
27. Muacevic A, Steiger HJ. Computer-assisted resection of cerebral arteriovenous malformations. *Neurosurgery* 1999;**45**:1164–70.
28. Russell SM, Woo HH, Joseffer SS, *et al.* Role of frameless stereotaxy in the surgical treatment of cerebral arteriovenous malformations: technique and outcomes in a controlled study of 44 consecutive patients. *Neurosurgery* 2002;**51**:1108–16.
29. Gonzalez LF, Albuquerque FC, Boom S, *et al.* Image-guided resection of embolized cerebral arteriovenous malformations based on catheter-based angiography. *Neurosurgery* 2010;**67**:471–5.
30. Schramm J, Mokrusch T, Fahlbusch R, *et al.* Detailed analysis of intraoperative changes monitoring brain stem acoustic evoked potentials. *Neurosurgery* 1988;**22**:694–702.
31. Jameson LC, Sloan TB. Neurophysiologic monitoring in neurosurgery. *Anesthesiol Clin* 2012;**30**:311–31.
32. Chalouhi N, Theofanis T, Jabbour P, *et al.* Safety and efficacy of intraoperative angiography in craniotomies for cerebral aneurysms and arteriovenous malformations: a review of 1093 consecutive cases. *Neurosurgery* 2012;**71**:1162–9.
33. Ng YP, King NK, Wan KR, *et al.* Uses and limitations of indocyanine green videoangiography for flow analysis in arteriovenous malformation surgery. *J Clin Neurosci* 2013;**20**:224–32.
34. Takagi Y, Sawamura K, Hashimoto N, *et al.* Evaluation of serial intraoperative surgical microscope-integrated intraoperative near-infrared indocyanine green videoangiography in patients with cerebral arteriovenous malformations. *Neurosurgery* 2012;**70**:34–42.
35. Solomon RA, Stein BM. Interhemispheric approach for the surgical removal of thalamocaudate arteriovenous malformations. *J Neurosurg* 1987;**66**:345–51.
36. Shi YQ, Chen XC. Surgical treatment of arteriovenous malformations of the striatothalamocapsular region. *J Neurosurg* 1987;**66**:352–6.
37. U HS, Kerber CW, Todd MM. Multimodality treatment of deep periventricular cerebral arteriovenous malformations. *Surg Neurol* 1992;**38**:192–203.
38. Tew JM, Jr., Lewis AI, Reichert KW. Management strategies and surgical techniques for deep-seated supratentorial arteriovenous malformations. *Neurosurgery* 1995;**36**:1065–72.
39. Lawton MT, Hamilton MG, Spetzler RF. Multimodality treatment of deep arteriovenous malformations: thalamus,

basal ganglia, and brain stem. *Neurosurgery* 1995;**37**:29–35.

40. de Oliveira E, Tedeschi H, Siqueira MG, *et al.* Arteriovenous malformations of the basal ganglia region: rationale for surgical management. *Acta Neurochir (Wien)* 1997;**139**:487–506.
41. Drake CG, Friedman AH, Peerless SJ. Posterior fossa arteriovenous malformations. *J Neurosurg* 1986;**64**:1–10.
42. Yaşargil MG (ed.) *Microneurosurgery*. New York: Thieme, 1998.
43. Solomon RA, Stein BM. Management of arteriovenous malformations of the brain stem. *J Neurosurg* 1986;**64**:857–64.

Chapter 16

Complications of arteriovenous malformations rupture and medical management of hemorrhage

Giuseppe Lanzino and Ross Puffer

Introduction and epidemiology

Arteriovenous malformations (AVMs) are responsible for only 1–2% of all strokes and 4% of primary intracerebral hemorrhages. However, patients with intracranial hemorrhage from an AVM are usually younger than most stroke victims and AVMs are responsible for one-third of intracranial hemorrhages in young adults [1].

The incidence of hemorrhage as a presenting symptom of an intracranial AVM varies among different series in relation to the time period considered (before or after the widespread availability of non-invasive imaging studies) and the type of setting: population-based study versus series of patients referred for tertiary specialized care. In a small retrospective but population-based study conducted between 1965 and 1992 in Olmsted County, 65% of patients with AVMs presented with hemorrhage [2]. With advances in imaging techniques and widespread availability of non-invasive imaging studies, the relative percentage of patients with AVMs presenting with hemorrhage is decreasing. In a prospective population-based study conducted in Scotland, 114 of 229 adults (50%) diagnosed with an intracranial parenchymal AVM between 1999 and 2003 suffered an intracranial hemorrhage as a presenting symptom [3]. Parenchymal hemorrhage is the most common mode of hemorrhagic presentation. In the Scottish Intracranial Vascular Malformations Study [4], 50% of the hemorrhages were strictly limited to the brain parenchyma and intraventricular hemorrhage (IVH) was present in 34%. Similarly in the study conducted in Olmsted County, intracerebral hemorrhage (ICH) was present in 41% of patients, subarachnoid hemorrhage (SAH) in 24%, IVH in 12%, and a combination of the different types in 23% [2]. In the Scottish study, location of the hematoma was lobar in 73%, deep in 11%, and infratentorial in 16% [1]. The median volume in 90 patients with ICH was 16 cm^3 [5], and IVH was present in 34%.

Of patients with AVMs who present with hemorrhage, 93% are from the AVM and the remainder are from associated intracranial aneurysms [3]. Median age of patients with ruptured AVMs is 47 years, with overall equal distribution between men and women [5].

Clinical presentation and initial evaluation

Presenting symptoms vary considerably based on the location of the hemorrhage, size of the corresponding hematoma, and the presence of intraventricular blood. Generally, symptoms progress over a period of minutes to hours, as opposed to the acute onset of headache that is more common in SAHs or acute ischemia. Symptoms from ICH may include multiple vascular territories, which may further help to delineate ICH as an underlying cause of symptoms instead of more common ischemic etiologies [6]. These symptoms may include focal neurological deficit, hemiplegia, or signs of raised intracranial pressure (ICP) such as headache, nausea, and vomiting. Lobar hemorrhages may cause clinical seizures in up to one-third of patients [7]. Focal deficits, such as visual field cuts, focal weakness, and aphasia may be indicative of a cortically based hemorrhage [6]. Deeper lesions, such as those in the thalamus, may present with hemisensory loss or complete hemiplegia if the hemorrhage affects the basal ganglia or internal capsule [6]. Cerebellar hemorrhages may cause ataxia and nystagmus. Depressed mental status and rapid decline in neurological status may be present if hematoma expansion is large enough to compress critical brainstem structures or cause significant supratentorial midline shift. Hydrocephalus may develop if ventricular drainage is impaired by hematoma expansion, even if no ventricular extension is present.

Management of the patient with a ruptured arteriovenous malformations

Initial management

Focal neurological symptoms with acute onset are commonly vascular in origin, so prompt recognition of these symptoms, initiation of cardiorespiratory support, and expedient transfer to an emergency department are mainstays of management by emergency services. Patients with a decreased level of consciousness and a Glasgow Coma Scale (GCS) score of ≤8 may benefit from intubation. As intubation may increase ICP, patients with a suspected or demonstrated intracranial bleed

Comprehensive Management of Arteriovenous Malformations of the Brain and Spine, ed. Robert F. Spetzler, Douglas S. Kondziolka, Randall T. Higashida, and M. Yashar S. Kalani. Published by Cambridge University Press.

may benefit from pretreatment with short-acting barbiturates and neuromuscular-blocking agents.

Medical management of AVM rupture follows the same treatment guidelines as primary ICH. Recommendations for the medical management of ICH are taken from the most recent American Heart Association/American Stroke Association guidelines for management of spontaneous ICH. Information regarding class of recommendation and level of evidence are presented in parentheses as they are reported in the initial guidelines [8].

After presentation to an emergency department, rapid neuroimaging with either CT or MRI is recommended to determine the etiology of stroke: ischemic or hemorrhagic (class I, level A) [8]. Catheter angiography remains the gold standard for identifying a possible underlying vascular malformations and defining its angioarchitecture after a hemorrhage is identified on initial imaging, and there is suspicion for an underlying structural cause for the ICH. However, CT angiography is very useful to identify the cause of the ICH and visualize the exact location of the AVM in patients who are in need of urgent hematoma evacuation (class IIa, level B) [8]. CT angiography can usually be obtained at the same time as the initial CT after the intracranial hemorrhage is diagnosed and an underlying vascular malformations suspected based on patient age, presentation, and location and pattern of the hemorrhage.

Once a patient is stabilized and the cause of the hemorrhage is suspected to be or identified as an AVM, a catheter angiography should be performed, preferably within the first 24 hours. Catheter angiography, more than other non-invasive diagnostic methodologies, is useful in the identification of possible offending feeding pedicles or other associated aneurysms, which can often be treated during the diagnostic angiography to prevent rebleeding (Fig. 16.1) [9].

Patients with ICH from a ruptured AVM should be treated in an intensive care unit as such patients are very often unstable, both medically and neurologically. They often require intensive care monitoring and cardiorespiratory support. It has been demonstrated that patients with ICHs have a lower mortality

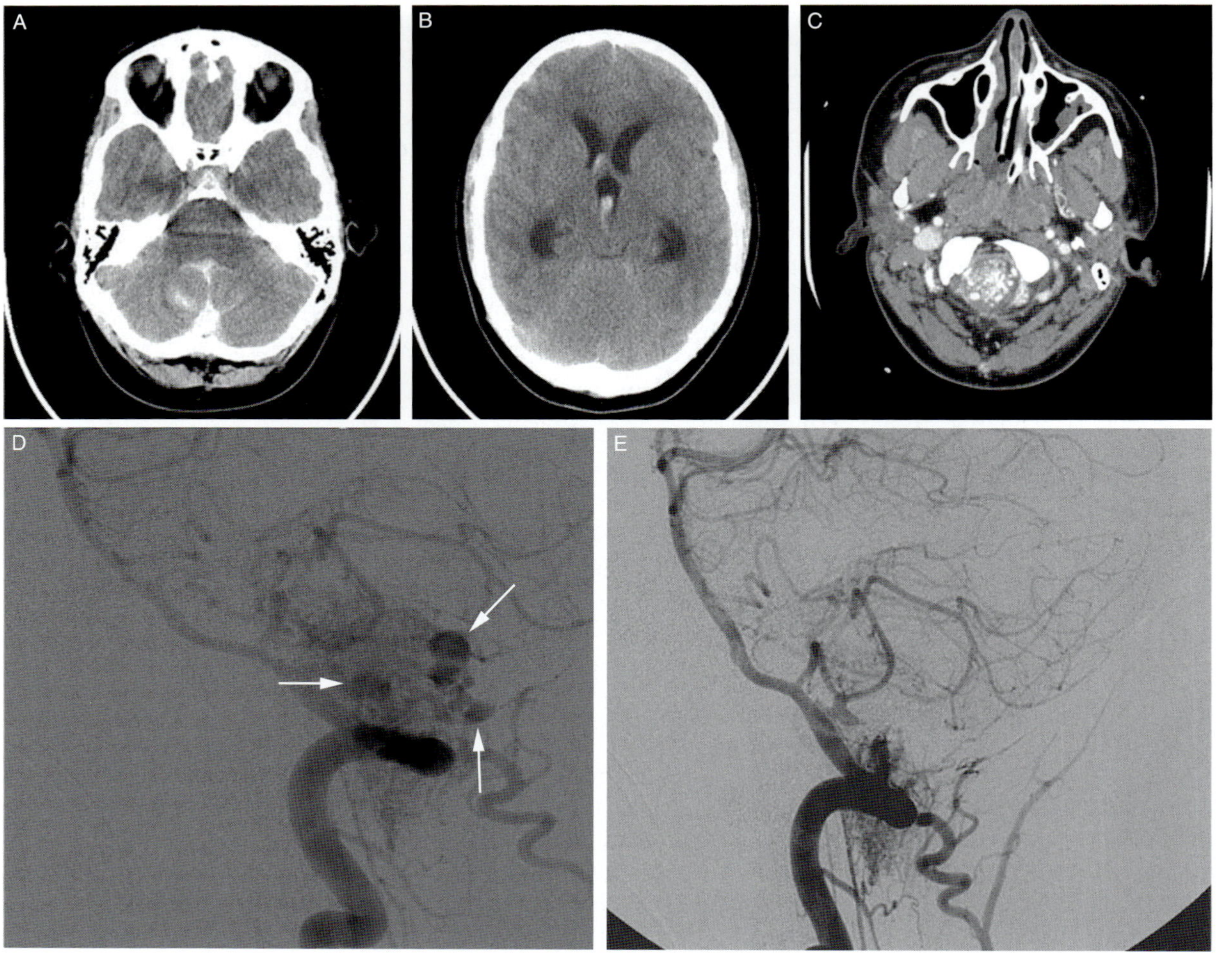

Fig. 16.1. A 15-year-old patient presented with sudden onset of headache followed by coma. There was subarachnoid hemorrhage and intraventricular hemorrhage from rupture of arteriovenous malformations (AVM)-associated aneurysms; target embolization was planned for the ruptured aneurysms. (A,B) Axial head CT demonstrated posterior fossa subarachnoid hemorrhage with intraventricular extension (A) and obstructive hydrocephalus (B). (C) Axial CT angiography showed a large brainstem AVM. (D) Catheter angiography (lateral vertebral artery injection) revealed multiple aneurysms (arrows) of the posterior inferior cerebellar artery feeding the AVM. (E) The offending aneurysms, which were felt to be the source of the bleed, were treated with selective *N*-butyl cyanoacrylate embolization as well as embolization of the feeding pedicle. Given the location and size, no treatment of the AVM was recommended. The patient made a full recovery except for a mild foot drop and remained well 4 years after the initial bleed.

when cared for in a dedicated neurointensive care setting with dedicated nursing staff (class I, level B) [8,10].

Neurological complications

Intraventricular hemorrhage and hydrocephalus

Patients with rapidly deteriorating neurological condition and level of consciousness may require urgent neurosurgical attention. If compromise of the level of consciousness is related to hydrocephalus and/or IVH, then placement of an external ventricular drain is a simple and usually safe life-saving measure. In this situation, if an external ventricular drain is placed, it is important to obtain vascular imaging (CT angiography). In such cases, the tract of the external ventricular drain must respect the location of the AVM as well as the pattern of venous drainage. In patients with coma secondary to acute hydrocephalus and/or IVH, placement of an external ventricular drain may result in dramatic improvement in their clinical condition (Fig. 16.1). In patients who may require urgent hematoma evacuation because of life-threatening mass effect and herniation, we prefer to resect the AVM in a delayed fashion and not at the time of the evacuation of the hematoma.

Vasospasm

Delayed cerebral vasospasm is a significant complication of aneurysmal SAH. Although symptomatic vasospasm is identified in 20–25% of patients, asymptomatic vasospasm can be identified in up to 70% of patients [11–13]. However, vasospasm after AVM rupture is rarely demonstrated and the incidence of asymptomatic vasospasm on delayed angiography after AVM rupture was 6.3% in a recent series [14]. Several factors may play a role in the lower incidence of vasospasm after AVM rupture compared with aneurysm rupture. These include the different hemodynamics of blood outflow after rupture, or a decreased concentration of oxyhemoglobin in extravasated blood since AVM rupture is often related to rupture of the venous outflow pathways.

Monitoring and management of intracranial pressure

In some instances of ICH caused by AVM rupture, ICP can be raised above physiological normal levels through a mass effect from hematoma expansion or extension of the blood clot into the ventricular system, eventually leading to hydrocephalus. Where there is a small hematoma and minimal IVH, ICP monitoring is likely not necessary. There are a number of invasive devices available for the monitoring and management of raised ICP, and the full discussion of their attributes, insertion techniques, and complication rates are beyond the scope of this chapter. Because of the limited amount of data regarding the ideal management of raised ICP in patients with ICH, recommendations are taken from traumatic brain injury guidelines. It is currently recommended that patients presenting with a GCS of ≤8, significant IVH, and evidence of herniation or hydrocephalus should be considered for monitoring and management of raised ICP. In this population, the goal should be maintaining the cerebral perfusion pressure between 50 and 70 mmHg (class IIb, level C) [8].

Seizures

Seizures may occur near ICH onset or within the first several weeks after the bleeding event; however, clinical seizure events have not increased mortality or led to a worsened neurological outcome after ICH [8]. A study on the use of phenytoin as a neuroprotective agent in ICH demonstrated that patients without a documented clinical seizure who were placed on phenytoin prophylaxis were significantly more likely to have died or have had a worse overall outcome than those not receiving prophylaxis at 90 days after the bleed [15,16]. The current guidelines for ICH recommend that clinical seizures should be treated with antiepileptic medications (class I, level A). Electroencephalography (EEG) can be used to diagnose potential seizure episodes in patients with depressed mental status out of proportion to the degree of injury from the ICH (class IIa, level B). Those patients with EEG findings of seizure should be treated with antiepileptic medications (class I, level C) [8]. There is currently a class III, level B recommendation against the use of prophylactic anticonvulsant medications in the setting of ICH [8]. However, we consider prophylactic anticonvulsants in patients with high-flow AVMs if surgery is contemplated.

Medical and systemic complications

Blood pressure management

In many instances of ICH, blood pressure is significantly elevated, potentially through activation of multiple signaling pathways induced by the stress of the bleeding event. In spontaneous, non-AVM-related ICH, several studies have suggested that systolic blood pressure >140 mmHg is associated with hematoma expansion as well as increased morbidity and mortality [17]. Classical teaching indicates that in patients with ICH, blood pressure control that is too aggressive may reduce blood flow in the regions surrounding the hematoma. However, this concept has been challenged by recent large, well-conducted studies. The Intracerebral Hemorrhage Acutely Decreasing Arterial Pressure Trial investigators have addressed the question of whether aggressive blood pressure control decreases peri-hematoma flow in a multicenter randomized trial [18]. Patients with spontaneous ICH <24 hours after onset and systolic blood pressure >150 mmHg were assigned to either a regimen targeting a systolic blood pressure of 150 mmHg, or to a group with a target of <180 mmHg [18]. The investigators concluded that rapid blood pressure lowering after ICH did not reduce peri-hematoma blood flow [18].

In the Intensive Blood Pressure Reduction in Acute Cerebral Haemorrhage Trial (INTERACT), patients with spontaneous ICH were randomly assigned to either an intensive blood pressure control group (target systolic blood pressure of <140 mmHg) or standard management (target systolic blood pressure of <180 mmHg) [19]. The INTERACT investigators found that early intensive lowering of blood pressure is safe and, at least in patients with spontaneous ICH, may be associated with better functional outcomes [19]. It is not known to what extent data obtained in patients with spontaneous ICH can be translated to patients with ICH from AVM rupture. It is reasonable to assume that aggressive lowering of blood pressure in the acute phase to a target systolic blood pressure of ≤140 mmHg is both safe and reasonable even in patients with ICH from AVM rupture.

Venous thromboembolism

There is a high risk of venous thromboembolism in patients who present with an ICH. Class I level B evidence supports the use of pneumatic compression devices, in addition to elastic stockings, to prevent this complication in patients with ICH [8]. The interesting medical dilemma revolves around the use of heparin anticoagulation in these patients. There have been two randomized controlled trials addressing this issue, demonstrating no increased risk of rebleeding and no difference in incidence of deep venous thrombosis in patients started on low-dose subcutaneous heparin on day 4 or day 10 after the bleed [20,21]. Current guidelines recommend documentation of cessation of bleeding, at which point low-dose subcutaneous low-molecular-weight heparin or unfractionated heparin can potentially be used for deep vein thrombosis prophylaxis in patients who are immobile one to four days from presentation (class IIb, level B) [8].

Hyperglycemia

Hyperglycemia can be predictive of poor outcome and higher rates of mortality in both diabetic and non-diabetic patients who experience an ICH [22–24]. Some studies recommend the use of insulin infusions to maintain tight glycemic control (glucose levels of 80–110 mg/dL) in patients with ICH; however, other studies have demonstrated a higher rate of hypoglycemia and poor outcomes in patients whose glucose levels are managed with insulin infusion [25–29]. Current recommendations regarding the monitoring and treatment of aberrant glucose levels state that glucose should be monitored in the setting of ICH and normoglycemia is recommended (class I, level C) [8]. There are no current recommendations regarding targeted therapy to normalize glucose levels, or what the ideal range of blood glucose levels is in the setting of ICH.

Special considerations

Hemorrhage during pregnancy

Management of intracranial hemorrhage from AVM rupture during pregnancy poses special challenges [30]. The goal of therapy is preservation of the mother's life while avoiding maneuvers that may jeopardize the fetus. Medical therapy and anesthetic management in this situation must be modified, particularly in the early phases of pregnancy, to minimize the potential teratogenetic effects on the fetus. Mannitol should be avoided unless necessary because of the potential for severe electrolyte anomalies in the fetus. We usually contemplate surgery during pregnancy for small ruptured AVMs that are easy to access. Otherwise, definitive treatment of the AVM is delayed until the completion of pregnancy. If surgery is contemplated, induced hypotension should also be avoided in this setting because of the risks of promoting fetal hypoxia. Similarly, utmost care should be paid to avoid significant blood loss.

Timing of surgery after intracranial hemorrhage from arteriovenous malformations

The annual risk of rehemorrhage in patients with parenchymal AVMs varies greatly and depends on the specific angioarchitectural features of the AVM [2,31–35]. Characteristics such as single venous outflow, stasis of the venous drainage pathways, and/or ectactic venous drainage seem to put an AVM at a higher risk of rebleeding. Overall, the risk of rebleeding over the short term in all patients is relatively low, and this has important implications for the timing of AVM treatment. Our philosophy on management of patients with AVMs presenting with ICH is similar to the strategy eloquently summarized by Heros in a recent commentary [36]. In patients who need urgent or emergency evacuation of the hematoma, the main goal is surgical decompression to resolve mass effect. In such a case, we attempt resection of the AVM only in those patients with superficial well-defined small AVMs. Otherwise, we prefer to delay definitive surgical treatment of the AVM to a few weeks later, when the residual hematoma is liquefied, the brain edema has resolved, and the AVM planes are more readily distinguishable. As shown by Hartmann and coworkers [37], many patients recover to a good level of function after ICH from an AVM. Therefore, care should be exercised during surgery for AVMs in the acute phase after rupture as even patients with severe neurological deficits may recover good function. In this setting, the lack of neurological recovery may indeed be related to the morbidity of AVM surgery rather than the damage of the ICH.

Several other situations merit special mention. Over the years, we have seen a subset of patients with a high risk of early rebleeding in the acute/hyperacute phase. In these patients, there is clear-cut outflow obstruction with increased resistance and venous stasis (Fig. 16.2). In these patients, consideration should be given to early surgical or endovascular intervention since they tend to suffer from early and often devastating rebleeds. Another important consideration in delayed treatment of ruptured AVM is to repeat a catheter angiography the day before surgical treatment. Such a delayed angiogram may show the real extent of the AVM or, in some cases, even spontaneous thrombosis of the entire AVM (Fig. 16.3).

Outcome after intracranial hemorrhage from arteriovenous malformations rupture

While it is unlikely that there are signs or symptoms that are specifically attributable to AVM rupture and not primary ICH, there may be an important difference in outcome after hemorrhage in patients with AVMs. Rupture of an AVM and

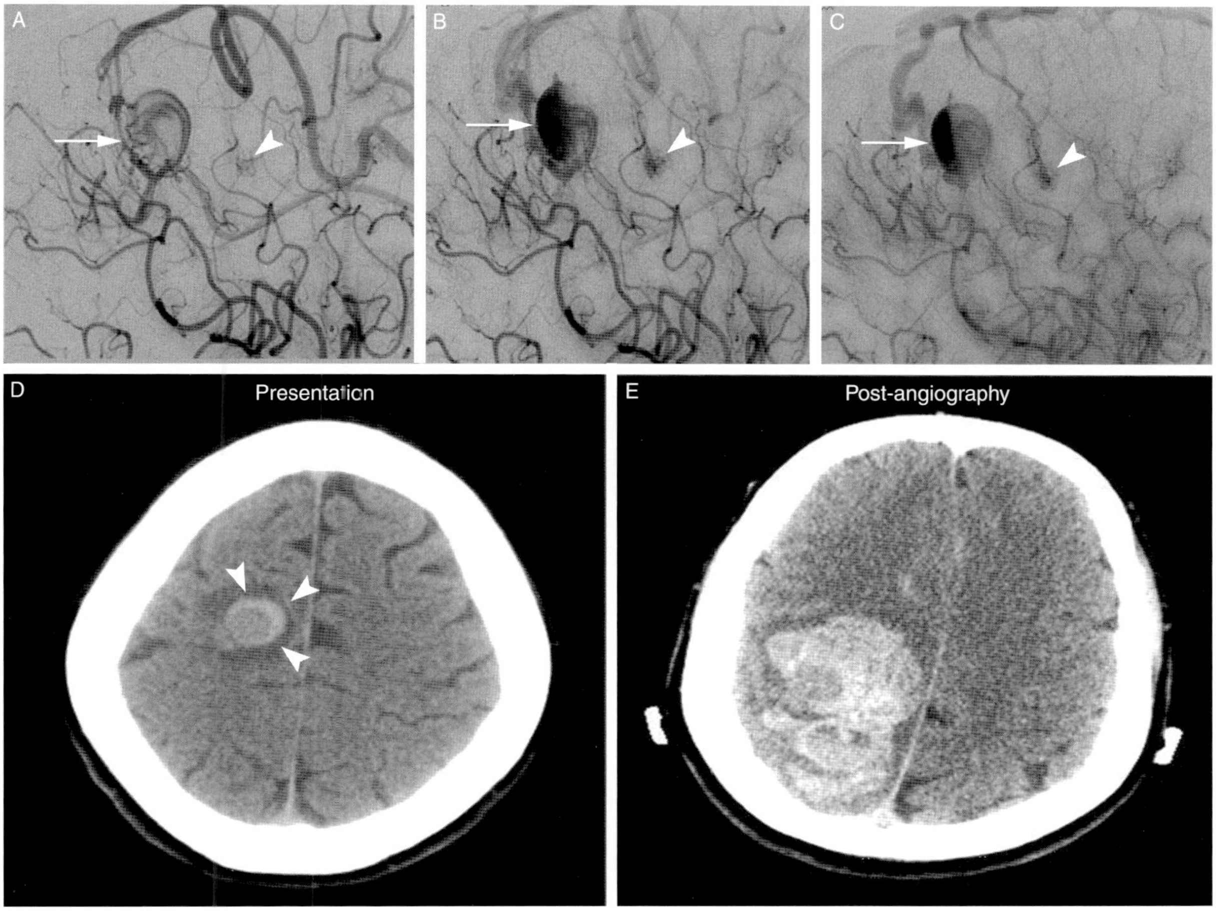

Fig. 16.2. A 52-year-old woman presented with sudden left leg weakness. Although the overall short-term risk of rebleeding after arteriovenous malformation (AVM) rupture is low, there is a subset a patients with obvious outflow restriction who are at high risk of early rebleeding. (A–C) Catheter angiography the day following admission demonstrated a small AVM nidus draining into a dilated venous varix with significant contrast stasis within the varix (arrows). Other adjacent micro-AVMs were identified (arrowheads). (D) CT at presentation showed a small crescent hemorrhage (arrowheads) surrounding a hyperdense round lesion with perilesional edema. The patient was diagnosed with hereditary hemorrhagic teleangectasia. (E) The patient experienced sudden headache and rapid neurological deterioration after angiography and a CT scan showed a new intraparenchymal hematoma. She underwent emergency clot evacuation and AVM resection.

corresponding ICH are most common in the second to fourth decades of life, compared with primary ICH, which tends to occur later into the fifth decade of life and beyond [6]. These and other factors may contribute to the potential for better outcomes in patients experiencing ICH from an AVM versus primary ICH. Several studies have aimed to determine if there is a difference in functional outcome in patients with AVMs compared with patients with primary ICH [37,38]. One study, which included 113 patients who had experienced parenchymal hemorrhage, compared outcomes at 30 days for patients who survived the primary parenchymal ICH. Significantly better outcomes based on National Institutes of Health Stroke Scale scores were demonstrated in patients with AVMs, with a mean score of 3.9 ± 6.2 compared with 13.6 ± 9.5 in patients without AVMs [38]. When the entire cohort of 241 patients was analyzed, 72% of patients with AVMs had a good functional outcome after the incident hemorrhage, defined as a modified Rankin Scale score of ≤2. Even in the 12% of untreated patients with AVMs who experienced rehemorrhage, 55% still were classified as having a good functional outcome [38]. This is compared with an overall 30-day mortality rate from all-cause ICH, which has been estimated to be 44–52% [6,39].

A study from Scotland confirmed these findings by showing that patients with AVM-related ICH are younger, have lower blood pressure at admission, and better GCS score than patients with spontaneous ICH [6]. Case fatality at one month was 50% for patients with spontaneous ICH and 11% for those with AVM-related ICH [6]. At two years, the risk of death was higher in spontaneous ICH. The median modified Rankin Scale score at one year after ICH was 2 after AVM-related ICH and 6 after spontaneous ICH [6]. The prognosis of AVM-related ICH is better than spontaneous ICH after adjustment for factors known to affect the outcome of ICH [5].

Recent population-based studies have shown that the overall prognosis of ICH after AVM rupture, although better than spontaneous ICH, is not quite as benign as some single center studies had suggested. In the Scottish study, the case fatality rate after ICH from an AVM was 11% at one month and 13% at two years [6]. The percentage of patients who were dead or dependent (modified Rankin Scale score, ≥3) at one year was 40% [6]. Case-fatality rate

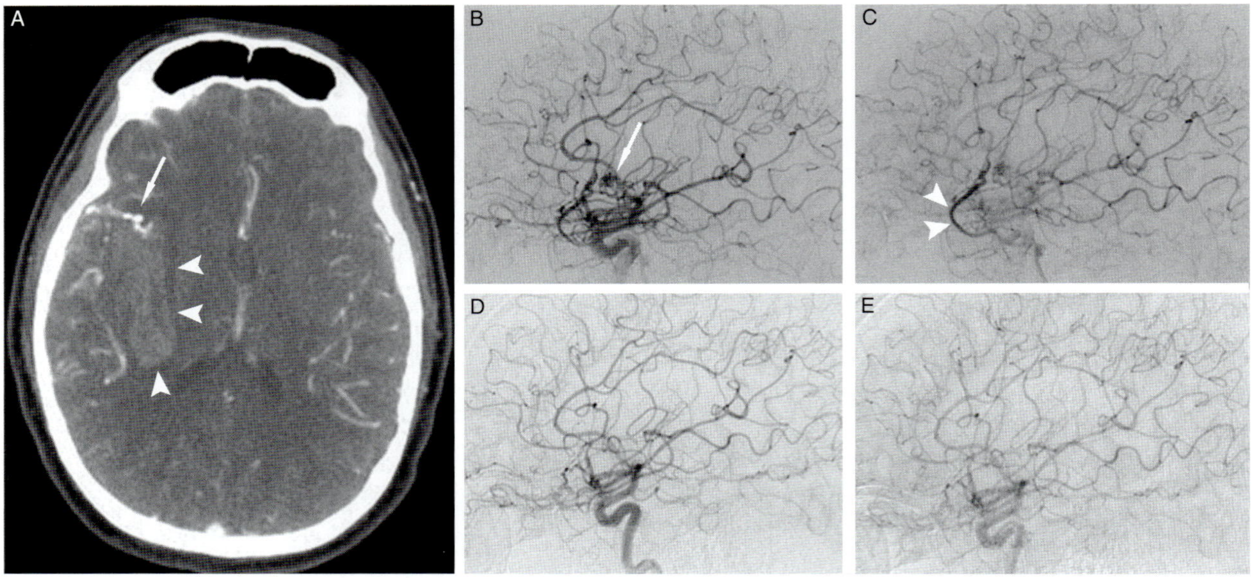

Fig. 16.3. A 44-year-old man presented with sudden left hemiparesis and headache from a right sylvian intracranial hemorrhage. If arteriovenous malformations (AVM) resection is delayed in a patient presenting with hemorrhage, catheter angiography should be repeated shortly before resection. In some cases of ruptured AVMs, the original angiography may not show the full extent of the AVM because the nidus may be compressed or partially thrombosed. Moreover, some AVMs may undergo spontaneous thrombosis after rupture. (A) Axial CT angiography demonstrated an area of hemorrhage (arrowheads) with associated AVM (arrow). (B,C) Catheter angiography (lateral internal carotid artery projection) showed a small right frontal AVM (B, arrow) with drainage through a right sylvian vein noted in the late arterial phase (C, arrowheads). (D,E) After a month of intense physical rehabilitation, the patient was referred to us and surgical resection was recommended. The day before the planned resection, a repeat catheter angiography (lateral internal carotid artery projection) showed spontaneous resolution of the AVM without filling of the sylvian vein in the late arterial phase.

is age dependent and was 9.2% at one month in patients younger than 60 years and 21% in those older than 60 years.

Conclusions

Hemorrhage from an AVM is a rare cause of ICH. Although the general management of patients with ICH from an AVM does not differ from that for those presenting with a spontaneous ICH, the natural history of AVM-associated ICH may be better. Regardless of cause, ICH should be managed with aggressive blood pressure control and resuscitation of the patient. When initial examination indicates, monitoring of the ICP may be needed. In significant mass effect or ICP refractory to medical therapy or the use of an external ventricular drain, surgical evacuation of the clot without resection of the AVM should be the goal. In most cases, patients with AVMs presenting with hemorrhage should be treated in a delayed fashion to provide time for clot resolution and a decrease in edema caused by the hemorrhage.

References

1. Al-Shahi R, Warlow C. A systematic review of the frequency and prognosis of arteriovenous malformations of the brain in adults. *Brain* 2001;**124**:1900–26.
2. Brown RD, Jr., Wiebers DO, Torner JC, *et al.* Frequency of intracranial hemorrhage as a presenting symptom and subtype analysis: a population-based study of intracranial vascular malformations in Olmsted Country, Minnesota. *J Neurosurg* 1996;**85**:29–32.
3. Cordonnier C, Al-Shahi SR, Bhattacharya JJ, *et al.* Differences between intracranial vascular malformation types in the characteristics of their presenting haemorrhages: prospective, population-based study. *J Neurol Neurosurg Psychiatry* 2008;**79**:47–51.
4. Al-Shahi R, Bhattacharya JJ, Currie DG, *et al.* Scottish Intracranial Vascular Malformation Study (SIVMS): evaluation of methods, ICD-10 coding, and potential sources of bias in a prospective, population-based cohort. *Stroke* 2003;**34**:1156–62.
5. van Beijnum J, Lovelock CE, Cordonnier C, *et al.* Outcome after spontaneous and arteriovenous malformation-related intracerebral haemorrhage: population-based studies. *Brain* 2009;**132**:537–43.
6. Hoffer A, Singer J, Bambakidis NC, Selman W. Spontaneous intracerebral hemorrhage. In Ellenbogen RG, Abdulrauf SI, Sekhar LN, eds. *Principles of Neurological Surgery,* 3rd edn. Philadelphia, PA: Elsevier, 2012, pp. 257–64.
7. Vespa PM, O'Phelan K, Shah M, *et al.* Acute seizures after intracerebral hemorrhage: a factor in progressive midline shift and outcome. *Neurology* 2003;**60**:1441–6.
8. Morgenstern LB, Hemphill JC, III, Anderson C, *et al.* Guidelines for the management of spontaneous intracerebral hemorrhage: a guideline for healthcare professionals from the American Heart Association/American Stroke Association. *Stroke* 2010;**41**:2108–29.

9. Zacharia BE, Vaughan KA, Jacoby A, *et al.* Management of ruptured brain arteriovenous malformations. *Curr Atheroscler Rep* 2012;**14**:335–42.
10. Diringer MN, Edwards DF. Admission to a neurologic/neurosurgical intensive care unit is associated with reduced mortality rate after intracerebral hemorrhage. *Crit Care Med* 2001;**29**:635–40.
11. Charpentier C, Audibert G, Guillemin F, *et al.* Multivariate analysis of predictors of cerebral vasospasm occurrence after aneurysmal subarachnoid hemorrhage. *Stroke* 1999;**30**:1402–8.
12. Ecker A, Riemenschneider PA. Arteriographic demonstration of spasm of the intracranial arteries, with special reference to saccular arterial aneurysms. *J Neurosurg* 1951;**8**:660–7.
13. Murayama Y, Malisch T, Guglielmi G, *et al.* Incidence of cerebral vasospasm after endovascular treatment of acutely ruptured aneurysms: report on 69 cases. *J Neurosurg* 1997;**87**:830–5.
14. Gross BA, Du R. Vasospasm after arteriovenous malformation rupture. *World Neurosurg* 2012;**78**:300–5.
15. Messe SR, Sansing LH, Cucchiara BL, *et al.* Prophylactic antiepileptic drug use is associated with poor outcome following ICH. *Neurocrit Care* 2009;**11**:38–44.
16. Naidech AM, Garg RK, Liebling S, *et al.* Anticonvulsant use and outcomes after intracerebral hemorrhage. *Stroke* 2009;**40**:3810–15.
17. Willmot M, Leonardi-Bee J, Bath PM. High blood pressure in acute stroke and subsequent outcome: a systematic review. *Hypertension* 2004;**43**:18–24.
18. Butcher KS, Jeerakathil T, Hill M, *et al.* The Intracerebral Hemorrhage Acutely Decreasing Arterial Pressure Trial. *Stroke* 2013;**44**:620–6.
19. Anderson CS, Huang Y, Arima H, *et al.* Effects of early intensive blood pressure-lowering treatment on the growth of hematoma and perihematomal edema in acute intracerebral hemorrhage: the Intensive Blood Pressure Reduction in Acute Cerebral Haemorrhage Trial (INTERACT). *Stroke* 2010;**41**:307–12.
20. Boeer A, Voth E, Henze T, *et al.* Early heparin therapy in patients with spontaneous intracerebral haemorrhage. *J Neurol Neurosurg Psychiatry* 1991;**54**:466–7.
21. Dickmann U, Voth E, Schicha H, *et al.* Heparin therapy, deep-vein thrombosis and pulmonary embolism after intracerebral hemorrhage. *Klin Wochenschr* 1988;**66**:1182–3.
22. Kimura K, Iguchi Y, Inoue T, *et al.* Hyperglycemia independently increases the risk of early death in acute spontaneous intracerebral hemorrhage. *J Neurol Sci* 2007;**255**:90–4.
23. Fogelholm R, Murros K, Rissanen A, *et al.* Long term survival after primary intracerebral haemorrhage: a retrospective population based study. *J Neurol Neurosurg Psychiatry* 2005;**76**:1534–8.
24. Passero S, Ciacci G, Ulivelli M. The influence of diabetes and hyperglycemia on clinical course after intracerebral hemorrhage. *Neurology* 2003;**61**:1351–6.
25. Finfer S, Chittock DR, Su SY, *et al.* Intensive versus conventional glucose control in critically ill patients. *N Engl J Med* 2009;**360**:1283–97.
26. van den Berghe G, Wouters P, Weekers F, *et al.* Intensive insulin therapy in critically ill patients. *N Engl J Med* 2001;**345**:1359–67.
27. Oddo M, Schmidt JM, Carrera E, *et al.* Impact of tight glycemic control on cerebral glucose metabolism after severe brain injury: a microdialysis study. *Crit Care Med* 2008;**36**:3233–8.
28. Vespa P, Boonyaputthikul R, McArthur DL, *et al.* Intensive insulin therapy reduces microdialysis glucose values without altering glucose utilization or improving the lactate/pyruvate ratio after traumatic brain injury. *Crit Care Med* 2006;**34**:850–6.
29. Vespa PM. Intensive glycemic control in traumatic brain injury: what is the ideal glucose range? *Crit Care* 2008;**12**:175.
30. Lanzino G, Jensen ME, Cappelletto B, *et al.* Arteriovenous malformations that rupture during pregnancy: a management dilemma. *Acta Neurochir (Wien)* 1994;**126**:102–6.
31. Stapf C, Labovitz DL, Sciacca RR, *et al.* Incidence of adult brain arteriovenous malformation hemorrhage in a prospective population-based stroke survey. *Cerebrovasc Dis* 2002;**13**:43–6.
32. Stapf C, Mast H, Sciacca RR, *et al.* The New York Islands AVM Study: design, study progress, and initial results. *Stroke* 2003;**34**:e29–e33.
33. Mast H, Young WL, Koennecke HC, *et al.* Risk of spontaneous haemorrhage after diagnosis of cerebral arteriovenous malformation. *Lancet* 1997;**350**:1065–8.
34. Hillman J. Population-based analysis of arteriovenous malformation treatment. *J Neurosurg* 2001;**95**:633–7.
35. ApSimon HT, Reef H, Phadke RV, *et al.* A population-based study of brain arteriovenous malformation: long-term treatment outcomes. *Stroke* 2002;**33**:2794–800.
36. Heros RC. Arteriovenous malformation-associated intracerebral hemorrhage. *World Neurosurg* 2012;**78**:586–7.
37. Hartmann A, Mast H, Mohr JP, *et al.* Morbidity of intracranial hemorrhage in patients with cerebral arteriovenous malformation. *Stroke* 1998;**29**:931–4.
38. Choi JH, Mast H, Sciacca RR, *et al.* Clinical outcome after first and recurrent hemorrhage in patients with untreated brain arteriovenous malformation. *Stroke* 2006;**37**:1243–7.
39. Broderick J, Brott T, Tomsick T, *et al.* Lobar hemorrhage in the elderly. The undiminishing importance of hypertension. *Stroke* 1993;**24**:49–51.

Chapter 17

Endovascular treatment of supratentorial arteriovenous malformations

Charles A. Bruno Jr., Philip M. Meyers, and Randall T. Higashida

Introduction

Arteriovenous malformations (AVMs; first described by Virchow in 1863) of the brain are rare, complex, vascular lesions that can result in significant morbidity and mortality. Current therapeutic modalities include microsurgical resection, radiosurgery (focused radiation), and endovascular embolization [1]. Endovascular embolization is primarily used as a preoperative adjuvant before microsurgery or radiosurgery. Endovascular treatment is directed at particularly "weak points" within the AVM, including flow-related aneurysms and high-flow fistulae, and to decrease lesion volume and establish more normal blood flow patterns within surrounding brain parenchyma [2]. For AVMs that are not amenable to surgery or radiosurgery because of patient factors or AVM features, palliative embolization has been used successfully to reduce the risk of hemorrhage, alleviate clinical symptoms, and preserve or improve neurological function [3–8]. Less frequently, embolization is used as "primary therapy" particularly for smaller, surgically difficult lesions. Treatment planning requires a multidisciplinary team with expertise in cerebrovascular neurosurgery, endovascular intervention, and radiation therapy in order to provide all therapeutic options and determine the most appropriate treatment regimen according to patient characteristics and AVM morphology.

Pathogenesis

Brain AVMs are focal, abnormal, intraparenchymal conglomerations of dilated arteries and veins that lack normal vascular organization at the subarteriolar level as well as a normal capillary bed, resulting in direct connections between the cerebral arterial and venous systems [9,10]. The intervening network of vessels between the distal aspects of the arterial feeders and the proximal aspects of the draining veins is called the nidus, the primary target of embolization. Gliotic brain parenchyma is found within and surrounding the nidus. On angiography, brain AVMs demonstrate arteriovenous shunting, which results in early opacification of the draining vein(s) and shortened arteriovenous transit time. Brain AVMs are classified as superficial or deep types. Superficial AVMs are further divided into sulcal, gyral, or mixed, while deep types, which are relatively rare, are subdivided into subarachnoid, deep parenchymal, plexal, and mixed types [11]. Traditionally, brain AVMs have been thought of as congenital vascular lesions, without the potential for de novo postnatal development, resulting from failure of capillary formation during embryonic development [12]. Although the majority of brain AVMs are congenital, cases of both de novo development in an adult and recurrent disease in children have been reported [13,14].

Epidemiology

Brain AVMs are relatively uncommon vascular malformations with a prevalence of < 1% and an incidence of between 0.01 and 0.001% [15–17]. The overwhelming majority of brain AVMs are sporadic, although familial occurrence has been described [18]. An increased prevalence of brain AVMs is seen with certain conditions, including Osler–Weber–Rendu disease and Sturge–Weber syndrome [19,20].

Natural history and clinical manifestations

The morbidity and mortality of brain AVMs is primarily related to their propensity to cause intraparenchymal hemorrhage and, to a lesser degree, subarachnoid and intraventricular hemorrhage [20]. Approximately 45–70% of patients with brain AVMs present with intracranial hemorrhage. Mortality rates after the first hemorrhage are between 10 and 30%, and morbidity rates of 25–60% have been reported [15,21]. Other less ominous presentations of brain AVMs include seizures, headache, and focal neurological deficits. Venous hypertension, arterial steal, and hydrocephalus are known complications of brain AVMs [17,22].

Brain AVMs are extremely heterogeneous with respect to their angioarchitecture and biological behavior (Fig. 17.1). Hemorrhage risk is related to angiographic appearance and other clinical features. It is generally accepted that brain AVMs carry an annual risk of hemorrhage of 1–3% and an annual mortality rate of 1% [16,23]. The risk of rebleeding during the first year following initial rupture has been reported

Comprehensive Management of Arteriovenous Malformations of the Brain and Spine, ed. Robert F. Spetzler, Douglas S. Kondziolka, Randall T. Higashida, and M. Yashar S. Kalani. Published by Cambridge University Press.

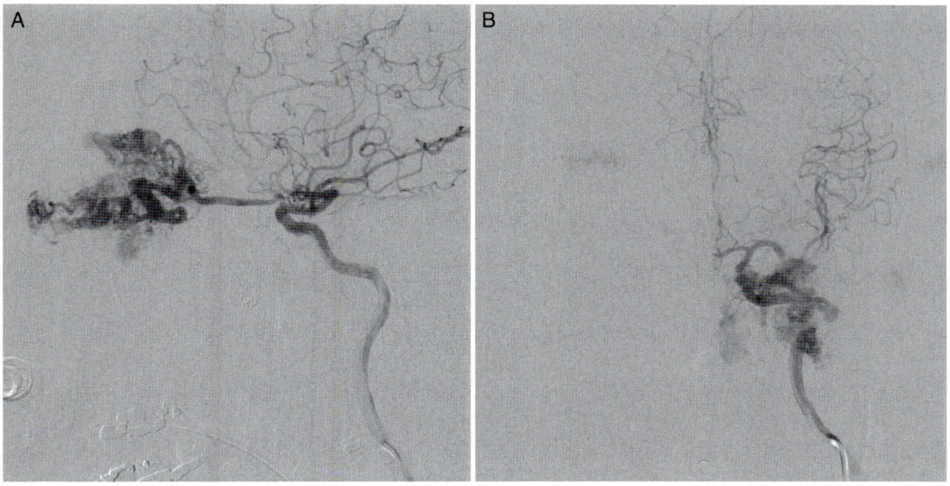

Fig. 17.1. A 56-year-old man presented with left eye redness, pain, and signs of venous congestion secondary to a left ophthalmic artery arteriovenous malformation (A, lateral view; B, anteroposterior view).

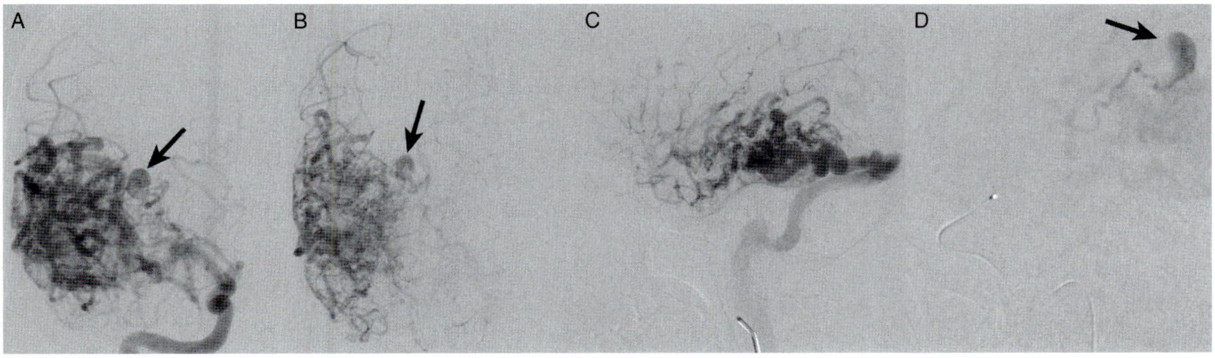

Fig. 17.2. A 28-year-old woman presented with diffuse intraventricular hemorrhage and hydrocephalus related to a posterior right temporal lobe arteriovenous malformation. (A–C) Angiography (A, anteroposterior view, arterial phase; B, anteroposterior view, late arterial phase; C, lateral view). (D) Superselective angiography, anterior choroidal artery. An intranical anterior choroidal artery aneurysm (arrows) was identified and felt to be the source of bleeding.

to be as high as 6–17%, subsequently declining to baseline, although this is not universally accepted [23,24]. Prognosis is particularly poor for patients with posterior fossa AVMs, which have mortality rates of up to 66.7% after the first hemorrhage and approaching 100% with recurrent hemorrhage. Reported risk factors for hemorrhage include [23,25–28]:

- previous hemorrhage
- deep venous drainage
- intraventricular or periventricular location
- intranidal aneurysms (Fig. 17.2)
- feeding by perforators
- feeding by the vertebrobasilar system
- location in the basal ganglia
- occlusive changes in the venous channel(s)
- male sex.

Pregnancy does not increase the risk of hemorrhage [29]. There is no evidence to suggest that a substantial undiagnosed reservoir of non-symptomatic brain AVMs exists in the general population. On the contrary, the great majority of brain AVMs will become symptomatic during a patient's lifetime, and the majority will bleed (Fig. 17.3). The risk of hemorrhage is lifelong and rises with age [30].

Grading systems

The ability to estimate the treatment risk for an individual patient with a brain AVM is extremely difficult as the variability in complexity of AVMs is so great. As a result, numerous grading systems have been developed in order to correlate specific AVM characteristics (anatomical, hemodynamic, and physiological properties) with surgical outcomes and define the degree of difficulty involved in safely removing AVMs surgically. The most widely utilized system for relative surgical risk analysis was reported by Spetzler and Martin in 1986 [31]. The grading system is based on three criteria: AVM size (small, < 3 cm; medium, 3–6 cm; large, >6 cm), pattern of venous drainage (superficial or deep), and neurological eloquence of adjacent brain regions (areas considered eloquent are sensorimotor, language, and visual cortex; hypothalamus and thalamus; internal capsule; brainstem; cerebellar peduncles; and deep cerebellar nuclei). Points are assigned for each of these three criteria and combined to give a total score of 1–5 (Table 17.1). Grades I and II lesions are generally considered safe for surgery, with very low incidence of surgically induced neurological deficits, while grades IV and V lesions are frequently accompanied by significant surgically induced neurological deficits. Grade VI lesions are considered

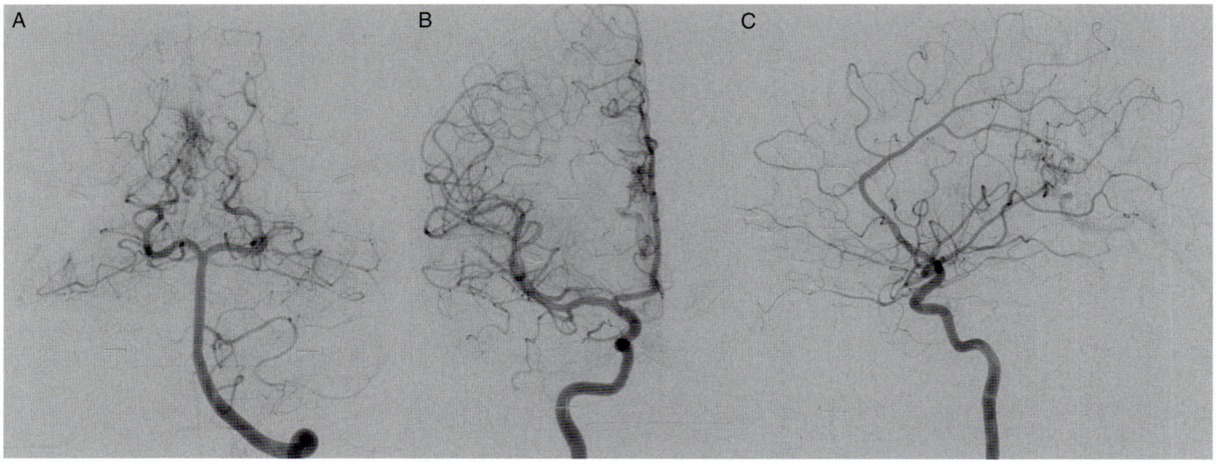

Fig. 17.3. A 15-year-old boy presented with intraventricular hemorrhage related to midline arteriovenous malformation at the level of the septum pellucidum. (A–C) Angiography (A, anteroposterior view, left vertebral injection; B, anteroposterior view, right internal carotid artery injection; C, lateral view, right internal carotid artery injection). The patient went on to have radiosurgery with complete resolution of the arteriovenous malformation (images not shown).

Table 17.1. Spetzler–Martin grading system for brain arteriovenous malformations[a]

Graded feature	Points assigned
Size	
Small (<3 cm)	1
Medium (3–6 cm)	2
Large (>6 cm)	3
Eloquence of adjacent brain	
Non-eloquent	0
Eloquent	1
Pattern of venous drainage	
Superficial only	0
Deep	1

[a] Total grade is based on size, eloquence of area affected, and venous drainage. *Source*: From Spetzler and Martin, 1986 [31], with permission.

inoperable [31]. A prospective evaluation of the Spetzler–Martin grading system examining 120 patients accurately correlated both new-temporary and new-permanent neurological deficits. Permanent major neurological deficits for grades I–III were 0%, increasing to 21.9% and 16.7% in patients with grade IV and grade V lesions, respectively [32].

Embolization of brain arteriovenous malformations

Therapeutic embolization of a brain AVM was first described in 1960 by Luessenhop and Spence utilizing flow-directed steel spheres covered with methylmethacrylate, and later Silastic spheres, injected directly into a surgically accessed cervical internal carotid artery [33]. This technique relied on the proportionately greater degree of blood flow to the AVM compared with normal cerebral branches in order to direct the embolic agents into the AVM nidus. Accidental embolization of normal cerebral vessels resulting in cerebral infarction was a potential problem. Additionally, occlusion of proximal arterial feeders could prevent entry into the nidus, leaving the nidus active. This often led to AVM recruitment of deep perforators, making surgery ultimately more challenging [34,35]. In 1974, Serbinenko reported on the use of a detachable balloon attached to a flexible flow-directed catheter. Similar to the problem seen with Silastic spheres, the detachable balloons sometimes occluded the proximal feeder pedicles, thus inducing the nidus to recruit deep perforators and making surgical resection more challenging [36]. In 1976, Kerber reported on the use of a microcatheter with a calibrated-leak balloon to superselectively catheterize the cerebral vasculature [37]. This novel device overcame the problems seen with the use of the diagnostic catheters: difficulty in placing the catheter precisely in the desired area and controlling the infusion of the occluding agent. In addition, Kerber used a liquid embolic agent, isobutyl-2-cyanoacrylate [37]. Since then, the development of smaller microcatheters, microguidewires, and novel embolic materials has led to technical achievements in AVM embolization and solidified its role as an important tool in the treatment of brain AVMs.

Indications for embolization

Although surgical resection remains the standard for the definitive eradication of most brain AVMs, endovascular embolization has the potential to enhance the safety and efficacy of AVM treatment when applied as adjuvant therapy before microsurgery [4–8]. Indications for AVM embolization include

- adjuvant therapy prior to microsurgery
- adjuvant therapy prior to radiosurgery
- palliative therapy for symptomatic but inoperable lesions
- primary therapy for smaller, surgically difficult, AVMs that contain few arterial feeders.

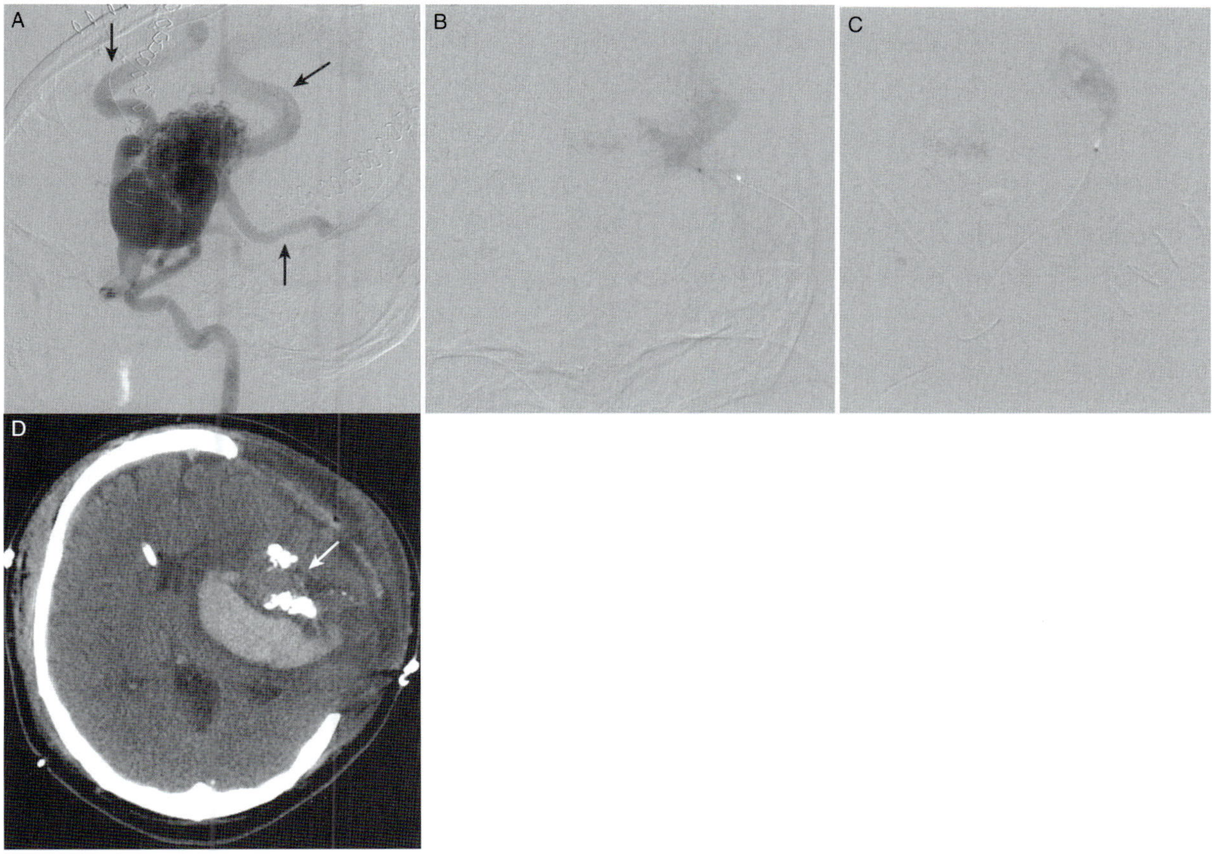

Fig. 17.4. A 32-year-old man presented with subarachnoid hemorrhage related to a large arteriovenous malformations involving the left frontal lobe, left basal ganglia, and left temporal lobe. (A) Angiography showed large veins (arrows) draining into the superior sagittal sinus and left transverse sinus (lateral view, left internal carotid artery injection). (B,C) Subtracted angiography with microcatheter injections of feeding pedicles. (D) *N*-Butyl cyanoacrylate in the nidus (arrow) on unenhanced CT image.

Preoperative embolization of AVMs has been shown to reduce operative time and intraoperative blood loss, with no difference in surgical complications or long-term neurological outcome [38]. In fact, Pasqualin *et al.* showed that patients treated with embolization prior to surgery experienced fewer postoperative neurological deficits, fewer deaths, and had a lower incidence of postoperative epilepsy when compared with patients who had surgery alone [39]. Embolization is also capable of converting lesions of high Spetzler–Martin grade to lower grades, thus turning potentially inoperable lesions into operable lesions [40]. Embolization improves surgical outcomes through several mechanisms, including: eliminating deep feeding arteries such as the anterior/posterior perforating vessels, choroidal vessels, and posterior cerebral vessels [41]; decreasing the size of the active nidus; and eliminating feeding pedicle or nidal aneurysms that have either bled or are at risk of rupture [42–44]. Additionally, presurgical embolization decreases the risk of postsurgical hemorrhage caused by changes in hemodynamics within the surrounding normal brain, and it can act as a surgical roadmap as embolized vessels are easily identifiable. Preoperative embolization in conjunction with surgery has also been shown to be cost effective when compared with surgery alone (Fig. 17.4) [45].

Another potential role of embolization is adjuvant therapy before radiotherapy, particularly for medium and large AVMs. Embolization in this setting has several theoretical benefits [46]. First, it has been shown to reduce AVM size so that the residual nidus is a smaller target that can be irradiated with a better cure rate and fewer side-effects. The cure rate increases with decreasing AVM volume, and smaller lesions (< 3 cm in diameter) carry lower rates of morbidity [47]. Preradiosurgical embolization may also be used to occlude arterial feeder or intranidal aneurysms to reduce the risk of bleeding while awaiting the delayed action of radiosurgery; to target large high-flow arteriovenous fistulae, which are less sensitive to radiosurgery [47–50]; and to reduce symptoms related to venous hypertension [4]. The risk–benefit ratio must be carefully considered in these patients. Untoward complications of embolization could precipitate the need for surgical extirpation of an inoperable AVM. There is also some evidence that embolization prior to radiosurgery may reduce the efficacy of radiotherapy to cure AVMs. Although the causes are not entirely clear, experienced authors have argued that radiopaque embolic material may “shield” the nidus from adequate radiation absorption or it may activate certain vascular growth factors [51]. Embolization has also been shown to be safe and effective in treating residual lesions that persist after radiosurgery. In six patients who underwent endovascular treatment of their brain AVMs after radiosurgery failed, one was cured with embolization alone, three underwent surgical resection for cure after embolization, and two went on to have successful repeat radiosurgery following embolization [52].

Palliative embolization of brain AVMs is typically employed in patients with large, symptomatic but inoperable cortical and subcortical lesions. The indication for palliative embolization is usually acute hemorrhage. Embolization under these circumstances should be used to treat specific high-risk AVM angioarchitectural features such as aneurysms, or to alleviate specific clinical signs and symptoms related to vascular steal and/or mechanical compression [4,53,54]. Partial embolization may also be beneficial in patients with medically refractory seizures or with progressive neurological deficits thought to be secondary to venous hypertension or arterial "steal" phenomenon causing ischemia. Palliative embolization is not recommended as a broad treatment strategy for inoperable lesions as it does not appear to produce better clinical results than medical management and there is no evidence to suggest that partial AVM embolization alters long-term hemorrhagic risk [4,55,56]. On the contrary, partial embolization has been shown to worsen the clinical course compared with the natural history of an untreated lesion [57].

Less frequently, embolization is used as "primary therapy," particularly for smaller, surgically difficult AVMs that contain few arterial feeders. Published cure rates in the literature vary considerably because of selection bias, varying goals of treatment, and differing technique. Although cure rates of up to 40% have been reported in some series [52,58,59], delayed recanalization seems to be a problem even for smaller AVMs. Furthermore, the AVMs that would have a high probability of cure with embolization are typically amenable to complete surgical resection or radiosurgical cure without the associated risks of embolization [60–62]. Deep central lesions with limited feeders are exceptions where embolization can play an important role in cure [63].

Embolic agents

Current embolic materials used to treat brain AVMs can be divided into solid and liquid agents. Solid agents consist of polyvinyl alcohol particles, fibers, coils, and balloons. Liquid agents, which are more commonly used, consist of cyanoacrylate monomers *N*-butyl cyanoacrylate (NBCA), as well as polymeric precipitates in solutions such as ethylene covinyl alcohol. Absolute (100% anhydrous) ethanol is an additional liquid embolic agent that is not commonly used now. The principle agents currently in use for treating brain AVMs include NBCA (Trufil; Codman, Raynham, MA, USA), Onyx (a copolymer of ethylene and vinyl alcohol; Covidien ev3 Neurovascular, Irvine, CA, USA), and to a lesser extent, polyvinyl alcohol particles and coils. The most commonly used agents are NBCA and Onyx and these will be discussed individually.

N-Butyl cyanoacrylate

Embolization with cyanoacrylate has evolved tremendously since its introduction in the mid 1970s because of the development of different adhesive formulations as well as advances in catheter and guidewire technologies. Isobutyl-2-cyanoacrylate has been replaced by NBCA, which was approved by the US Food and Drug Administration for brain embolization in 2000 because of NBCA's more predicable polymerization qualities, ease of surgical resection, and lack of toxicity [64]. Use of NBCA for the treatment of brain AVMs is predicated on its liquid character, which allows it to penetrate nidal vessels where it ultimately polymerizes to a solid state upon contact with blood and endothelial cells via an anionic mechanism, causing thrombosis and vessel occlusion [65]. The polymerized product is an adhesive, non-biodegradable solid material that induces an inflammatory response within the walls of embolized vessels, which is believed to play an important role in the permanence of the occlusion created with this agent [66].

As NBCA is not radiopaque, it must be opacified to monitor its flow during injection (Fig. 17.5). Ethiodol, and to a lesser extent tantalum powder, is mixed with NBCA to make the solution radiopaque. Ethiodol also acts as a retarding agent to slow the polymerization rate, as pure NBCA polymerizes almost immediately at the catheter tip. The objective is to create a mixture of glue/ethiodol that will prevent early polymerization within the feeding artery but also late polymerization within the draining vein(s). Concentrations of 25% glue and higher are typically used to achieve nidal penetration. Concentrations below 25% will usually polymerize too slowly [65]. Because of the importance that mastery of this process represents, there is a learning curve to assure its safe and proper use.

Embolization with NBCA facilitates surgical resection by helping to identify the embolized vessels, differentiating them from normal vessels, as well as providing a distinct boundary between the AVM and normal brain parenchyma. Vessels embolized with NBCA are compressible and easily cut with microscissors [38].

Onyx

Onyx is one of the newest non-adhesive liquid embolic agents available for treatment of brain AVMs [67]. It consists of an ethylvinyl alcohol copolymer dissolved in dimethyl sulfoxide. Tantalum powder is added for radiopaque visualization. Onyx is available in 1.5 mL ready-to-use vials in three different viscosities: Onyx 18, 20, and 34 contain ethylvinyl alcohol copolymer at 6%, 6.5%, and 8%, respectively. The Onyx vials must be shaken for at least 20 minutes prior to use in order to obtain a homogeneous solution consisting of the embolic component and the tantalum powder [68].

Unlike NBCA, which polymerizes almost immediately, Onyx has a very slow solidification rate and this allows for a more prolonged and controlled injection, albeit under increased pressure. This, in theory, enables larger parts of the AVM to be occluded with each microcatheterization. The slow polymerization rate and lack of adherence allows for prolonged

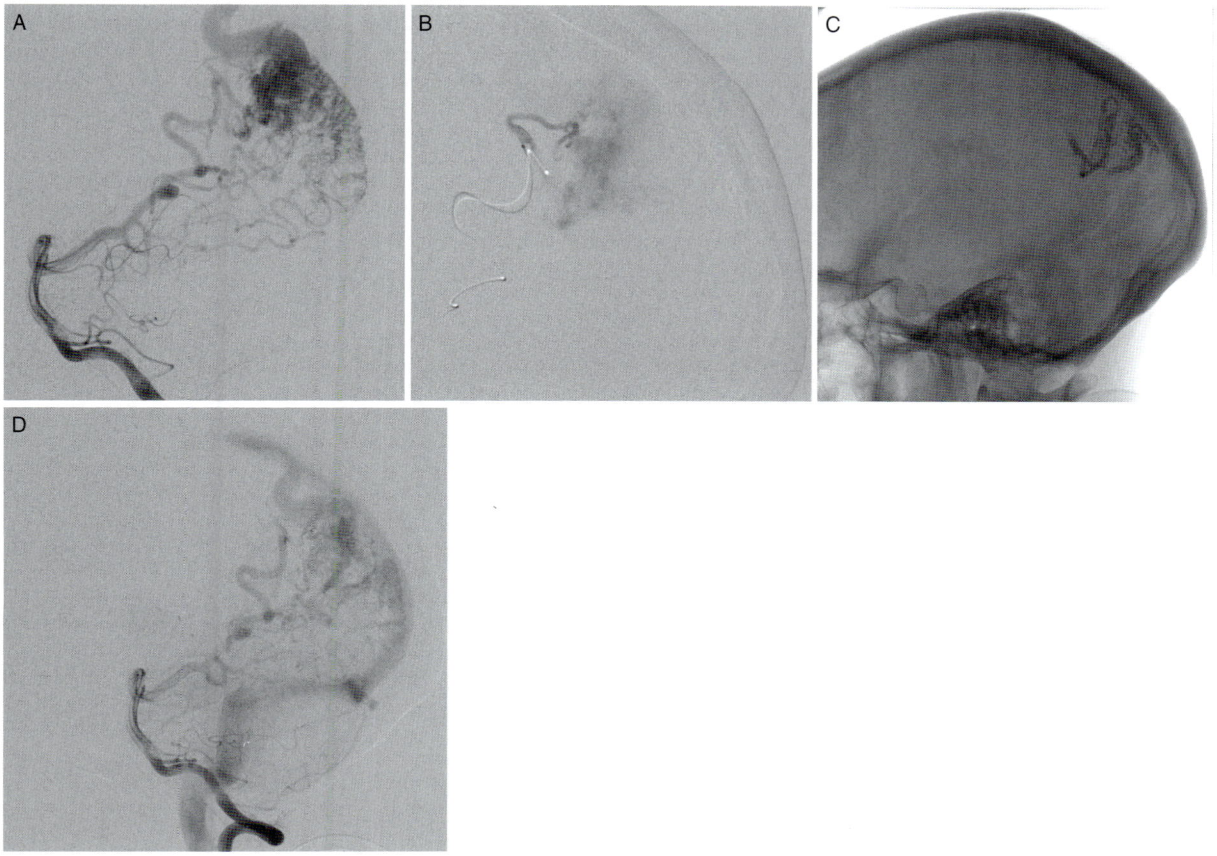

Fig. 17.5. Preoperative embolization of a left occipital arteriovenous malformations in a 35-year-old woman. (A) Angiography (lateral view, left internal carotid artery injection). (B) Subtracted angiography with microcatheter injection of feeding pedicle. (C) *N*-Butyl cyanoacrylate in nidus on unsubtracted lateral image. (D) Final postembolization digital subtraction angiography showed satisfactory reduction in size and flow.

and repeated injections from the same point, resulting in deeper penetration into a larger part of the nidus [68–70]. However, it should be noted that these are theoretical advantages as there is currently no published evidence confirming this. Some peer-reviewed publications describe longer fluoroscopy times and higher complication rates [71].

One other disadvantage or limitation of Onyx is its high radiopacity. It may be difficult or impossible to visualize the distribution of the material once it is injected in large AVMs previously treated with Onyx because of overprojection. This can potentially result in untoward injection of collateral arteries or the venous outflow system, with catastrophic results. Another disadvantage of Onyx is its poor visualization during reflux in very small vessels [70].

Risks and outcomes

Embolization of brain AVMs is not without risk, with large clinical series reporting morbidity rates of up to 16% and mortality rates of up to 4% [3,8,61,65,68–70,72–81]. Rates of morbidity and mortality vary greatly as they are dependent on many factors, including patient selection, embolic agent(s) used, goals of embolization, time of outcome assessment, and pre-existing neurological morbidity [8]. The following summarizes the largest and most recent clinical series to date regarding AVM embolization outcomes.

In 1995, Frizzel and Fisher published data on 1246 patients from 32 brain AVM embolization series performed over a 35-year period from 1969 to 1993 [81]. Temporary morbidity from embolization was 10%, and permanent morbidity was 8%. Overall mortality was 1%. Embolization resulted in cure in 5% of AVMs. They found no difference in these rates prior to or after 1990.

Debrun *et al.* reported on 54 brain AVMs treated with NBCA from April 1994 to December 1995 [65]. A mortality rate of 3.7% and morbidity rate of 5.6% (two minor and one severe permanent neurological deficit) were seen. Three patients (5.6%) were cured with embolization alone while 11 patients (20%) were cured after surgical resection. Three patients underwent radiosurgery, with one cure after one year.

Hartmann *et al.* evaluated 233 consecutive patients who underwent 545 embolization procedures between 1991 and 1998 [72]. Treatment-related neurological deficits were seen in 33 patients (14%), including five with disabling deficits (2%). There were two deaths, both secondary to parenchymal hemorrhage with ventricular extension. The five patients with disabling complications had treatment-induced ischemic strokes. Factors statistically associated with new deficits included increasing age, number of embolizations, and normal neurological status at baseline. Neither the total score of the Spetzler–Martin grading system nor any of its three components predicted treatment complications [72].

Taylor *et al.* reviewed 339 AVM embolization procedures performed in 201 patients from June 1992 to May 2003 [3]. A variety of embolic agents were used including polyvinyl alcohol particles (260 procedures [80.2%]), NBCA (43 procedures [13.3%]), detachable coils (30 procedures [9.3%]), and Onyx (5 procedures [1.5%]). Four patients (2%) died; 18 (9%) developed permanent neurological deficits; 7 (3.5%) had temporary neurological deficits, and 18 (9%) had a vascular complication without neurological compromise. Analysis of numerous variables including patient age, sex, AVM location (supratentorial or infratentorial), and the type of embolic agent used was performed. None of the variables tested was a statistically significant predictor of poor outcome, although there was a trend toward poorer outcome with increasing patient age [3].

In 2006, Haw and colleagues reported on 306 patients who underwent 513 brain AVM embolizations: 62 complications occurred in 56 patients [61]. Eight deaths were reported, six secondary to hemorrhage and two secondary to ischemic stroke. Location of the AVM in an eloquent part of the brain, presence of a fistula, and venous deposition of glue cast were all statistically associated with complications.

In 2009, Starke *et al.* reported the results of 377 embolizations in 202 patients [8]. There were 29 new clinical deficits after embolization (8% of procedures; 14% of patients), 19 of which were moderate or significant. Interestingly, on long term follow-up at 43.3 ± 34.6 months after embolization, clinical deficits had resolved in a significant number of patients, with only five having persistent neurological deficits, of which four were moderate and one was significant. Factors statistically associated with new deficits were staged embolization using more than one procedure, AVM diameter < 3 cm, AVM diameter >6 cm, deep venous drainage, and eloquent location. Patients with medium-sized lesions were less likely to develop postprocedural deficits. Similar to prior reports, there were 10 periprocedural hemorrhages (2.6% of procedures; 4% of patients). Six cerebral infarctions were also reported [8].

Sahlein *et al.* reported in 2012 a retrospective review spanning eight years from January 1997 to December 2006 and including 130 patients with 131 brain AVMs [76]. Their report is novel in that they largely used a single-stage approach for embolization as opposed to the multiple-stage embolization strategy typically employed at most institutions. An average of 1.28 embolization sessions per AVM were used, with 105 lesions treated with a single embolization (80%). The reduction in embolization sessions per patient occurred without an increase in untoward events or compromise in degree of devascularization. Permanent and/or significant morbidity and mortality rates were 0.8%. Additionally, a higher rate of angiographically complete occlusion (33%) was seen compared with that reported in most other similarly sized studies [3,8,61,65,68–70,72–81].

Studies using Onyx have shown similar rates of morbidity and mortality. Panagiotopoulos *et al.* retrospectively reviewed 82 consecutive patients with brain AVMs treated with Onyx between July 2002 and January 2008; 119 embolization procedures were performed (1.45 per patient) [68]. The authors report complete obliteration in 20 patients (24.4%); 16 (20%) developed new neurological deficits following embolization; 10 (12%) experienced non-disabling neurological deficits, and 6 (7%) experienced disabling neurological deficits. The causes of periprocedural deficits included intracerebral hemorrhage (six patients), intraventricular hemorrhage (one patient), subarachnoid hemorrhage (three patients), and infarcts/perfusion deficits (three patients). In three patients, the cause was not identified. Two patients died secondary to intraparenchymal hemorrhage [68].

Pierot *et al.* prospectively studied 50 patients from May 2003 to March 2005 to evaluate the efficacy and safety of Onyx in treating brain AVMs [79]. In all, 149 embolization procedures were performed (mean 3.0 sessions/patient) with 116 (77.9%) performed with Onyx and the others performed with a combination of Onyx and glue. At one month after treatment, morbidity and mortality rates were 8% and 2%, respectively. Cure was reported in four patients (8.3%) [79].

In 2008 Katsaridis *et al.* reported on 101 patients who underwent a total of 219 embolization sessions with Onyx [70]. There were three deaths, and eight patients had permanent neurological deficits. Complete AVM obliteration was reported in 28 patients.

Complications

As with all neurointerventional procedures, any step in the embolization process from gaining arterial access to achieving hemostasis involves risk to the patient, including groin complications (hematoma, dissection), contrast reactions, and nephrotoxicity. Periprocedural complications that are particularly relevant to brain AVM embolization include intracerebral hemorrhage and ischemia/infarction, leading to transient or permanent neurological deficits.

Periprocedural hemorrhage can have many causes, including both technical factors and physiological changes brought about by the embolization [61,82]. Technical factors include arterial perforation/dissection by the microwire or microcatheter, rupture of an aneurysm, and vascular injuries during retrieval of the catheter after glue injection [83]. Periprocedural hemorrhage can also be seen with inadvertent compromise of outflow veins and subsequent elevation of intranidal pressure. It is extremely important to avoid embolization of draining veins particularly early in the process. Although proximal arterial pressure elevation after nidus embolization has been raised as a potential cause of periprocedural hemorrhage, the changes are very small and unlikely to result in hemorrhagic complications [84].

However, the risk of normal perfusion breakthrough phenomenon (postprocedural edema and hemorrhage in cerebral tissue adjacent to the AVM nidus) [61] is more compelling as a cause of periprocedural hemorrhage. High flow through the nidus of AVMs elevates venous pressures and results in chronically low cerebral perfusion pressure, which can impair cerebral autoregulation within the brain parenchyma surrounding an AVM. Originally described by Spetzler *et al.*

[82], the idea of normal perfusion breakthrough argues that the sudden increase in perfusion pressure resulting from embolization of the nidus disrupts the chronically ischemic capillary bed within the surrounding brain parenchyma. Without normal autoregulatory mechanisms in place, this can result in cerebral edema and hemorrhage. This phenomenon can be minimized by staging endovascular procedures [42,85].

Causes of acute cerebral ischemia/infarction include arterial dissection and thromboembolic disease related to catheter or guidewire manipulation, reflux of embolic material into normal cerebral vessels, and showering of glue droplets during retrieval of the microcatheter. Retrograde thrombosis of feeding arteries is another potential cause of cerebral infarction reported in the literature [86] and venous infarction can result from delayed venous thrombosis [87].

The decision to perform embolization of a brain AVM should take into consideration the Spetzler–Martin grade of the lesion as well as inherent risk of embolization. In general, Spetzler–Martin grade II or III lesions may be embolized before surgery or radiosurgery. Grade IV or V lesions should not be embolized unless this is to be done in conjunction with other treatment modalities (surgery or radiosurgery) for the goal of complete cure. The only exception to this may be in a patient with a grade IV or V lesion with venous outflow obstruction in whom embolization is used to reduce arterial inflow to control edema, or in a patient with true "steal," in whom embolization is used to relieve the amount of shunting through the AVM.

Conclusions

Modern treatment of brain AVMs is a multimodality endeavor, requiring a multidisciplinary team with expertise in cerebrovascular neurosurgery, endovascular intervention, and radiation therapy in order to provide all therapeutic options and determine the most appropriate treatment regimen depending on patient characteristics and AVM morphology. Transarterial embolization has become a major component of AVM management, either as a stand-alone curative method or, more commonly, as an adjunct to microsurgery or radiosurgery. As newer embolic agents become available and as microcatheter technology improves, the role of endovascular treatment for brain AVMs will likely expand.

References

1. Richling B, Killer M, Al-Schameri AR, *et al.* Therapy of brain arteriovenous malformations: multimodality treatment from a balanced standpoint. *Neurosurgery* 2006;**59**:S148–57.
2. Morgan MK, Zurin AA, Harrington T, *et al.* Changing role for preoperative embolisation in the management of arteriovenous malformations of the brain. *J Clin Neurosci* 2000;**7**:527–30.
3. Taylor CL, Dutton K, Rappard G, *et al.* Complications of preoperative embolization of cerebral arteriovenous malformations. *J Neurosurg* 2004;**100**:810–12.
4. Ogilvy CS, Stieg PE, Awad I, *et al.* AHA Scientific Statement: recommendations for the management of intracranial arteriovenous malformations – a statement for healthcare professionals from a special writing group of the Stroke Council, American Stroke Association. *Stroke* 2001;**32**:1458–71.
5. Deruty R, Pelissou-Guyotat I, Mottolese C, *et al.* The combined management of cerebral arteriovenous malformations. Experience with 100 cases and review of the literature. *Acta Neurochir (Wien)* 1993;**123**:101–12.
6. Deruty R, Pelissou-Guyotat I, Amat D, *et al.* Multidisciplinary treatment of cerebral arteriovenous malformations. *Neurol Res* 1995;**17**:169–77.
7. Hartmann A, Mast H, Mohr JP, *et al.* Determinants of staged endovascular and surgical treatment outcome of brain arteriovenous malformations. *Stroke* 2005;**36**:2431–5.
8. Starke RM, Komotar RJ, Otten ML, *et al.* Adjuvant embolization with *N*-butyl cyanoacrylate in the treatment of cerebral arteriovenous malformations: outcomes, complications, and predictors of neurologic deficits. *Stroke* 2009;**40**:2783–90.
9. Friedlander RM. Clinical practice. Arteriovenous malformations of the brain. *N Engl J Med* 2007;**356**:2704–12.
10. Berman MF, Sciacca RR, Pile-Spellman J, *et al.* The epidemiology of brain arteriovenous malformations. *Neurosurgery* 2000;**47**:389–96.
11. Valavanis A. The role of angiography in the evaluation of cerebral vascular malformations. *Neuroimaging Clin N Am* 1996;**6**:679–704.
12. Mullan S, Mojtahedi S, Johnson DL, *et al.* Embryological basis of some aspects of cerebral vascular fistulas and malformations. *J Neurosurg* 1996;**85**:1–8.
13. Friedman JA, Pollock BE, Nichols DA. Development of a cerebral arteriovenous malformation documented in an adult by serial angiography. Case report. *J Neurosurg* 2000;**93**:1058–61.
14. Kader A, Goodrich JT, Sonstein WJ, *et al.* Recurrent cerebral arteriovenous malformations after negative postoperative angiograms. *J Neurosurg* 1996;**85**:14–18.
15. Ondra SL, Troupp H, George ED, *et al.* The natural history of symptomatic arteriovenous malformations of the brain: a 24-year follow-up assessment. *J Neurosurg* 1990;**73**:387–91.
16. Crawford PM, West CR, Chadwick DW, *et al.* Arteriovenous malformations of the brain: natural history in unoperated patients. *J Neurol Neurosurg Psychiatry* 1986;**49**:1–10.
17. Laakso A, Hernesniemi J. Arteriovenous malformations: epidemiology and clinical presentation. *Neurosurg Clin N Am* 2012;**23**:1–6.
18. van Beijnum J, van der Worp HB, Schippers HM, *et al.* Familial occurrence of brain arteriovenous malformations: a systematic review. *J Neurol Neurosurg Psychiatry* 2007;**78**:1213–17.
19. Kikuchi K, Kowada M, Sasajima H. Vascular malformations of the brain in hereditary hemorrhagic telangiectasia (Rendu–Osler–Weber disease). *Surg Neurol* 1994;**41**:374–80.

20. Laufer L, Cohen A. Sturge–Weber syndrome associated with a large left hemispheric arteriovenous malformation. *Pediatr Radiol* 1994;**24**:272–3.
21. Mast H, Young WL, Koennecke HC, *et al.* Risk of spontaneous haemorrhage after diagnosis of cerebral arteriovenous malformation. *Lancet* 1997;**350**:1065–8.
22. Graf CJ, Perret GE, Torner JC. Bleeding from cerebral arteriovenous malformations as part of their natural history. *J Neurosurg* 1983;**58**:331–7.
23. Fults D, Kelly DL, Jr. Natural history of arteriovenous malformations of the brain: a clinical study. *Neurosurgery* 1984;**15**:658–62.
24. Zacharia BE, Vaughan KA, Jacoby A, *et al.* Management of ruptured brain arteriovenous malformations. *Curr Atheroscler Rep* 2012;**14**:335–42.
25. Marks MP, Lane B, Steinberg GK, *et al.* Hemorrhage in intracerebral arteriovenous malformations: angiographic determinants. *Radiology* 1990;**176**:807–13.
26. Turjman F, Massoud TF, Vinuela F, *et al.* Correlation of the angioarchitectural features of cerebral arteriovenous malformations with clinical presentation of hemorrhage. *Neurosurgery* 1995;**37**:856–60.
27. Vinuela F, Nombela L, Roach MR, *et al.* Stenotic and occlusive disease of the venous drainage system of deep brain AVMs. *J Neurosurg* 1985;**63**:180–4.
28. Mansmann U, Meisel J, Brock M, *et al.* Factors associated with intracranial hemorrhage in cases of cerebral arteriovenous malformation. *Neurosurgery* 2000;**46**:272–9.
29. Horton JC, Chambers WA, Lyons SL, *et al.* Pregnancy and the risk of hemorrhage from cerebral arteriovenous malformations. *Neurosurgery* 1990;**27**:867–71.
30. ApSimon HT, Reef H, Phadke RV, *et al.* A population-based study of brain arteriovenous malformation: long-term treatment outcomes. *Stroke* 2002;**33**:2794–800.
31. Spetzler RF, Martin NA. A proposed grading system for arteriovenous malformations. *J Neurosurg* 1986;**65**:476–83.
32. Hamilton MG, Spetzler RF. The prospective application of a grading system for arteriovenous malformations. *Neurosurgery* 1994;**34**:2–6.
33. Luessenhop AJ, Spence WT. Artificial embolization of cerebral arteries. Report of use in a case of arteriovenous malformation. *J Am Med Assoc* 1960;**172**:1153–5.
34. Wolpert SM, Stein BM. Catheter embolization of intracranial arteriovenous malformations as an aid to surgical excision. *Neuroradiology* 1975;**10**:73–85.
35. Luessenhop AJ, Rosa L. Cerebral arteriovenous malformations. Indications for and results of surgery, and the role of intravascular techniques. *J Neurosurg* 1984;**60**:14–22.
36. Serbinenko FA. Balloon catheterization and occlusion of major cerebral vessels. *J Neurosurg* 1974;**41**:125–45.
37. Kerber C. Balloon catheter with a calibrated leak. A new system for superselective angiography and occlusive catheter therapy. *Radiology* 1976;**120**:547–50.
38. Jafar JJ, Davis AJ, Berenstein A, *et al.* The effect of embolization with *N*-butyl cyanoacrylate prior to surgical resection of cerebral arteriovenous malformations. *J Neurosurg* 1993;**78**:60–9.
39. Pasqualin A, Scienza R, Cioffi F, *et al.* Treatment of cerebral arteriovenous malformations with a combination of preoperative embolization and surgery. *Neurosurgery* 1991;**29**:358–68.
40. Spetzler RF, Martin NA, Carter LP, *et al.* Surgical management of large AVMs by staged embolization and operative excision. *J Neurosurg* 1987;**67**:17–28.
41. Debrun G, Vinuela F, Fox A, *et al.* Embolization of cerebral arteriovenous malformations with bucrylate. *J Neurosurg* 1982;**56**:615–27.
42. Martin NA, Khanna R, Doberstein C, *et al.* Therapeutic embolization of arteriovenous malformations: the case for and against. *Clin Neurosurg* 2000;**46**:295–318.
43. Rosenblatt S, Lewis AI, Tew JM. Combined interventional and surgical treatment of arteriovenous malformations. *Neuroimaging Clin N Am* 1998;**8**:469–82.
44. Perata HJ, Tomsick TA, Tew JM, Jr. Feeding artery pedicle aneurysms: association with parenchymal hemorrhage and arteriovenous malformation in the brain. *J Neurosurg* 1994;**80**:631–4.
45. Jordan JE, Marks MP, Lane B, *et al.* Cost-effectiveness of endovascular therapy in the surgical management of cerebral arteriovenous malformations *AJNR Am J Neuroradiol* 1996;**17**:247–54.
46. Dion JE, Mathis JM. Cranial arteriovenous malformations. The role of embolization and stereotactic surgery. *Neurosurg Clin N Am* 1994;**5**:459–74.
47. Deruty R, Pelissou-Guyotat I, Amat D, *et al.* Complications after multidisciplinary treatment of cerebral arteriovenous malformations. *Acta Neurochir (Wein)* 1996;**138**:119–31.
48. Pollock BE, Flickinger JC, Lunsford LD, *et al.* Factors associated with successful arteriovenous malformation radiosurgery. *Neurosurgery* 1998;**42**:1239–44.
49. Gobin YP, Laurent A, Merienne L, *et al.* Treatment of brain arteriovenous malformations by embolization and radiosurgery. *J Neurosurg* 1996;**85**:19–28.
50. Friedman WA, Bova FJ. Radiosurgery for arteriovenous malformations. *Neurol Res* 2011;**33**:803–19.
51. Mamalui-Hunter M, Jiang T, Rich KM, *et al.* Effect of liquid embolic agents on GammaKnife surgery dosimetry for arteriovenous malformations. *J Neurosurg* 2011;**115**:364–70.
52. Marks MP, Lane B, Steinberg GK, *et al.* Endovascular treatment of cerebral arteriovenous malformations following radiosurgery. *AJNR Am J Neuroradiol* 1993;**14**:297–303.
53. Konan AV, Roy D, Raymond J. Endovascular treatment of hemifacial spasm associated with a cerebral arteriovenous malformation using transvenous embolization: case report. *Neurosurgery* 1999;**44**:663–6.
54. Sugita M, Takahashi A, Ogawa A, *et al.* Improvement of cerebral blood flow and clinical symptoms associated with embolization of a large arteriovenous malformation: case report. *Neurosurgery* 1993;**33**:748–51.
55. Kwon OK, Han DH, Han MH, *et al.* Palliatively treated cerebral arteriovenous malformations: follow-up results. *J Clin Neurosci* 2000;7(Suppl 1):69–72.

56. Lv X, Wu Z, Li Y, *et al.* Hemorrhage risk after partial endovascular NBCA and Onyx embolization for brain arteriovenous malformation. *Neurol Res* 2012;**34**:552–6.

57. Miyamoto S, Hashimoto N, Nagata I, *et al.* Posttreatment sequelae of palliatively treated cerebral arteriovenous malformations. *Neurosurgery* 2000;**46**:589–94.

58. Fournier D, terBrugge KG, Willinsky R, *et al.* Endovascular treatment of intracerebral arteriovenous malformations: experience in 49 cases. *J Neurosurg* 1991;**75**:228–33.

59. Valavanis A, Yaşargil MG. The endovascular treatment of brain arteriovenous malformations. *Adv Tech Stand Neurosurg* 1998;**24**:131–214.

60. Schaller C, Schramm J. Microsurgical results for small arteriovenous malformations accessible for radiosurgical or embolization treatment. *Neurosurgery* 1997;**40**:664–72.

61. Haw CS, terBrugge K, Willinsky R, *et al.* Complications of embolization of arteriovenous malformations of the brain. *J Neurosurg* 2006;**104** 226–32.

62. Willinsky R, Goyal M, terBrugge K, *et al.* Embolisation of small (< 3 cm) brain arteriovenous malformations. Correlation of angiographic results to a proposed angioarchitecture grading system. *Interv Neuroradiol* 2001;**7**:19–27.

63. Hurst RW, Berenstein A, Kupersmith MJ, *et al.* Deep central arteriovenous malformations of the brain: the role of endovascular treatment. *J Neurosurg* 1995;**82**:190–5.

64. Brothers MF, Kaufmann JC, Fox AJ, *et al.* *N*-Butyl 2-cyanoacrylate: substitute for IBCA in interventional neuroradiology – histopathologic and polymerization time studies. *AJNR Am J Neuroradiol* 1989;**10**:777–86.

65. Debrun GM, Aletich V, Ausman JI, *et al.* Embolization of the nidus of brain arteriovenous malformations with *N*-butyl cyanoacrylate. *Neurosurgery* 1997;**40**:112–20.

66. Vinters HV, Lundie MJ, Kaufmann JC. Long-term pathological follow-up of cerebral arteriovenous malformations treated by embolization with bucrylate. *N Engl J Med* 1986;**314**:477–83.

67. Taki W, Yonekawa Y, Iwata H, *et al.* A new liquid material for embolization of arteriovenous malformations. *AJNR Am J Neuroradiol* 1990;**11**:163–8.

68. Panagiotopoulos V, Gizewski E, Asgari S, *et al.* Embolization of intracranial arteriovenous malformations with ethylene-vinyl alcohol copolymer (Onyx). *AJNR Am J Neuroradiol* 2009;**30**:99–106.

69. Weber W, Kis B, Siekmann R, *et al.* Endovascular treatment of intracranial arteriovenous malformations with Onyx: technical aspects. *AJNR Am J Neuroradiol* 2007;**28**:371–7.

70. Katsaridis V, Papagiannaki C, Aimar E. Curative embolization of cerebral arteriovenous malformations (AVMs) with Onyx in 101 patients. *Neuroradiology* 2008;**50**:589–97.

71. Velat GJ, Reavey-Cantwell JF, Sistrom C, *et al.* Comparison of *N*-butyl cyanoacrylate and Onyx for the embolization of intracranial arteriovenous malformations: analysis of fluoroscopy and procedure times. *Neurosurgery* 2008;**63**:ons73–8.

72. Hartmann A, Pile-Spellman J, Stapf C, *et al.* Risk of endovascular treatment of brain arteriovenous malformations. *Stroke* 2002;**33**:1816–20.

73. Meisel HJ, Mansmann U, Alvarez H, *et al.* Effect of partial targeted *N*-butyl-cyanoacrylate embolization in brain AVM. *Acta Neurochir (Wien)* 2002;**144**:879–87.

74. Jayaraman MV, Marcellus ML, Hamilton S, *et al.* Neurologic complications of arteriovenous malformation embolization using liquid embolic agents. *AJNR Am J Neuroradiol* 2008;**29**:242–6.

75. Ledezma CJ, Hoh BL, Carter BS, *et al.* Complications of cerebral arteriovenous malformation embolization: multivariate analysis of predictive factors. *Neurosurgery* 2006;**58**:602–11.

76. Sahlein DH, Mora P, Becske T, *et al.* Nidal embolization of brain arteriovenous malformations: rates of cure, partial embolization, and clinical outcome. *J Neurosurg* 2012;**117**:65–77.

77. n-BCA Trial Investigators. *N*-butyl cyanoacrylate embolization of cerebral arteriovenous malformations: results of a prospective, randomized, multi-center trial. *AJNR Am J Neuroradiol* 2002;**23**:748–55.

78. Mounayer C, Hammami N, Piotin M, *et al.* Nidal embolization of brain arteriovenous malformations using Onyx in 94 patients. *AJNR Am J Neuroradiol* 2007;**28**:518–23.

79. Pierot L, Januel AC, Herbreteau D, *et al.* Endovascular treatment of brain arteriovenous malformations using onyx: results of a prospective, multicenter study. *J Neuroradiol* 2005;**36**:147–52.

80. van Rooij WJ, Jacobs S, Sluzewski M, *et al.* Curative embolization of brain arteriovenous malformations with onyx: patient selection, embolization technique, and results. *AJNR Am J Neuroradiol* 2012;**33**:1299–304.

81. Frizzel RT, Fisher WS, III. Cure, morbidity, and mortality associated with embolization of brain arteriovenous malformations: a review of 1246 patients in 32 series over a 35-year period. *Neurosurgery* 1995;**37**:1031–9.

82. Spetzler RF, Wilson CB, Weinstein P, *et al.* Normal perfusion pressure breakthrough theory. *Clin Neurosurg* 1978;**25**:651–72.

83. Purdy PD, Batjer HH, Samson D. Management of hemorrhagic complications from preoperative embolization of arteriovenous malformations. *J Neurosurg* 1991;**74**:205–11.

84. Henkes H, Gotwald TF, Brew S, *et al.* Pressure measurements in arterial feeders of brain arteriovenous malformations before and after endovascular embolization. *Neuroradiology* 2004;**46**:673–7.

85. Alexander MD, Connolly ES, Meyers PM. Revisiting normal perfusion pressure breakthrough in light of hemorrhage-induced vasospasm. *World J Radiol* 2010;**2**:230–2.

86. Sipos EP, Kirsch JR, Nauta HJ, *et al.* Intra-arterial urokinase for treatment of retrograde thrombosis following resection of an arteriovenous malformation. Case report. *J Neurosurg* 1992;**76**:1004–7.

87. Duckwiler GR, Dion JE, Vinuela F, *et al.* Delayed venous occlusion following embolotherapy of vascular malformations in the brain. *AJNR Am J Neuroradiol* 1992;**13**:1571–9.

Chapter 18

Endovascular treatment of arteriovenous malformations of the posterior fossa

Travis M. Dumont, L. Nelson Hopkins, and Elad I. Levy

Introduction

Arteriovenous malformations (AVMs) located in the infratentorial compartment make up less than 15% of brain AVMs in large series [1–3]. Despite their relative paucity in number, infratentorial AVMs represent an important subset for treatment because as many as 85% of patients with these lesions present with hemorrhage [1,4–7], with a propensity toward poor outcome after rupture compared with their supratentorial counterparts [4]. Hemorrhage as a presenting symptom of infratentorial AVMs may in part be explained by a relatively high incidence of prenidal aneurysms [7–9] and deep venous drainage [7,10]. Consequently, a newly diagnosed infratentorial AVM should be strongly considered for treatment given the unclear natural history and tendency toward poor outcome after rupture.

Presentation and natural history

Mass effect from an infratentorial AVM is most frequently associated with a cerebellopontine angle or brainstem location, typically with a cranial neuropathy [1,11–14]. Presentation with hydrocephalus has been described [15,16]. Neuralgia is an uncommon presentation and has resolved after AVM treatment [17–19]. Seizure is relatively absent as a presenting symptom in infratentorial AVMs, compared with AVMs of the supratentorial compartment [8,10,11]; consequently, unruptured AVMs are more likely to be clinically silent.

Anatomical considerations

Approximately 70% of infratentorial AVMs are located in the cerebellum and 25% within the brainstem [20]. Location of the AVM nidus is of principal importance in determination of risk associated with endovascular treatment. The AVMs of the brainstem carry significantly more morbidity with endovascular embolization than do those of the cerebellum [20]. Unlike supratentorial AVMs, the size of AVM nidus is less important as a predictive variable for perioperative morbidity associated with treatment of infratentorial AVMs. This is because larger infratentorial AVMs are typically located in the hemisphere of the cerebellum, which is a more forgiving location for endovascular embolization compared with the cerebellopontine angle or brainstem, regardless of AVM size. Because of this, infratentorial AVMs do not stratify well into the classification system of Spetzler–Martin [20]. We have routinely relied on pedicle size and number and nidus location in making the determination of preoperative risk for endovascular treatment of all intracranial AVMs.

An understanding of the arterial pedicle anatomy of infratentorial AVMs is critical when considering endovascular embolization. Six-vessel cerebral angiography (bilateral vertebral arteries, as well as internal and external carotid arteries) is performed on all patients with newly diagnosed AVMs. Contribution from the internal carotid arteries would be extraordinarily rare; however, approximately 10% of infratentorial AVMs are fed by one or both external carotid arteries [11]. Holohemispheric cerebellar AVMs typically have input from all three ipsilateral cerebellar arterial trunks [21]; selective angiography may be necessary to visualize all pedicles in this high-flow environment. Because prenidal aneurysms are more frequently encountered with infratentorial AVMs than with supratentorial AVMs [7–9], the performance of selective angiography to assess for an aneurysm in such patients is strongly advised.

Embolization agents and devices

Most infratentorial AVM embolization procedures are performed with liquid embolic agents. We use one of two commercially available liquid embolics for all arterial pedicle embolization procedures. The most frequently used is a copolymer of ethylene and vinyl alcohol dissolved in dimethyl sulfoxide (DMSO) (Onyx; Covidien ev3 Neurovascular, Irvine, CA, USA). When infused into the bloodstream, this agent precipitates to form a non-adhesive, spongy solid. Onyx is available in three increasing viscosities: Onyx 18, 20, and 34 containing the ethylvinyl alcohol copolymer at 6%, 6.5%, and 8%, respectively. As Onyx precipitates from solution, it behaves in a predictable manner that allows the surgeon to control penetration of the embolysate into the nidus and to minimize embolization into draining venous structures and unwanted proximal reflux. *N*-Butyl cyanoacrylate (NBCA) is a commercially available

Comprehensive Management of Arteriovenous Malformations of the Brain and Spine, ed. Robert F. Spetzler, Douglas S. Kondziolka, Randall T. Higashida, and M. Yashar S. Kalani. Published by Cambridge University Press.

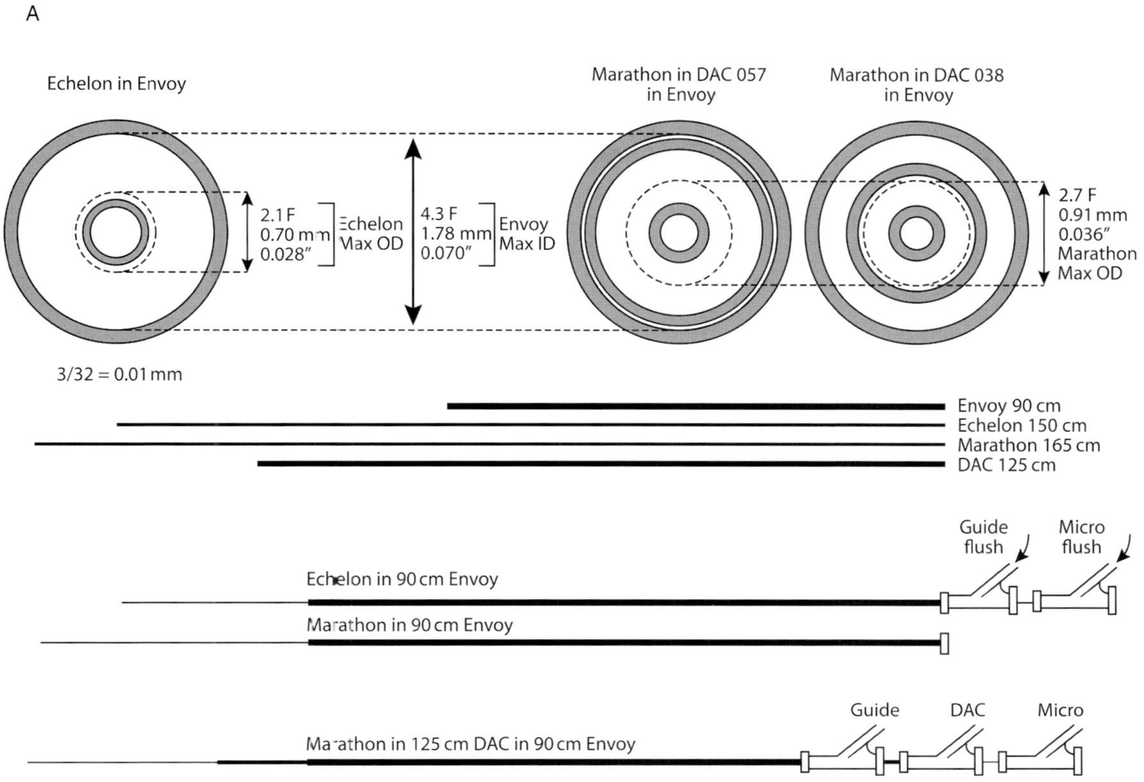

Fig. 18.1. Commonly employed catheter systems for infratentorial arteriovenous malformation embolization. (A) The typical guide catheter–microcatheter setup. The two-catheter system is employed most frequently; rarely, a three-catheter system is employed. (B) Two-catheter system. An Onyx-compatible microcatheter is threaded through a 6F guide catheter. In this case, the 150 cm Echelon microcatheter is within a 90 cm 6F angled-tip Envoy catheter. With continuous flush hemostatic valves, a maximum of 24 cm of working length distal to the guide catheter is available. A cross-section displays the capacious working space within the guide catheter lumen for this simple system. (C) Three-catheter system. A triaxial catheter system, with a 165 cm Onyx-compatible Marathon microcatheter delivered through a 125 cm distal access catheter (DAC 038 or DAC 057), delivered through a 90 cm 6F Envoy catheter. With continuous flush hemostatic valves on each catheter, a maximum of 24 cm of working length distal to the guide catheter is available. Cross-sections of the triaxial system with either DAC is shown. With the DAC 038, angiographic runs are performed through the guide catheter. With the DAC 057, angiographic runs are performed through the DAC. ID, internal diameter; OD, outside diameter.

glue polymer (Trufill, DePuy Synthes-Codman, Raynham, MA, USA) packaged with ethiodized oil that we use with less frequency for embolization procedures. Trufill has a rapid polymerization time once infused into the selected arterial pedicle and forms a dense cast of the AVM nidus. The short polymerization time makes it more difficult to control the behavior of this embolysate compared with Onyx. We employ a 1:2 NBCA:ethiodized oil ratio, which simplifies preparation and allows a predictable result. We then add glacial acetic acid (2–6 drops) to further delay polymerization as necessary and produce a more reliable embolization with improved penetration of the embolysate cast into the AVM nidus. A higher ratio of ethiodized oil will have a similar effect. With high-magnification angiography, we find it unnecessary to add tantalum powder as an opacifying agent.

Embolization of infratentorial AVMs requires a relatively simple catheter system (Fig. 18.1), with only a guide catheter and microcatheter required. For most patients, we use an angled-tip 6 French (F) guiding catheter (Envoy, DePuy Synthes-Codman), which may be guided directly into the dominant vertebral artery without an exchange technique. For patients in which more tortuous anatomy is encountered, we use a 6F guiding catheter with a more flexible distal segment (Envoy DA [DePuy Synthes-Codman], Neuron [Penumbra, Alameda, CA, USA], or Navien [formerly ReFlex; ev3-Covidien]). Because these catheters have a very soft distal end, they are most easily directed into position within the vertebral artery over a soft exchange-length wire (0.88 mm [0.035″]) positioned in the vessel of interest with any 5F diagnostic catheter. Each of these guiding catheters has advantageous characteristics (specifications of our most frequently used catheters are summarized in Table 18.1). The Envoy provides the greatest support but may be more likely to initiate trauma (iatrogenic vertebral dissection) in a tortuous vessel. For tortuous vessels, we find the Envoy DA catheter to be the most versatile as it can be delivered to a safe distal position within the target vessel with relative ease. The Navien catheter has a slightly larger inner diameter than similar catheters, which is more useful if a larger distal access catheter (DAC 057; Concentric Medical, Freemont, CA, USA) is employed; and the Neuron 070 has the softest distal tip but provides good stability only when proximal vertebral tortuosity is encountered.

Although a variety of over-the-wire or flow-directed microcatheters are available, we generally employ DMSO-compatible microcatheters, which allow the surgeon the flexibility to use Onyx. Unless the targeted vessel is very small or in a very distal location, we prefer to use the steerable Echelon-10

B

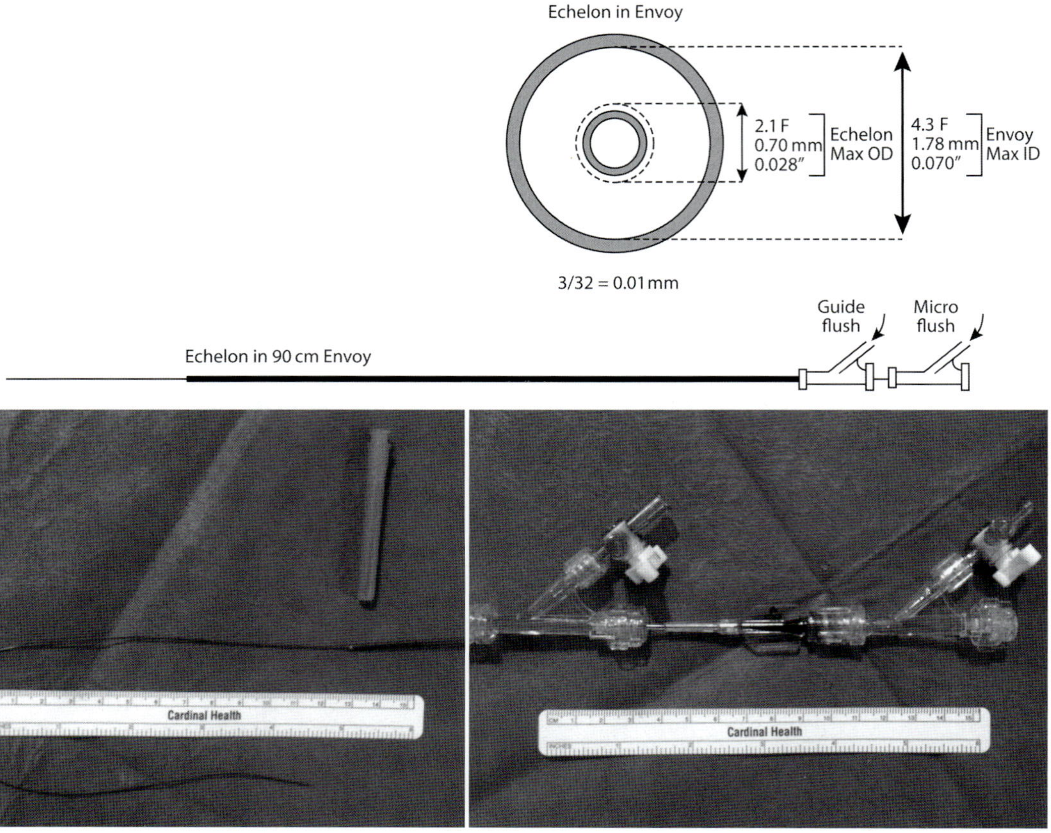

C

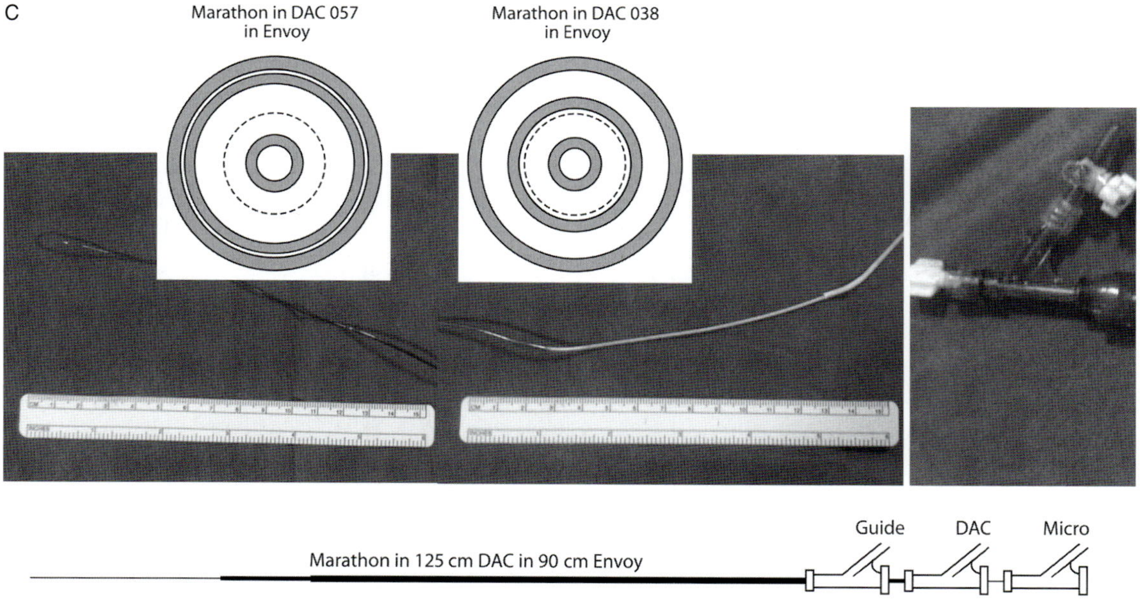

Fig. 18.1. (cont.).

Table 18.1. Commonly used catheters for infratentorial arteriovenous malformations embolization

	Length (cm)			French gauge diameter (mm [inches])			Dead space (mL)
	Total	Proximal support length	Flexible distal length	Proximal outer	Distal outer	Inner	
Guide catheters							
Envoy	90 or 100	85 or 95	N/A	6F, 2.00 (0.079)	Same as proximal	5.3F, 1.78 (0.070)	–
Envoy DA	95 or 105	85 or 95	8	6F, 2.00 (0.079)	Same as proximal	5.4F, 1.80 (0.071)	–
Navien (formerly ReFlex)	105 or 115	96 or 106	8	6.4F, 2.12 (0.084)	6.2F, 2.06 (0.081)	5.5F, 1.83 (0.072)	–
Neuron 070	95 or 105	81 or 91	6	6.2F, 2.08 (0.082)	5.9F, 1.98 (0.078)	5.3F, 1.78 (0.070)	–
Distal access catheters							
DAC 038	125 or 136	N/A	N/A	3.9F, 1.30 (0.051)	Same as proximal	2.9F, 0.97 (0.038)	–
DAC 057	115 or 125	N/A	N/A	5.2F, 1.75 (0.069)	Same as proximal	4.3F, 1.45 (0.057)	–
Dimethyl sulfoxide-compatible microcatheters							
Marathon (partially flow-directed)	165	N/A	25	2.7F, 0.91 (0.036)	1.5F, 0.51 (0.020)	1.0F, 0.33 (0.013)	0.25
Echelon-10 (not flow directed)	150	N/A	N/A	2.1F, 0.70 (0.028)	1.7F, 0.57 (0.022)	1.3F, 0.43 (0.017)	0.34

N/A, not applicable; –, information not provided by manufacturers.

microcatheter (ev3-Covidien), which hastens embolization because of its larger capacity than the other available Onyx-compatible microcatheter, the Marathon (ev3-Covidien). In addition, truly steerable microwires (0.35 mm [0.014″]) can be used for selection of tortuous arterial pedicles, including those found in relatively low-flow areas. We rarely use the Echelon-14 microcatheter, which is stiffer than the Echelon-10 but has the same inner diameter. The Marathon microcatheter is flow directed, although less so than other flow-directed microcatheters. We use a steerable microwire (0.25 mm [0.010″]) for this system, which offers some navigability in small vessels. The Marathon microcatheter is significantly longer than the Echelon-10, which is useful when the target position for embolization is very distal (e.g., in the setting of a very tortuous superior cerebellar artery pedicle). The Marathon microcatheter is quite soft, to a degree that it may be difficult to navigate tortuous anatomy without employing a distal access catheter.

A distal access catheter of intermediate diameter is generally not required for infratentorial AVM embolization. However, when multiple embolization sessions are planned at a distally located target, a distal access catheter may hasten the procedure. An additional benefit to this type of catheter is the ability to perform more selective angiographic runs, which may offer the surgeon more clarity of the anatomical detail of a targeted arterial pedicle. This is particularly true for pedicles of the superior cerebellar arteries, where ipsilateral imaging simplifies navigation in the lateral plane. We use one of two distal access catheters, DAC 038 or DAC 057 [21]. The DAC 038 is smaller and much more easily navigated to branches of the vertebrobasilar system, but selective angiographic runs must be performed with the microcatheter removed because of the smaller inner lumen of this catheter (2.9F; compared with the maximum outer diameter of the Marathon microcatheter of 2.7F). The DAC 057 is larger and more difficult to navigate into distal vertebrobasilar branches, such as the superior cerebellar artery or posterior cerebral artery. This catheter is a better choice for pedicles of the posterior inferior cerebellar artery or anterior inferior cerebellar artery and, given its maximum outer diameter (5.2F), it is best used with a larger 6F guide catheter, such as the Navien (inner diameter, 5.5F).

Perioperative risk assessment

Endovascular treatment of infratentorial AVMs is predicated on several factors. These include symptomatology, location, and vascular anatomy. Careful assessment of these factors should be performed when a new diagnosis of AVM is encountered. Treatment of AVMs involves consideration of a multimodal management strategy, including endovascular embolization, surgical resection, and stereotactic radiosurgery.

Because the role for obliteration of unruptured AVMs remains somewhat unclear [22,23], incidentally noted and asymptomatic AVMs, including those of the infratentorial compartment, may be considered for observational management. Typically, we recommend endovascular treatment for asymptomatic AVMs when anatomical features that portend a higher risk for hemorrhage are encountered. This includes prenidal aneurysm, large size, exclusively deep venous drainage, and venous varices [5,24–26]. Such features, particularly prenidal aneurysm and exclusively deep venous drainage, are more frequent in infratentorial AVMs [7–9]. Symptomatic patients should be counseled on the unique risks of infratentorial AVMs when expectant management is planned.

Although widely applied for perioperative risk assessment, the components of the Spetzler–Martin grading scheme [27] are of less relevance to infratentorial AVMs, particularly with respect to endovascular treatment. Location of AVM nidus within functional tissue is of much greater relevance than venous drainage pattern and size. Size is of less relevance in determining treatment morbidity because infratentorial AVMs are less likely to have a large diameter because of their anatomical confinement. Large AVMs encompassing an entire cerebellar hemisphere may be encountered, but these tend to be associated with neurological complications much less often than AVMs of the brainstem, despite their size. Large AVMs of the brainstem are uncommon. Drainage pattern is of less relevance in determining endovascular-treatment-related morbidity because most infratentorial AVMs are deep draining. A four-tier grading system for infratentorial AVMs has been suggested that is based primarily on location and venous drainage patterns and accords less importance to nidus size (Table 18.2), but this system has not been validated [20]. The three-tier modification of the original Spetzler–Martin classification system [28] (Table 18.3) has been validated to be predictive for perioperative complications after surgical resection of cerebellar AVM [29] but not for endovascular treatment. Similarly, a supplementary AVM grading scale to be applied with the conventional Spetzler–Martin score has been introduced [30] and is more accurate in prediction of perioperative complications for posterior fossa AVM than the conventional Spetzler–Martin score [29], but it has not been validated for endovascular treatment of AVMs.

In our experience, functional distribution of vascular pedicles or en passage vessels are of primary importance for endovascular treatment of infratentorial AVMs, and no embolization should be performed if the superselective Wada test is positive [31]. When considering preoperative risk of endovascular treatment, we have considered the number, diameter, and functional distribution of arterial pedicles to be of greatest value in assessment of perioperative risk (Table 18.4). More arterial pedicles imply more microcatheter manipulations and potential for intraoperative complications, such as arterial dissection and displaced embolysate. Smaller arterial pedicles are more difficult to catheterize, and this correlates with greater risk of intraoperative complication. In our experience, the greatest predictor of postoperative complications is a positive Wada test [31]; therefore, functional distribution of arterial pedicles is of greatest importance. We recommend superselective Wada testing of each arterial pedicle prior to embolization, and all procedures are performed with conscious sedation, rather than general anesthesia, for this purpose. Endovascular operative risk can only truly be assessed after microcatheterization of individual arterial pedicles (Fig. 18.2).

Table 18.2. Grading scale for arteriovenous malformations by George *et al.*

Grade	Features
i	Medial AVM with main supply from either the posterior inferior cerebellar artery or the superior cerebellar artery and draining medially into the vein of Galen, the straight sinus, or the transverse sinus
ii	Lateral AVM with main supply from the anterior inferior cerebellar artery and draining laterally toward the petrosal vein and sigmoid sinus
iii	Deep AVM supplied by perforating branches of the basilar artery and draining into ependymal and periaxial veins
iv	Extensive AVMs combining at least two of the above types

AVM, arteriovenous malformations. *Source*: from George *et al.* 1992 [20].

Table 18.3. Three-tier modifications of Spetzler–Martin classification system for arteriovenous malformations

Class	Spetzler–Martin grade
A	I and II
B	III
C	IV and V

Source: Spetzler and Ponce, 2011 [28].

Table 18.4. Buffalo endovascular treatment grading scale for arteriovenous malformations

Graded feature	Points assigned[a]
No. arterial pedicles	
1 or 2	1
3 or 4	2
≥5	3
Diameter of most arterial pedicles (mm)	
>1	0
≤1	1
Location	
Non-functional tissue	0
Functional tissue	1

[a] Grade is given by the sum of the points for the three features.

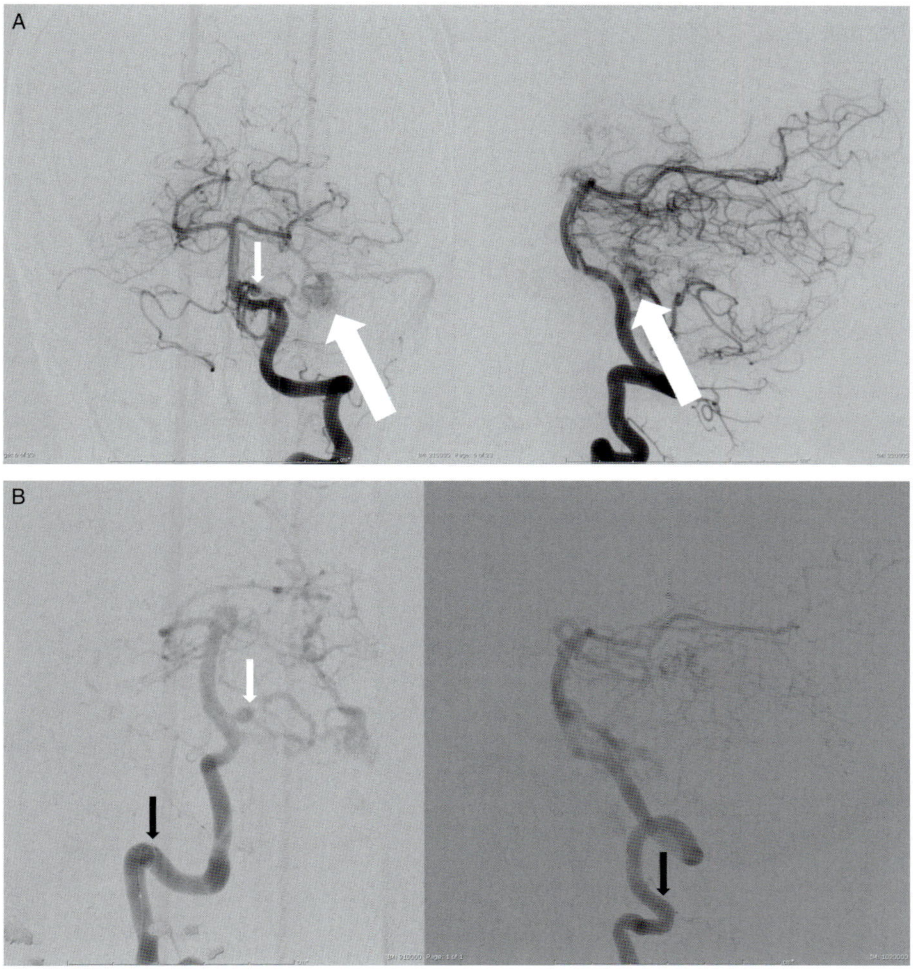

Fig. 18.2. A 53-year-old woman presented with sudden thunderclap headache and was found to have an infratentorial arteriovenous malformations (AVM) on non-invasive imaging. On presentation, evaluation was negative for subarachnoid hemorrhage. (A) Left vertebral artery cerebral angiography showed a deep draining AVM with a single arterial pedicle and small nidus (large arrow), with an associated prenidal aneurysm of anterior inferior cerebellar artery origin (small arrow) (left, anteroposterior view; right, lateral view). (B) Based on high-risk features for rupture (prenidal aneurysm) and favorable characteristics for endovascular embolization (single large pedicle), endovascular treatment was planned and this roadmap view was used to catheterize the anterior inferior cerebellar artery-based arterial pedicle. The aneurysm is seen clearly on the anteroposterior view (white arrow), and the microwire (black arrow) within the right vertebral artery is visualized in anticipation of navigation into the arterial pedicle. (C) Microcatheter run (the magnification is similar to that of B) showed a blush of contrast material within the AVM nidus (white arrows in anteroposterior (left) and lateral (right) views). The distal end of the microcatheter within the arterial pedicle is best appreciated on the anteroposterior view and highlighted with the black arrow. Wada testing was performed with the microcatheter within the arterial pedicle distal to the aneurysm. After infusion of amobarbital and lidocaine, the patient developed dysarthria and dysmetria. With the failed Wada test, no embolization was performed. (D) As the prenidal aneurysm represented a high-risk feature for subsequent hemorrhage, this was embolized with detachable coils. Left vertebral artery injection after coil embolization of the aneurysm showed no residual filling of the aneurysm (small arrow) with persistent filling of the AVM (large arrow) (left, anteroposterior view; right, lateral view). Because of the small nidus size, this patient was subsequently treated with stereotactic radiosurgery.

Treatment strategy

Treatment is recommended for patients with symptomatic and ruptured infratentorial compartment AVMs. Presentation with a large hemorrhage typically necessitates urgent craniotomy for hematoma evacuation to minimize neurological compromise from a mass effect. Consideration for AVM embolization is performed only after stabilization of the neurological examination. For patients not presenting in extremis, the treatment strategy should be tailored to the vascular lesion encountered.

In our experience, treatment of cerebellar AVMs is most frequently performed first with endovascular embolization and then followed by surgical resection or stereotactic radiosurgery as adjunctive treatments when endovascular "cure" is not possible. We approach endovascular treatment of infratentorial AVMs with the purpose of cure, although because of location or unfavorable angioarchitecture, infratentorial AVM are frequently not amenable to endovascular cure. With endovascular AVM embolization, the goal should be to obliterate arterial pedicles to reduce flow through the AVM nidus while minimizing risk of hemorrhage and neurological complication by any means possible. Prenidal aneurysms are typically treated prior to pedicle embolization. An AVM without an arterial pedicle of sufficient caliber and functional distribution should not be considered for embolization.

We have found that small AVMs of the cerebellar hemisphere with few large pedicles are most suitable for complication-free endovascular cure (Fig. 18.3). In contrast, endovascular cure is typically not possible for AVMs with many (over five) pedicles or primarily small pedicles with a diffuse nidus, and endovascular treatment should be directed toward making adjunctive treatments more safe. Compared with cerebellar AVMs, endovascular cure of brainstem or cerebellopontine angle AVMs is less likely because of the presence of en passage vessels and proximity to vital brain structures. Treatment with resection or stereotactic radiosurgery is likely the best treatment option for brainstem AVM. Those AVMs located primarily within the brainstem may be suitable for endovascular embolization if one or two large pedicles without en passage vessels are encountered. Even in such optimal circumstances, cure of a brainstem AVM with endovascular embolization is not typical. Published clinical experience is limited, with a less than 50% complete obliteration rate in patients deemed suitable candidates for endovascular treatment of brainstem AVMs, with frequent embolic complications

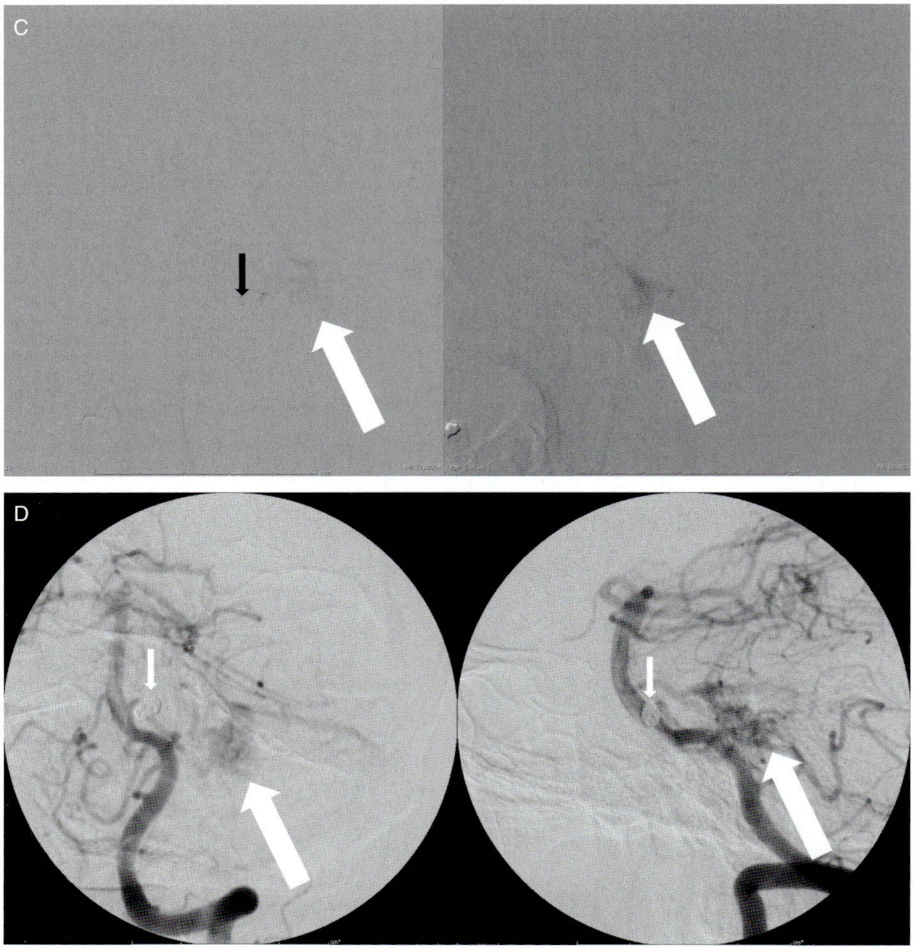

Fig. 18.2. (cont.).

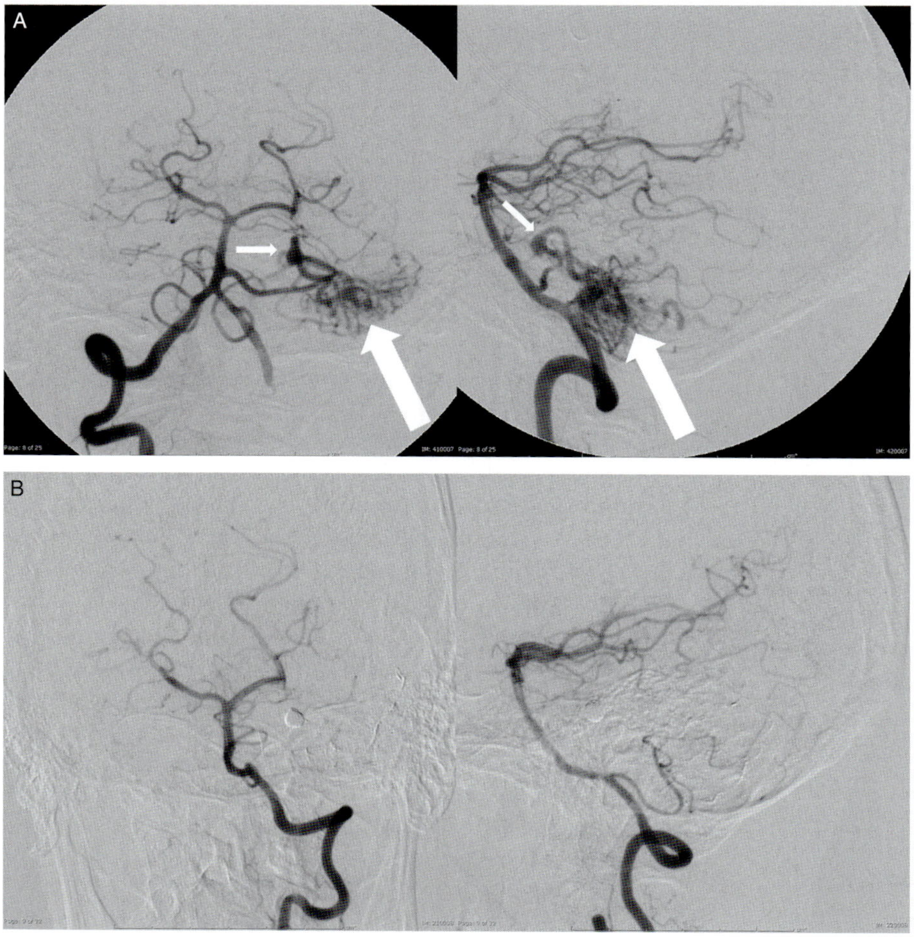

Fig. 18.3. A 43-year-old man presented with Hunt–Hess grade II and Fisher grade 2 subarachnoid hemorrhage. Non-invasive imaging was suggestive of an infratentorial anterior inferior cerebellar artery arteriovenous malformation (AVM), and cerebral angiography was performed on presentation. (A) Diagnostic angiography confirmed an infratentorial AVM with a small cerebellar-based nidus (large arrows) and a prenidal aneurysm (small arrow) (left, anteroposterior view; right, lateral view). Given the hemorrhagic presentation, high-risk features for intraprocedural hemorrhage (prenidal ruptured aneurysm), and favorable features for endovascular treatment (single large pedicle in non-eloquent tissue), endovascular embolization was planned at the time of presentation. The single anterior inferior cerebellar artery-based pedicle was embolized with Onyx after coil embolization of the aneurysm and negative superselective Wada testing. (B) Upon completion of the procedure, angiography displayed no residual flow into the AVM (left, anteroposterior view; right, lateral view). The patient had an uncomplicated hospitalization after treatment, with discharge on hospital day 13 after recovery from the subarachnoid hemorrhage.

resulting in neurological deficit [32,33]. Larger AVMs that cannot be completely obliterated with endovascular techniques may be suitable for either resection or stereotactic radiosurgery, although we favor definitive treatment only after embolization of major arterial pedicles (Fig. 18.4). Based on this, lesions most suitable for stereotactic radiosurgery are treated in an attempt to shrink the lesion diameter to reduce the morbidity of radiosurgery [34], and lesions most suitable for resection are embolized to simplify the surgical approach by targeting arterial pedicles less accessible by surgery [21]. For AVMs suitable for stereotactic radiosurgery, obliterating part of the nidus to diminish the largest diameter from >3 to ≤3 cm may limit morbidity associated with that approach [34]. For AVMs suitable for craniotomy, obliterating deep feeding arterial pedicles may vary, based on the surgical approach. For example, if an AVM is superiorly located within the vermis or cerebellar hemisphere, obliterating pedicles from the superior cerebellar artery may be of greatest value intraoperatively. For an inferiorly

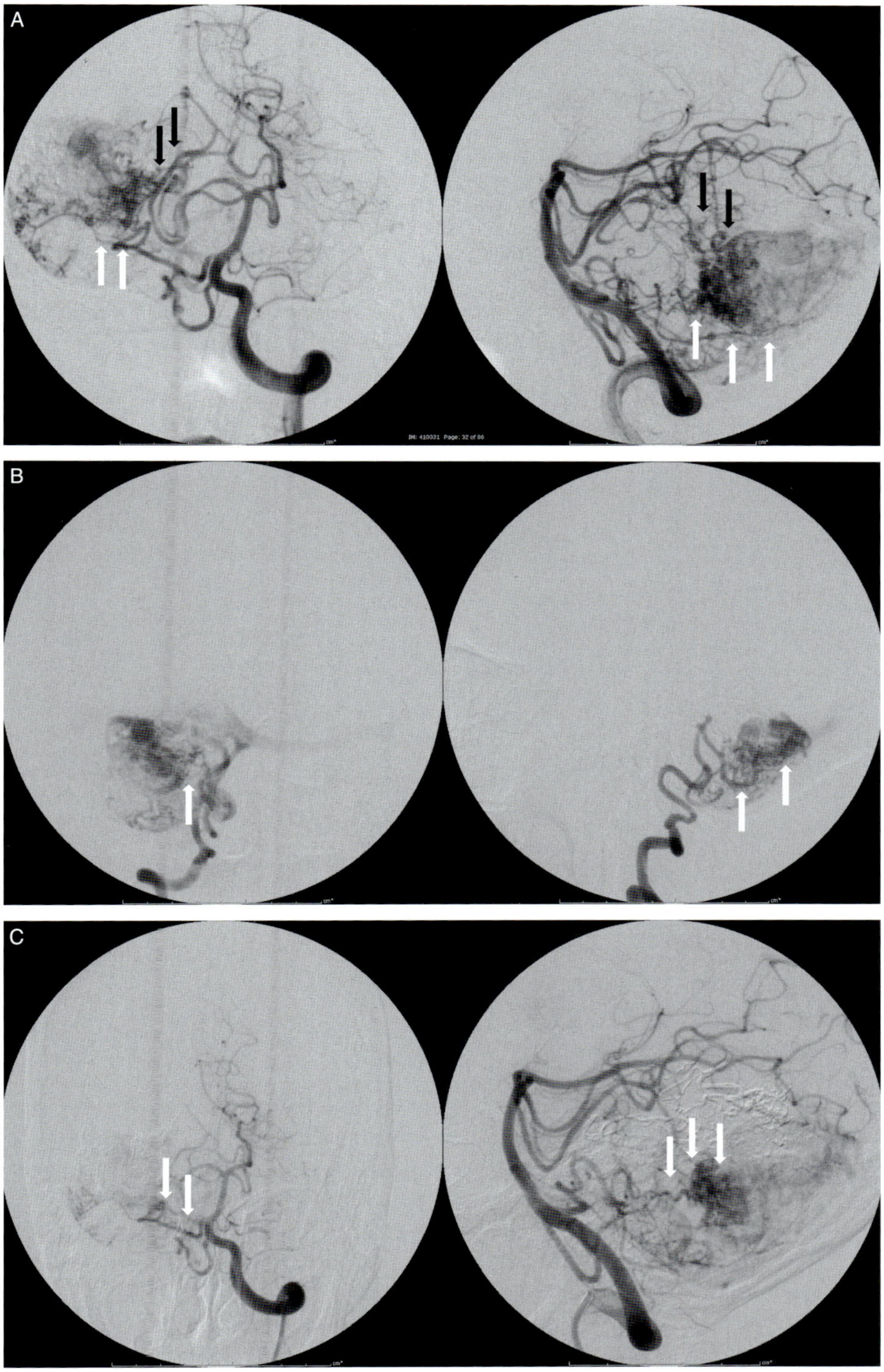

Fig. 18.4. A 43-year-old man presented with a small right cerebellar intraparenchymal hemorrhage and was found to have an arteriovenous malformation (AVM) of the right cerebellar hemisphere, with multiple arterial pedicles from the posterior inferior cerebellar artery (PICA), anterior inferior cerebellar artery (AICA), and superior cerebellar artery (SCA). Given the presentation with hemorrhage, AVM obliteration was planned. (A) Left vertebral artery injection on presentation showed arterial pedicles from the AICA (white arrows) and SCA (black arrows) (left, anteroposterior view; right, lateral view). (B) Right vertebral artery injection on presentation showed arterial pedicles from the PICA (white arrows). The AVM nidus encompassed the entire cerebellar hemisphere with both deep and superficial drainage (Spetzler–Martin grade IV and class C [Table 18.3]; left, anteroposterior view; right, lateral view). With multiple large arterial pedicles from the PICA, AICA, and SCA and non-eloquent position (Buffalo score 3 [Table 18.4]; George *et al.* grade iv [Table 18.2]), treatment options for obliteration were not optimal with surgical, radiosurgical, or endovascular techniques. After extensive discussion of treatment options, endovascular exploration with purpose of embolization was planned. Multiple endovascular embolizations were performed at intervals of four to six weeks to reduce nidus filling with the goal of obliteration. With each embolization procedure, a superselective Wada test was performed with no neurological findings. (C) Left vertebral artery injection after Onyx embolization of three SCA-based pedicles. Persistent flow into the AVM nidus through AICA-based arterial pedicles can be seen (white arrows) (left, anteroposterior view; right, lateral view). (D) Left vertebral artery injection, after Onyx embolization of two AICA-based pedicles. A blush of flow into the nidus is appreciated best on the anteroposterior view (black arrows) (left, anteroposterior view; right, lateral view). (E) Right vertebral artery injection after Onyx embolization of a single PICA-based arterial pedicle. Compared with the pre-embolization injection (B), there is diminished flow with some residual nidus filling (black arrows) (left, anteroposterior view; right, lateral view). (F) Left vertebral artery injection six weeks after PICA-based pedicle embolization with Onyx, and roughly 6 months after initial SCA-based pedicle embolization. There is minimal residual filling of the AVM nidus (black arrows). The residual arterial pedicles are not large enough in caliber to allow for catheterization and embolization. The right vertebral artery, AICA, and SCA have atrophied because of the diminished flow after embolization (left, anteroposterior view; right, lateral view). The residual AVM nidus was treated with stereotactic radiosurgery. (G,H) Left (G) and right (H) vertebral artery injections 2 years after radiosurgery, showing no residual AVM (left, anteroposterior view; right, lateral view).

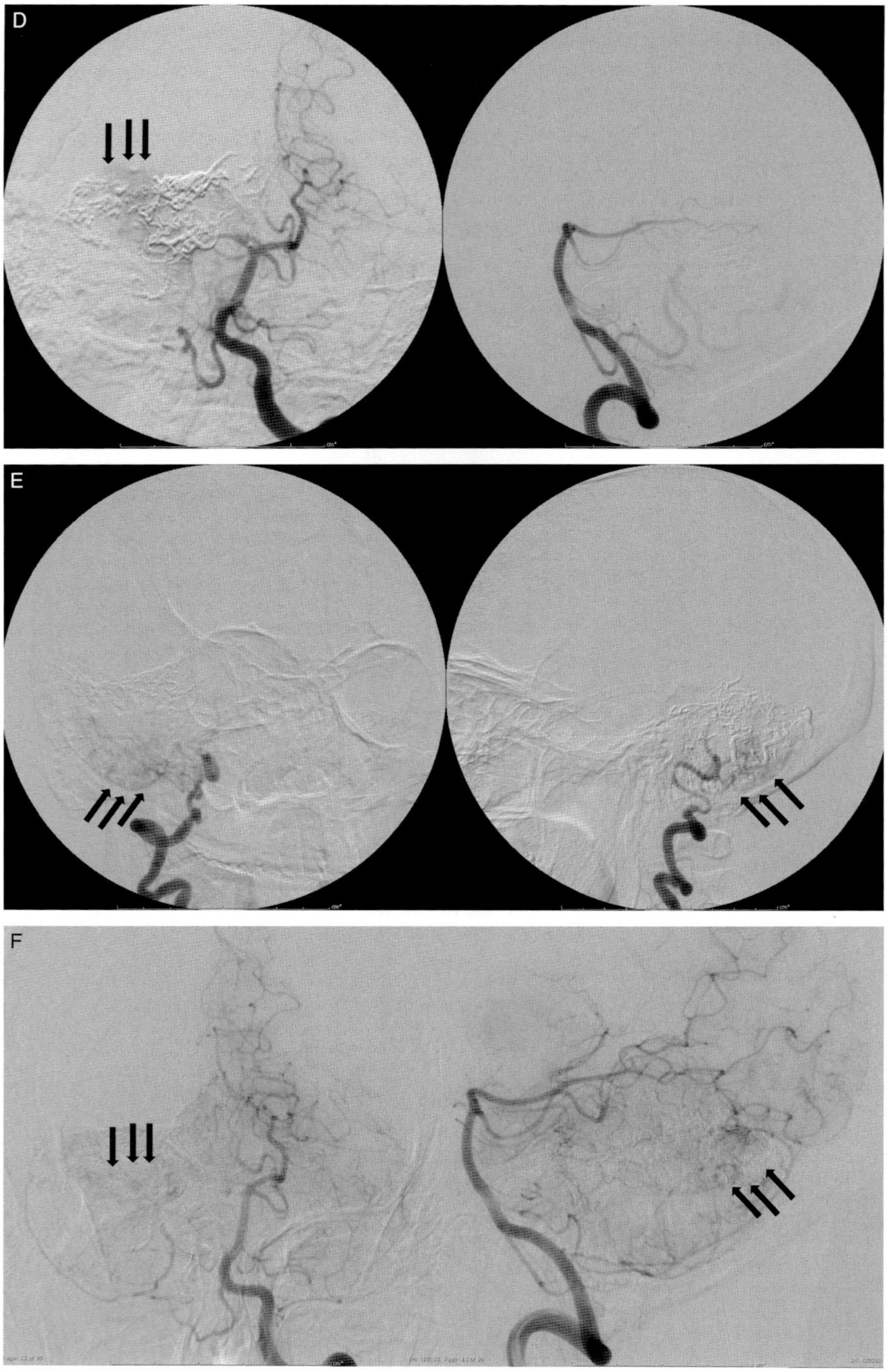

Fig. 18.4. (cont.).

situated AVMs, obliterating pedicles from the anterior or posterior inferior cerebellar arteries is likely to be of greatest value.

The number of arterial pedicles embolized in one setting may vary, based on treatment goals. Early experience with endovascular embolization of large AVMs showed anecdotal evidence of increased hemorrhage risk with large-volume embolization in a single setting [35–37]. Although the related mechanism remains unclear, theoretically, a large-volume embolization could produce a significant change in flow through an AVM, leading to hemorrhage. With this in mind, we attempt to perform embolization of arterial pedicles at intervals of four to six weeks and limit the embolization volume to approximately one-third of the total nidus volume during one embolization procedure. Ideally, the highest-risk pedicles are treated first, followed by the largest or higher flow pedicles. This practice allows for minimization of radiation exposure associated with endovascular embolization procedures, as well as prevention of dramatic hemodynamic changes to the brain following pedicle embolization. If surgical excision is planned and the goal of endovascular treatment is to minimize

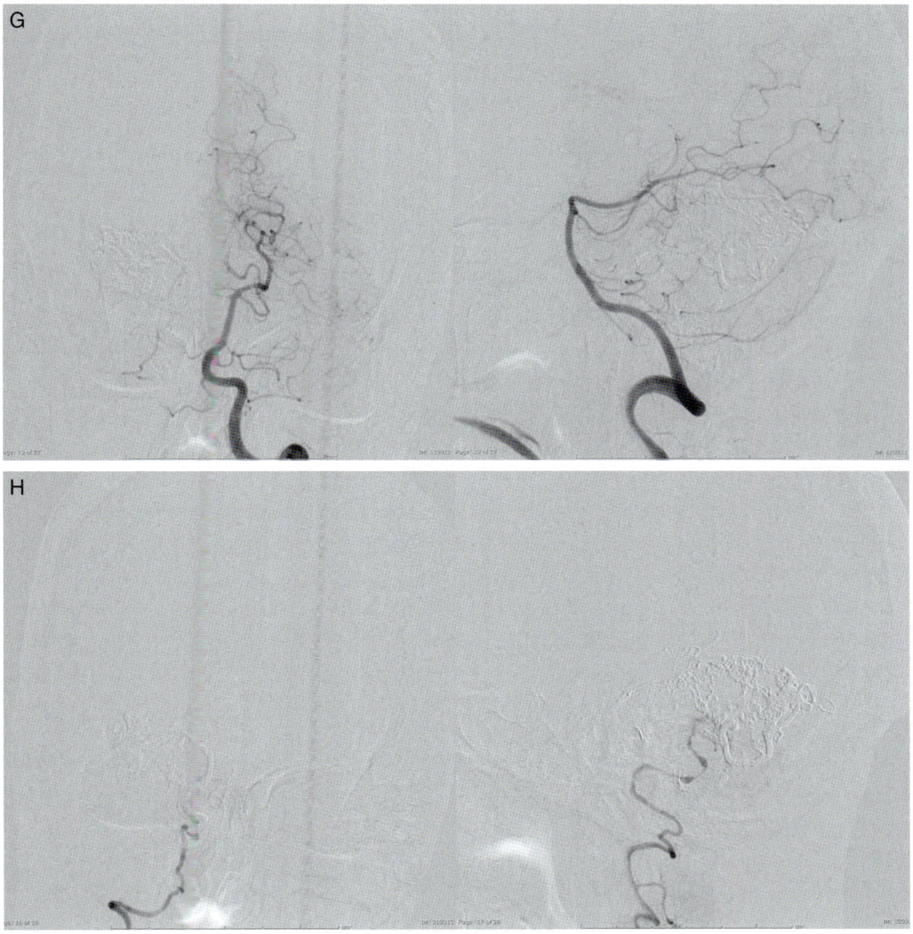

Fig. 18.4. (cont.).

intraoperative bleeding, the treatment strategy is different; we embolize as many pedicles as is safely possible in one session and plan craniotomy within 24 hours (Fig. 18.5).

Endovascular embolization technique

Endovascular embolization is performed only after six-vessel angiography has been performed and studied. An arterial pedicle of interest should be identified prior to commencing the procedure. Ideally, features at highest risk for hemorrhage (associated aneurysm or high-flow arterial pedicles) are the first targeted in order to minimize hemorrhage risk. Prenidal aneurysms are generally able to be treated with endovascular techniques and may involve standard coil embolization or glue embolization in which the entire arterial pedicle, in addition to the aneurysm, is embolized. In the absence of high-risk features, the largest arterial pedicle is typically targeted first.

The functional distribution of an arterial AVM pedicle is of greatest importance for treatment of infratentorial AVMs. Therefore, conscious sedation enabling a superselective Wada test is of extreme importance to limit perioperative neurological morbidity with endovascular treatment of infratentorial AVMs [31]. We also perform the endovascular embolization procedures with conscious sedation. Catheterization of the bladder is recommended, as AVM embolization procedures may be time consuming. Generally, fentanyl and midazolam are administered at a modest dose (50–100 μg and 1–4 mg, respectively) once patients are placed on the angiography suite table in supine position with a semi-rigid headrest to minimize motion during the procedure. A non-compliant patient or child who is unable to participate with Wada testing is offered treatment with general anesthesia; when appropriate (e.g., a lesion located within the brainstem), a variant of the superselective Wada test in which electrophysiology is used may be performed. Embolization procedures are performed using biplane angiography.

Standard femoral artery access with a 6F sheath is obtained after the patient has been sedated. Generally, the dominant vertebral artery is selected with roadmap visualization, and a 6F guide catheter placed within the vertebral artery in a non-occlusive position. Typically, the guide catheter is advanced to a position at least at the first 90 degree turn encountered at the level of the C2 vertebrae. If the vessel is of sufficient caliber such that occlusion is not problematic, soft-tipped guide catheters should be advanced to a more distal position, and occasionally are navigated safely cephalad to the C1 vertebra. Once the guide catheter is in position within the vertebral artery, microcatheterization is performed.

Both c-arm units of the biplane angiography table are adjusted to an ideal position for proper visualization of arterial anatomy to select the pedicle of interest. Because of the

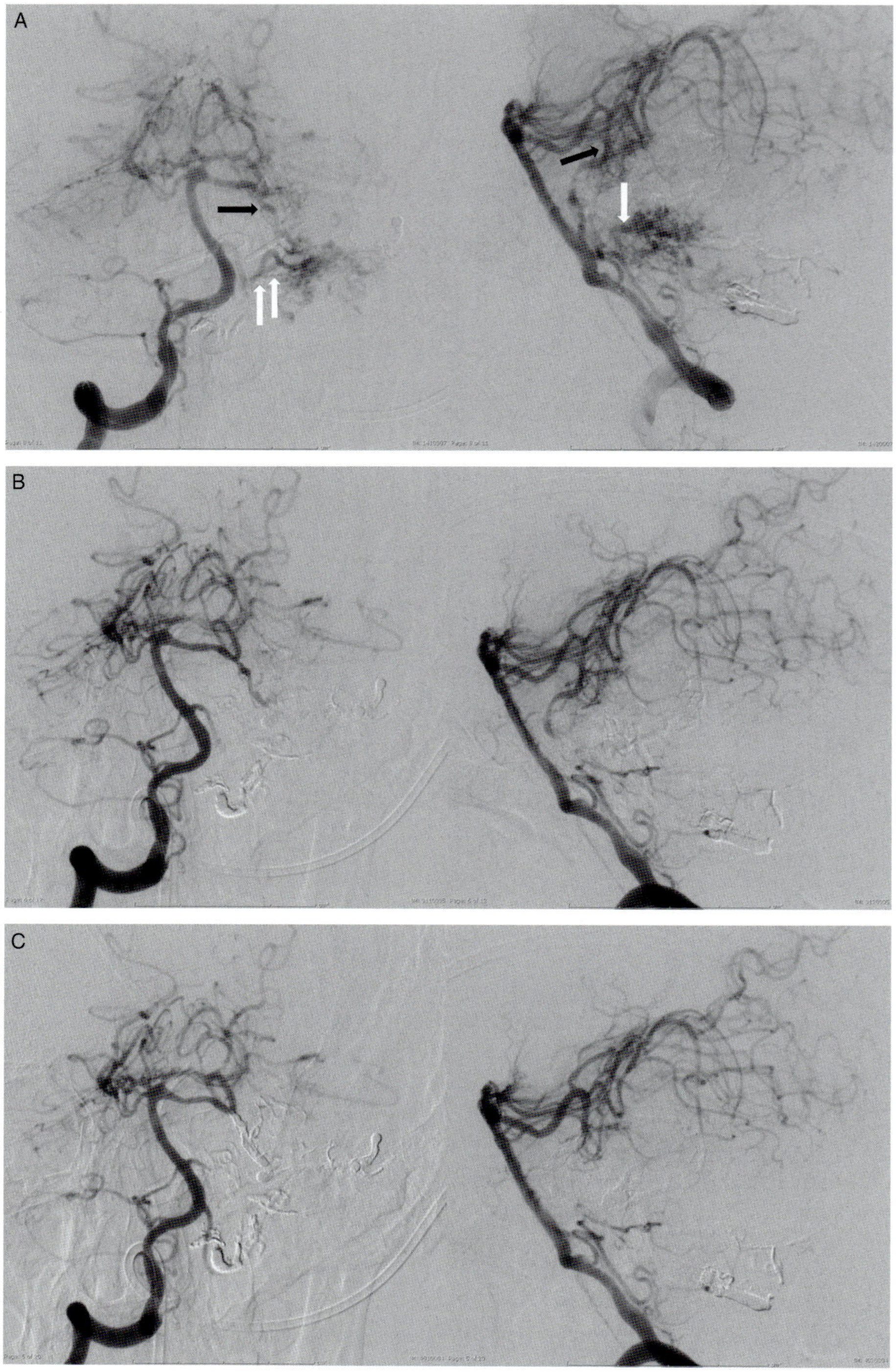

Fig. 18.5. A 45-year-old man harbored a partially treated arteriovenous malformation (AVM) with arterial pedicles from the posterior inferior cerebellar artery (PICA), anterior inferior cerebellar artery (AICA), and superior cerebellar artery (SCA) with deep and superficial drainage (Spetzler–Martin grade IV and class C [Table 18.3]; Buffalo score 3 [Table 18.4]; George *et al.* grade iv [Table 18.2]). He was previously treated with Onyx embolization of a PICA-based arterial pedicle before being lost to follow up. He presented with a large posterior fossa hemorrhage, at which point urgent craniectomy was performed with subtotal resection of the AVM. (A) Postoperative angiography confirmed residual filling of the AVM nidus via arterial pedicles of the SCA (black arrow) and AICA (white arrow). Aneurysm clip and liquid embolic cast from his previous embolization and craniotomy can be appreciated as artifact from the subtracted image (left, anteroposterior view; right, lateral view). Embolization of both arterial pedicles was performed during one procedure to minimize arterial flow to the AVM nidus prior to definitive resection performed the same day. In this case, because of a poor baseline neurological examination, no Wada testing was performed. (B) Left vertebral artery injection after Onyx embolization of the AICA-based pedicle. (C) Left vertebral artery injection after Onyx embolization of the SCA-based pedicle. A distal access catheter placed at the vertebrobasilar junction simplified access to both the AICA and SCA. Unfortunately, the patient did not survive the complications of the surgery, despite a complete resection after this embolization.

inherent complexity of most AVMs, multiple views may be required to direct the microcatheter into a desired position within the targeted arterial pedicle. As many arterial pedicles of infratentorial AVMs are tortuous, a distal access catheter may be employed to stabilize the microcatheter system and allow better control of a steerable microwire to direct the microcatheter to the desired position within the targeted pedicle and into the AVM nidus. When a distal access catheter is used, we employ the triaxial technique described above, advancing the distal access catheter over the microcatheter to a non-occlusive position. If the vessel caliber is sufficiently capacious such that occlusion is not a problem, the distal access catheter may be advanced to a position just distal to the ostium within the superior cerebellar artery, anterior inferior cerebellar artery, or posterior inferior cerebellar artery, where selective angiography may be performed and used as a roadmap for microcatheter manipulation.

Microcatheterization is performed with a flow-directed or steerable microwire. The microcatheter is advanced over the microwire using direct fluoroscopic visualization with roadmap guidance. We curve the tip of the microwire and advance it through the basilar artery keeping the microwire tip looped to avoid inadvertent selection of perforating vessels. For optimal control and safety, the microwire is advanced ahead of the microcatheter by at least 1–2 cm but typically not more than 3 or 4 cm. Once the microcatheter is positioned at the ostium of the targeted vessel or arterial pedicle, the microwire is retracted back into the microcatheter and advanced, without a looped tip, directly into the selected vessel. The microwire is then directed toward the AVM nidus with the aid of roadmap technique. We generally advance the microcatheter with an over-the-wire technique, although in high-flow AVMs, a microcatheter may be advanced without the microwire with reasonable safety if no resistance is encountered. To minimize unwanted movement of embolysate to functional vessels, the microcatheter tip is positioned as close as possible to the AVM nidus. Once the microcatheter tip is in an acceptable position, angiography is performed through the microcatheter to confirm position within the AVM nidus and ensure no extravasation of contrast material is present.

After positioning of the microcatheter is complete, a superselective Wada test is performed. A focused neurological examination is performed to serve as a baseline. Amobarbital (75 mg) and lidocaine (30 mg) are administered though the microcatheter into the selected arterial pedicle, and the neurological examination is repeated. For infratentorial AVMs, a focused examination on cranial nerve and cerebellar function is of critical importance to assess for potential neurological sequelae after pedicle embolization.

Once a suitable target (arterial pedicle) has been identified, embolization is performed. The microcatheter is disconnected from the flush system for embolization. With infusion of the embolysate, a slow injection is performed under fluoroscopic visualization to assess for unwanted anterograde flow into venous elements and retrograde flow into proximal (and potentially functional) arteries. For Onyx embolization, a bolus of DMSO is delivered into the microcatheter to flush saline and contrast material (volume 0.23 mL for Marathon and 0.34 mL for Echelon microcatheters) prior to introduction of the Onyx embolysate. The Onyx is delivered via a 1 mL syringe directly into the microcatheter at a rate of 0.1 mL/min. No fluoroscopic visualization is required for the first 0.2 or 0.3 mL for the Marathon or Echelon catheters, respectively. We prefer to deliver the Onyx with continuous small pulsations under direct fluoroscopic visualization. A roadmap is useful to assess for Onyx penetration into the nidus and ensure that anterograde flow into venous outlet structures is minimized. Once retrograde flow is appreciated, delivery is paused for 1–2 minutes. In our experience, allowing a pause once retrograde flow is appreciated before continuing the embolization procedure may allow additional anterograde flow of Onyx into the AVM nidus. As long as little or no retrograde flow is appreciated, we continue to administer the Onyx embolysate at a rate of approximately 0.1 mL/min with care to avoid anterograde flow into venous structures. The amount of Onyx delivered will vary widely based on the size of the arterial pedicle and AVM nidus (in our experience, an injection of more than 2 mL of Onyx into one arterial pedicle is uncommon). If a significant amount of resistance is encountered with injection, the wise surgeon will avoid excessive efforts to continue embolization because excessive pressure may cause embolic material to break through the sidewall of the microcatheter, causing unwanted embolization.

Other suitable embolysate options include NBCA and detachable coils. With liquid embolics available for embolization procedures, use of detachable coils in our practice is limited to treatment of prenidal aneurysms. Where the AVM nidus is diffuse or in patients where an optimal distal position of the microcatheter cannot be achieved, NBCA may be employed. The NBCA embolysate infusion technique is similar to that of Onyx, with some exceptions. The microcatheter is flushed with dextrose 5% in water (rather than DMSO), which may be delivered at a more rapid rate than 0.1 mL/min. When preparing and handling the prepared NBCA, we change gloves and use a separate back table to avoid contact with blood or saline, which may initiate or hasten polymerization of the NBCA. The NBCA is delivered directly through the flushed microcatheter under fluoroscopic visualization to assess for reflux. In our experience, once reflux of NBCA is noted, anterograde flow of this embolysate into the AVM nidus is less likely than when Onyx is used, and embolization is typically terminated at this point. With hydrophilic microcatheters, such as the Marathon or Echelon, we have found it is unusual for the catheter tip to become attached to delivered embolysate, although (as with Onyx) this will occur if a significant amount (1–2 cm of catheter length) of reflux is encountered.

After arterial pedicle embolization is complete, the microcatheter must be removed with care to avoid damage to the artery itself or unwanted migration of the embolysate from the microcatheter. To minimize risk and patient discomfort, we typically administer an additional bolus of fentanyl. The microcatheter is gently retracted with fluoroscopic visualization over the course of 0.5–2 minutes, while the microcatheter is gently aspirated with a 1 mL syringe. The patient typically experiences discomfort as tension builds within the microcatheter system and straightens the affected blood vessel. Once the tip of the microcatheter detaches, it is removed with haste; and aspiration is continued with the attached 1 mL syringe to prevent embolysate from leaving the microcatheter. If a significant amount of proximal reflux of embolysate has been encountered with the procedure, the surgeon may find significant difficulty in withdrawal of the microcatheter. We strongly caution against aggressive maneuvers to remove the microcatheter as vessel rupture or microcatheter tearing may occur. We employ several strategies to subvert this and safely remove the microcatheter. First, the microcatheter may be retracted a small amount (1–2 cm) and then clamped in place at the point where it exits the hemostatic valve to allow continuous negative pressure. We then wait 3–5 minutes before repeating this process. This gradual retraction typically is sufficient to release the microcatheter within 10–20 minutes. Second, a small amount of embolic material may be advanced through the microcatheter as the catheter is withdrawn, effectively "releasing" the seal with more liquid embolic material (although more reflux of liquid embolic will occur). Third, if a distal access catheter is employed, this may be advanced over the microcatheter to provide a fulcrum against which the microcatheter may be withdrawn with less force to the site at which the microcatheter is affixed. In the rare situation where these strategies are not successful, the microcatheter should be trapped in position with a suture at the access site to prevent its embolization and large vessel occlusion.

Upon completion of the embolization procedure, postoperative angiography in standard views serves as a new baseline. The AVM is studied for potential signs of unstable hemodynamics, such as new venous outflow stenosis or delayed nidus draining (Fig. 18.6). Such findings may be a harbinger of increased rupture risk, and patients are counseled to consider urgent resection. In the absence of evident complications or unstable hemodynamic findings, the guiding catheter is removed and the arteriotomy closed in standard fashion.

Postoperative course

Patients are observed in a neurosurgical intensive care unit for at least 12 hours after an embolization procedure and have hourly neurological examinations. Patients may complain of mild headache after embolization, which typically remits with administration of oral corticosteroid (dexamethasone, 2–4 mg two to six times daily). Generally, the administration of narcotics is not required. Routine postoperative intervention includes strict blood pressure control to 80% of the patient's baseline (or systolic blood pressure 90–130 mmHg for otherwise healthy patients), and basic laboratory tests to ensure no dramatic change in the patient's hematocrit level and no compromise of renal function in conjunction with contrast material administration. After unremarkable elective procedures, most patients are discharged home on the first postoperative day.

Estimation of complications after endovascular infratentorial AVM obliteration is difficult because of limited reported series and irregular reporting of complications. Perioperative and technical complications would not be expected to be significantly different from that of combined AVM treatment (5–6% of patients in series with Onyx embolization) [38,39]. With superselective Wada testing performed in most cases, neurological complications after infratentorial AVM embolization are uncommon in our experience. Post-treatment AVM ruptures are likely under-reported. We have encountered hemorrhage from intraoperative vessel perforation and delayed postoperative hemorrhage has been described; the resulting posterior fossa hemorrhage typically results in dramatic neurological decline requiring urgent craniectomy.

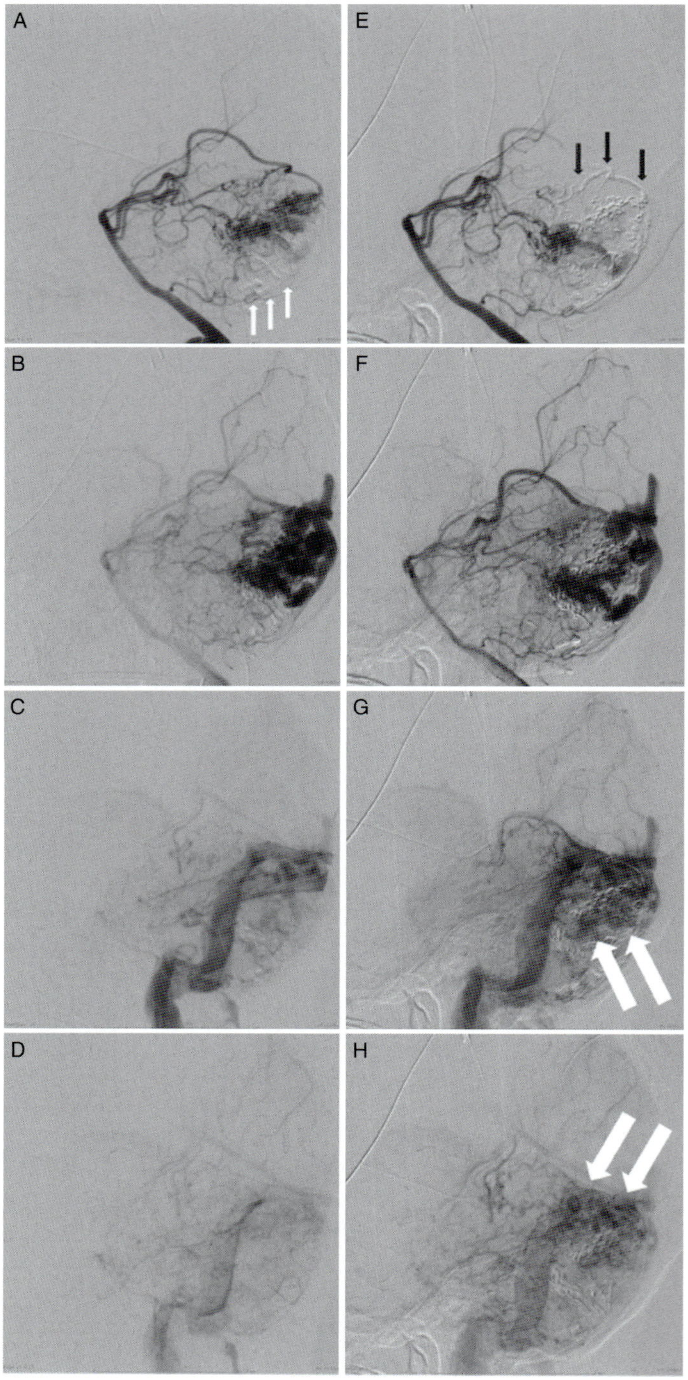

Fig. 18.6. An example of delayed draining of an arteriovenous malformation (AVM) nidus after embolization. (A–D) Lateral view angiography showed arterial, capillary, venous, and late venous phases prior to embolization of a superior cerebellar artery (SCA) branch. Previous embolization of a posterior inferior cerebellar artery-based arterial pedicle had been performed (white arrows). (E–H) Arterial, capillary, venous, and late venous phase lateral view angiography after embolization of an SCA branch (black arrows) showed stasis of contrast material within the AVM nidus consistent with delayed drainage or venous outlet obstruction (white arrows). This may represent a high-risk feature for subsequent hemorrhage, and definitive treatment with complete embolization and resection was considered.

Conclusions

Endovascular embolization represents an important modality for treatment of infratentorial AVMs. Anatomical considerations are of utmost importance when considering endovascular treatment of these lesions. An AVM located in the cerebellum (rather than in the brainstem or cerebellopontine angle) with few (one or two) arterial pedicles is most likely to be cured with endovascular treatment. Infratentorial AVMs with features unfavorable for cure with endovascular techniques should be considered for adjunctive endovascular embolization to minimize the mortality associated with definitive treatment strategies. A simple catheter system is capable of performing most infratentorial endovascular AVM embolization procedures. Procedures should be performed under conscious sedation when possible, as superselective Wada testing prior to pedicle embolization will diminish neurological compromise with embolization.

References

1. Arnaout OM, Gross BA, Eddleman CS, *et al.* Posterior fossa arteriovenous malformations. *Neurosurg Focus* 2009;**26**:E12.
2. Neacsu A, Ciurea AV. General considerations on posterior fossa arteriovenous malformations clinics, imaging and therapy. Actual concepts and literature review. *J Med Life* 2010;3:26–35.
3. Sinclair J, Kelly ME, Steinberg GK. Surgical management of posterior fossa arteriovenous malformations. *Neurosurgery* 2006;**58**:ons189–201.
4. Fults D, Kelly DL, Jr. Natural history of arteriovenous malformations of the brain: a clinical study. *Neurosurgery* 1984;**15**:658–62.
5. Hernesniemi JA, Dashti R, Juvela S, *et al.* Natural history of brain arteriovenous malformations: a long-term follow-up study of risk of hemorrhage in 238 patients. *Neurosurgery* 2008;**63**:823–9.
6. Kader A, Young WL, Pile-Spellman J, *et al.* The influence of hemodynamic and anatomical factors on hemorrhage from cerebral arteriovenous malformations. *Neurosurgery* 1994;**34**:801–7.
7. Khaw AV, Mohr JP, Sciacca RR, *et al.* Association of infratentorial brain arteriovenous malformations with hemorrhage at initial presentation. *Stroke* 2004;**35**:660–3.
8. Schmidt NO, Reitz M, Raimund F, *et al.* Clinical relevance of associated aneurysms with arteriovenous malformations of the posterior fossa. *Acta Neurochir Suppl* 2011;**112**:131–5.
9. Westphal M, Grzyska U. Clinical significance of pedicle aneurysms on feeding vessels, especially those located in infratentorial arteriovenous malformations. *J Neurosurg* 2000;**92** 995–1001.
10. da Costa L, Thines L, Dehdashti AR, *et al.* Management and clinical outcome of posterior fossa arteriovenous malformations: report on a single-centre 15-year experience. *J Neurol Neurosurg Psychiatry* 2009;**80**:376–9.
11. Batjer H, Samson D. Arteriovenous malformations of the posterior fossa. Clinical presentation, diagnostic evaluation, and surgical treatment. *J Neurosurg* 1986;**64**:849–56.
12. Drake CG, Friedman AH, Peerless SJ. Posterior fossa arteriovenous malformations. *J Neurosurg* 1986;**64**:1–10.
13. Kelly ME, Guzman R, Sinclair J, *et al.* Multimodality treatment of posterior fossa arteriovenous malformations. *J Neurosurg* 2008;**108**:1152–61.
14. Stahl SM, Johnson KP, Malamud N. The clinical and pathological spectrum of brain-stem vascular malformations. Long-term course stimulates multiple sclerosis. *Arch Neurol* 1980;**37**:25–9.
15. Pribil S, Boone SC, Waley R. Obstructive hydrocephalus at the anterior third ventricle caused by dilated veins from an arteriovenous malformation. *Surg Neurol* 1983;**20**:487–92.
16. Hoi SU, Kerber C. Ventricular obstruction secondary to vascular malformations. *Neurosurgery* 1983;**12**:572–5.
17. Lesley WS. Resolution of trigeminal neuralgia following cerebellar AVM embolization with Onyx. *Cephalalgia* 2009;**29**:980–5.
18. Simon SD, Yao TL, Rosenbaum BP, *et al.* Resolution of trigeminal neuralgia after palliative embolization of a cerebellopontine angle arteriovenous malformation. *Cent Eur Neurosurg* 2009;**70**:161–3.
19. Wanke I, Dietrich U, Oppel F, *et al.* Endovascular treatment of trigeminal neuralgia caused by arteriovenous malformation: is surgery really necessary? *Zentralbl Neurochir* 2005;**66**:213–16.
20. George B, Celis-Lopez M, Kato T, *et al.* Arteriovenous malformations of the posterior fossa. *Acta Neurochir (Wien)* 1992;**116**:119–27.
21. O'Shaughnessy BA, Getch CC, Bendok BR, *et al.* Microsurgical resection of infratentorial arteriovenous malformations. *Neurosurg Focus* 2005;**19**:E5.
22. Stapf C. The rationale behind "A Randomized Trial of Unruptured Brain AVMs" (ARUBA). *Acta Neurochir Suppl* 2010;**107**:83–5.
23. Stapf C, Mohr JP, Choi JH, *et al.* Invasive treatment of unruptured brain arteriovenous malformations is experimental therapy. *Curr Opin Neurol* 2006;**19**:63–8.
24. Lv X, Wu Z, Jiang C, *et al.* Angioarchitectural characteristics of brain arteriovenous malformations with and without hemorrhage. *World Neurosurg* 2011;**76**:95–9.
25. Stapf C, Mast H, Sciacca RR, *et al.* Predictors of hemorrhage in patients with untreated brain arteriovenous malformation. *Neurology* 2006;**66**:1350–5.
26. Stefani MA, Porter PJ, terBrugge KG, *et al.* Large and deep brain arteriovenous malformations are associated with risk of future hemorrhage. *Stroke* 2002;**33**:1220–4.
27. Spetzler RF, Martin NA. A proposed grading system for arteriovenous malformations. *J Neurosurg* 1986;**65**:476–83.

28. Spetzler RF, Ponce FA. A 3-tier classification of cerebral arteriovenous malformations. *J Neurosurg* 2011;**114**:842–9.

29. Rodriguez-Hernandez A, Kim H, Pourmohamad T, *et al.* Cerebellar arteriovenous malformations: anatomical subtypes, surgical results, and increased predictive accuracy of the supplementary grading system. *Neurosurgery* 2012;**71**:1111–24.

30. Lawton MT, Kim H, McCulloch CE, *et al.* A supplementary grading scale for selecting patients with brain arteriovenous malformations for surgery. *Neurosurgery* 2010;**66**:702–13.

31. Tawk RG, Tummala RP, Memon MZ, *et al.* Utility of pharmacologic provocative neurological testing before embolization of occipital lobe arteriovenous malformations. *World Neurosurg* 2011;**76**:276–81.

32. Liu HM, Wang YH, Chen YF, *et al.* Endovascular treatment of brain-stem arteriovenous malformations: safety and efficacy. *Neuroradiology* 2003;**45**:644–9.

33. Thines L, Dehdashti AR, da Costa L, *et al.* Challenges in the management of ruptured and unruptured brainstem arteriovenous malformations: outcome after conservative, single-modality, or multimodality treatments. *Neurosurgery* 2012;**70**:155–61.

34. Gobin YP, Laurent A, Merienne L, *et al.* Treatment of brain arteriovenous malformations by embolization and radiosurgery. *J Neurosurg* 1996;**85**:19–28.

35. Han PP, Ponce FA, Spetzler RF. Intention-to-treat analysis of Spetzler–Martin grades IV and V arteriovenous malformations: natural history and treatment paradigm. *J Neurosurg* 2003;**98**:3–7.

36. Ovalle F, Shay SD, Mericle RA. Delayed intracerebral hemorrhage after uneventful embolization of brain arteriovenous malformation is related to volume of embolic agent administered: multivariate analysis of 13 predictive factors. *Neurosurgery* 2012;**70**:313–20.

37. Wikholm G, Lundqvist C, Svendsen P. Embolization of cerebral arteriovenous malformations Part I. Technique, morphology, and complications. *Neurosurgery* 1996;**39**:448–57.

38. Lv X, Wu Z, Jiang C, *et al.* Complication risk of endovascular embolization for cerebral arteriovenous malformation. *Eur J Radiol* 2011;**80**:776–9.

39. Weber W, Kis B, Siekmann R, *et al.* Endovascular treatment of intracranial arteriovenous malformations with onyx: technical aspects. *AJNR Am J Neuroradiol* 2007;**28**:371–7.

Chapter

19 Endovascular treatment of arteriovenous fistulae of the brain

Omar Choudhri and Michael P. Marks

Introduction

Arteriovenous fistulae of the brain are rare acquired lesions that form 10–15% of all intracranial vascular malformations [1], representing 6% of supratentorial and 35% of infratentorial vascular malformations [2]. Endovascular neurosurgery has evolved over the years with improvements in microcatheters, liquid embolics, and coils and this has allowed most intracranial fistulae to be treated by an endovascular approach. Dural arteriovenous fistulae (DAVFs) and carotid–cavernous fistulae (CCFs) are the major subtypes of intracranial fistulae.

In DAVFs, there is an abnormal communication between arterial and venous systems involving one or more dural sinuses and branches of the external carotid artery (ECA), internal carotid artery (ICA), and/or vertebral arteries. The fistulous connection is often present within leaves of dura mater and involves a dural sinus or an adjacent cortical vein. A DAVF is usually supplied by dural arteries from the ECA although pial arterial supply may also be commonly seen [3].

The CCFs are lesions with fistulous arterial drainage specifically into the cavernous sinus and they may be direct, secondary to a tear in the wall of cavernous ICA, or indirect, with dural arterial supply to the cavernous sinus [4].

This chapter will briefly discuss the pathophysiology, clinical presentation, and natural history of these lesions. It will review classification systems used to assist with management decisions and then focus on management with an emphasis on what has become first-line management of these lesions, endovascular therapy.

Pathophysiology

There is no clear consensus regarding the pathogenesis of DAVFs but a number of hypotheses have been proposed [5]. The most common hypothesis is the thrombosis and venous hypertension pathway [6]. This suggested mechanistic pathway involves three steps: (1) dural sinus thrombosis, leading to impaired sinus drainage; (2) development of fistulous channels between the thrombosed sinus and dural arteries; and (3) recanalization of the dural sinus, which allows direct arterial shunting into the sinus from dural arteries. Venous hypertension appears to be the trigger for the formation of a DAVF. This has been demonstrated in rodent models with creation of carotid artery to external jugular vein fistulae [7,8].

Angiogenic factors likely play a role in the pathophysiological development of DAVFs. Basic fibroblast growth factor is a powerful angiogenic growth factor that is found in increased amounts in surgical DAVF specimens [9]. Increased proangiogenic factors are also identified in rodent models of DAVF [10]. It is hypothesized that venous hypertension and resultant ischemia triggers the formation of pro-angiogenic substances by dura and brain [9]. This may alter the balance between pro- and antiangiogenic agents, leading to an increased number of arteriovenous fistulous connections. Other vascular growth factors such as vascular endothelial growth factor and ephrin-B2 may also play a role in this pro-angiogenic cascade [11]. A similar underlying process is seen in patients with moyamoya and ischemia, who have increased basic fibroblast growth factor in cerebrospinal fluid [12].

There have been some limited studies on the histopathology of DAVF surgical specimens [5]. Thickening of intimal lining of involved sinuses, arteries, and veins and obliteration of internal elastic lamina were seen in a study of transverse–sigmoid DAVF specimens [13]. Hamada *et al.* found that the essential abnormality was a connection between dural arteries and veins within the venous sinus wall. They described these fistulous vessels in the sinus wall as "crack-like" venules measuring 30 μm or less [14].

Historical perspective and diagnosis

The first anatomical description of a DAVF was in 1881 by Rizzoli, although it was a scalp arteriovenous fistula draining intracranially through a torcular emissary vein [15]. The first angiographic description came from Ernest Sachs Sr. (1879–1958) in 1931, who trained under Sir Victor Horsley. Subsequently, Bergstrand and colleagues published the first two angiographic demonstrations in 1936 [16]. Newton and Cronqvist provided some good early angiographic descriptions in 1969 [2]. With the evolving field of neuroangiography, brain arteriovenous fistulae became better characterized and

Comprehensive Management of Arteriovenous Malformations of the Brain and Spine, ed. Robert F. Spetzler, Douglas S. Kondziolka, Randall T. Higashida, and M. Yashar S. Kalani. Published by Cambridge University Press.

diagnosed. Currently diagnosis of these lesions may utilize CT, MRI, and cerebral angiography.

Although CT often demonstrates features suggestive of venous hypertension and hemorrhage in patients with DAVF, it is rarely diagnostic. Findings such as cortical edema, subarachnoid hemorrhage, subdural hematoma, or intraparenchymal hemorrhage may be seen in advanced cases. Contrast-enhanced CT and CT angiography can sometimes show dilated cortical veins, enlarged ECA branches, and, rarely, the fistula site.

Use of MRI has significantly advanced non-invasive diagnosis of DAVF and has helped to select patients who may need cerebral angiography. The sensitivity of CT angiography to diagnose DAVF is only 15.4% while MRI/MR angiography can have sensitivity up to 50% [17]. Basic MRI can show parenchymal changes seen in the setting of DAVF while MR angiography can improve depiction of the fistula site and feeding arteries. The latter, however, is limited, given low spatial resolution, restricted field of coverage, and presence of saturation artifact. Some three-dimensional time of flight MRI and MR digital subtraction angiography protocols can provide dynamic images that can help in the detection of early venous filling of some of these fistulae [18]. Venous arterial spin labeling signal on MRI is frequently used at our center in early evaluation in patients with DAVFs. Le *et al.* reported sensitivity and specificity of 78% and 85% for venous arterial spin labeling (ASL) to identify DAVFs and small arteriovenous malformations (AVMs) diagnosed on formal cerebral angiography [19].

Some studies have used positron emission tomography to demonstrate abnormal hemodynamic and metabolic parameters in the areas of involved cortical draining veins. Significant improvement in regional cerebral blood flow, regional cerebral blood volume, and regional cerebral metabolic rate for oxygen was noted in these regions after treatment [20].

Even with advancements in non-invasive imaging, detailed cerebral angiography remains the cornerstone for diagnosis and evaluation of DAVFs. A complete angiographic study should involve selective injections of both ECAs and ICAs and vertebral arteries. The venous phase of the angiographic run is particularly crucial to allow appreciation of the fistula point, drainage pattern, and alternative venous drainage pathways available. Appreciation of cortical venous drainage, venous outflow stenosis, and venous hypertension is also important to characterize the severity of these lesions and to make recommendations for treatment. During angiographic workup of a direct CCF, the common carotid artery may be compressed during ICA (Mehringer maneuver) or vertebral artery (Huber maneuver) injections to delineate the exact site of tear in the cavernous ICA [4].

Clinical presentation

While DAVFs present at a mean patient age of 50–60 years, a wide age range at the time of diagnosis is seen across studies [21]. They often present in perimenopausal women, suggesting an underlying hormonal etiology [2], while hemorrhagic presentation is more common in men [22]. Although DAVFs are often idiopathic, in many patients they can be traced to trauma, venous thrombosis, infection, hypercoagulable state, tumors (meningiomas), and prior neurosurgical procedures.

Although patients with DAVFs are often asymptomatic, they frequently present with headaches and pulsatile tinnitus. Tinnitus is pulsatile secondary to shunting occurring with each systolic arterial phase. The tinnitus is most often present in patients with fistulae around the temporal bone and middle ear and can often be functionally debilitating. A unilateral bruit is often heard at physical examination. The tinnitus can often improve with pressure on the scalp or turning the head, or with maneuvers reducing arterial shunting into the fistula. The headache is often more severe on the side of the fistula and is aggravated by changes in head elevation, physical activity, stress, and elevated blood pressure during a Valsalva maneuver.

Symptoms are also intrinsically related to the location of the DAVF, patterns of venous drainage, and extent of the fistula. Clinical manifestations could include encephalopathy, gait ataxia, seizures, cranial nerve deficits, and myelopathy. Patients with a CCF may present with ophthalmoplegia, proptosis, chemosis, pain, and reduced visual acuity given venous hypertension in the cavernous sinus [23]. If patients develop venous hypertension, they may present with cerebral edema, intracranial hemorrhage, seizures, ischemia, or hydrocephalus [3]. A DAVF is a dynamic entity and it can progress to alter its drainage pattern. Any change in a patient's clinical symptoms, including worsening headaches, change in pattern of tinnitus, or new deficits, should trigger repeat evaluation.

Classification systems

The natural history of DAVFs correlates with the pattern of venous drainage particularly as it relates to reflux into pial or cortical veins. All DAVF classification schemes are based on the anatomical pattern of venous drainage, with a spectrum from normal sinus drainage to retrograde sinus drainage to cortical venous reflux with venous hypertension (Table 19.1) [21,24,25].

Djindjian *et al.* were the first to propose a classification system for DAVFs (Table 19.1) [24]. They described a three-level system with type I draining to the ipsilateral sinus, type II toward the contralateral sinus, and type III draining into cortical veins. Patients with type I DAVFs were felt to be at low risk for hemorrhage and were often asymptomatic but could present with headaches and tinnitus. Patients with type II DAVFs were felt to be at higher risk for hemorrhage and could develop increased intracranial pressure particularly if the contralateral sinus was stenotic. Patients with type III were thought to be the highest risk and could develop brain edema or infarction and hemorrhage with greater frequency.

Cognard *et al.* proposed a modification of the original Djindijan–Merland classification scheme based on the clinical presentation of 205 patients over an 18-year period (Table 19.1) [21]. This is a five-tiered classification system that takes into account patterns of venous drainage into a sinus or cortical veins and the presence or absence of venous ectasia. The strength of this classification lies in its correlation between angiographic characteristics and clinical presentation [15].

Table 19.1. Grading scales for dural arteriovenous fistulae

Study	Grade/type	Description
Djindjian *et al.* (1973) [24]	I	Venous drainage to the ipsilateral sinus
	II	Venous drainage to the contralateral sinus
	III	Venous drainage to the cortical veins
Cognard *et al.* (1995) [21]	I	Anterograde drainage into the main sinus
	IIa	Drainage into the main sinus with reflux into the other sinus(es)
	IIb	Drainage into the main sinus with reflux into cortical veins
	IIa+b	Drainage into the main sinus with reflux into other sinuses + cortical veins
	III	Direct cortical venous drainage without venous ectasia
	IV	Direct cortical venous drainage with venous ectasia (>5 mm and three times larger than diameter of the draining vein)
	V	Drainage into spinal perimedullary veins
Borden *et al.* (1995) [25]	I	Anterograde drainage into dural sinus/meningeal vein
	II	Anterograde drainage into dural sinus plus retrograde cortical venous drainage
	III	Isolated retrograde cortical venous drainage

Type I involves normal anterograde sinus drainage. Type IIa has partial or complete retrograde sinus drainage. Retrograde sinus drainage can occur with outflow stenosis/obstruction of the involved sinus or with high-volume arteriovenous shunting. Types IIb to IV have varied degrees of retrograde cortical venous drainage into pial veins. Types III and IV have exclusive cortical pial venous drainage while type IV demonstrates enlarged venous varix or ectasia. Cognard *et al.* defined a venous varix as a segment >5 mm or larger than three times the diameter of the draining vein. Type V DAVFs are cranial lesions with drainage into spinal perimedullary veins, often leading to myelopathy. In the original Cognard clinical series, intracranial hemorrhage was seen in 10% of patients with type II and 65% with type IV [21]. Aggressive symptoms, including hemorrhage, seizures, intracranial hypertension, and focal neurological deficits, were as high as 97% in their series.

Borden *et al.* devised a similar classification system in 1995 with an effort to unify classification of spinal and cranial DAVFs (Table 19.1) [25]. It is a simplified classification with type I having anterograde sinus drainage only, type II with anterograde sinus drainage and some retrograde pial venous drainage, while type III has purely pial or cortical venous drainage and these patients have a high risk for hemorrhage, venous hypertension, and neurological deficits. Lesions are subclassified as having a single fistula (subtype a) or multiple fistulae (subtype b). The Borden and Cognard classifications are the most commonly used in routine clinical practice. Both schemes were used across a series of 102 intracranial DAVFs in 98 patients that confirmed the validity of these classifications [26].

Two studies have shown that cortical venous drainage may not be the only prognostic factor for DAVF hemorrhage [27,28]. These studies suggested that symptomatic venous hypertension has an equally important role to play in the future behavior of the DAVF. Soderman *et al.* performed a retrospective review of 85 patients with Borden type II/III DAVFs [28]. Annual hemorrhage risk was 7.4% for patients presenting with intracerebral hemorrhage compared with 1.5% for those who did not. Strom *et al.* analyzed 28 patients with Borden type II/III DAVFs and found an annual hemorrhage risk of 7.6% in patients with symptomatic cortical venous drainage compared with 1.4% in patients with asymptomatic cortical venous drainage [27]. Therefore symptomatic venous hypertension has a higher risk of future neurological events than does the asymptomatic hypertension incidentally found with cortical venous drainage. Zipfel *et al.* have proposed a modified classification system that stratifies symptomatic and asymptomatic cortical venous drainage [22]. Immediate treatment is recommended for symptomatic cortical venous drainage in patients with Borden type II/III DAVFs. The reason for this observation is that angiographic cortical venous drainage may not necessarily indicate symptomatic venous hypertension.

Barrow *et al.* proposed a four-tiered classification system for CCF based on anatomical and radiographic characteristics: type A is a direct fistula between the ICA and the cavernous sinus; type B is an indirect shunt between meningeal branches from the ICA and the cavernous sinus; type C is an indirect CCF between meningeal branches of the ECA and the cavernous sinus; while type D is a shunt between meningeal branches of both ICA and ECA and the cavernous sinus [29].

Management

Generally the decision to treat a patient with DAVF is based on a combination of angiographic classification of the fistula, which strongly influences the natural history of the lesion, and the clinical presentation of the patient. Patients with acute presentations such as intracranial hemorrhage, infarction, and visual loss with cortical venous drainage may warrant immediate treatment. Patients with low-grade fistulae with no evidence of cortical venous drainage should be treated if the clinical symptoms are bothersome to the patient. This could include severe headaches or tinnitus, which are functionally debilitating. The treatment approach is based on angiographic characteristics of the fistula, including size and number of arterial feeders, venous drainage pattern, native venous drainage, site of the fistula, and number of accessible venous pathways. This mandates a detailed angiographic study and thoughtful understanding of arterial and venous anatomy.

Conservative management

Most low-grade DAVFs (Borden type I) with benign symptoms can be managed conservatively. In absence of cortical venous drainage, patients are treated only if headaches or tinnitus are bothersome and impairing functioning. Kim *et al.* studied the natural history of DAVFs in 112 patients and found that 12.5% showed spontaneous occlusion while 4% showed progression to a higher grade [30].

Compression therapy

Direct compression therapy to obliterate the arterial supply to an arteriovenous fistula can be done in the highly motivated patient with mild symptoms and absence of cortical venous drainage [5]. It can be recommended for indirect CCF where the patient can complete compression of the lateral carotid–jugular area over 30 minutes or so. There should be no evidence of cervical carotid atherosclerosis before this treatment is recommended. Similarly the occipital artery can be manually compressed when supplying a transverse–sigmoid DAVF. Higashida *et al.* demonstrated that it could promote thrombosis in up to 30% patients with indirect CCF and 17% with direct CCF [31]. Anecdotally, we have not found that this therapeutic approach yields as high a rate of thrombosis in our patients.

Endovascular techniques

Endovascular embolization can help to obliterate most arteriovenous fistulae using either transarterial or transvenous embolization [32]. Improvements in microcatheters and liquid embolics have allowed safe treatment of cerebral arteriovenous fistulae. It is crucial to understand the easiest access to the fistula to allow adequate closure of the fistulous connection.

The angioarchitecture seen on the cerebral angiogram is reviewed to evaluate the following critical factors: (1) arterial feeders, (2) fistulous connection, (3) venous outflow, (4) normal dural sinuses, (5) venous anomalies (i.e., venous pouches), (6) potential extracranial to intracranial anastomoses, and (7) potential anastomoses to cranial nerve vasculatures.

Transarterial embolization

Transarterial embolization of DAVFs involves obliteration of the fistula via the arterial route, usually using liquid embolic agents. Platinum coils, silk sutures, collagen, silastic spheres, and a multitude of other agents have been used historically for parent artery occlusion [33,34]. However these agents have been abandoned because they sacrifice the parent vessel and do not penetrate the fistula, which results in high rates of recanalization [3].

Most DAVFs have supply from the ECA circulation and could include supply from the middle meningeal artery, superficial temporal artery, ascending pharyngeal artery, and occipital artery. There are several important considerations before a transarterial embolization route is selected. First, proximal arterial embolization should be avoided. Once the arterial feeder to the DAVF has been catheterized, an attempt should be made to advance the microcatheter as close as possible to the fistula to allow the liquid embolic agent to penetrate the fistula. Second, any anastomosis of extracranial vessels with the intracranial circulations must be identified. Any embolization material that crosses these anastomoses could place these patients at risk for stroke. These may include anastomoses between meningohypophyseal or inferolateral trunks of the ICA and branches of the internal maxillary artery as well as anastomoses between the vertebral artery and branches of the ascending pharyngeal and occipital arteries. A full discussion of the dangerous anastomoses is beyond the scope of this chapter and the reader is referred to additional references [35,36]. Third, branches of middle meningeal, ascending pharyngeal, occipital, and posterior auricular artery supply multiple cranial nerves and these arterial feeders should be tested with lidocaine and methohexital once an acceptable catheter position is reached and before embolization is started [37]. Intraoperative monitoring may also be considered if the patient is under general anesthesia; otherwise awake neurological testing should be done during the procedure.

Embolic agents for arterial approach

Polyvinyl alcohol particles (multiple vendors) and Embospheres (Merit Medical, South Jordan, UT, USA) are particle embolic agents that can penetrate small feeders involved in DAVF but do not necessarily occlude the actual fistula site. The embolic plug formed usually degrades over days to weeks, leading to high rates of recurrence and also to secondary recruitment of new arterial feeders [38]. The new collaterals on recurrence are smaller, tortuous, and often not amenable to embolization. Given the short-term effects of these agents, they might be considered as an adjunct before operative obliteration of a DAVF. McConnell *et al.* have suggested using polyvinyl alcohol particles in combination with liquid embolics in multipedicle fistula by providing a safer conduit for liquid embolics [1].

N-Butyl cyanoacrylate (NBCA) (Trufill, DePuy Synthes-Codman, Neurovascular, Raynham, MA, USA) is a frequently used liquid embolic agent for transarterial embolization of DAVF. It is a clear, free-flowing monomer mixed with different proportions of ethiodized oil (Ethiodol) for radiopacity and polymerizes on contact with ionic fluid. Increasing the amount of Ethiodol delays the polymerization time and allows the glue mixture use to be modified to vary the rate of polymerization. The mixture of Ethiodol to NBCA will vary depending upon the distance between the catheter tip and the actual fistula site, as well as the size and the flow rate of the artery supplying the fistula. Given its rapid polymerization time, NBCA may be used with high-flow arteriovenous shunts. It can be safely used in combination with a wedged microcatheter technique, creating a flow arrest condition in the feeding vessel and allowing adequate glue penetration [39]. Balloon-assisted glue embolization has been reported in some patients with high-flow fistulae such as vein of Galen malformations. Balloon inflation affords more control in the glue injection and prevents distal embolization [40]. Simultaneous perfusion of dextrose 5% through the guiding catheter during NBCA injection dramatically improves the distal progression of glue through the small, tortuous arterial feeders of a DAVF [41]. The NBCA forms a discrete plug rather than a confluent cast and the plug can fragment and embolize distally. It also only allows single pedicle selection, and injection and rapid withdrawal of catheter is required. In experienced hands, acrylic glue can have excellent obliteration rates [42]. Guedin *et al.* reported glue embolization in 38 patients with DAVFs with an obliteration rate of 89.5% and durability of >30 years [43].

Ethylene vinyl alcohol copolymer (Onyx Liquid embolic system, Covidien ev3 Neurovascular, Irvine, CA, USA) is a newer liquid embolic available in varying viscosities: Onyx 18 and 34 contain 6% and 8% ethylene vinyl alcohol, respectively. Tantalum powder added to the suspension provides radiopacity. Onyx is dissolved in dimethyl sulfoxide (DMSO) and it precipitates in blood to form a solid cast from the exterior to the interior [3]. Onyx acts as a non-adhesive precipitate and layers concentrically within the artery. It forms a continuous cast, allows for slower controlled injections, and a larger volume can be injected. The concentric flow of Onyx allows it to seek multiple small feeders as part of the DAVF fistulous site. Manipulation of flow by interrupting and reinitiating the injection can redirect the path of the forming embolus. Care should be taken to avoid feeders supplying cranial nerves as Onyx can percolate vasa nervosum and lead to cranial nerve palsies [44]. Onyx injections are also associated with longer fluoroscopy times. There have been multiple reports demonstrating efficacy of Onyx use in DAVFs even in the presence of cortical venous drainage [45]. Appropriate positioning of the DMSO-compatible catheter adjacent to the fistula site is a crucial determining factor in complete DAVF obliteration. Occlusion rates of DAVF with Onyx can range from 62.5% to 100% according to different reports [46–53]. Onyx has also been successfully used in CCFs, with successful casting of the cavernous sinus and obliteration of the fistula [54,55]. Cognard *et al.* suggested Onyx was the preferred liquid embolic for DAVF, demonstrating complete fistula obliteration in 23 of 25 treated patients [48]. Onyx 34 can be used in combination with Onyx 18 to help in the formation of a better Onyx plug, particularly in a high-flow shunt. Use of a DMSO-compatible balloon catheter obviates the need for an Onyx plug and hence large amounts of Onyx can be injected safely without concern of reflux [56]. Complications with any liquid embolic can include catheter breakage, radiation injury, and cranial nerve palsies [57].

Transvenous embolization

Transvenous embolization involves occluding the fistula pocket from the venous route. This technique generally involves packing or occluding the venous drainage immediately adjacent to the fistula. It is crucial to understand the location of the fistula site in relation to the venous system and whether or not the transvenous embolization involves obliterating the sinus. Transvenous embolization may be preferred in DAVFs with supply from arterial feeders supplying cranial nerves, or when the transarterial approach is a high risk. Patients with venous sinus occlusion or high-grade venous stenosis may be poor candidates for appropriate access for transvenous embolization. The access to the venous system could be transfemoral or percutaneous. Transvenous treatment may be advantageous in middle fossa DAVFs with multiple small arterial feeders where arterial embolization may not be feasible. Klisch *et al.* reported a high rate of occlusion with transvenous embolization in their series of 31 patients [58].

There are several important considerations with transvenous treatment. First, the segment of sinus to be occluded should be draining the fistula entirely. Second, the sinus to be occluded should not be the dominant sinus contributing to the venous drainage of the native brain. Most sinuses occluded are already defunctionalized and hence do not affect native drainage and the risk of venous infarcts and hemorrhage. Third, the fistula and associated sinus should be occluded entirely to avoid skipped sinus areas; diversion of the fistula into associated anastomotic venous channels, including cortical veins, risks stroke and hemorrhage.

Once appropriate venous access is obtained, we leave a catheter in a large arterial feeder supplying the fistula to allow imaging of the fistula during the process of venous embolization. A number of agents can be used for transvenous embolization, including metallic coils, detachable balloons, and liquid embolics (glue or Onyx). There have been some studies employing angioplasty and subsequent placement of self-expanding stents to obliterate the fistula pocket involving the sinus wall, with encouraging results [59].

Platinum coils, particularly fibered coils with high thrombogenic properties, are often used. Detachable platinum coils are useful as the initial coils when filling the fistula pocket. Detachable platinum coils can give accurate placement and frame before pushable fibered coils are injected. Given sinus compliance properties, coils are generally oversized to allow adequate packing. Forming a compact coil mass that completely occludes the fistulae and the associated "defunctionalized" sinus is crucial.

Liquid embolics such as NBCA and Onyx can be employed as adjunctive agents to occlude the fistula pocket and involved sinus. These agents allow improved penetration of the septated fistula pockets [55].

A direct percutaneous approach may be employed for transvenous embolization, particularly for cavernous sinus access via the pterygoid plexus and superior ophthalmic vein [60]. Direct puncture of the superior or inferior ophthalmic veins, facial veins, or frontal veins for appropriate venous access have been well described [3].

Treatment of direct carotid–cavernous fistulae

Direct CCF were historically treated with ligation of the common carotid artery or ICA. Wallace Hamby, an American neurosurgeon, was first to ligate the ICA in 1932 as part of a trapping procedure for CCF [16]. Sacrifice of the ICA is still an option in some situations, particularly if the patient has good intracranial collaterals, which is determined after performing a balloon test occlusion.

The balloon catheter technique, introduced by Serbinenko, advanced the treatment of CCFs. Detachable balloons can be used to perform a transarterial transfistula balloon embolization. The balloon is passed through the tear in the ICA and

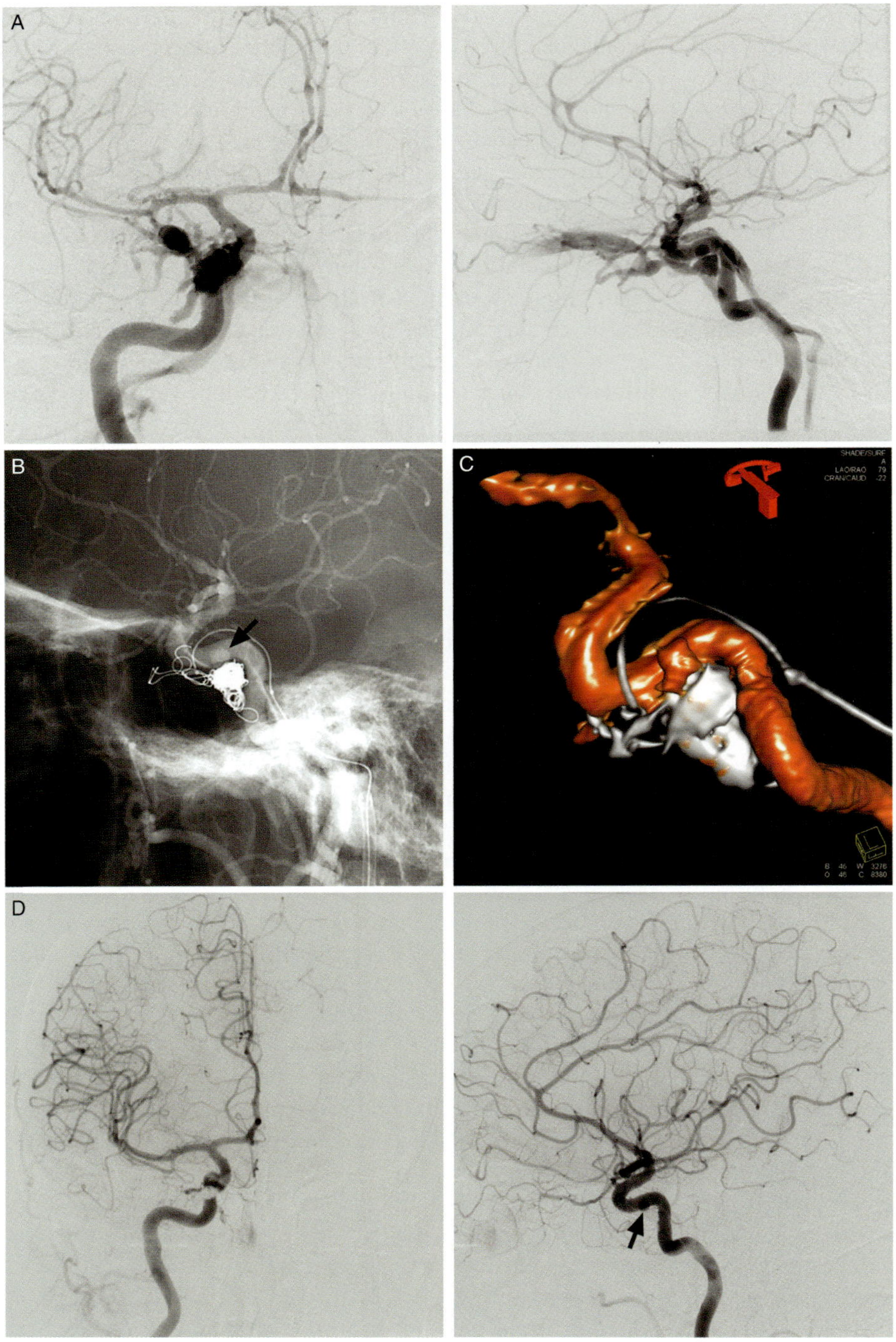

Fig. 19.1. Direct carotid–cavernous fistula (CCF; Barrow type A) from a ruptured cavernous internal carotid artery (ICA) aneurysm in a 67-year-old woman with sudden-onset chemosis and proptosis of right eye. (A) Arterial phase angiography from right ICA demonstrated the right cavernous sinus, right superior ophthalmic vein, and inferior petrosal sinus, consistent with a direct CCF (left, anteroposterior view; right, lateral view). (B) Lateral unsubtracted skull base view demonstrated a coil mass in the right cavernous sinus, and a cavernous ICA aneurysm (arrow) that had ruptured. (C) Treatment was performed with transvenous coil embolization. Rotational three-dimensional angiography demonstrated the cavernous sinus coil mass, microcatheter, and the cavernous ICA aneurysm. (D) Angiography of right ICA after treatment demonstrated obliteration of the fistula and the small cavernous ICA aneurysm (arrow) (left, anteroposterior view; right, lateral view).

inflated to occlude the fistula while maintaining artery patency before it is detached [4]. Detachable balloons are no longer available in the USA.

Transvenous coil embolization of the cavernous sinus is a more common approach, where the cavernous sinus is accessed through the inferior petrosal sinus or another route. Coils are then placed into the cavernous sinus while avoiding prolapse into the ICA from the fistula site (Fig. 19.1)

Stent-assisted treatment of a direct CCF has been discussed in the literature by laying a covered stent across the site of fistula. Stent-assisted coil embolization of a direct CCF has also been described [61].

Combined arterial and venous approaches

A combination of transarterial and transvenous techniques may be employed in some DAVFs to achieve occlusion of a complex fistula. Occasionally, a direct craniotomy over the fistula site may be needed to allow direct packing with coils, such as in the torcular DAVF [62].

Additional treatment options

Microsurgery

In the 1970s and 1980s, primary treatment of most cranial DAVFs was microsurgical disconnection and associated

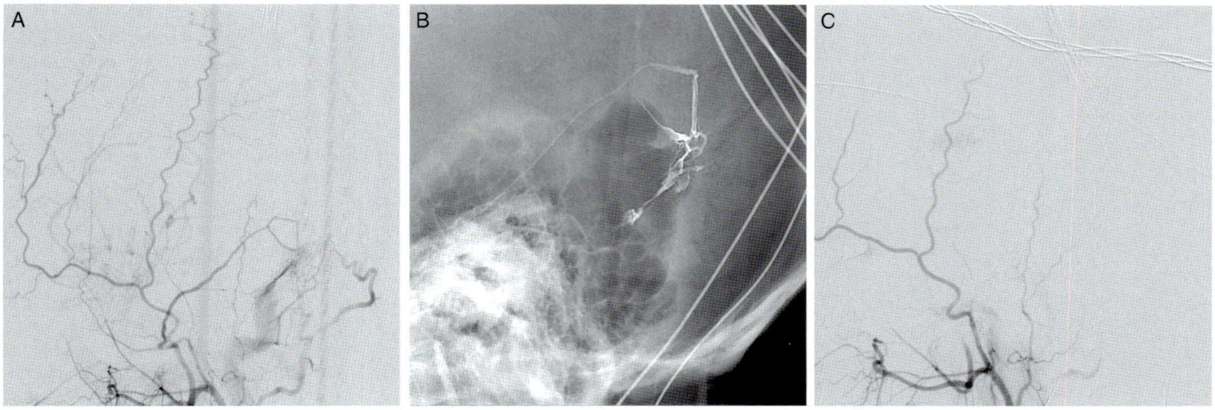

Fig. 19.2. Transverse sigmoid dural arteriovenous fistula in a 30-year-old woman presenting with headaches and tinnitus. (A) Lateral right external carotid artery injection demonstrated a Cognard I fistula supplied by right middle meningeal artery and occipital artery draining into the transverse–sigmoid junction. (B) Lateral unsubtracted view after transarterial Onyx embolization demonstrated a microcatheter advanced into the distal middle meningeal artery and Onyx-18 cast penetrating the fistula. (C) Right lateral external carotid artery injection after treatment showed obliteration of fistula. The transverse–sigmoid sinus is not visualized.

removal of dura/sinuses. Surgical procedures are often technically challenging, have high morbidity, and can involve significant blood loss. There is a small subset of patients for whom aggressive endovascular embolization of DAVF fails and who are treated with surgery. Intraoperative angiography is a useful tool in the treatment of these patients and can significantly help in guiding surgical treatment in definitive treatment of DAVF [63]. A hybrid operative–angiography suite can help to achieve a high rate of cure for these patients requiring a surgical approach.

Combined surgical and endovascular approaches can be used to treat some DAVFs. We have found this to be useful for treatment of torcular DAVFs that are inaccessible from both transverse sinuses. The torcula can be exposed after a craniotomy, and the fistula site can then be packed with coils and embolic material. There have been other reports using surgical exposures for endovascular treatment of DAVFs.

Radiation

Radiation therapy, including radiosurgery with gamma knife and CyberKnife, is another known modality for treatment of DAVFs. It is usually employed as a salvage primary therapy in patients who have exhausted endovascular and surgical therapies or as an adjunctive therapy. It allows a slow controlled obliteration of a fistula and has a latency period of at least six months before the fistula is obliterated. Obliteration rates can vary from 50 to 100% for indirect CCF and from 20 to 100% for non-CCF DAVF [64].

Dural arteriovenous fistulae by anatomical location

Transverse and sigmoid sinus

The transverse–sigmoid junction is the most common site of DAVF in most reported clinical series [5]. Patients frequently present with tinnitus given the proximity of the sinuses to the middle ear. Hemorrhage, myelopathy, stroke, and venous hypertension can be experienced by patients with high-grade fistulae. The arterial supply is most often seen from occipital artery, middle meningeal artery, ascending pharyngeal artery, posterior meningeal branches off the vertebral artery, and tentorial branches off the meningohypophyseal trunk. Transvenous embolization is preferred where the sinus is defunctionalized. Transarterial embolization with Onyx (Fig. 19.2) or NBCA (Fig. 19.3) glue may be performed by catheterization of distal arterial feeders and distal penetration of the embolic agent.

Cavernous sinus

Cavernous sinus DAVFs are seen more commonly in women (Figs. 19.1 and 19.4). A direct CCF with a tear in the wall of the ICA can be spontaneous or acquired [61]. Causes could include closed head injury, rupture of intracavernous ICA, iatrogenic injury during trans-sphenoidal surgery, or collagen vascular diseases such as Marfan syndrome. Indirect CCFs usually have supply from branches of the ECA: the internal maxillary arteries and middle meningeal arteries with contribution from the meningohypophyseal trunk and the inferolateral trunk. There is reversal of flow in the superior ophthalmic veins and the angular facial veins and patients often present with chemosis, proptosis, and oculomotor palsies. Most are grade I on presentation given early ocular symptoms and are treated with transvenous embolization.

Tentorial

Tentorial DAVFs or superior petrosal DAVFs involve the petrous ridge and are aggressive lesions. There is >90% incidence of aggressive neurological symptoms on presentation, including intracranial hemorrhage [3]. Tentorial DAVFs derive their arterial supply from the meningohypophyseal trunk, occipital artery, ascending pharyngeal artery, middle meningeal artery, and posterior meningeal arteries from the vertebral artery. The majority of these patients have leptomeningeal or spinal perimedullary drainage. These lesions are treated with transarterial embolization and may require microsurgical obliteration.

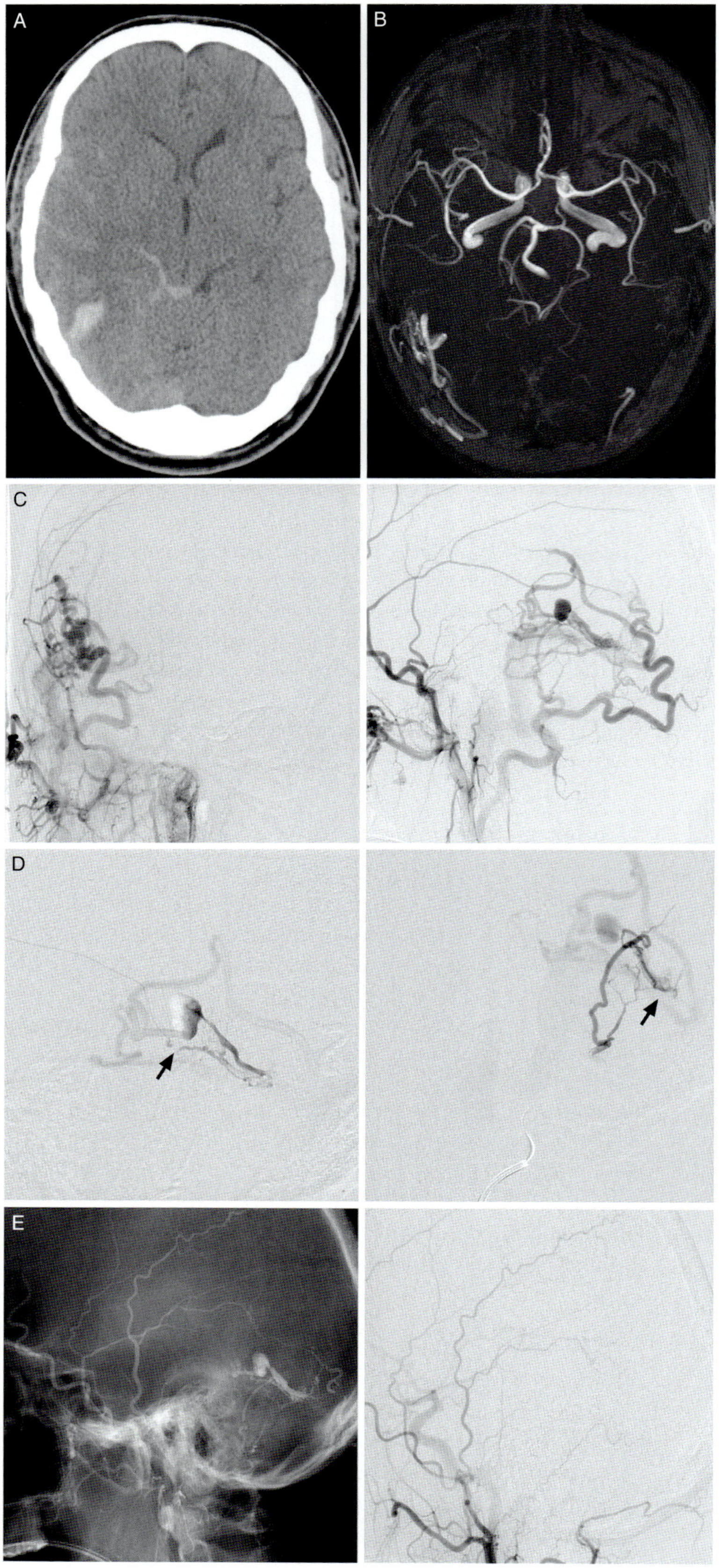

Fig. 19.3. Transverse sigmoid dural arteriovenous fistula (DAVF) with hemorrhage in a 50-year-old man presenting with severe headache. (A) Non-contrast CT revealed hemorrhage along the right tentorium and basal cisterns. (B) MR angiography showed a prominent right occipital artery and external circulation. (C) Angiography of external carotid artery projections demonstrated a Cognard IV transverse–sigmoid DAVF supplied by right middle meningeal artery and occipital artery (left, anteroposterior view; right, lateral view). (D) Microcatheter injection into the distal right middle meningeal artery demonstrated the fistula (arrow) and the venous varix. *N*-Butyl cyanoacrylate glue was injected transarterially through the microcatheter to occlude the fistula. (E). Unsubtracted lateral image (left panel) showed the glue cast along the fistula pocket and venous varix and a post-treatment right external carotid artery lateral view (right panel) demonstrated no evidence of early venous filling and the obliteration of the middle meningeal artery and occipital artery supply to the fistula.

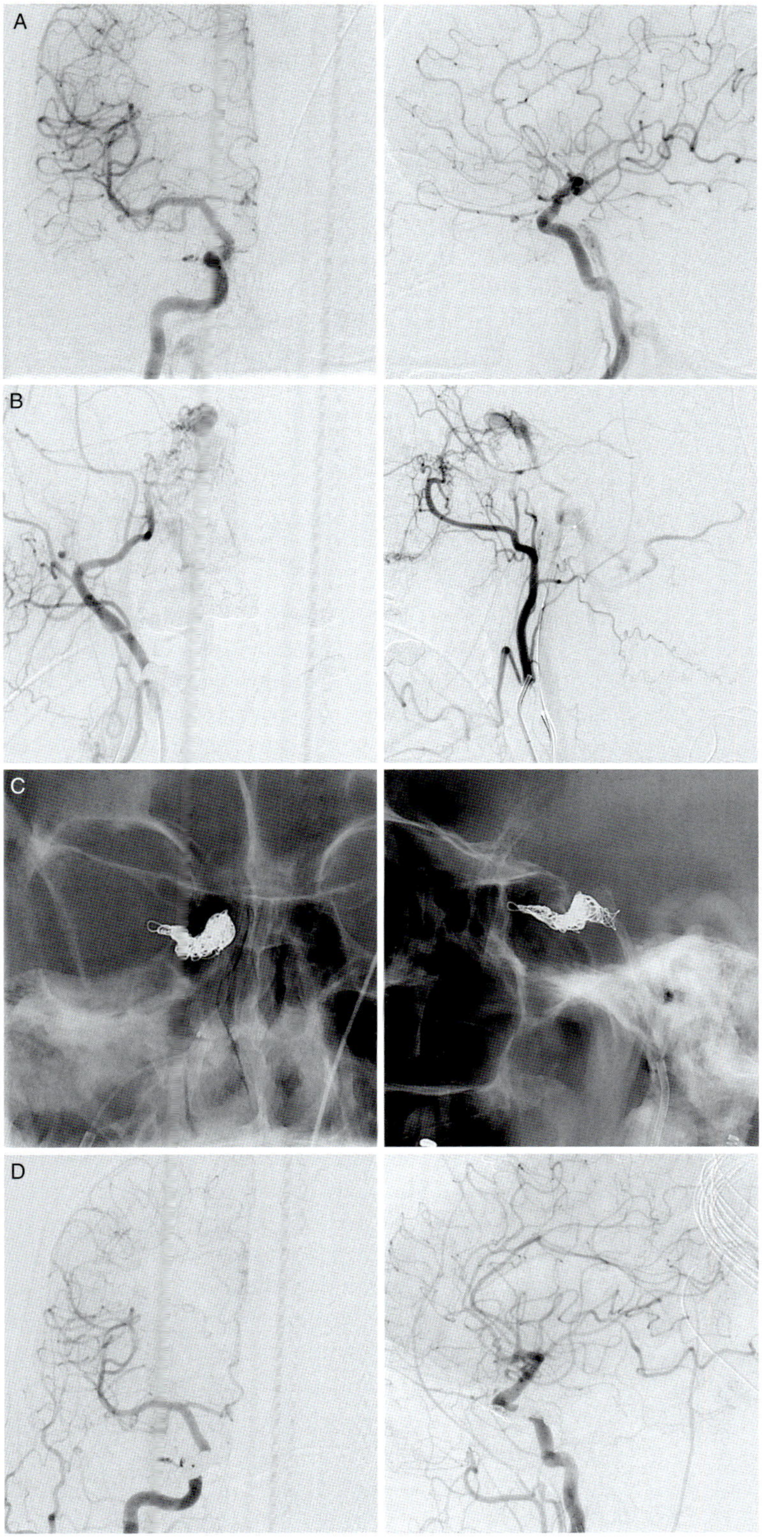

Fig. 19.4. Indirect carotid–cavernous fistula (CCF; Barrow type D) in a 66-year-old man with right orbital proptosis and discomfort who presented for evaluation. (A) Angiography of right internal carotid artery injection demonstrated early venous drainage into right cavernous sinus with supply from the meningohypophyseal trunk (left, anteroposterior view; right, lateral view). (B) Angiography of right external carotid artery demonstrated supply from the internal maxillary artery (left, anteroposterior view; right, lateral view). (C) Transvenous coil embolization of the right cavernous sinus was completed to occlude the fistula. Unsubtracted skull base views demonstrated the coil mass in place, conforming to the right cavernous sinus morphology (left, anteroposterior view; right, lateral view). (D) Angiography of right internal carotid artery injection 6 months after treatment demonstrate complete CCF occlusion and improvement of proptosis (left, anteroposterior view; right, lateral view).

Superior sagittal sinus

Middle meningeal arteries often feed superior sagittal sinus DAVFs and patients often present with headaches and cognitive impairment (Fig. 19.5). There can be bilateral arterial feeders and sacrifice of the superior sagittal sinus is usually not an option particularly in the posterior two-thirds of the sinus. Transarterial embolization is the preferred therapy with the aim of penetrating the fistula; Onyx is particularly useful for these patients [65]. The fistula is usually in the wall of the superior sagittal sinus and patency of the sinus proper is maintained with transarterial embolization. These parasinus pockets are difficult to catheterize from the transvenous route but some cases have been described in literature.

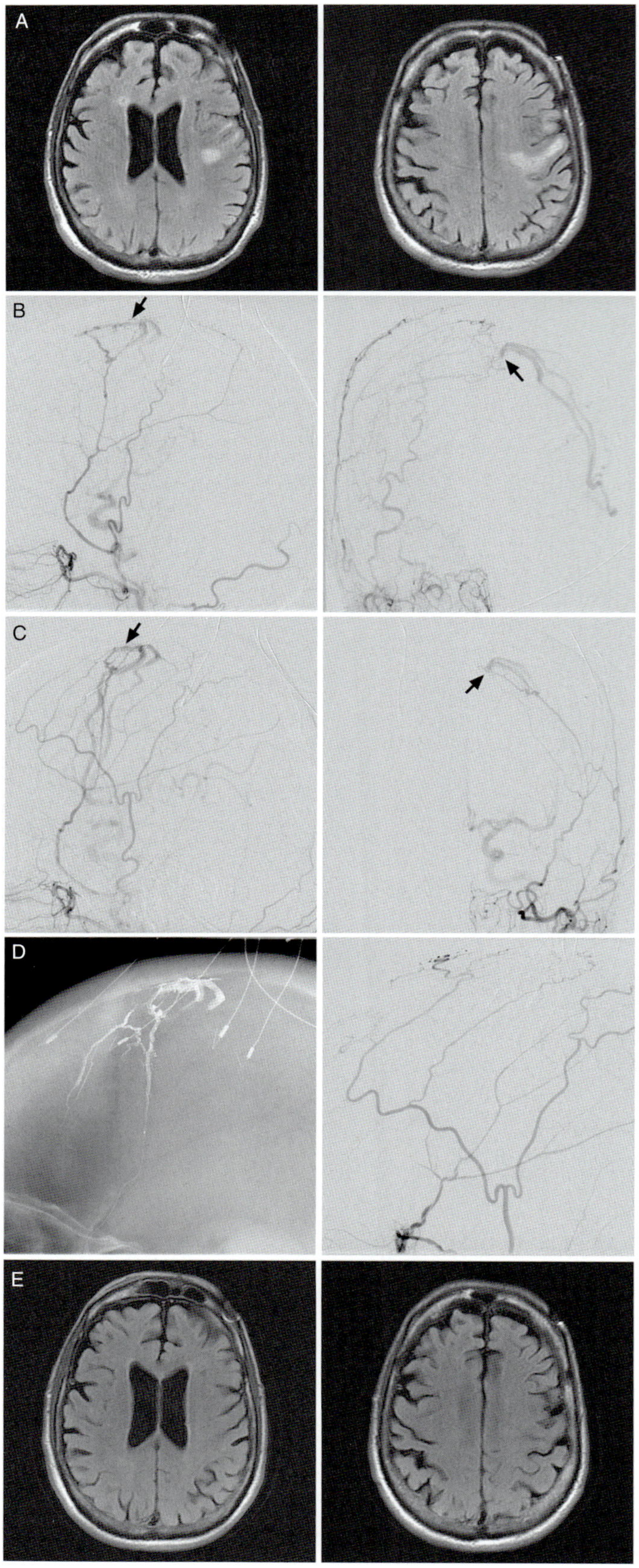

Fig. 19.5. A superior sagittal sinus (SSS) dural arteriovenous fistula in an 82-year-old man presenting with progressive cognitive decline and seizures. (A) Fluid attenuated inversion recovery (FLAIR) images demonstrated edema in the left frontal lobe. (B) Right external carotid artery injection demonstrated a Cognard III SSS fistula supplied by the right middle meningeal artery (left, anteroposterior view; right, lateral view). A fistula (arrow) at the SSS with subsequent cortical venous drainage in left hemisphere could be seen. (C) Left external carotid artery demonstrated a left middle meningeal artery supply to the fistula (arrow) (left, anteroposterior view; right, lateral view). (D) The fistula was treated with Onyx 18 injection into the left middle meningeal artery, with penetration into the fistula pocket. Unsubtracted lateral image (left panel) showed the Onyx cast. A right external carotid artery injection (right panel) demonstrated obliteration of fistula and lack of venous shunting. (E) Follow-up FLAIR MRI at 3 months demonstrated complete resolution of the initial left frontal lobe changes. The patient made a complete recovery with improvement of mental status and seizures.

Anterior cranial fossa/ethmoid

Anterior cranial fossa DAVFs develop at the cribriform plate and are usually fed by branches of the bilateral ethmoidal arteries and branches of the middle meningeal and internal maxillary arteries. There is a strong male preponderance and most ethmoidal DAVFs are symptomatic with leptomeningeal venous drainage. Given the small size of the ethmoidal vessels and difficulty with adequate penetration of liquid embolics, tortuous leptomeningeal venous drainage embolization may not yield good results. These lesions may be best treated with microsurgery involving coagulation of draining vein and fistula. Additionally there is a high risk of retinal infarction with attempts to catheterize the ophthalmic artery [66].

Other locations: torcular, inferior petrosal sinus, marginal, condylar

Torcular and marginal sinus DAVFs are rare but aggressive subtypes that are treated with transvenous embolization [67]; DAVFs involving the anterior condylar confluence form another rare subtype and can often be confused with DAVF of the marginal sinus. The neuromeningeal trunk of the ascending pharyngeal artery supplies the anterior condylar DAVF. Transarterial embolization may be high risk given supply to the vasa nervosum of cranial nerves IX–XII from the neuromeningeal trunk [68]. Transvenous embolization of the anterior condylar venous complex is the preferred route for treatment (Fig. 19.6).

Conclusions

Evolution and improvements in endovascular technology have immensely impacted DAVF treatment. Most fistulae can now be treated with endovascular embolization using coils and liquid embolics. Microsurgical treatment is still indicated for ethmoidal DAVF. Microsurgery and radiation is important multimodality treatment for complex fistulae. A multidisciplinary approach spearheaded by endovascular therapies can help to cure most patients with symptomatic or high-grade fistulae with relatively low risk. A thorough knowledge of vascular anatomy is crucial in understanding and treating arteriovenous fistulae in the brain.

Fig. 19.5. (cont.).

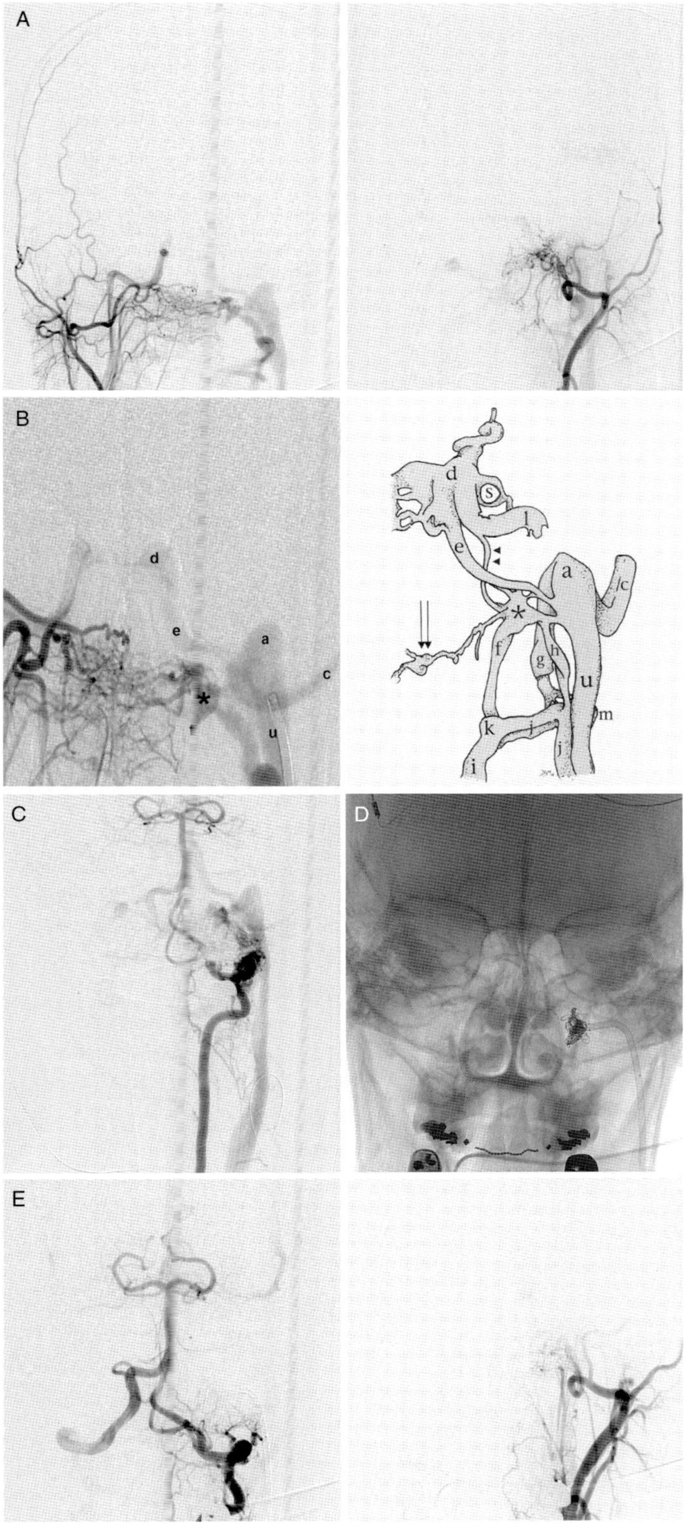

Fig. 19.6. Anterior condylar confluence (ACC) dural arteriovenous fistula in a 47-year-old woman with severe headaches, left eye pulsation, and pulsatile tinnitus who presented for evaluation. (A) Anteroposterior projection of the right external carotid artery (left panel) and left external carotid artery (right panel) demonstrated a Cognard I fistula with early venous drainage into the anterior condylar complex. Supply from bilateral ascending pharyngeal arteries could be seen. (B) Magnified anteroposterior view of the right external carotid artery (left panel) and illustrative schematic (right panel) show the venous anatomy of the ACC and its connections: anterior condylar vein (f), lateral condylar vein (h), internal jugular vein (u), inferior petrosal sinus (e), cavernous sinus (d), emissary vein of the foramen ovale (s), superior jugular bulb (a), sigmoid sinus (c), posterior condylar vein (g), anastomosis between anterior internal vertebral venous plexus and vertebral artery venous plexus (k), vertebral artery venous plexus (j), deep cervical vein (m), anterior internal vertebral venous plexus (i), venous plexus of Rektorzik (double arrowhead), and the prevertebral venous plexus (double arrow). (C) Anteroposterior view of the left vertebral artery demonstrated supply to the ACC fistula via posterior meningeal branches as well as the jugular bulb and internal jugular vein. (D) Transvenous coil embolization of the ACC resulted in complete occlusion of the fistula; the anteroposterior unsubtracted view after treatment demonstrated the coil mass conforming to the ACC morphology. (E) Post-treatment anteroposterior views of the left vertebral artery (left panel) and left external carotid artery (right panel) demonstrated complete obliteration of the fistula without evidence of early venous drainage into ACC. The patient had complete resolution of symptoms. (The schematic in (B) was adapted with permission from San Millan Ruiz D, Gailloud P, Rufenacht DA, *et al.* The craniocervical venous system in relation to cerebral venous drainage. *AJNR Am J Neuroradiol* 2002;23:1500–8.)

References

1. McConnell KA, Tjoumakaris SI, Allen J, *et al.* Neuroendovascular management of dural arteriovenous malformations. *Neurosurg Clin N Am* 2009;**20**:431–9.
2. Newton TH, Cronqvist S. Involvement of dural arteries in intracranial arteriovenous malformations. *Radiology* 1969;**93**:1071–8.
3. Narayanan S. Endovascular management of intracranial dural arteriovenous fistulas. *Neurol Clin* 2010;**28**:899–911.
4. Ng PP, Higashida RT, Cullen S, *et al.* Endovascular strategies for carotid cavernous and intracerebral dural arteriovenous fistulas. *Neurosurg Focus* 2003;**15**:E1.
5. Malek AM, Halbach VV, Higashida RT, *et al.* Treatment of dural arteriovenous malformations and fistulas. *Neurosurg Clin N Am* 2000;**11**:147–66.
6. Kutluk K, Schumacher M, Mironov A. The role of sinus thrombosis in occipital dural arteriovenous malformations: development and spontaneous closure. *Neurochirurgia (Stuttg)* 1991;**34**:144–7.
7. Lawton MT, Jacobowitz R, Spetzler RF. Redefined role of angiogenesis in the pathogenesis of dural arteriovenous malformations. *J Neurosurg* 1997;**87**:267–74.
8. Terada T, Higashida RT, Halbach VV, *et al.* Development of acquired arteriovenous fistulas in rats due to venous hypertension. *J Neurosurg* 1994;**80**:884–9.
9. Uranishi R, Nakase H, Sakaki T. Expression of angiogenic growth factors in dural arteriovenous fistula. *J Neurosurg* 1999;**91**:781–6.
10. Terada T, Tsuura M, Komai N, *et al.* The role of angiogenic factor bFGF in the development of dural AVFs. *Acta Neurochir (Wien)* 1996;**138**:877–83.
11. Tirakotai W, Bian LG, Bertalanffy H, *et al.* Immunohistochemical study in dural arteriovenous fistula and possible role of ephrin-B2 for development of dural arteriovenous fistula. *Chin Med J (Engl)* 2004;**117**:1815–20.
12. Takahashi A, Sawamura Y, Houkin K, *et al.* The cerebrospinal fluid in patients with moyamoya disease (spontaneous occlusion of the circle of Willis) contains high level of basic fibroblast growth factor. *Neurosci Lett* 1993;**160**:214–16.
13. Nishijima M, Takaku A, Endo S, *et al.* Etiological evaluation of dural arteriovenous malformations of the lateral and sigmoid sinuses based on histopathological examinations. *J Neurosurg* 1992;**76**:600–6.
14. Hamada Y, Goto K, Inoue T, *et al.* Histopathological aspects of dural arteriovenous fistulas in the transverse–sigmoid sinus region in nine patients. *Neurosurgery* 1997;**40**:452–6.
15. Gomez J, Amin AG, Gregg L, *et al.* Classification schemes of cranial dural arteriovenous fistulas. *Neurosurg Clin N Am* 2012;**23**:55–62.
16. Colby GP, Coon AL, Huang J, *et al.* Historical perspective of treatments of cranial arteriovenous malformations and dural arteriovenous fistulas. *Neurosurg Clin N Am* 2012;**23**:15–25.
17. Cohen SD, Goins JL, Butler SG, *et al.* Dural arteriovenous fistula: diagnosis, treatment, and outcomes. *Laryngoscope* 2009;**119**:293–7.
18. Coley SC, Romanowski CA, Hodgson TJ, *et al.* Dural arteriovenous fistulae: noninvasive diagnosis with dynamic MR digital subtraction angiography. *AJNR Am J Neuroradiol* 2002;**23**:404–7.
19. Le TT, Fischbein NJ, Andre JB, *et al.* Identification of venous signal on arterial spin labeling improves diagnosis of dural arteriovenous fistulas and small arteriovenous malformations. *AJNR Am J Neuroradiol* 2012;**33**:61–8.
20. Kuroda S, Furukawa K, Shiga T, *et al.* Pretreatment and posttreatment evaluation of hemodynamic and metabolic parameters in intracranial dural arteriovenous fistulae with cortical venous reflux. *Neurosurgery* 2004;**54**:585–91.
21. Cognard C, Gobin YP, Pierot L, *et al.* Cerebral dural arteriovenous fistulas: clinical and angiographic correlation with a revised classification of venous drainage. *Radiology* 1995;**194**:671–80.
22. Zipfel GJ, Shah MN, Refai D, *et al.* Cranial dural arteriovenous fistulas: modification of angiographic classification scales based on new natural history data. *Neurosurg Focus* 2009;**26**:E14.
23. Kobayashi N, Miyachi S, Negoro M, *et al.* Endovascular treatment strategy for direct carotid–cavernous fistulas resulting from rupture of intracavernous carotid aneurysms. *AJNR Am J Neuroradiol* 2003;**24**:1789–96.
24. Djindjian R, Cophignon J, Theron J, *et al.* Embolization by superselective arteriography from the femoral route in neuroradiology. Review of 60 cases. 1. Technique, indications, complications. *Neuroradiology* 1973;**6**:20–6.
25. Borden JA, Wu JK, Shucart WA. A proposed classification for spinal and cranial dural arteriovenous fistulous malformations and implications for treatment. *J Neurosurg* 1995;**82**:166–79.
26. Davies MA, terBrugge K, Willinsky R, *et al.* The validity of classification for the clinical presentation of intracranial dural arteriovenous fistulas. *J Neurosurg* 1996;**85**:830–7.
27. Strom RG, Botros JA, Refai D, *et al.* Cranial dural arteriovenous fistulae: asymptomatic cortical venous drainage portends less aggressive clinical course. *Neurosurgery* 2009;**64**:241–7.
28. Soderman M, Pavic L, Edner G, *et al.* Natural history of dural arteriovenous shunts. *Stroke* 2008;**39**:1735–9.
29. Barrow DL, Spector RH, Braun IF, *et al.* Classification and treatment of spontaneous carotid–cavernous sinus fistulas. *J Neurosurg* 1985;**62**:248–56.
30. Kim DJ, terBrugge K, Krings T, *et al.* Spontaneous angiographic conversion of intracranial dural arteriovenous shunt: long-term follow-up in nontreated patients. *Stroke* 2010;**41**:1489–94.
31. Higashida RT, Hieshima GB, Halbach VV, *et al.* Closure of carotid cavernous sinus fistulae by external compression of the carotid artery and jugular vein. *Acta Radiol Suppl* 1986;**369**:580–3.
32. Kiyosue H, Hori Y, Okahara M, *et al.* Treatment of intracranial dural arteriovenous fistulas: current strategies based on location and hemodynamics, and alternative techniques of transcatheter embolization. *Radiographics* 2004;**24**:1637–53.
33. Halbach VV, Higashida RT, Hieshima GB, *et al.* Treatment of dural arteriovenous malformations involving the superior sagittal sinus. *AJNR Am J Neuroradiol* 1988;**9**:337–43.

34. Halbach VV, Higashida RT, Hieshima GB, *et al.* Dural fistulas involving the cavernous sinus: results of treatment in 30 patients. *Radiology* 1987;**163**:437–42

35. Siddiqui AH, Chen PR. Intracranial collateral anastomoses: relevance to endovascular procedures. *Neurosurg Clin N Am* 2009;**20**:279–96.

36. Geibprasert S, Pongpech S, Armstrong D, *et al.* Dangerous extracranial–intracranial anastomoses and supply to the cranial nerves: vessels the neurointerventionalist needs to know. *AJNR Am J Neuroradiol* 2009;**30**:1459–68.

37. Deveikis JP. Sequential injections of amobarbital sodium and lidocaine for provocative neurologic testing in the external carotid circulation. *AJNR Am J Neuroradiol* 1996;**17**:1143–7.

38. Nichols DA, Rufenacht DA, Jack CR, Jr., *et al.* Embolization of spinal dural arteriovenous fistula with polyvinyl alcohol particles: experience in 14 patients. *AJNR Am J Neuroradiol* 1992;**13**:933–40.

39. Nelson PK, Russell SM, Woo HH, *et al.* Use of a wedged microcatheter for curative transarterial embolization of complex intracranial dural arteriovenous fistulas: indications, endovascular technique, and outcome in 21 patients. *J Neurosurg* 2003;**98**:498–506.

40. Andreou A, Ioannidis I, Nasis N. Transarterial balloon-assisted glue embolization of high-flow arteriovenous fistulas. *Neuroradiology* 2008;**50**:267–72.

41. Moore C, Murphy K, Gailloud P. Improved distal distribution of *N*-butyl cyanoacrylate glue by simultaneous injection of dextrose 5% through the guiding catheter: technical note. *Neuroradiology* 2006;**48**:327–32.

42. Saraf R, Shrivastava M, Siddhartha W, *et al.* Evolution of endovascular management of intracranial dural arteriovenous fistulas: single center experience. *Neurol India* 2010;**58**:62–8.

43. Guedin P, Gaillard S, Boulin A, *et al.* Therapeutic management of intracranial dural arteriovenous shunts with leptomeningeal venous drainage: report of 53 consecutive patients with emphasis on transarterial embolization with acrylic glue. *J Neurosurg* 2010;**112**:603–10.

44. Chen J, Crane B, Niparko J, *et al.* Direct intraoperative confirmation of penetration of ethylene vinyl alcohol copolymer (Onyx) into the vasa nervosa of the facial nerve. *J Neurointerv Surg* 2012;**4**:435–7.

45. Chew J, Weill A, Guilbert F, *et al.* Arterial Onyx embolisation of intracranial DAVFs with cortical venous drainage. *Can J Neurol Sci* 2009;**36**:168–75.

46. Natarajan SK, Ghodke B, Kim LJ, *et al.* Multimodality treatment of intracranial dural arteriovenous fistulas in the Onyx era: a single center experience. *World Neurosurg* 2010;**73**:365–79.

47. De Keukeleire K, Vanlangenhove P, Kalala Okito JP, *et al.* Transarterial embolization with ONYX for treatment of intracranial non-cavernous dural arteriovenous fistula with or without cortical venous reflux. *J Neurointerv Surg* 2011;**3**:224–8.

48. Cognard C, Januel AC, Silva NA, Jr., *et al.* Endovascular treatment of intracranial dural arteriovenous fistulas with cortical venous drainage: new management using Onyx. *AJNR Am J Neuroradiol* 2008;**29**:235–41.

49. Carlson AP, Taylor CL, Yonas H. Treatment of dural arteriovenous fistula using ethylene vinyl alcohol (onyx) arterial embolization as the primary modality: short-term results. *J Neurosurg* 2007;**107**:1120–5.

50. Abud TG, Nguyen A, Saint-Maurice JP, *et al.* The use of Onyx in different types of intracranial dural arteriovenous fistula. *AJNR Am J Neuroradiol* 2011;**32**:2185–91.

51. Ghobrial GM, Marchan E, Nair AK, *et al.* Dural arteriovenous fistulas: a review of the literature and a presentation of a single institution's experience. *World Neurosurg* 2013;**80**:94–102.

52. Macdonald JH, Millar JS, Barker CS. Endovascular treatment of cranial dural arteriovenous fistulae: a single-centre, 14-year experience and the impact of Onyx on local practise. *Neuroradiology* 2010;**52**:387–95.

53. Nogueira RG, Dabus G, Rabinov JD, *et al.* Preliminary experience with onyx embolization for the treatment of intracranial dural arteriovenous fistulas. *AJNR Am J Neuroradiol* 2008;**29**:91–7.

54. Gandhi D, Ansari SA, Cornblath WT. Successful transarterial embolization of a Barrow type D dural carotid–cavernous fistula with ethylene vinyl alcohol copolymer (Onyx). *J Neuroophthalmol* 2009;**29**:9–12.

55. Zhang J, Lv X, Jiang C, *et al.* Transarterial and transvenous embolization for cavernous sinus dural arteriovenous fistulae. *Interv Neuroradiol* 2010;**16**:269–77.

56. Shi ZS, Loh Y, Duckwiler GR, *et al.* Balloon-assisted transarterial embolization of intracranial dural arteriovenous fistulas. *J Neurosurg* 2009;**110**:921–8.

57. Pei W, Huai-Zhang S, Shan-Cai X, *et al.* Isolated hypoglossal nerve palsy due to endovascular treatment of a dural arteriovenous fistula with Onyx-18. *Interv Neuroradiol* 2010;**16**:286–9.

58. Klisch J, Huppertz HJ, Spetzger U, *et al.* Transvenous treatment of carotid cavernous and dural arteriovenous fistulae: results for 31 patients and review of the literature. *Neurosurgery* 2003;**53**:836–56.

59. Levrier O, Metellus P, Fuentes S, *et al.* Use of a self-expanding stent with balloon angioplasty in the treatment of dural arteriovenous fistulas involving the transverse and/or sigmoid sinus: functional and neuroimaging-based outcome in 10 patients. *J Neurosurg* 2006;**104**:254–63.

60. Caragine LP, Jr., Halbach VV, Dowd CF, *et al.* Intraorbital arteriovenous fistulae of the ophthalmic veins treated by transvenous endovascular occlusion: technical case report. *Neurosurgery* 2006;**58**:onsE170.

61. Gemmete JJ, Ansari SA, Gandhi DM. Endovascular techniques for treatment of carotid–cavernous fistula. *J Neuroophthalmol* 2009;**29**:62–71.

62. Spiotta AM, Sivapatham T, Hussain MS, *et al.* Combined surgical and endovascular approach to a complex dural arteriovenous fistula involving the superior sagittal sinus and torcula. *J Stroke Cerebrovasc Dis* 2012;**21**:283–8.

63. Pandey P, Steinberg GK, Westbroek EM, *et al.* Intraoperative angiography

for cranial dural arteriovenous fistula. *AJNR Am J Neuroradiol* 2011;**32**:1091–5.

64. Loumiotis I, Lanzino G, Daniels D, *et al.* Radiosurgery for intracranial dural arteriovenous fistulas (DAVFs): a review. *Neurosurg Rev* 2011;**34**:305–15.

65. Arat A, Inci S. Treatment of a superior sagittal sinus dural arteriovenous fistula with Onyx: technical case report. *Neurosurgery* 2006;**59**:onsE169–70.

66. Lawton MT, Chun J, Wilson CB, *et al.* Ethmoidal dural arteriovenous fistulae: an assessment of surgical and endovascular management. *Neurosurgery* 1999;**45**:805–10.

67. Evans AJ, Kallmes DF, Jensen ME, *et al.* The marginal sinus normal anatomy and involvement with arteriovenous fistulae. *Interv Neuroradiol* 1996;**2**:215–21.

68. Abiko M, Ikawa F, Ohbayashi N, *et al.* Endovascular treatment for dural arteriovenous fistula of the anterior condylar confluence involving the anterior condylar vein. A report of two cases. *Interv Neuroradiol* 2008;**14**:313–17.

Chapter 20

Endovascular management of vein of Galen malformations

Sasikhan Geibprasert, Peter Dirks, Karel terBrugge, and Timo Krings

Introduction

Vein of Galen aneurysmal malformations (VGAMs) are arteriovenous malformations (AVMs) of the choroidal system that develop in the early embryonic stage and have been recognized as possibly the only embryonic vascular malformations. Unlike pial AVMs, the actual shunt lies in the subarachnoid space. Raybaud *et al.* were the first to recognize that the ectatic vein in a VGAM is, in fact, not the vein of Galen but rather the median vein of the prosencephalon, the embryonic precursor of the vein of Galen itself [1]. Additionally, there is persistence of alternative routes for deep venous drainage as most often the choroidal vein and the thalamostriate vein fail to connect to the torcula owing to the arterialization and missing development of the vein of Galen and the straight sinus [2]. The clinical presentation of VGAM and its natural history vary significantly from pial AVMs. The management options, timing of intervention, and potential complication make it imperative that this condition be recognized precisely and accurately and managed at an experienced center at the optimal moment in time in order to achieve a normally developing child.

Angioarchitecture

It is possible to distinguish the angioarchitectural differences between an AVM involving the vein of Galen forerunner (the median vein of the prosencephalon) and an AVM with venous drainage into a dilated vein of Galen (VGAD). The first involves the choroidal fissure and extends from the interventricular foramen rostrally to the atrium laterally [3]. The arterial supply usually involves all the choroidal arteries, including subfornical and anterior choroidal contributions; it may also receive significant contribution from the subependymal network from the posterior circle of Willis. Involvement of transmesencephalic arteries (which are easy to identify on MRI) would exclude the diagnosis of VGAM [4]. Subependymal and transcerebral contributions appear as accessory in the supply to the shunt, possibly created by the venous-sump effect [5]. As they are secondarily triggered by the VGAM, they will spontaneously disappear after proper treatment of the major supply to the shunt. A persistent limbic arterial arch is often seen that bridges the posterior cerebral artery with the pericallosal artery through the choroidal arteries. The nidus of the lesion is usually located in the midline and, therefore, usually receives bilateral and symmetrical supply [3].

True VGAM can be phenotypically divided into two types on the basis of the angioarchitecture: choroidal and mural [5]. The choroidal type (Fig. 20.1A) corresponds to a very primitive condition, with the contribution of all the choroidal arteries and an interposed network before opening into the large venous pouch. It is mostly encountered in neonates with poor clinical scores. On the other hand, mural types of VGAM (Fig. 20.1B) represent direct anteriovenous fistulae within the wall of the median vein of the prosencephalon. These fistulae can be single or multiple and either converge into a single venous chamber or into multiple venous lobulations located along the anterior aspect of the pouch. This form is more often encountered in infants with better clinical scores. Transitional forms exist between these two types (Fig. 20.1C).

The venous drainage, by definition, is toward the dilated median vein of the prosencephalon, and no communication exists between this vein and the deep venous system of the brain, necessitating alternative routes of drainage for the choroidal, septal, and thalamostriate veins. Thalamostriate veins open into the posterior and inferior thalamic veins, which occurs normally during the third month in utero. They secondarily join either the lateral perimesencephalic or a subtemporal vein, demonstrating a typical epsilon shape on lateral angiography. The remainder of the venous drainage is variable, with the straight sinus being absent in almost all patients, an angiographic feature that differentiates the VGAM from AVMs that drain into the vein of Galen, which will subsequently appear dilated (VGADs).

A major differential diagnosis for VGAMs is the VGAD, a pial AVM draining into the deep venous system with an acquired dilatation of the vein of Galen confluence caused either by stenosis at the venodural junction or by thrombosis of the straight sinus. The dilated vein drains the normal brain in addition to the malformations. The presence of primary opening of the shunt into a non-choroidal vein or demonstration of reflux into normal cerebral venous tributaries that open into the

Comprehensive Management of Arteriovenous Malformations of the Brain and Spine, ed. Robert F. Spetzler, Douglas S. Kondziolka, Randall T. Higashida, and M. Yashar S. Kalani. Published by Cambridge University Press.

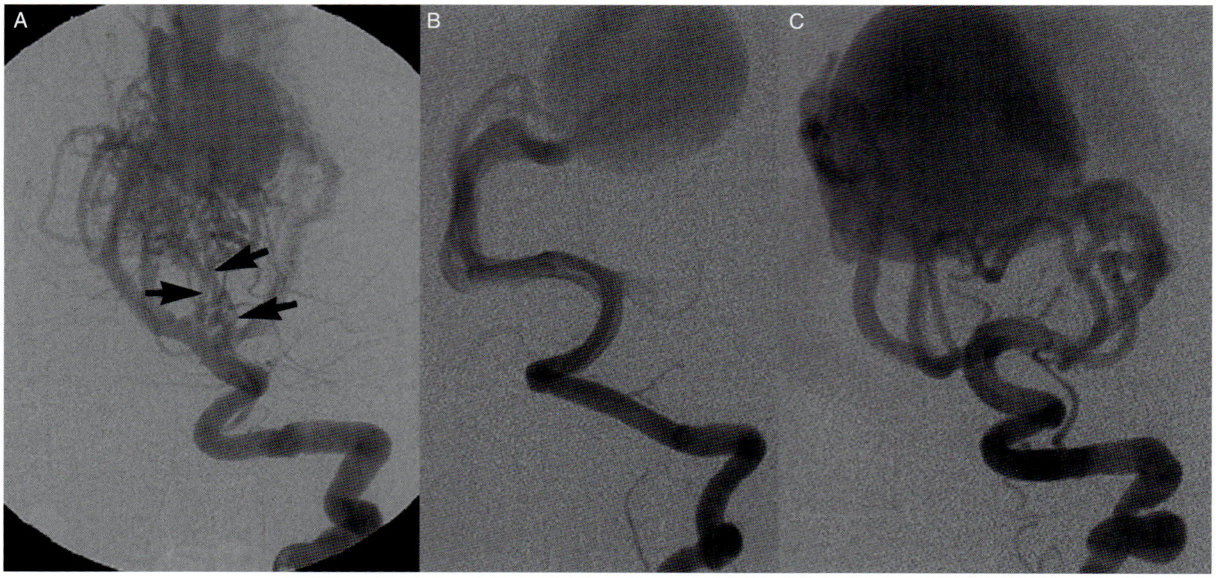

Fig. 20.1. The nidus of a vein of Galen arteriovenous malformation can be choroidal type (A), mural type (B), or mixed (C).

venous pouch confirms the diagnosis of VGAD. These lesions are typically found in older children with clinical presentations resembling other pial AVMs [6]. Dural arteriovenous contributions into these shunts, when present, are usually secondary lesions resulting from the sump effect and thrombosis of the outflow sinuses.

Clinical presentation

The prenatal incidental diagnosis of VGAM on screening antenatal ultrasound can be made by visualization of a dilated, often roundish, vascular midline structure, representing the dilated median prosencephalic vein; however, sufficient dilatation of the vein is required before it can be seen. In the recent description of the Toronto series, there was no correlation between early prenatal diagnosis of VGAM and the follow-up outcome; therefore, an in utero diagnosis of VGAM without any signs of multiorgan failure or brain parenchymal changes is, in our opinion, not an indication for therapeutic termination of the pregnancy [7]. However, obtaining a diagnosis prenatally will help in deciding the facilities needed for neonatal care after delivery.

Congestive heart failure is the most common presentation in the neonatal group and is probably related to a lower cardiovascular volume of these patients. The prognosis of the neonate with VGAM is related to the severity of heart failure [8] and in many cases, the diagnosis of VGAM is obtained only after an investigation for congestive heart failure [9].

Many of the severely affected patients have progression to pulmonary hypertension with respiratory distress and multiorgan failure, which is why the Hôpital Bicêtre group have introduced a scoring system to gauge the severity of the clinical presentation based on the assessment of multiple organs (Table 20.1) [10].

The initial management of VGAM with congestive heart failure in the neonatal group consists of medical stabilization of the heart failure, typically with inotropic drugs, diuretics, mechanical ventilation, or inhaled nitric oxide [11]. If medical management fails, early partial embolization is recommended to decrease the shunting volume [8]. There have been reports that the use of prostaglandin E may be helpful in some situations to stabilize the patient while awaiting treatment of the VGAM [11].

Lasjaunias *et al.* [10] suggested that the treatment decision should be based upon the total neonatal score in the scoring system described in Table 20.1. However, in our recent study, we have found that in addition to a medium-to-low overall total neonatal score (<12), a score of ≤2 in a single category and certain imaging findings also predict a poor outcome and, therefore, should also be taken into consideration [7].

Clinical presentation with hydrodynamic disorders, such as hydrocephalus and macrocrania, are more frequent in the infantile group. The presence of the high-flow arteriovenous shunt causes increased venous pressure within the straight sinus and torcula. If the sutures are open, adaptation to the increased pressure occurs by expansion of the intracranial volume, resulting in macrocrania. This expansion of the cranial vault, together with the presence of a high-flow shunt, interferes with the normal skull base development and likely results in secondary stenosis of the jugular foramen [10]. In addition, the induced intimal hyperplasia from increased shear stress to the venous wall in the high-flow shunt may also play a role in the so-called jugular dysmaturation, and is also seen in changes in peripheral veins in patients with hemodialysis grafts [12]. A combination of these two factors will result in varying degrees of jugular bulb stenosis, which will lead to improvement of the cardiac overload (and, therefore, a paradoxical amelioration of cardiac symptoms) but will also lead to further increased intracranial venous pressure (Fig. 20.2A). If in these patients the cranial vault fails to expand (which is the similar pathomechanism seen in patients with severe craniosynostosis [13]), decompensation occurs. When combined with the compression of the

Table 20.1 Neonatal evaluation score from the Hôpital Bicêtre

Points	Cardiac function	Cerebral function	Respiratory function	Hepatic function	Renal function
5	Normal	Normal	Normal	N/A	N/A
4	Overload, no medical treatment	Subclinical isolated electroencephalography abnormal	Tachypnea, finishes bottle of food	N/A	N/A
3	Failure, stable with medical treatment	Non-convulsive intermittent neurological signs	Tachypnea, does not finish bottle of food	No hepatomegaly, normal function	Normal
2	Failure, not stable with medical treatment	Isolated convulsion	Assisted ventilation, normal saturation FiO_2 <25%	Hepatomegaly, normal function	Transient anuria
1	Ventilation necessary	Seizures	Assisted ventilation, normal saturation FiO_2 >25%	Moderate or transient hepatic insufficiency	Unstable diuresis with treatment
0	Resistant to medical treatment	Permanent neurological signs	Assisted ventilation, desaturation	Abnormal coagulation, elevated enzymes	Anuria

FiO_2, fraction of inspired oxygen; N/A, not applicable.

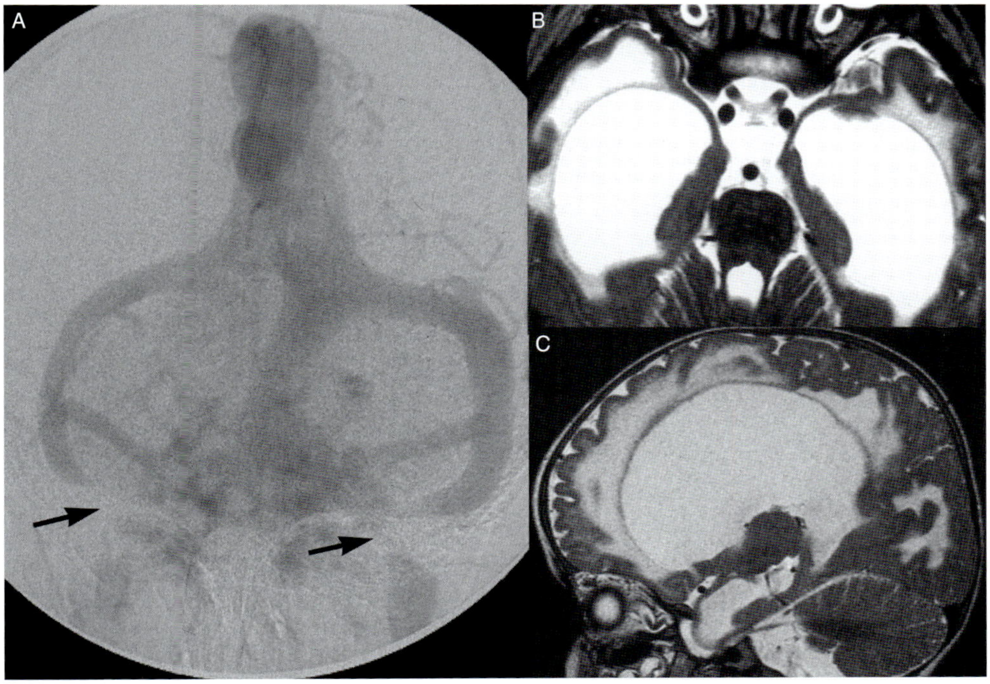

Fig. 20.2. Jugular bulb stenosis (see text for details of the possible mechanisms). (A) Angiography showing bilateral jugular bulb stenosis (arrows). (B,C) T_2-weighted MRI in axial (B) and sagittal (C) views showing significant hydrocephalus associated with venous hyperpressure.

aqueduct by the enlarged venous pouch, subsequent ventricular dilatation will ensue (Fig. 20.2B,C). The hydrocephalus then results in compression of the medullary veins, which further decreases reabsorption of cerebrospinal fluid and further worsens the hydrocephalus and increases intracranial pressure. As a result, tonsillar herniation can occur. Most patients with significant jugular bulb stenosis have associated hydrocephalus, proving the role of increased venous pressure in the pathomechanism of hydrocephalus. Management of hydrocephalus should be directed at reducing the arteriovenous shunt as the underlying cause. Embolization will decrease the venous pressure and improve the chance for a better outcome. Early ventricular shunting in these patients is known to have a poor outcome [14,15]; therefore, ventricular drainage should be kept only for those patients who do not improve after embolization or have a hydrocephalus unrelated to the VGAM.

Clinical presentation in children is related to long-standing venous hypertension, caused by the hydrovenous disorder described above, and will lead to neurocognitive delay since there will be interference with normal myelination. In deep hydrovenous watershed failure, which can occur when the compliance of the medullary veins lose their normal ventricular–cortical gradient, calcifications occur that will lead to epilepsy [5]. These calcifications are usually bilateral and symmetrically located, preferentially in the frontal region. Calcifications in the striatum and in particular the caudate and putamen bilaterally are an expression of the subacute ischemia in the region of the prominent collateral circulation system, after the cortical veins become unable to drain the cerebral white substance, or when the persisting thalamic pathways are overloaded with the drainage of the parieto-occipital regions. The calcifications are not produced by arterial steal [16].

Implications/indications of clinical manifestations for treatment

The clinical manifestations of VGAM can be broadly classified into three groups: (1) neonates with congestive cardiac failure and/or multiorgan failure, (2) infants with hydrocephalus related to hydrovenous disorder, and (3) children with neurocognitive delay.

The appropriate management at each of these stages differs and each will be considered individually. Obviously, a considerable overlap exists in these scenarios where decision making is based on the underlying pathophysiology. Emergency management should be limited to specific situations.

Neonates presenting with congestive cardiac failure

Congestive cardiac failure is mainly encountered in neonates with choroidal forms of VGAM, which are the most frequent arteriovenous shunts diagnosed at that age. Severe congestive cardiac failure is associated with persistence of the fetal type of circulation. Septal communications and ductus arteriosus are often noted during cardiac ultrasound. These should not be considered as associated cardiac malformations and, like most of the disorders encountered under these circumstances, they disappear spontaneously following endovascular management of the VGAM itself. Renal and hepatic damage may further aggravate congestive cardiac failure and the function of these organs may be transiently impaired. After VGAM is suspected clinically, pretherapeutic evaluations should be obtained. These include (1) clinical evaluation and documentation of all possible events that have occurred since birth, including presence of convulsions; (2) evaluation of renal and liver function; (3) transcranial ultrasound to evaluate for the presence of encephalomalacia; (4) cardiac ultrasound to assess cardiac tolerance and to diagnose associated conditions; (5) a good-quality MRI to provide all the necessary morphological information regarding the lesion itself and to evaluate the status of myelinization and the presence of hypoxic–ischemic changes related to true arterial steal; and (6) electroencephalography if the child is in the intensive care unit.

Angiography is not indicated in the neonatal workup and not recommended. In neonates, the immediate goal is to restore a satisfactory systemic physiology in order to have the baby feeding normally, thus gaining time [10]. The first few months of clinical assessment are crucial in order to be able to predict the future neurological state of the child. The goal is to have a baby who is stable on medication for cardiac insufficiency and to gain time for easier technical management. It is important to recognize the presence of significant developmental delay, as well as early features of hydrocephalus and macrocrania. The presence of encephalomalacia and moyamoya pattern predicts poor clinical outcome in our experience [17]. A decrease in head circumference is probably the worst finding to be noted, since it indicates loss of brain substance and early suture fusion.

Emergency management in the neonate should be restricted to very specific situations. In the scoring system proposed by Lasjaunias *et al.*, a score between 8 and 12 should indicate emergency endovascular management [10], basically to reduce the degree of shunting to some degree to allow the child to come out of heart failure. We usually embolize one or two major pedicles. The aim of management at this stage is not necessarily to obliterate the shunt completely.

Additionally, the management team should direct its attention to the management of congestive cardiac failure. This would include two strategies: to reduce oxygen consumption and to improve oxygen delivery. This can be achieved by tracheal intubation, mechanical ventilation, or the use of drugs, such as diuretic, given in conjunction with expert advice from a pediatric cardiologist.

In conclusion, management at the neonatal stage is directed toward gaining time to allow for improved treatment circumstances by management of the congestive cardiac failure, recognition and exclusion of neonates in whom irreversible brain damage has already occurred, and partial endovascular embolization in a select group of patients to reduce the degree of arteriovenous shunting.

Ventricular enlargement and increasing head size

As opposed to congestive cardiac failure, disorders of cerebrospinal fluid circulation can manifest themselves at any age: in utero, as neonates, and as infants. Choroidal and mural types of VGAM may equally give rise to these kinds of manifestation. They result from the abnormal hemodynamic condition present in the torcular venous sinus confluence, the posterior conversion of the venous drainage of the brain, and the immaturity of the pacchionian granulation (arachnoid granulation) system. Compression of the aqueduct by the dilated vein is rarely a contributing factor [14,18]. This is evident by actual demonstration of patency of the aqueduct itself, and by the presence of prominent cerebrospinal fluid spaces in relation to the cerebral sulci. Spontaneous stabilization of an enlarging head and dilatation of the ventricles can occur with cavernous sinus capture of the sylvian veins. At that time, a new low-pressure venous system offers an alternative pathway for water resorption and, therefore, improved hydration status of the cerebral tissue.

Ventricular shunting in VGAM carries an additional risk of morbidity. It does not deal with the problem created by the hydrodynamic disorders but only transiently and incompletely resolves the emergency situation at the ventricular level. Various series have consistently shown poor clinical results in infants with shunts [15,19]. The deficits, seizures, and hemorrhage seen following ventricular shunting have been so well accepted that they have even been considered as part of the natural history of VGAM. Endovascular management in the same situation has been clearly shown to stop the progression of these disorders. Complete obliteration of the fistula is usually not necessary, and even partial embolization often results in rapid reversal of the overhydration of brain tissue. If the increase in head circumference appears to be too rapid, if there is preclinical MRI evidence of intraventricular hyperpressure, or if the clinical follow-up demonstrates a significant developmental delay, then urgent embolization should be carried out. Ventricular shunting should be avoided unless there is clear demonstration of raised pressure within the ventricles in spite of an adequate attempt at embolization.

Developmental delay

Development delay is part of the natural history of most patients with untreated VGAMs. Careful evaluations of neurocognitive performances show that most children with increasing head size present with some degree of mental retardation. In infancy, assessment of neurocognitive delay is not easy and requires collaboration with a specialist. Consistent and uniform well-established grading scales should be used. The major aim of such tests should not be to compare children but are intended to act as an aid to follow one child's ongoing development. From the point of view of management, it is important to recognize irreversible brain damage and potentially treatable or preventable situations. The presence of venous infarcts or calcifications as well as encephalomalacia would suggest irreversible brain damage, while presence of hydrovenous disorders and hydrocephalus are potentially treatable conditions. As mentioned above, treatment of hydrovenous disorders should be achieved with eradication of the fistula itself, rather than placement of a shunt [5]. With increasing head size, obstruction of venous outflow by narrowing of the jugular veins tends to become apparent.

Chronic vein of Galen aneurysm malformations with patent sinuses

A patient who does not undergo decompensation, either because of the presence of congestive cardiac failure at neonatal age or the presence of cerebrospinal fluid hydrodynamic disorders, will subsequently enter into a stage of chronicity. At this stage, the clinical manifestation as well as the prognosis is primarily dependent on the patency of the draining dural sinuses. If there is patency of draining sinuses, the prognosis is generally good. Seizures and mental retardation are the main symptoms if the correction of the arteriovenous shunt is not done in time. Morphological sequelae express themselves in the form of calcifications, subependymal atrophy, and eventually the stigmata of previous acute accidents, with cortical and subcortical atrophy. Since in classical VGAM there cannot be any pial or subpial reflux, focal venous infarcts or parenchymal hemorrhages are not common. The insult to the brain is a slow and permanent one and is usually demonstrated in the form of calcifications and atrophy. The timing of intervention is, therefore, important, and most of these sequelae can be prevented by early occlusion of the shunt. However, it is important to realize that the clinical outcome of children with patent sinuses is relatively good compared with those with secondary occluded sinuses.

Dural sinus occlusion and supratentorial congestion and reflux

Evolution of a VGAM to dural sinus occlusion and supratentorial congestion and reflux is very common and presumably related to abnormal skull base growth and maturation caused by increased head size, as well as by venous high-flow angiopathy. It is usually progressive and may develop slowly without symptoms over a long period of time. The development of jugular bulb stenosis protects the heart but it exposes the brain to congestion, venous infarcts, and hemorrhagic manifestations. The capture of the sylvian veins by the cavernous sinus would have a significant positive influence in the overall course of events.

Overall, there is little understanding at present of the cause of occlusion of the dural sinuses. Neither has it been possible to precisely predict the patients who are going to evolve toward this occlusive phenomenon. Subsequent to the occlusion, the overall prognosis remains guarded and little can be done in terms of management. Hence identification of the therapeutic window prior to the onset of this occlusive phenomenon is important.

The infratentorial impact and consequence of the dural sinus occlusion is tonsillar prolapse. It is secondary to posterior fossa venous congestion and usually disappears with correction of the arteriovenous shunt. Syringomyelia has also been described as a consequence of this tonsillar prolapse [20].

Endovascular management

Goals

In our experience, endovascular management of VGAM is clearly beneficial over other forms of treatment. The transarterial approach with undiluted *N*-butyl cyanoacrylate as the embolic agent is in our practice the typical approach (Fig. 20.3). Limited case reports exist in the literature of using a transvenous approach to reach the dilated sac. Conceptually, the aim of treatment is to exclude the malformations from the circulation. Hence, theoretically, the ultimate result should be similar whether the arterial or the venous route is used to achieve this. However, the limited experience of intervention using the venous route and the lack of published outcome analysis data do not seem to support this and we, therefore, feel that the results are better using the transarterial route [10,17,21–25]. Possible reasons for poor results from the venous approach may be related to poor overall understanding of the anatomy and pathophysiology. In a mural type of VGAM with a single hole, excellent results should be possible by either of the two routes. However, if there is a possibility of reflux into secondarily recruited arteries of the brain parenchyma, created as a consequence of the sump effect, the venous approach may lead to complications, such as hemorrhage. We also strongly believe that for the choroidal type of VGAM, the venous approach would not be suitable given the interspersed nidus, which will lead to hemorrhage when occluding only the dilated venous sac.

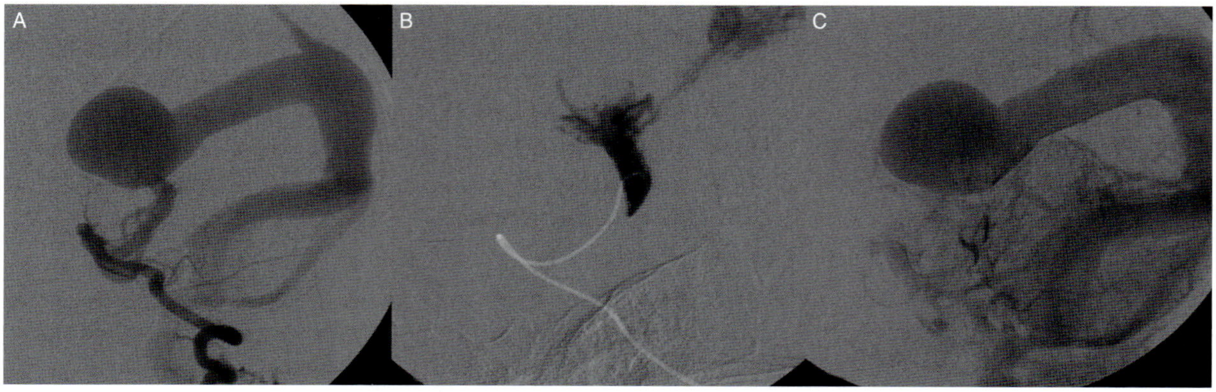

Fig. 20.3. A 4-month-old baby in mild heart failure who was responding to medical management and without other systemic failure and with normal brain on imaging. (A) Angiography with left vertebral artery injection showed evidence of the mural type of vein of Galen malformations in frontal view. (B) The main choroidal feeding artery was catheterized and embolized with pure glue. (C) The immediate postembolization left vertebral artery angiography in lateral view demonstrated significantly decreased flow through the lesion and ameliorated perfusion of the cerebellar parenchyma. In addition, baby's tachycardia normalized and systemic blood pressure increased.

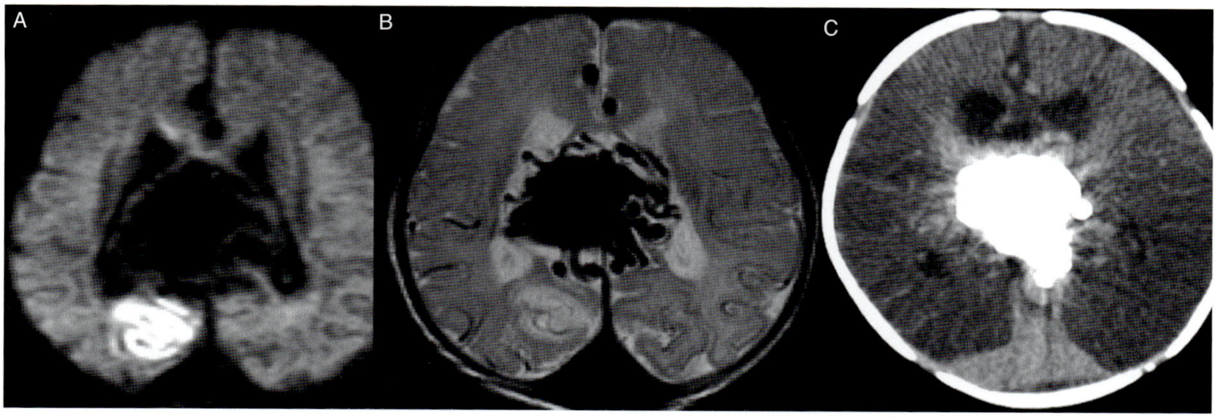

Fig. 20.4. This baby was born in severe congestive heart failure that was unresponsive to medical therapies. (A) Diffusion-weighted MRI showed signal changes with evidence of arterial steal from branches of the middle cerebral artery and the beginning of changes in apparent diffusion coefficient. These changes should mitigate against any kind of management as it indicates arterial steal, often triggering apoptotic cascades (melting brain syndrome). (B) T_2-weighted MRI showed evidence of arterial steal from the middle cerebral artery. (C) Despite successful embolization (without procedure-related complications), diffuse ischemia was seen on follow-up imaging and the baby subsequently died.

Identification of irreversible brain damage is exceedingly important. Changes in the apparent diffusion coefficient with restriction on diffusion-weighted MRI should mitigate against any kind of management as it indicates arterial steal, which often triggers apoptotic cascades (melting brain syndrome; Fig. 20.4) [5]. Emergency management should be limited to a few situations, such as non-resolving congestive cardiac failure that cannot be stabilized by medication, growing head circumference because of altered cerebrospinal fluid hydrodynamics, and impending occlusion of jugular veins without sufficient rerouting of blood to the facial venous system. Our approach has been to perform multiple staged arterial embolizations aimed at slowly reducing the flow across the arteriovenous fistulae [7].

Results

The natural history of VGAM described in previous literature varies with the age group, clinical presentation, and management given in each series. Although the outcome of patients has been improving through the years, the overall outcome is still considered poor [10,26–28]. In the largest series (317 patients) reported so far [10], approximately 19% (57/300; 17 lost to follow up) were considered to be in too bad a clinical condition to be treated. Of the 216 treated patients, 73 (34%) had a bad outcome, ranging from permanent neurological symptoms and mental retardation to death. According to these numbers, the overall poor outcome is approximately 46%.

Despite the increasing understanding of the pathophysiology of VGAMs over the years, the questions of whether and when to treat a patient still remain unanswered.

In our recently published experience [7], we found that a subgroup of carefully selected patients had a good outcome with conservative management and close follow-up. The criteria for selection of these patients were (1) a high neonatal (>17) or admission score (>3); (2) clinical symptoms of only mild congestive heart failure well controlled with medication and no neurological symptoms; (3) imaging findings with no parenchymal loss, calcifications, hydrocephalus, tonsillar herniation, or evidence of arterial steal; and (4) angioarchitecture findings of low-flow shunts (i.e., two or less enlarged arterial feeder groups), lack of deep venous drainage, lack of jugular bulb stenosis.

The presence of severe congestive heart failure with multi-organ failure (seen as a neonatal score of <8) is probably the only single criteria indicating withholding treatment in a patient. However, a combination of other factors, most of which represent permanent brain damage, were also shown in our recent series to be associated with a poor outcome: an overall poor clinical status (neonatal score of <12), evidence of a single organ failure (neonatal score of ≤2 in a single category), neurological symptoms at presentation, parenchymal changes, arterial steal, or subcortical calcifications on imaging.

For the remaining patients, in whom treatment is considered or is indicated, timing is still uncertain. It has been proposed that the optimal timing for embolization of a VGAM is at four to five months of age since this waiting period is not enough to develop permanent brain damage while offering enough benefit concerning arterial access and contrast limitation problems. A case report by Cherif *et al.* questions this waiting period, since the patient developed congestive heart failure resulting in death after being stable for two weeks [29]. Since we did not find a statistically significant difference between waiting period or average age at treatment and outcome, we think that this case report highlights the necessity of closely observing the patient and adapting the treatment strategy based on the patient's individual evolution. In our practice, the following clinical conditions speak in favor of a more urgent treatment: deterioration of cardiac function (uncontrolled by medication), evidence of arterial steal, progressive occlusion of the venous outflow (jugular bulb stenosis), developing macrocrania/hydrocephalus, and, for older children, psychomotor developmental arrest or delay of more than two months. This necessitates close clinical observation (cardiac status, Denver developmental milestones, head circumference), and imaging follow-up (MRI at birth, at six weeks, and prior to treatment at three to five months in our practice). If the patient remains stable during the follow-up period, then starting the treatment at three to five months may be sufficient to avoid permanent brain damage.

Given the rarity of the disease, the individual patient's condition, the parents' decision, and the operator's personal experience, no general guidelines can be given, particularly since it is psychologically difficult to withhold treatment in the acute setting of a newborn and since even patients with evidence of brain damage may eventually recover in part given the plasticity and adaptability of the brain in the childhood period. However, if treatment is to be contemplated, it has to be kept in mind that these patients are in a high-risk group; a good outcome can, therefore, not necessarily be hoped for and a higher risk of treatment-related complications can be expected.

Complications

Non-neurological complications related to the embolization procedure and the technical difficulties of injecting glue are rare; Lasjaunias *et al.* found a 4% complication rate [10]. This was related to glue causing an asymptomatic occlusion of the internal iliac artery or the microcatheter getting glued in place. Our experience has been very similar, with an exceedingly low non-neurological complication rate [17]. Repeated punctures of the femoral artery do not seem to cause any significant problems.

The risk of venous passage of glue is obvious, particularly in inexperienced hands. The malformations is typically high flow and we usually use a very high concentration of glue during embolization in these patients. Tantulum powder is typically added to the mixture to increase opacification. The injection can be made under induced hypotension. Care must be taken with catheter positioning, which should ideally be against the vessel wall in order to have a slower flow and a shorter polymerization time. Venous infarction as a consequence of venous passage of glue has been described but is rare. The phenomenon of perfusion breakthrough has not occurred in our experience or that of Lasjaunias *et al.* Acute closure of these high-flow fistulae does not, therefore, seem to cause any problems if performed by arterial embolization. Also, in the experience of Lasjaunias *et al.* [10], as well as our own experience, consumption coagulopathy has not been observed. Overall, in experienced hands with a staged procedure approach to VGAMs, arterial embolizations can be performed with a low complication rate.

The stenosis of the jugular foramina and the timing of capture of the cavernous sinus affect the overall prognosis. At present, these cannot be predicted. Stenosis of the jugular foramina after capture of the cavernous sinuses allows an alternative route of drainage for the brain. However, if it occurs prior to capture of cavernous sinuses, the outcome is dismal.

Conclusions

Major progress has been made since the mid 1990s in the understanding and management of neonates, infants, and children presenting with VGAMs. The apparent dismal prognosis of these patients some 20 years ago has now changed to a more optimistic outlook. While significant challenges in the management of patients with VGAMs continue to exist, their positive response to endovascular treatment are now widely recognized.

Patient selection and the timing of treatment are essential in the decision-making process and when done properly by an experienced team will result in a favorable outcome and a normally developing child. We recommend the arterial approach as the method of choice for embolization therapy since its published results compare favorably with those treated with venous approach and surgical intervention. Ventricular shunting should be avoided as it has a negative impact on the vein of Galen malformation itself and, as opposed to arterial embolization, it does not reduce the venous hyperpressure phenomenon responsible for most of the clinical symptomatology. Management of patients with VGAMs, more than any other vascular disorder affecting the CNS, depends on the presence and coordination of an entire multidisciplinary treatment team, which must consist of an experienced pediatric interventionalist and neurosurgeon with pediatric expertise, neuroimaging, and development assessment teams. If such a team is not available, then patients with this disorder should be sent to a specialized treatment center for improved decision making and care.

References

1. Raybaud CA, Strother CM, Hald JK. Aneurysms of the vein of Galen: embryonic considerations and anatomical features relating to the pathogenesis of the malformation. *Neuroradiology* 1989;**31**:109–28.
2. Lasjaunias P, Garcia-Monaco R, Rodesch G, *et al.* Deep venous drainage in great cerebral vein (vein of Galen) absence and malformations. *Neuroradiology* 1991;**33**:234–8.
3. Lasjaunias P. *Vascular Diseases in Neonates, Infants and Children: Interventional Neuroradiology Management*. Berlin: Springer, 1997.
4. Krings T, Geibprasert S, terBrugge K. Classification and endovascular management of pediatric cerebral vascular malformations. *Neurosurg Clin N Am* 2010;**21**:463–82.
5. Alvarez H, Garcia MR, Rodesch G, *et al.* Vein of Galen aneurysmal malformations. *Neuroimaging Clin N Am* 2007;**17**:189–206.
6. Ozanne A, Alvarez H, Krings T, *et al.* [Pediatric neurovascular malformations: vein of Galen arteriovenous malformations (VGAM), pial arteriovenous malformations (pial AVM), dural sinus malformations (DSM).] *J Neuroradiol* 2007;**34**:145–66.
7. Geibprasert S, Krings T, Armstrong D, *et al.* Predicting factors for the follow-up outcome and management decisions in vein of Galen aneurysmal malformations. *Childs Nerv Syst* 2010;**26**:35–46.
8. Chevret L, Durand P, Alvarez H, *et al.* Severe cardiac failure in newborns with VGAM. Prognosis significance of hemodynamic parameters in neonates presenting with severe heart failure owing to vein of Galen arteriovenous malformation. *Intensive Care Med* 2002;**28**:1126–30.
9. Hartung J, Heling KS, Rake A, *et al.* Detection of an aneurysm of the vein of Galen following signs of cardiac overload in a 22-week old fetus. *Prenat Diagn* 2003;**23**:901–3.
10. Lasjaunias PL, Chng SM, Sachet M, *et al.* The management of vein of Galen aneurysmal malformations. *Neurosurgery* 2006;**59**:S184–94.
11. Karam O, da Cruz E, Rimensberger PC. VGAM induced high-flow congestive heart failure responsive to PGE1 infusion. *Int J Cardiol* 2009;**132**: e60–e62.
12. Misra S, Fu AA, Puggioni A, *et al.* Increased shear stress with upregulation of VEGF-A and its receptors and MMP-2, MMP-9, and TIMP-1 in venous stenosis of hemodialysis grafts. *Am J Physiol Heart Circ Physiol* 2008;**294**: H2219–30.
13. Rollins N, Booth T, Shapiro K. MR venography in children with complex craniosynostosis. *Pediatr Neurosurg* 2000;**32**:308–15.
14. Zerah M, Garcia-Monaco R, Rodesch G, *et al.* Hydrodynamics in vein of Galen malformations. *Childs Nerv Syst* 1992;**8**:111–17.
15. Johnston IH, Whittle IR, Besser M, *et al.* Vein of Galen malformation: diagnosis and management. *Neurosurgery* 1987;**20**:747–58.
16. Yu YL, Chiu EK, Woo E, *et al.* Dystrophic intracranial calcification: CT evidence of "cerebral steal" from arteriovenous malformation. *Neuroradiology* 1987;**29**:519–22.
17. Li AH, Armstrong D, terBrugge KG. Endovascular treatment of vein of Galen aneurysmal malformation: management strategy and 21-year experience in Toronto. *J Neurosurg Pediatr* 2011;**7**:3–10.
18. Diebler C, Dulac O, Renier D, *et al.* Aneurysms of the vein of Galen in infants aged 2 to 15 months. Diagnosis and natural evolution. *Neuroradiology* 1981;**21**:185–97.
19. Quisling RG, Mickle JP. Venous pressure measurements in vein of Galen aneurysms. *AJNR Am J Neuroradiol* 1989;**10**:411–17.
20. ApSimon HT, Ives FJ, Khangure MS. Cranial dural arteriovenous malformation and fistula: radiological diagnosis and management. Review of thirty four patients. *Australas Radiol* 1993;**37**:2–25.
21. Casasco A, Lylyk P, Hodes JE, *et al.* Percutaneous transvenous catheterization and embolization of vein of Galen aneurysms. *Neurosurgery* 1991;**28**:260–6.
22. Dowd CF, Halbach VV, Barnwell SL, *et al.* Transfemoral venous embolization of vein of Galen malformations. *AJNR Am J Neuroradiol* 1990;**11**:643–8.
23. Halbach VV, Dowd CF, Higashida RT, *et al.* Endovascular treatment of mural-type vein of Galen malformations. *J Neurosurg* 1998;**89**:74–80.
24. Lylyk P, Vinuela F, Dion JE, *et al.* Therapeutic alternatives for vein of Galen vascular malformations. *J Neurosurg* 1993;**78**:438–45.
25. Mickle JP, Quisling RG. The transtorcular embolization of vein of Galen aneurysms. *J Neurosurg* 1986;**64**:731–5.
26. Staberg M, Jonsbo F. [Vein of Galen aneurysm diagnosed in the perinatal period. A retrospective assessment.] *Ugeskr Laeger* 2007;**169**:3190–3.
27. Jones BV, Ball WS, Tomsick TA, *et al.* Vein of Galen aneurysmal malformation: diagnosis and treatment of 13 children with extended clinical follow-up. *AJNR Am J Neuroradiol* 2002;**23**:1717–24.
28. Fullerton HJ, Aminoff AR, Ferriero DM, *et al.* Neurodevelopmental outcome after endovascular treatment of vein of Galen malformations. *Neurology* 2003;**61**:1386–90.
29. Cherif A, Neji K, Sebai L, *et al.* [Vein of Galen aneurysmal malformation: a neonatal case with unusual evolution.] *Arch Pediatr* 2007;**14**:893–6.

Chapter 21

Endovascular treatment of spinal arteriovenous malformations and fistulae

Kiron Thomas and In Sup Choi

Introduction

The spectrum of spinal vascular lesions encompasses a wide range of etiological, pathophysiological, histological, and topographical diversity, with lesions involving the spinal cord, its meninges, and the spine. Arteriovenous shunt disorders may involve any part of the spinal axis including paraspinal structures. Those located outside the spinal canal but with hemodynamic and clinical consequences to the neural elements within, have been categorized by Berenstein *et al.* as parachordal arteriovenous fistulae (AVFs) and include extracranial, vertebro-vertebral, paraspinal, extradural, and extraspinal AVFs [1]. Arteriovenous shunts can be complex and diverse and have the propensity to compromise the structure and functioning of the neural constituents, sometimes with devastating results. Previously, these uncommon disorders were primarily observational findings at autopsies and surgeries, without any specific available therapy. With the development of superselective spinal angiography, and advances in endovascular and microsurgical techniques, these lesions, which may be acquired or congenital, are now considered potentially curable.

Vascular lesions have been long recognized as possible etiologies for spinal and spinal cord pathologies, including spinal intramedullary and subarachnoid hemorrhage, and myelopathy [2,3]. The spinal cord, phylogenically, is the most evolved structure in vertebrates. Its vascular anatomy, since the first description by Adamkiewicz in 1882, has been recognized to be complex and highly variable [4]. However, the configuration follows a basic rule of segmental arrangement with evolutionary changes. Ever since the first intraoperative observation of a spinal vascular lesion in the late 1800s (identified as a vascular malformations at autopsy) and the recognition that these lesions can cause intraspinal hemorrhage [2,5,6], numerous descriptions and classifications have been proposed to describe vascular malformations of the extracranial CNS. Early nomenclature schemes and classifications based on micro- and macrostructure of the lesion, its topographic arrangement, and generalizations based on vascular pathologies in other biological systems, in retrospect were often incomplete and inaccurate. The advent of spinal angiography, particularly selective spinal angiography in the mid 1960s [7], revolutionized the understanding of vascular pathologies of the spine and the spinal cord. Angiographically derived information integrated with knowledge of functional and developmental anatomy resulted in more accurate terminological description and organization/classification.

Vascular anatomy

Development

The spine and spinal cord develop from the embryonic mesoderm and ectoderm, respectively [8]. During early organogenesis in vertebrate embryos, the ectodermal layer develops a central, longitudinal thickening, termed the neural plate. The ectoderm then invaginates along the neural plate, converging and apposing the lateral margins together over it to form the neural tube, which separates from the overlying ectoderm and becomes the precursor of the CNS. Cells at the margins of the neural plate separate from the neural tube into two bundles, forming the neural crest, which later differentiates into components of the peripheral nervous system. Just ventral to the neural tube is the notochord, a rod of specialized mesodermal tissue that constitutes the defining characteristic in chordate development. The notochord signals for and synchronizes the development of surrounding tissues during organogenesis, particularly the neural tube [9]. The mesodermal layer underlying the ectoderm would by then have divided to flank the neural tube on either side. As the development of the neural tube progresses, the notochord signals for segmentation of the adjacent para-axial mesoderm into somites, 42–44 pairs in total rostrocaudally. Some of these at the caudal end regress; some at the rostral end are destined to develop into cephalic structures [10–12]. The remaining somites form the segmental substrates for future vertebrae (sclerotome), somatic muscles (myotome), and skin (dermatome), thus defining the future relationship of these structures with the spinal cord. Each somite and its corresponding segment of the neural tube receive blood supply through ventral and dorsal channels from paired segmental arteries that arise from the dorsal aorta. These

Comprehensive Management of Arteriovenous Malformations of the Brain and Spine, ed. Robert F. Spetzler, Douglas S. Kondziolka, Randall T. Higashida, and M. Yashar S. Kalani. Published by Cambridge University Press.

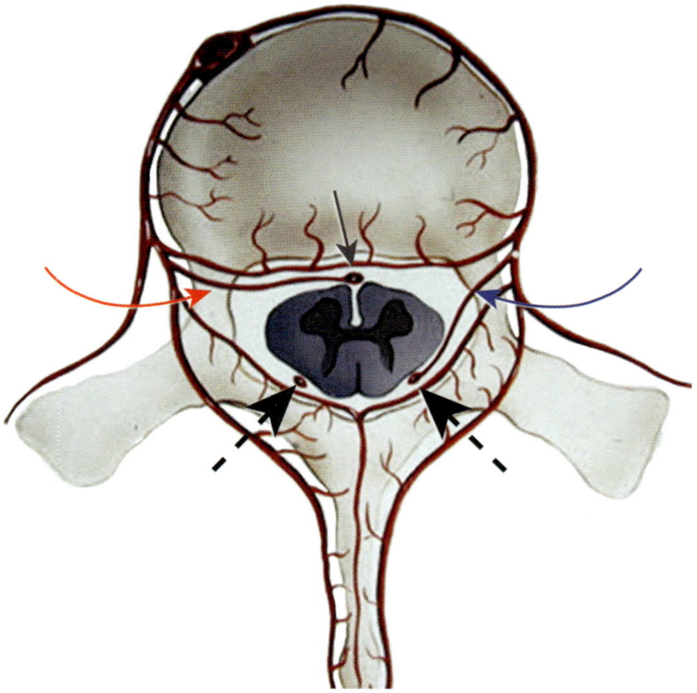

Fig. 21.1. The arterial supply to the spine and spinal cord, demonstrating segmental, radiculomedullary (red curved arrow), radiculopial (purple curved arrow), anterior spinal (black arrow), and posterior spinal (black broken arrows) arteries.

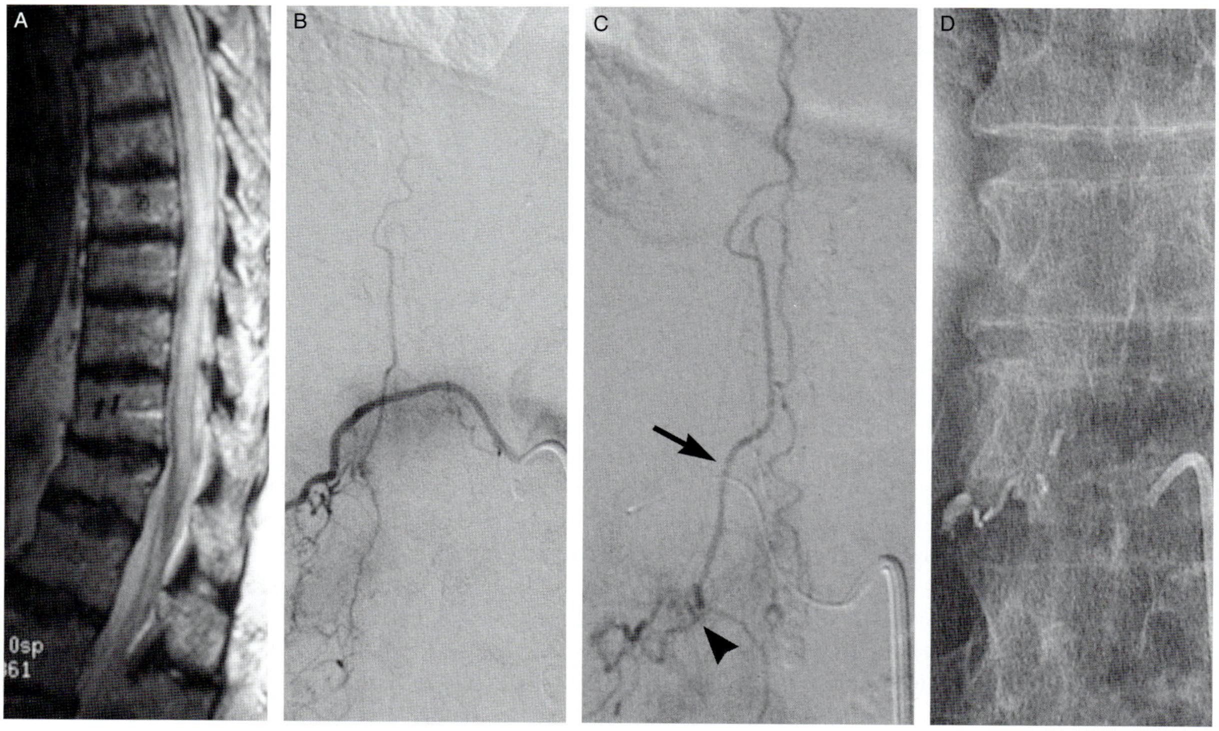

Fig. 21.2. Spinal dural arteriovenous fistula in a 76-year-old woman with slowly progressive lower extremity weakness. (A) MRI of the thoracic spine showed extensive T_2 signal change in the thoracic cord. (B) Anteroposterior projection of selective angiogram of right T12 segmental artery in early arterial phase demonstrated the arteriovenous shunt and proximal draining vein from the radiculomeningeal artery. (C) Magnified view of right distal T12 segmental artery microcatheter injection. The arteriovenous fistula (arrowhead) and the proximal draining vein (arrow) have been opacified. Cephalad and caudal venous drainage can be seen. The fistula was then embolized with *N*-butyl cyanoacrylate–Ethiodol. (D) Plain anteroposterior radiograph of the thoracic spine demonstrated the *N*-butyl cyanoacrylate cast in the fistula and proximal draining vein. Following endovascular treatment, the patient experienced substantial improvement in her symptoms.

metameric arteries form the basic vascular unit and supply the mesenchymal and ectodermal derivatives. Each half of the neural tube is supplied by the ipsilateral radiculospinal artery (Figs. 21.1 and 21.2) via dorsal and ventral branches.

Around the sixth week of development, the paired ventral branches of the segmental radiculospinal artery anastomose with the levels above and below, forming a longitudinal network, and later fuse in midline, forming the anterior spinal axis (anterior spinal artery [ASA]). In a similar fashion, the posterior branches of the radiculospinal arteries fuse to form two posterior longitudinal axes (posterior spinal artery [PSA]) (Fig. 21.1). These, unlike their ventral unpaired counterpart, are discontinuous channels. Most of the segmental feeders then regress to become radicular arteries supplying the nerve roots, dura, and the mesenchymal derivatives. The branches of the radiculospinal segmental arteries that persist to supply the spinal longitudinal axes are termed radiculomedullary when feeding the anterior spinal, and radiculopial when connected to posterior spinal arteries (Fig. 21.1.). At the conclusion of spinal neurovascular evolution, only 2–14 (average of 6) radiculomedullary and 11–16 radiculopial arteries remain [13,14]. The radial supply design thus gradually loses prominence and is replaced by the longitudinal axes of blood vessels. Vascular insults at this stage of development may result in involvement of all metameric components, as in Cobb syndrome (Fig. 21.3) or cutaneovertebromedullary angiomatosis, collectively termed spinal arteriovenous metameric syndrome (SAMS) [15].

Spinal arterial supply in adults

The arterial supply of the spinal cord comprises a system of three distinct longitudinal anastomotic channels – one ASA and two PSAs – receiving numerous segmental or radicular feeders mainly from vertebral, intercostal segmental, and lumbar segmental arteries. Segmental arteries may also arise from thyrocervical and costocervical trunks of the subclavian arteries. The radiculospinal artery enters the spinal canal through the intervertebral foramen, piercing the dural sleeve of the spinal nerve. The levels and the number of segmental arterial tributaries to the longitudinal systems are highly variable, resulting in perhaps the most important aspect related to spinal endovascular interventional procedures. In addition to the longitudinal axes, there are anastomotic arterial networks around the surface of the spinal cord (pial plexus, vasa corona), as well as within the parenchyma – both radial and longitudinal [14,16]. The anterior two-thirds of the spinal cord parenchyma is supplied by the ASA, including the anterior horns and spinothalamic and corticospinal tracts. Hence, the critical need for mapping and preserving the ASA and its radiculomedullary supply during spinal angiographic procedures cannot be overemphasized.

Venous drainage

Spinal venous systems may be organized into intrinsic, extrinsic, and epidural and paraspinal veins [14,16]. The intrinsic venous system of the spinal cord comprises a network of symmetric, radially arranged intramedullary venules with axial as well as longitudinal anastomoses, and small pial veins. These, in turn, are connected to extramedullary longitudinal channels, of which two may be prominent – ventral and dorsal median veins. The anterior channel is non-dominant, unlike its arterial counterpart. The longitudinal veins have extensive anastomoses, including transmedullary connections, and largely follow the arterial course. Radicular distributaries from the longitudinal network follow the nerve root to connect with the epidural plexus and extraspinal venous network. There can be emissary veins that do not follow the radicular nerves but rather connect with the epidural venous plexus independently. The epidural venous system is a plexiform venous lake without valves and, therefore, could be easily influenced by gravity and changes in pressure within the thoracic and abdominal cavities. It has been proposed that dural leaflets at the point of exit of the radicular vein may serve as a functional valve to impede the reflux from extraspinal veins into the intradural compartment [17,18]. The extensive transmedullary anastomoses and the triplication of the thoracic longitudinal venous channels leave room for stagnation at these levels with alteration of flow dynamics. The characteristic serpiginous appearance of a spinal dural AVF (SDAVF) is distinctly related to spinal venous anatomy (Fig. 21.4). These are attributed to the effects of increased flow and pressure within the longitudinally oriented perimedullary venous plexus of the cord. This condition leads to congestion and stagnation within the intrinsic venous system of the lower thoracic levels of the cord, resulting in edema and tissue hypoxia.

Classification and epidemiology

Virchow classified systemic vascular pathology into angioma cavernosum, an absence of parenchyma between the abnormal blood vessels; angioma racemosum (hamartoma), parenchyma interspersed with the abnormal vessels; telangiectasiae; and tumors [19]. This system was frequently used when referring to spinal vascular lesions until Wyburn-Mason's monograph in 1943, which described three types of spinal vascular lesion: venous, arteriovenous, and true tumors [20]. Following the introduction of selective spinal angiography, which delineated the vascularization of these lesions with clarity not known before, numerous classifications have been proposed to organize spinal vascular malformations on the basis of arterial supply, location, and nidus architecture. Anson and Spetzler classified spinal cord vascular malformations into four groups [21]. Group I refers to fistulae from the radiculomeningeal artery draining into radicular and perimedullary veins. Group II, also called glomus arteriovenous malformations (AVMs), are intramedullary shunts with a tightly coiled nidus and multiple medullary arterial feeders. Group III, or juvenile malformations, are extensive lesions that can have intra- and extramedullary components, and group IV are pial or perimedullary fistulae between a spinal cord artery and vein, first designated as a separate class of AVM by Heros *et al.* [22].

Berenstein and Lasjaunias described a simple classification that incorporated clinical and pathological differentiation as well as offering prognostic value and this was adopted by consensus among various expert groups in surgical neuroangiography [23]. This broad classification categorizes primary vascular disorders of the spine and spinal cord into spinal vascular lesions, which include SDAVFs and spinal extradural or paraspinal AVFs, and spinal cord vascular lesions, which include spinal cord AVMs, spinal cord telangiectasiae, and cavernous malformations [23]. From a review of 155 patients with spinal intradural AVMs, the gross and histological appearance of the lesions and consideration of possible metameric or

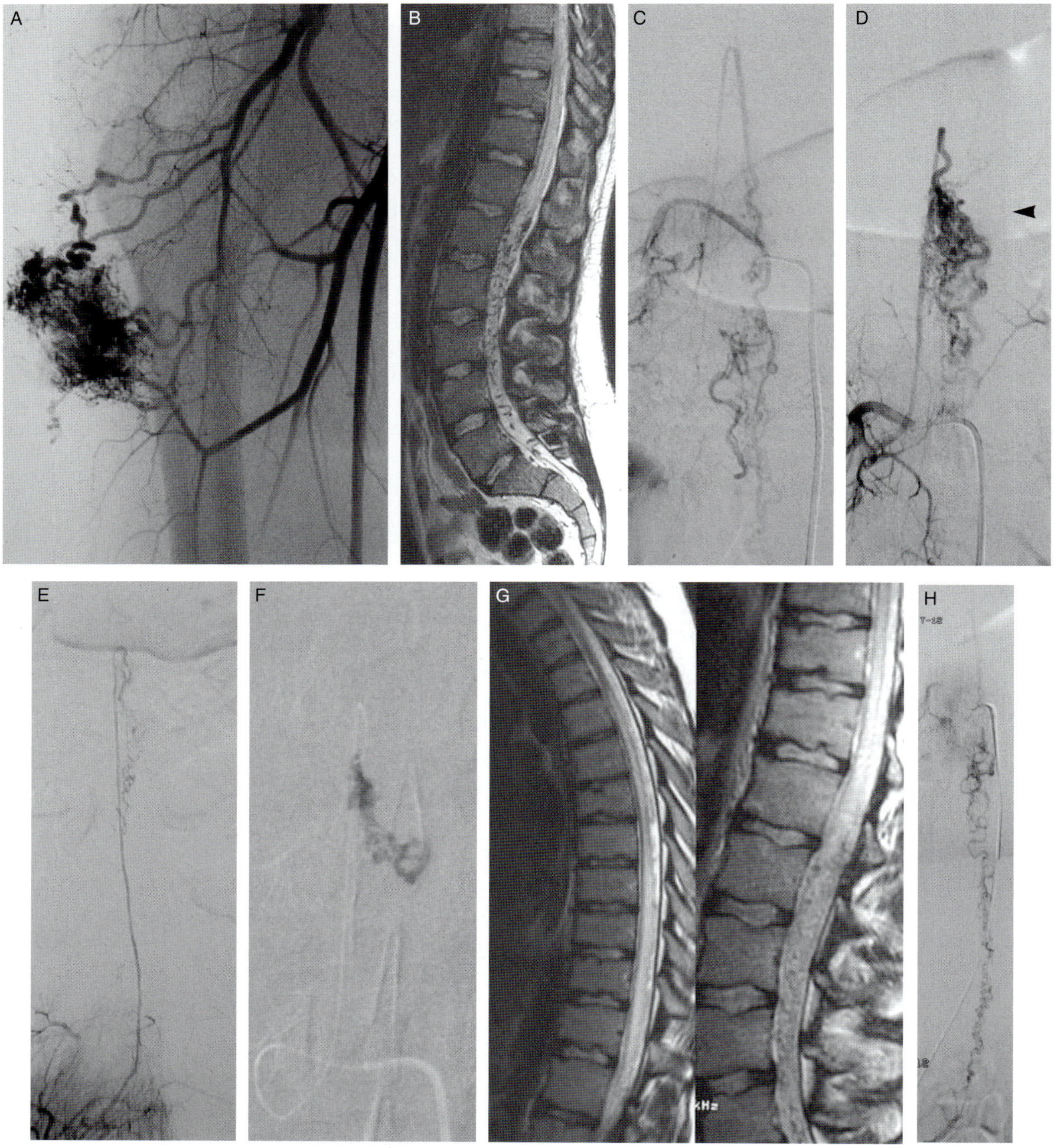

Fig. 21.3. Spinal arteriovenous metameric syndrome in a 17-year-old man with gradually increasing, hemorrhagic, serpiginous lump on the posterolateral aspect of the gluteal region. Selective angiography revealed a high-flow arteriovenous malformation (AVM) in the posterior compartment of the upper thigh, which was embolized with particles. A few months later, he developed progressive ipsilateral foot drop, which was initially presumed to be from compressive neuropathy. Following a second round of particle embolization of the gluteal vascular malformations, he went on to develop progressive paraparesis. (A) Right common iliac injection opacified an arteriovenous nidus in the posterolateral aspect of the thigh, corresponding to the L5 myotome. (B) MRI of the spine then revealed intramedullary signal change involving the lower cord with serpiginous vascular flow voids in the lumbosacral canal. Selective spinal angiography was then performed. (C) The radiculomedullary artery was opacified on right T12 injection. The descending limb was enlarged in caliber. A small nidus was opacified in the conus region. The descending portion of a large draining vein can be seen. (D) A large right posterior spinal artery can be seen filling from right L2 injection and feeding a large vessel at the L5 myelomere. Note the collateral filling of the left posterior spinal artery (arrowhead) of left L1. Dilated draining veins (not shown) were seen ascending and descending from the malformations. (E) Right iliolumbar artery filled the L5 radicular artery, which entered the (L5) foramen and ascended along the cauda and opacified a small network of vascular malformations, presumably along the L5 nerve root. (F) *N*-Butyl cyanoacrylate cast in the feeding pedicle from right L2 radiculopial artery. The patient experienced significant improvement of his lower extremity strength. However, symptoms returned and progressed 9–10 months after the initial therapy, along with new bladder dysfunction. (G) MRI of the spine at that time showed progression of the intramedullary T_2-weighted signal change and persistence of flow voids. Spinal angiography was repeated. (H) Late arterial phase of right T12 injection redemonstrated the arteriovenous shunt at the conus level, with delayed emptying of prominent ascending and descending draining veins, indicating venous hypertension and congestion. (I) Microcatheter injection of the anterior spinal artery from right T12 showed two feeding branches: one circumferential branch going around the posterior surface of the conus and another supplying the shunt through the arterial basket of the conus. Reduction of flow through the AVM, in preparation for surgical resection, was achieved with polyvinyl alcohol particle embolization from the distal anterior spinal artery. (J) Intraoperative photograph of the AVM located on the posterior surface of the conus. (K) MRI at follow-up 2 years later showed resolution of the T_2 signal changes. The patient's paraparesis and bladder dysfunction gradually improved, albeit not completely.

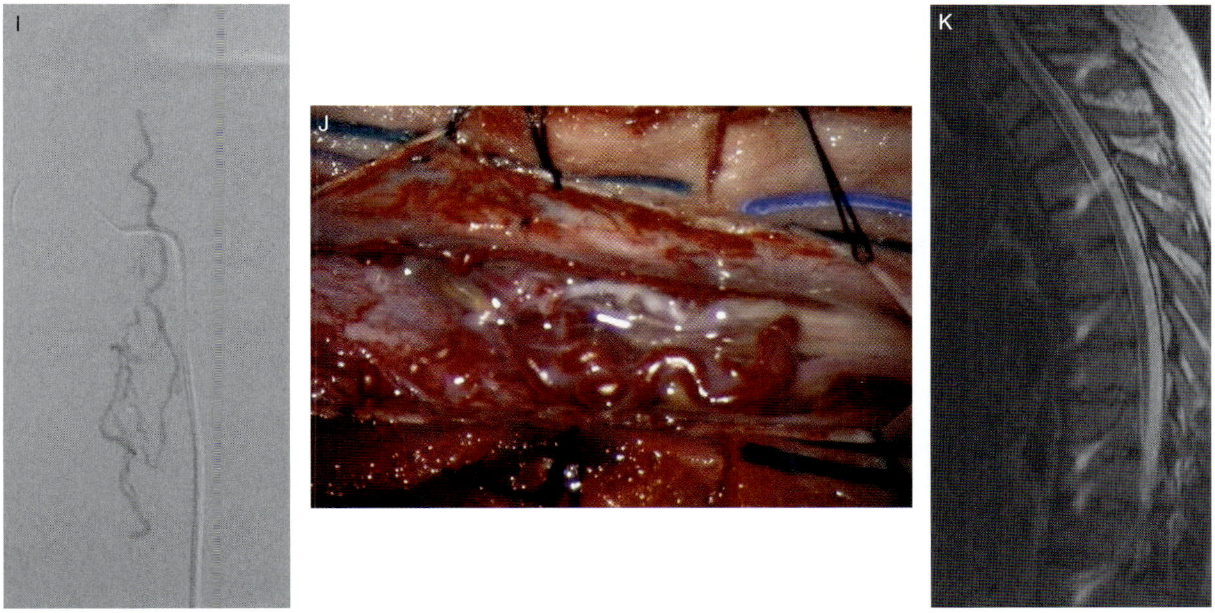

Fig. 21.3. (cont.).

genetic associations allowed a further classification of spinal cord AVMs into three groups: group 1, single shunts with genetic basis and hereditary transmission; group 2, multiple shunts with genetic basis without hereditary pattern and with either metameric involvement (2A, e.g., Cobb syndrome) or without demonstrable metameric involvement (2B); and group 3, single shunts without proven genetic basis [1,24]. Hereditary links have been established in hereditary hemorrhagic telangiectasia (Osler–Weber–Rendu syndrome) [25]. This disorder, which is inherited as an autosomal dominant trait with heterogenous expression, may manifest with spinal arteriovenous shunts in addition to more common mucocutaneous telangiectasiae and pulmonary, hepatic, cerebral, and other systemic arteriovenous shunts. It constitutes the primary disorder in group 1 [1,24]. Group 2A (i.e., non-hereditary multiple metameric shunts) can be etiologically explained by the vascular dysgenesis that occurs during the embryonic stage prior to differentiation and migration of the germinal layers into their respective phenotypic fates (Fig. 21.3). Radicular and myelomeric congruence is essential to demonstrate metameric disposition of spinal vascular malformations. Group 2B contains lesions in which metameric relationships are not evident, but may be suspected. Given the multiplicity of shunts and organs involved, these are designated as "syndromic arteriovenous shunts" [24]. Spinal AVMs that may occur with Klippel–Trénaunay–Weber and Parkes-Weber syndromes are classified under this group.

This classification [23], while addressing the phenotype and dynamicity of spinal intradural arteriovenous shunts, also broadly categorizes them by angioarchitecture and is key to understanding the lesional characteristics and etiopathology of the lesions [1,24]. However, it is also critical to be able to separate spinal arteriovenous shunts angiographically into distinct categories that aid diagnosis, prognosis, and treatment planning, based on readily available radiopathological data at the time of angio-examination. From a segmental perspective, arterialization of the spinal cord can be organized by the location and circumferential relationship of the vessels to the cord, as (1) extramedullary supply via the paired segmental radiculospinal arteries, which branch into the radiculopial artery and radiculomedullary arteries; (2) perimedullary vessels consisting of the ventral (anterior) spinal artery and the pial (posterior spinal) network; and (3) intramedullary branches from the perimedullary vessels, consisting of sulcal arteries from the ASA, which supply nearly two-thirds of the spinal cord, the radial perforating arteries, and the intrinsic anastomoses between the two.

Hence, angio-anatomically, vascular abnormalities of the spinal cord associated with arteriovenous shunting may be considered as the following distinct entities: (1) spinal cord AVMs, including metameric vascular lesions of the spine and spinal cord; (2) SDAVFs, including both dural and epidural fistulae; and (3) paraspinal AVFs.

Based on the relationship and location of the shunt to the cord surface, further division can be made into intramedullary AVMs (referred to as SCAVMs) and perimedullary AVFs and AVFs of the filum terminale (collectively referred to as spinal cord AVFs [SCAVFs]). This broad generalization is useful in angiographic identification of the lesion and in endovascular treatment planning. A comprehensive review of the entire range of spinal vascular malformations is beyond the scope of this chapter and only the most clinically significant entities, SDAVFs and spinal cord AVMs, will be discussed here.

Incidence

Even as SDAVFs are being more frequently recognized in older populations, spinal vascular malformations in general are uncommon and statistically fewer than cerebral vascular

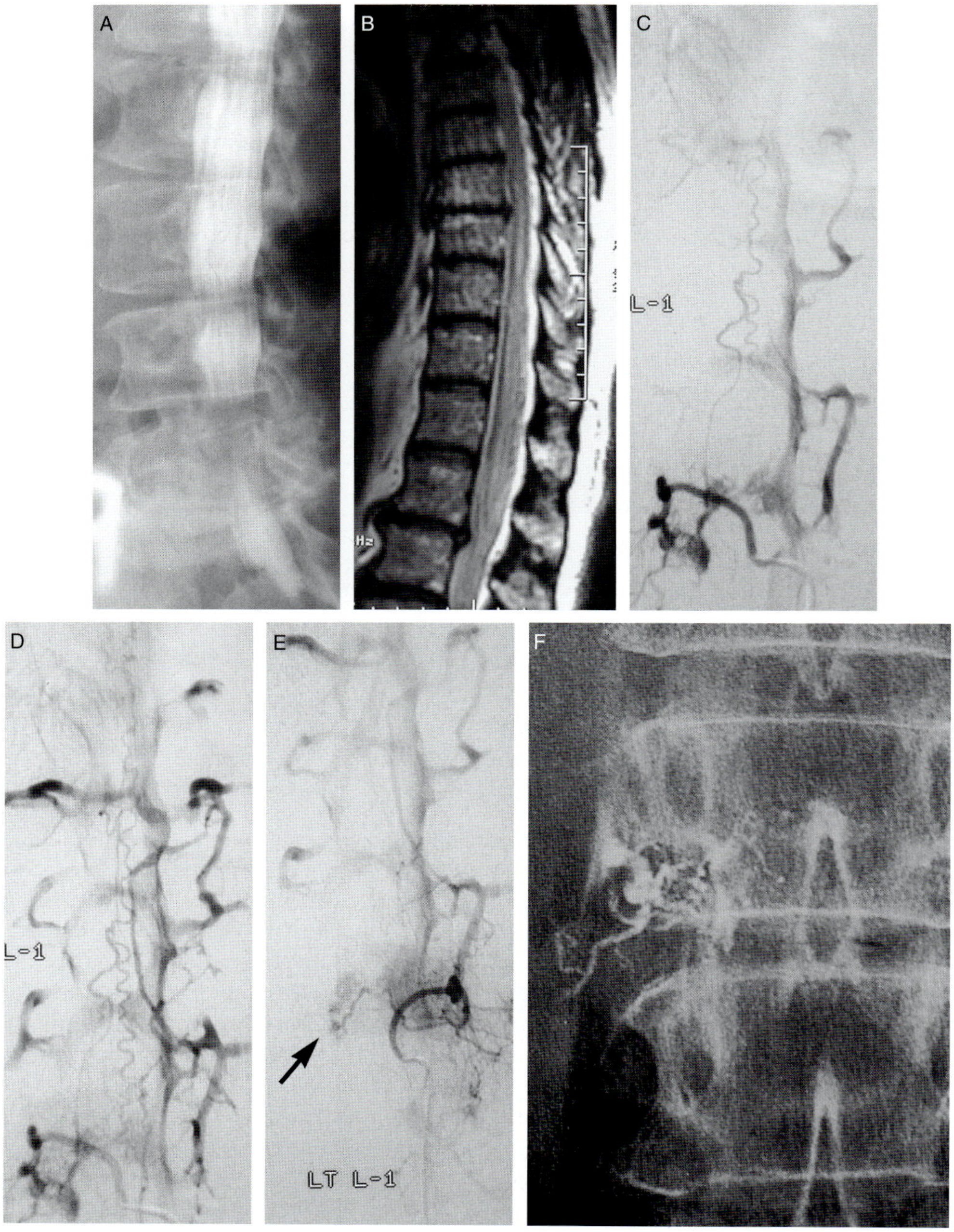

Fig. 21.4. Spinal epidural arteriovenous fistula in a 63-year-old woman with back pain, progressive lower extremity weakness, and urinary retention. (A) Myelography showed partial block at L5–S1. She then underwent laminectomy without any significant improvement in her symptoms. (B) MRI of the spine was then repeated and showed T_2 hyperintense signal involving the thoracic cord and conus. (C,D) Anteroposterior selective angiography in midarterial phase of the right L1 segmental artery. A prominent extradural arterial feeder can be seen supplying a shunt draining into epidural veins and then into the perimedullary venous network. (E) Left L1 injection demonstrated a prominent extradural artery crossing midline and supplying the shunt (arrow). Embolization of the fistula and arterial feeder from left L1 and then right L1 was successfully performed with *N*-butyl cyanoacrylate–Ethiodol. (F) Plain radiograph of lumbar spine in anteroposterior projection demonstrated the glue cast in the fistula and feeding branches from right and left L1 segmental artery. The patient had improvement of her sensorimotor function within a month of the procedure.

malformations. However, on volumetric comparison of these tissues and the respective incidence of neoplastic lesions in them, it seems that spinal and cerebral vascular malformations have comparable incidences [23]. Even though the true prevalence of spinal vascular malformations in the general population is difficult to estimate, some available statistics do define the incidence of spinal vascular lesions in symptomatic patients. In 78 patients with myelopathy of undetermined cause, 22 (28%) had angiograms that confirmed an AVM (Spetzler–Martin grade I in 19, grade II in 1, and grade IV in 2) [26]. Pooled data from three large series of 296 patients estimated the incidence of SDAVFs and spinal cord AVMs (including SCAVFs) at 35 and 59%, respectively [23]. The reversal of incidence between SDAVFs and spinal cord AVMs in the above report likely reflects a referral bias, as we now know that SDAVFs are far more common than spinal cord AVMs. Metameric lesions accounted for 6% in that series. An analysis of spinal angiography for 132 patients showed SDAVFs in 66 of

97 (68%) spinal arteriovenous lesions identified [27]. The annual incidence of SDAVF is estimated to be 5 to 10 per million people [28].

It is clear that SDAVFs have a clear male predilection. Berenstein and Lasjaunias reported on collective analysis of five series comprising 172 patients with SDAVFs; men (85%) were affected five times more than women (15%) [23]. By comparison, spinal cord AVMs have only a slight male to female preponderance. In a series of 155 patients with spinal cord AVMs, 81 (52%) were men and 74 (48%) were women [1]. In children in the same series, there was a more striking sex predilection pattern for spinal cord AVMs, with 80% boys and 20% girls. The mean ages of the patients with SDAVF at the time of diagnosis in these five series ranged from 49 to 59 years [23]. In a series of 81 patients, the age of patients with intradural AVMs ranged from 4 to 58 years, with a mean age of 27 [29]. In the report by Berenstein and Lasjaunias of 81 patients, the ages of patients with SDAVF ranged from 35 to 87 years, with a mean age of 56 [23]. In that series, SCAVMs were diagnosed in patients between the ages of 2 and 42, with a mean age of 22. In another series of 55 patients with SDAVFs, ages of affected individuals ranged from 29 to 75, with a mean age of 57; the ages of patients with SCAVMs ranged from 14 to 40, with a mean of 31 [30]. From these results, it is reasonable to infer that SDAVFs are more commonly recognized in the sixth decade of life or later, whereas spinal cord AVMs commonly present in the second and third decades. The spinal cord AVMs will contain both SCAVMs and intradural AVFs. The latter, which are leptomeningeal fistulae between a medullary artery and vein, account for 10–20% of all spinal cord AVMs [31]. The nidi of the intramedullary type may be located partially outside the cord surface and may also harbor AVFs within, whereas large intradural AVFs always present outside the cord surface [1,32]. In two series of 97 patients [23,29] with spinal intradural AVMs, 79 (81%) had true AVMs with nidus or intramedullary lesions, and 18 (19%) had SCAVFs [23]. This is consistent with the later reported series of Rodesch *et al.* of 155 patients with SCAVMs in which 30 (19%) patients had intradural AVFs and 125 (81%), intradural AVMs [24]. In our experience of 85 patients (mean age 62 years; male:female ratio of 63:22) who underwent spinal angiography for myelopathic symptoms and were found to have spinal AVMs, 67 (79%) had SDAVFs (or epidural AVFs) and 16 (19%) SCAVMs. Two (2%) patients had metameric lesions. One patient, who initially had a negative spinal angiogram, was noted to have an SDAVF on a study repeated a year later.

Spinal dural arteriovenous fistula

In populations in their sixth decade and beyond, SDAVFs are the most commonly encountered vascular malformations. There is a clear sex preponderance, with men being affected nearly five times more than women. Historically, these were referred to as "slow flow arteriovenous malformations" or "corkscrew type malformations" from myelographic and angiographic impressions. In 1977, Kendall and Logue reported the location of the arteriovenous shunts to be "situated on or adjacent to the outer surface of the dura mater" and drained by "one or more veins which pierced the dura to join the coronal spinal venous plexus" [33]. The lesions mostly involve the thoracolumbar spine and are rarely seen in the cervical spine. Tadie *et al.* observed that venous drainage of the lumbar and lower thoracic spinal cord was cephalad into smaller radicular spinal veins, rendering it vulnerable to hemodynamic variations [34]. By comparison, cervical cord venous drainage is divergent and enjoys relatively free flow even in the presence of some hindrances. From angiographic and histological observations, venous congestion from arteriovenous shunting appears to be the pathological mechanism of myelopathy and symptoms. In fact, Willinsky *et al.* have suggested that a normal venous phase of the spinal circulation effectively rules out the presence of an SDAVF [35]. In spinal angiographic practice, radiculomedullary arterial injections should opacify the venous outflow from the spinal cord within usually 15 seconds, and no later than 22 seconds [36]. Delayed opacification of the veins is indicative of venous congestion, possibly from arterial shunting into the venous network.

The most frequent and striking initial presenting symptom is numbness and weakness of the lower extremities. In combined data from three series comprising 172 patients, lower extremity paresis was the presenting complaint in 69 (40%), followed in frequency by back pain, and bladder and bowel dysfunction [23]. In the same group, paraparesis with pyramidal findings was present in 151 patients (88%). In our series of 67 patients with SDAVFs, 58 (87%) presented with lower extremity weakness. These symptoms are slowly progressive in over 70% of patients. Stepwise, progressive with interspersed remissions, as well as acute presentations with rapid progression have also been reported. Intraspinal hemorrhage has not been reported with SDAVFs [29]. Patients would also often report diurnal aggravation of symptoms as the day progresses, which may also be explained by gravity- and posture-associated venous congestion in the intraspinal compartment. Neurological examination may reveal mixed upper and lower motor neuron signs. As a rule, a constellation of myelopathy and symptoms of conus syndrome in anyone in the fifth or sixth decade of life should warrant evaluation for SDAVF (Figs. 21.4 and 21.5) [37].

From demographic, angiographic, and histological evidence, as well as longitudinal follow up, these lesions are now deemed acquired rather than congenital [23,29]. Several mechanisms have been proposed as the etiology of SDAVFs, including spontaneous thrombosis, trauma, spinal stenosis, degenerative disc disease, infections, and previous surgery or instrumentation. The pathology in SDAVF is commonly a single, frequently microscopic, fistula located on the surface of the dura, usually at the level of the intervertebral foramen. However, unlike radicular arteries, the draining venous counterpart may pierce the dura away from the nerve root, resulting in bimetameric involvement [23]. The feeding artery is usually a dural branch of the radicular artery. The arterial supply, which is seemingly a single vessel on angiography, may in fact consist of multiple, small, collateral feeding arteries (microfistulae), which may coalesce prior to dural penetration [38]. The shunt

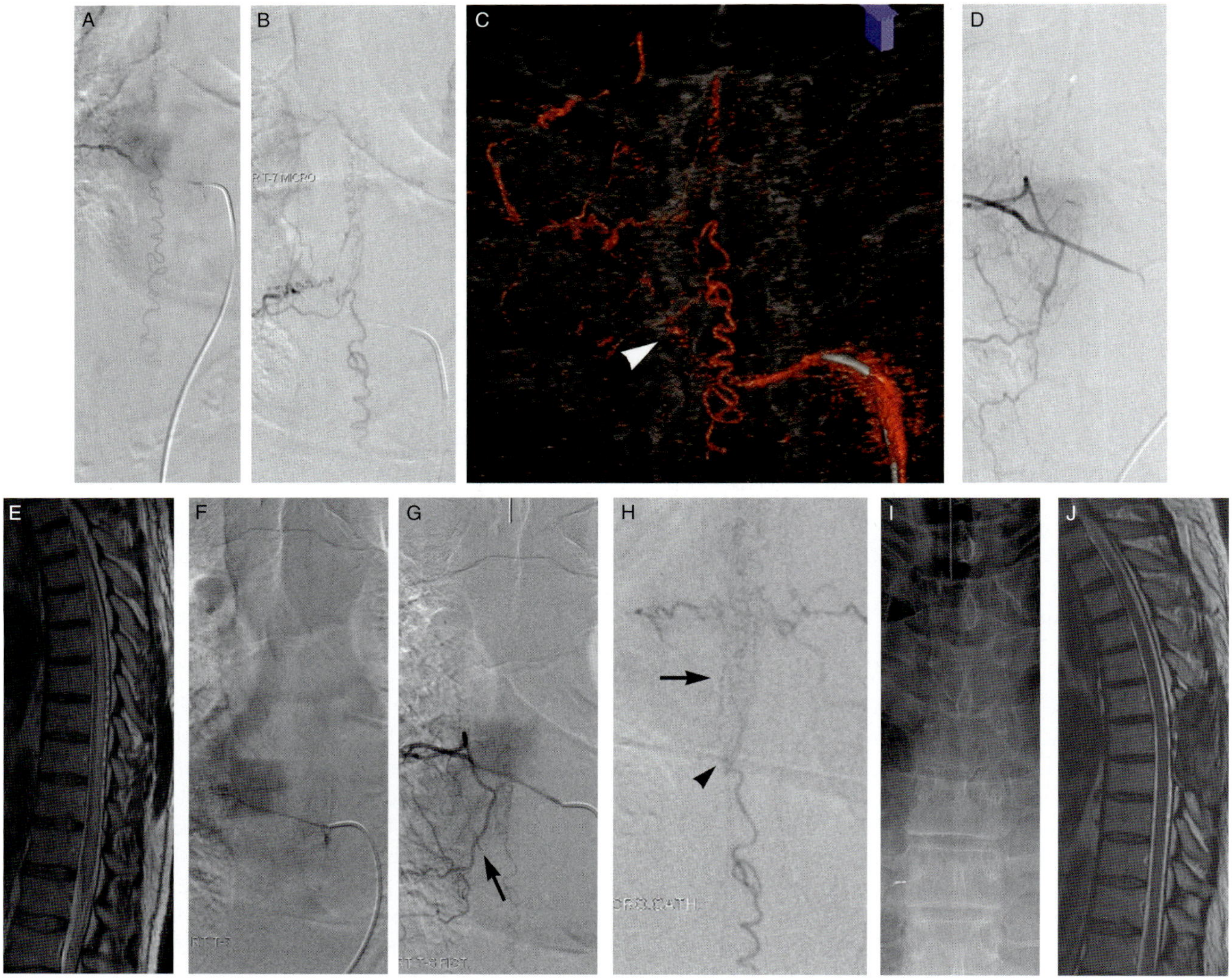

Fig. 21.5. Spinal dural arteriovenous fistula in a 54-year-old man with progressive lower extremity weakness and urinary urgency. MRI of spine was suggestive of dilated vessels on the cord surface with intramedullary edema. (A) Midarterial phase of right T7 intercostal artery injection; arteriovenous shunting and prominent descending draining vein could be seen. (B) Microcatheter injection of right T7 radiculospinal artery identified the shunt with two small venous channels draining cephalad. There is also a prominent descending draining vein. (C) Three-dimensional reconstruction of rotational angiography from right T7 injection demonstrated the fistula (arrowhead) in the subpedicular region. The fistula was successfully embolized with *N*-butyl cyanoacrylate–Ethiodol. (D) Postembolization selective angiography of right T6 intercostal artery injection did not demonstrate any supply to the shunt. The patient had excellent clinical improvement shortly after the treatment. (E) Sagittal T_2-weighted MRI of the thoracic spine was carried out as there was recurrence of symptoms about 3 months after the embolization procedure; this showed persistent intramedullary spinal cord signal increase. (F) Spinal angiography was repeated. Right T7 injection did not demonstrate any residual shunt. (G) Right T6 injections showed arteriovenous shunting through the previously known fistula at the level of T7 (arrow). (H) Microcatheter injection of right T6 radiculospinal artery showed the fistula (arrowhead) now being fed by a dural branch (arrow) of T6, with prominent ascending and descending veins. (I) Plain radiography (anteroposterior) of the thoracic spine showed the coils to mark the level for surgical localization. The patient had excellent recovery following surgical excision of the shunt. (J) Sagittal T_2-weighted MRI of the thoracic spine at follow-up showed complete resolution of the increased intramedullary signal and flow voids.

itself may be tiny and have the appearance of an abnormal vessel that has features of both artery and vein [39]. The draining vein is frequently single, often tortuous, and reaches the perimedullary venous system, often causing engorgement of the network. Manelfe *et al.* observed glomerulus-like vascular structures located along the dorsal extradural surface of the spinal dura, consisting of an afferent arterial mesh from a tortuous single capillary channel draining intradurally through an efferent vein [23,40]. The distinct similarity between this glomerulus-like structure and SDAVFs was noted by Merland *et al.* [41]. However, despite the striking morphological similarity to an arteriovenous shunt, its physiological role and its relation to pathological SDAVFs have not been demonstrated.

On histological examination, the venous wall may appear congested and thickened with sclerotic changes [39]. Various stages of neoangiogenesis, focal hemorrhage, thrombosis, and reorganization may be observed, explaining the symptomatology and pathophysiology. The cord may exhibit hypoxic and demyelinative changes, depending on the duration and severity of the hemodymamic insult. Congestive venopathy may cause extensive changes related to ischemia and hypoxia in the cord parenchyma. The pathophysiological changes appear to have a predilection for motor tracts, explaining the higher incidence of weakness as a presenting symptom, but they may progress to involve the entire gray matter and posterior columns. In advanced cases, degenerative changes are evident throughout the cord, particularly in the dependent portions. The two patients with subacute necrotizing myelopathy described by Foix and Alajouanine in 1926 are now believed to have been likely to have advanced congestive myelopathy from SDAVF [3,42].

With the development and advances in MRI, spinal vascular malformations can now be demonstrated with remarkable sensitivity (up to 97% when spinal AVF is considered as a possible, although not exclusively, primary diagnosis) and specificity. Findings include intramedullary T_2 hyperintensity, particularly in the conus and lower thoracic cord, flow voids on the cord surface, and cord expansion and enhancement. Newer techniques may even identify the site of the fistula. When simultaneously present, increased cord signal on T_2-weighted images and flow voids are remarkably specific, with a high likelihood ratio averaging 22.5 [43]. Catheter angiography remains the gold standard for both ruling out arteriovenous shunts and for understanding the angioarchitecture and planning treatment.

Principles of management

An SDAVF causes progressive myelopathy and disability, sometimes with little warning. The therapeutic approach to SDAVFs is based on the assumption that myelopathy, at least in the early stages, is related to reversible venous congestion and edema. It may become irreversible in its later stages when it has progressed to necrotizing myelopathy or cord degeneration. Spontaneous closure of an SDAVF without surgical or endovascular obliterative treatment is very unlikely [44]. Hence endovascular or surgical treatment should be considered in all patients with SDAVFs, even in those with mild or static symptoms. With the development of superselective catheterization and the demonstration of safe use of liquid embolic agents for arteriovenous shunt occlusion, endovascular therapy may be the first line of treatment for SDAVFs, subject to each group's practices. Surgery for SDAVF consists of the interruption of the draining vein by coagulation and disconnection from the dura at the site of fistula. Abnormal vessels may be visualized on the inner aspect of the dura at the time of surgery. In our practice, in patients undergoing spinal angiography for suspected SDAVF, embolization is planned and attempted in all patients with fistula or fistulae amenable to endovascular therapy.

Endovascular management

The goal of intervention in SDAVFs is to interrupt the AVF, which generally reverses the venous congestion and neurological symptoms [45]. Numerous types of embolic material, including stainless steel pellets, muscle fragments, and dura, have been historically used for this purpose [46]. With the development of superselective angiographic techniques and of various embolic agents, SDAVFs have been treated effectively by transarterial endovascular approaches. Occlusion of the draining vein, within a few millimeters of the arteriovenous shunt, results in complete obliteration of the fistulae and arrest of congestive venopathy. Just as the principle in surgical treatment of SDAVFs, a cure by endovascular method is achieved only when the embolic agent is lodged within the fistula itself and the proximal part of the draining vein, and not just proximal to the fistula. Selective catheterization is important to exclude the ASA or PSA from the same radicular branch, which would preclude endovascular treatment. Such patients should be referred for surgical excision. Spinal angiography, with or without endovascular intervention, is often significantly time consuming. An exhaustive diagnostic spinal angiogram may take in the order of 3–4 hours or more. General anesthesia is preferred to maximize diagnostic yield and accuracy in studying these submillimeter size vessels and shunts, and also to minimize patient discomfort. At our center, all spinal angiograms are, unless contraindicated, performed under general anesthesia.

Permanent angioembolic materials in current use are liquid adhesives such as *N*-butyl cyanoacrylate (NBCA [Trufill]; DePuy Synthes-Codman, Raynham, MA, USA) and a copolymer of ethylene and vinyl alcohol (Onyx; Covidien ev3 Neurovascular, Irvine, CA, USA). Particulate embolic material cannot sufficiently penetrate into the nidus of an SDAVF that harbors microfistulae, usually in the range of 40–60 μm. Consequently, embolization with particulate materials invariably results in re-establishment of shunt flow and clinical relapse. Embolization material with liquid adhesives such as NBCA and Onyx can reach the target to achieve a result comparable to surgical treatment and, hence, have become the agent of choice in transarterial embolization of SDAVFs [47,48]. Venous approaches have been described in the treatment of spinal epidural and paraspinal AVFs, but do not have any role in the treatment of SDAVFs [49–51].

Following meticulous selective spinal angiography performed in an orderly fashion and mapping of the fistula(e), as well as possible radiculomedullary and radiculopial tributaries in neighboring segments, the guide catheter is engaged in the proximal segmental branch that harbors the fistulous feeder. The stability of the guide catheter in the segmental artery is vital to navigating the microcatheter through the dural branch that supplies the shunt. Again, the goal is to reach as close to the shunt as possible with the microcatheter, and to deliver the embolic agent within the proximal part of the draining vein and fistula. We prefer to use NBCA mixed with ethiodized oil, which prevents premature polymerization of the acrylic agent, and tantalum powder, which serves as a radiopaque marker. Roadmapping technique enhances the ability to track the delivery of NBCA within the fistulous segment and thereby permits carefully controlled injections to match with previously gauged flow through the fistula. Filling the microcatheter with 5% dextrose solution prior to acrylic injection will prevent polymerization of NBCA in the catheter. Ventilator-managed apnea during angiographic runs reduces motion artifacts and improves diagnostic yield. Following satisfactory deposition of the acrylic embolus, selective angiography of the involved as well as neighboring segmental arteries is performed to document complete obliteration of the shunt. Systemic anticoagulation is reserved for patients suspected to have, or be at risk for, worsening myelopathy from progressive venous thrombosis. It is customary in our center to monitor patients in hospital for neurological deterioration for 24–48 hours following spinal endovascular embolization treatments.

Results of endovascular treatment

Success with endovascular embolization for SDAVFs varies from 25% to 90% in the literature; Berenstein and Lasjaunias achieved radiographic success in 25 (86%) of 29 patients with SDAVFs treated by the endovascular method [23]. Good radiographic results correlated with favorable clinical outcome in 24 of the 25 patients treated exclusively with endovascular embolization in that series of 31 patients. Of the four patients in whom endovascular treatment was unsuccessful, three responded to surgery. In our series of 67 patients with SDAVFs, embolization was attempted in 53 (79.1%); 13 (19.4%) were referred for surgery because of unfavorable vascular anatomy and 1 was not treated. Complete angiographic obliteration of the shunt was achieved in 38 (71.7%) patients treated by the endovascular technique. Embolization was not successful in 15 (28.3%) patients, who then underwent surgery with success. Sustained and substantial clinical improvement was noted in 32 (84.2%) of the patients treated exclusively by endovascular route. Improvement was modest or absent in six (15.8%). Two patients who underwent endovascular treatment, and one patient who underwent surgery, were later found to have recanalization of the shunt. These patients responded to surgery. Needless to say, detailed mapping of the lesion and its possible collateral supply is key to successful embolization. Release of venous vascular congestion is easily demonstrated in many patients, and dramatic clinical improvement may be seen in patients who have had less advanced and shorter duration of neurological deficits. In a series of 55 patients with SDAVFs, surgical treatment led to improvement of disabled gait in 20 (65%) of 31 severely affected patients and the clinicians suggested that good results are most likely in those patients who have mild or moderate neurological deficits preoperatively [30]. It was also suggested that neurological dysfunction of longer duration was more likely to be irreversible. In our experience, the likelihood of improvement is well correlated with the duration of symptoms rather than the severity of dysfunction: dramatic response to endovascular treatment was noted in six of our patients with acute-onset severe paraplegia.

In our experience, clinical improvement occurred primarily in motor function and deep sensory function. Superficial sensory and sphincter improvement was noted later in the follow-up period and was less satisfactory. Our overall results are comparable to the 72% clinical improvement noted in 26 patients following surgery for SDAVF reported by Rosenblum *et al.* [29]. Complications of endovascular therapy include injury to neural elements from distal migration of embolic agents. Our patients have not experienced any major complications from endovascular treatment of SDAVFs. Clinical deterioration, after initial improvement following treatment of SDAVFs, warrants thorough re-evaluation to rule out recurrence from collateralization or recanalization. On rare occasions, a second fistula may develop or be recognized on follow-up angiographic studies. Many of these patients are amenable to repeat embolization treatment or may be referred for surgical excision if the situation so warrants.

Spinal cord arteriovenous malformations

In contrast to SDAVFs, spinal cord AVMs may occur at any level of the spinal axis but are still more prevalent in the thoracolumbar region [23]; they may include both the SCAVM with distinct nidi as well as high-flow SCAVFs. The prevalence of spinal cord AVMs in the asymptomatic population is not known. While it is known that even extensive intramedullary lesions can be clinically silent, the incidence is best estimated from autopsies of myelopathic patients and from comparative data on reported series of patients with angiographically diagnosed spinal vascular lesions. An analysis of two series of 97 patients with spinal cord AVMs found 79 (81%) SCAVMs and 18 (19%) SCAVFs [23]. In 210 patients reported by Mourier *et al.*, 80 (38%) had SDAVFs, 94 (45%) had SCAVMs, and 36 (17%) had SCAVFs [31]. In contrast to SDAVFs, SCAVMs have only a slight male preponderance [1,52]. Patients typically present young, with over 50% manifesting symptoms prior to the age of 16 [1,37,53]. Muscle weakness almost invariably occurs with progression of the disease and time, but, unlike SDAVFs, such weakness may be the initial symptom in only a third of the patients. Radicular pain, erectile or ejaculatory dysfunction, bowel or bladder function disturbances, and sensory changes may accompany paresis at the time of diagnosis but are unusual as the initial symptoms. Myeloradiculopathic symptoms are often indistinguishable from those of SDAVF. Rosenblum *et al.* reported an average delay of 2.7 and 4.2 years from the time of initial symptoms to diagnosis of SDAVF and SCAVM, respectively [29]. Spinal bruit, if present, would be suggestive of a shunt but is seldom the primary reason for suspicion of SCAVM, possibly because of underevaluation. In our series of 18 patients with spinal cord AVMs, six had intradural AVMs, six perimedullary AVFs, and four AVFs of filum terminale (Fig. 21.6).

A further difference between SCAVMs and SDAVFs is that the former can cause (and is the most common etiology of) intraspinal hemorrhage: hematomyelia and epidural, subdural, and subarachnoid hemorrhage. In a series of 54 patients with intradural AVMs, subarachnoid hemorrhage caused the initial symptomatology in 17 (31%), exceeding those with paresis (9 [16%]) [29]. In the same series, more than 90% of patients with intradural AVMs developed paresis over time. The incidence of hemorrhage in spinal cord AVMs is higher in children and with cervical lesions [53]. Spinal hemorrhage can be intraparenchymal, subarachnoid, or even intracranial–subarachnoid when profuse or from cervical lesions. Spinal subarachnoid hemorrhage may manifest as sudden, severe pain – usually interscapular with associated meningismus, termed "coup de poignard" or "dagger thrust" [54]. In our experience of 18 patients with intradural lesions, 15 (83%) had developed weakness of the extremities by the time of diagnosis. Three (17%) had radiographic evidence of prior spinal cord hemorrhage. Patients may also describe acute pain involving the back, chest, or abdomen. Patients with high-flow fistulous lesions commonly present

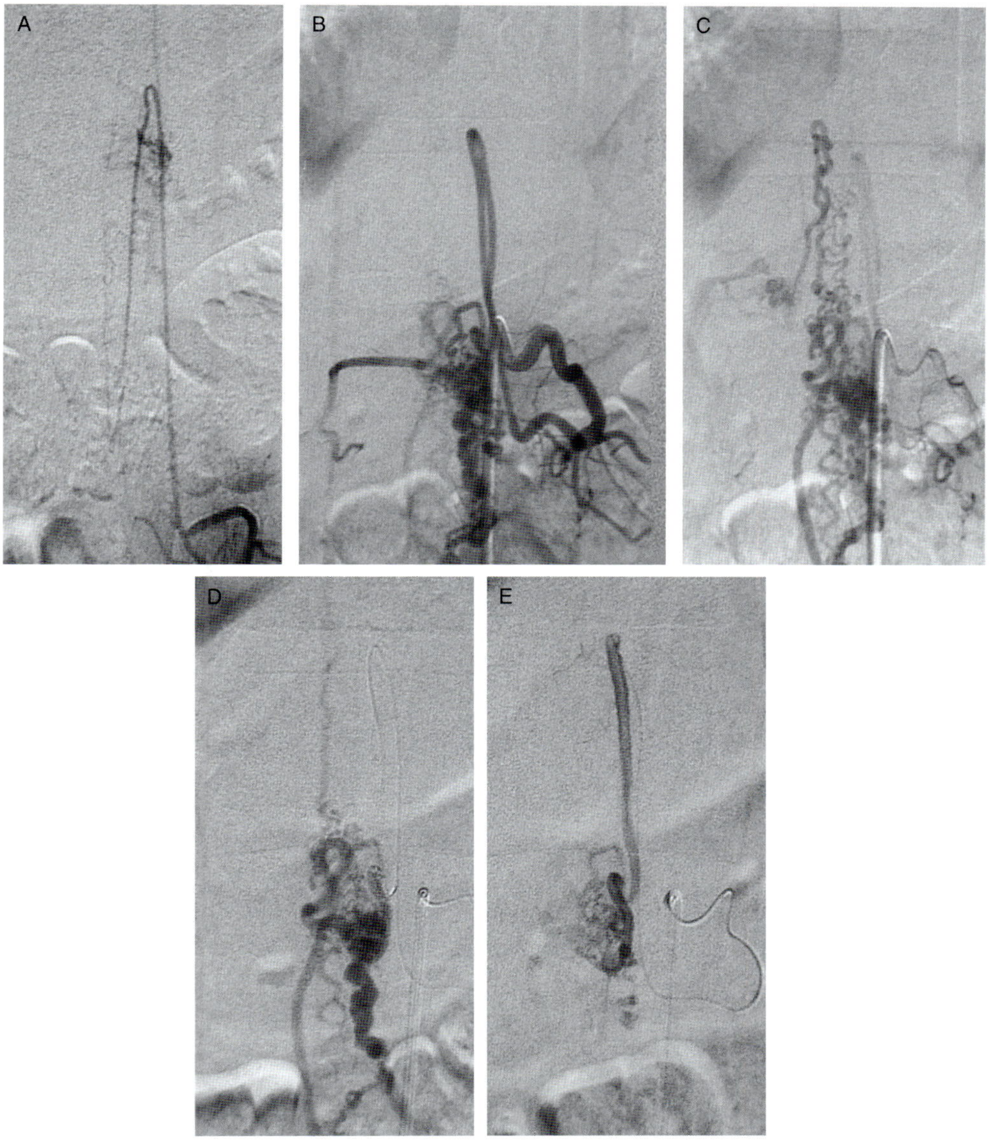

Fig. 21.6. Intramedullary arteriovenous fistula of the spinal cord in a 23-year-old man presenting with radicular back pain and paresthesiae. MRI of lumbar spine (not shown) revealed large intradural flow voids. (A) Selective angiography of left L3 segmental artery demonstrated a radiculomedullary artery. A small arteriovenous shunt was opacified at the left posterolateral aspect of the conus. Descending limb of the anterior spinal artery was displaced to the right, disproportionately to the size of the shunt. (B,C) Early arterial phase of left T6 injection. A hypertrophied radiculopial artery filled a large fistulous nidus at the level of L1. Midarterial phase demonstrated dilated perimedullary venous plexus. (D) Microcatheter injection in the distal left posterior spinal artery from left T6 opacified the shunt. (E) Microcatheter injection in the distal posterior spinal artery from left T6 following embolization with polyvinyl alcohol particles demonstrated reduction in flow through the shunt. The patient then underwent surgical resection of the shunt. Following surgery, he had transient exacerbation of lower extremity paresthesiae but improved significantly later.

with hemorrhage; in contrast, low-flow lesions manifest with symptoms of ischemia from venous congestion, as in SDAVFs. The five-year cumulative rebleed rate could be as high as 54% [1,53,55,56]. Neurological deterioration frequently occurs following intraspinal hemorrhage, but good clinical recovery is generally the rule. As with SDAVFs, MRI has replaced all other neuroimaging modalities as the non-invasive test of choice in evaluating patients with suspected spinal cord AVMs. This modality is useful in demonstrating intramedullary hemorrhage, presence of vascular flow voids, spinal cord signal changes, and associated extraspinal lesions in metameric syndromes. The presence of intramedullary hemorrhage effectively excludes SDAVFs as the etiology of shunt. MRI is also useful for longitudinal follow-up of the lesions and myelopathy.

Medullary arterial supply (ASA, PSA, or combined) to the arteriovenous shunt and medullary venous drainage constitute the pathological hallmark of spinal cord AVMs. Cervical SCAVMs may be supplied by the lateral spinal artery from intracranial circulation [1]. As in cerebral AVMs, it is possible to have dural feeders to the SCAVM; however, these may be difficult to separate angiographically from radiculomedullary and radiculopial supply. Dural adhesions following repeated hemorrhages may also be confused for primary dural supply to the SCAVM, which, if present, always follow metameric vascular arrangement [1]. Given the limitations of angiographic technique, angioarchitectural mapping of SCAVMs is more difficult and less complete compared with SDAVFs. Mapping of the lesion in relationship to the neural elements – to differentiate between intra- and extramedullary components – is essential for treatment planning. The presence of normal medullary supply from a feeding artery, rather than compromising location of the lesion, forms the limiting factor in endovascular treatment of SCAVMs (Fig. 21.7).

Subgroups of spinal cord arteriovenous malformations

Historically, numerous classifications and subclassifications of SCAVMs have been proposed based on lesional location and

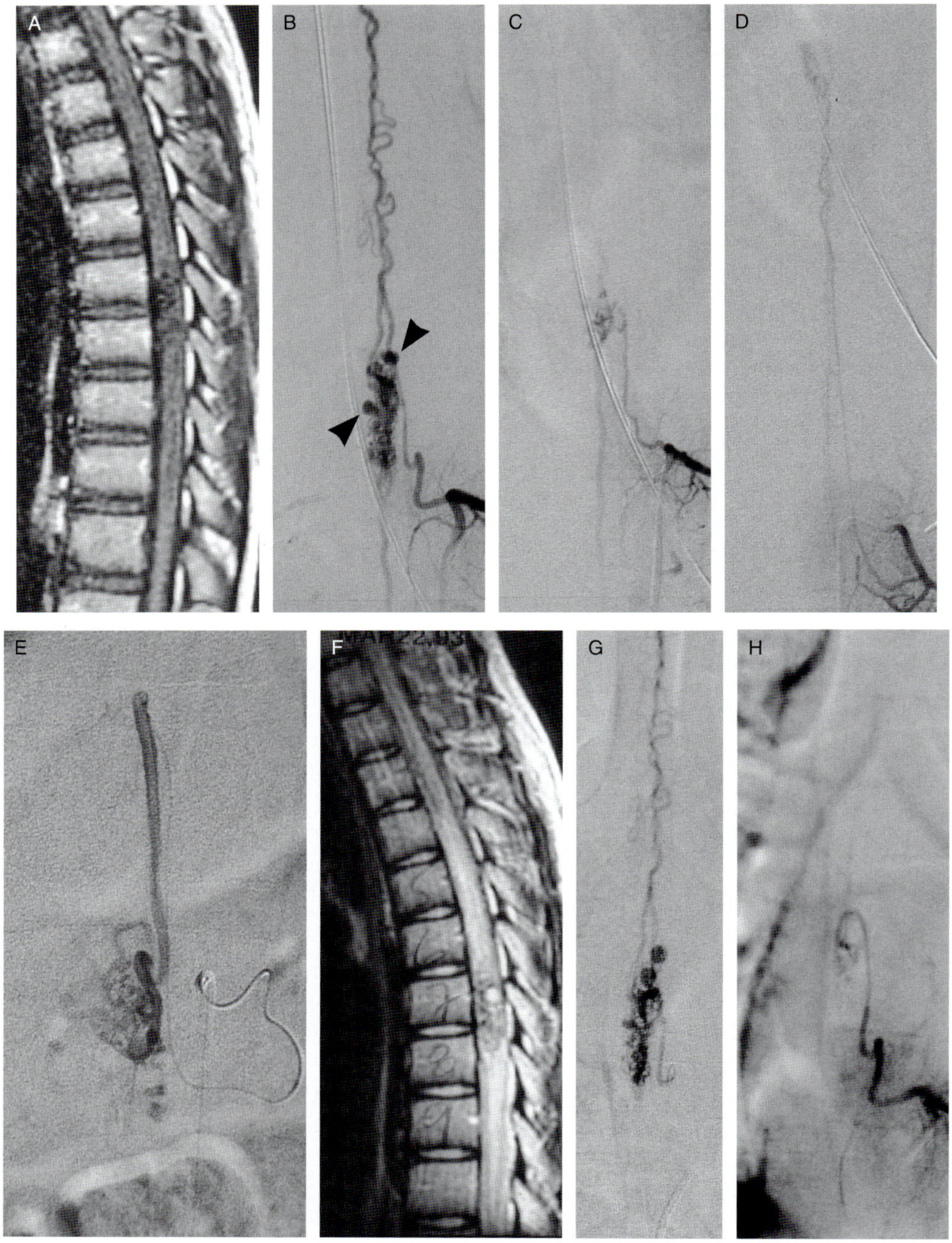

Fig. 21.7. Intramedullary arteriovenous malformations (AVM) of the spinal cord in a patient who presented at the age of 14 years with sudden paraparesis. (A) Sagittal T_1-weighted MRI of the thoracic spine showed intramedullary flow voids. (B) Selective spinal angiography was performed. Anteroposterior projection of left T8 intercostal artery injection in early arterial phase demonstrated a hypertrophied radiculomedullary contributor feeding a large nidus type intramedullary AVM with two intranidal aneurysms (arrowheads). Venous drainage is predominantly cephalad. (C) The radiculopial artery can be seen from left T9 injection, supplying the anterior–superior compartment of the nidus. (D) Left T12 injections opacified the anterior spinal artery supplying a small compartment of the AVM superiorly. (E) Oblique projection of left T8 injection in midarterial phase demonstrated anterior and posterior venous drainage. The patient recovered gradually but had sudden worsening a few months later. (F) Sagittal T_2-weighted MRI of the thoracic spine demonstrating hematomyelia. (G) The patient then underwent spinal angiography. Microcatheter injection from left T8 radiculopial artery filled the AVM nidus and redemonstrated the pseudoaneurysms. Embolization with polyvinyl alcohol particles was performed from this location since the microcatheter could not be advanced any further. (H) Postembolization selective angiography of left T8 intercostal artery showed significant reduction in opacification of the nidus and near-complete obliteration of the intranidal aneurysms. Following embolization treatment, the patient experienced slow improvement in his lower extremity strength and later plateaued.

angioarchitecture. The classification by Lasjaunias *et al.* described earlier in the chapter defines and organizes spinal cord AVMs on their genetic basis, metameric disposition, shunt plurality, and lesional characteristics [1,24]. Some spinal cord AVMs are considered to have a genetic basis; others may also have syndromic associations such as SAMS and Osler–Weber–Rendu, Klippel–Trénaunay–Weber, and Parks–Weber syndromes. For simplification, spinal cord AVMs may be further organized into intramedullary AVMs (SCAVMs) and the perimedullary AVFs and AVFs of the filum terminale (collectively referred to as SCAVFs).

Intramedullary arteriovenous malformations

The AVMs with a true nidus located, at least partially, within the parenchyma, account for approximately 80% of all spinal cord AVMs [1,24,31,55]. These correspond to group II malformations or glomus AVM and group III malformations or juvenile AVM described by Anson and Spetzler [21]. The nidus in the SCAVM is distinct with interspersed neural tissue and usually consists of tightly packed sinusoidal vessels fed by multiple branches from ASA, PSA, and, occasionally, dural vessels. The group III, juvenile AVM, malformations harbors a more expansive nidus spanning longer segments of the cord and extending often to adjacent non-neural elements such as bone and dura, corresponding to the metameric lesions described by Lasjaunias and colleagues [1,24]. The SCAVMs are more common than SCAVFs [24,31]. Male predilection for this disease is modest and patients usually present in the second or third decade of life [23,24,29,30]. Multiple arterial feeders to the nidus are usually present. The intrathecal feeding arteries frequently have a tortuous appearance. The draining veins undergo secondary thickening and appear hyalinized. The nidus often has an extramedullary or pial constituent and drains into the perimedullary venous plexus [57]. Intraspinal hemorrhage is frequently the initial symptom and may herald acute neurological deficits. In a series of 155 patients with intradural AVMs, Rodesch *et al.* noted approximately a 31.6% incidence of arterial aneurysms [24]. When present, arterial aneurysms are invariably associated with subarachnoid hemorrhage [55]. Aneurysms may be flow-related in cervical lesions, explaining the higher incidence of hemorrhage in that location, or may result from underlying dysplasia and structural abnormalities of the vessels. The cord itself may exhibit sequelae of congestive venopathy, necrosis, hematomyelia, and Wallerian degeneration. Neurological recovery following the initial hemorrhage is likely and spontaneous, but recurrent hemorrhage is common and may occur in up to 40% of patients in the first year following the initial hemorrhagic event [1,24,53,55,56]. Myelopathic symptoms frequently show slow progression and MRI may show myelomalacia, gliosis, cord expansion and edema, evidence of prior subarachnoid hemorrhage, hematomyelia, venous ectasia, or aneurysms.

Perimedullary arteriovenous fistulae

Perimedullary AVFs, group IV in the Anson and Spetzler classification [21], correspond to SCAVFs in the classification of spinal cord AVMs by Lasjaunias and colleagues [1,24]. They were first described by Djindjian *et al.* as intradural–extramedullary spinal AVMs [58] and Heros *et al.* designated them as a separate type of intradural AVM [22]. These lesions are extramedullary but within the leptomeninges, and consists of a high-flow fistulae between anterior or posterior spinal arteries and the spinal cord veins. Berenstein *et al.* noted that the shunts are subpial when ventrally located and fed by the ASA, and subarachnoid when dorsal and supplied by radiculopial arteries [1]. These are usually thoracolumbar and may range from a single low-flow fistula to extensive shunts in the ventral perimedullary space. They frequently cause spinal subarachnoid hemorrhage. Arterial aneurysms and venous ectasia can cause compressive myeloradiculopathy from mass effect within the spinal canal. The perimedullary AVFs constitute approximately 20% of all spinal intradural AVMs [24,31]. The age of patients at presentation is younger than that of those with SDAVFs, frequently in the second to fourth decade. A majority of these patients develop symptoms prior to 25 years of age. Male sex preponderance is evident in a series of 32 patients [59]. In addition to spinal hemorrhage and compressive myelopathy as mentioned above, patients can be present with progressive myelopathy with interspersed acute declines. Prognosis is dismal in untreated symptomatic patients, who may develop spinal cord transective symptoms in a few years. Radicular compression from giant venous dilatations can be present with asymmetric findings that may be confounding and further delay diagnosis. The pathology in a perimedullary AVF can vary in size and angioarchitecture, from small, single-hole fistula fed by a single vessel to larger fistulae fed by multiple feeders arising from the ASA and PSA, and giant, high-flow fistulae with dilated and ectatic veins that may harbor venous aneurysms or variceal pouches. The last have a higher incidence in children and occur frequently in association with hereditary hemorrhagic telangiectasia (Osler–Weber–Rendu syndrome) [59]. Spinal subarachnoid hemorrhage, when it occurs, is commonly of posterior spinal venous origin, whereas anterior spinal vein rupture results usually in hematomyelia [59]. MRI may reveal large, serpiginous, perimedullary flow voids; however, it is non-specific in distinguishing between various types of spinal vascular shunt. In our experience of 18 patients with spinal cord AVMs, six (33%; four men and two women) were found to have perimedullary AVFs. All of our patients presented with lower extremity weakness (Fig. 21.8).

Arteriovenous fistulae of the filum terminale

Arteriovenous fistulae involving the filum terminale form a distinct entity from other spinal cord AVMs because of the unique vascular anatomy of the filum, a filament of connective tissue extending from the conus medullaris to the terminus of the dural tube at the second sacral level [60]. The arterial supply is derived from caudal extension of the anterior spinal axis, forming the so-called vascular basket at the conus. Despite the absence of exiting nerve roots from the filum, radicular feeding vessels may arise from the lateral sacral artery to supply the coccygeal nerve, which runs closely with the filum. The artery of filum terminale runs on the ventral surface of the filum, just anterior to a longitudinal venous channel, which itself may drain into the extradural sacral venous plexus, allowing both

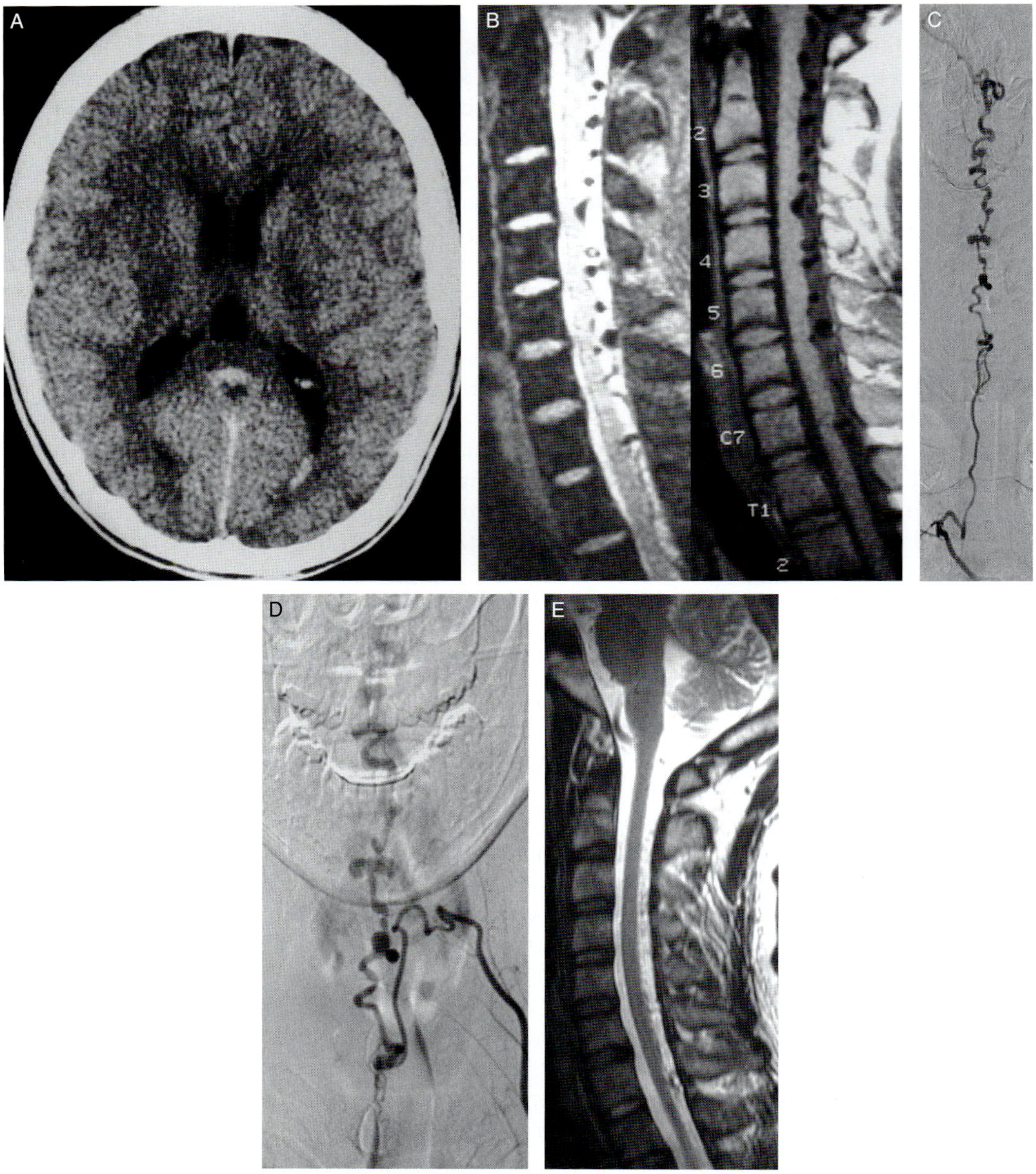

Fig. 21.8. Perimedullary arteriovenous fistula of the cervical spinal cord in a 20-year-old man. The disease first manifested as subarachnoid hemorrhage when he was 16 years of age. (A) Non-enhanced CT of the brain showed layering of blood in the occipital horn of the left lateral ventricle. Extensive cerebrovascular imaging, including cerebral catheter angiography, did not identify the source of hemorrhage. (B) Three years later, T_2-weighted (left) and T_1-weighted (right) MRI of the cervical spine revealed dilated serpiginous vessels on the posterior surface of the cord. (C) Selective spinal angiography was then performed. Right T4 intercostal artery injection showed a dilated radiculopial contributor bifurcating at the level of T1–T2, with both branches supplying an arteriovenous fistula at the level of C7. A large ectatic vein, harboring multiple variceal pouches, could be seen draining cephalad extending intracranially, opacifying the vein of Galen. (D) Injection of the left thyrocervical trunk demonstrated additional supply to the fistula from the radiculopial branch of the ascending cervical artery. The fistula was then embolized with *N*-butyl cyanoacrylate–Ethiodol mixture from right T3 and left ascending cervical supply. (E) Follow-up sagittal T_2-weighted MRI showed resolution of the abnormal vessels.

cephalad and caudal flow. Vascular malformations in the filum terminale are relatively rare and usually consist of a single-hole fistula between the artery of the filum and the draining vein. Congestive myelopathy ensues as with other spinal AVFs, but, atypically, urinary symptoms may precede motor weakness [60]. A 3.2% prevalence of AVF of filum terminale was seen in a series of 155 patients with spinal cord AVMs [24]. In our experience of 18 patients with spinal cord AVMs, four (22%; two men and two women) were discovered to have an AVF of filum terminale. All four patients presented with lower extremity weakness.

Principles of management

Spinal cord AVMs include both SCAVMs and SCAVFs. The principles of management of spinal cord AVMs differ from those of SDAVFs. Many factors must be taken into account in determining treatment options, including neurological symptoms and status; accessibility of the lesion; potential for substantial spinal cord collateral injury; presence of lesions that may pose a hemorrhagic risk, such as arterial aneurysms and venous varices; and patient age. Hence, it is not uncommon to attempt partial obliteration of the malformation with the intent to alleviate the most hemodynamically significant shunt and minimize hemorrhagic risk. The hemorrhagic risk, at times, mandates aggressive treatment of these lesions. As a rule, younger patients and those with a higher spinal level of the lesion (i.e., cervical or thoracic) are more aggressively treated.

Complete angiographic mapping of the malformations is paramount to delineate the arterial supply, regions of vulnerability, venous drainage pattern, and constraints if any, and to identify safely accessible feeding pedicles. It is also important to differentiate between direct and indirect feeders to the lesion, the latter being indicative of AVMs with a true nidus rather than the so-called "sump effect" [1]. Indirect supply usually consists of smaller caliber vessels supplying territory adjacent to the lesion. These may regress with occlusion of the primary supplying pedicle or gain prominence to become the residual supply to the shunt. Arterial and intranidal aneurysms, if present, are associated with high risk of subarachnoid hemorrhage or hematomyelia, and may by themselves be an indication for treatment [24,55]. These aneurysms can be seen as an irregular dilatation proximal to the AVM nidus [1]. Variceal dilatation of a draining vein is relatively common and may infrequently cause mechanical compression of neural elements in the spinal canal. These are seen distal to the arteriovenous junction and should be differentiated from intranidal aneurysms. Despite the variability in nidus architecture and compartmentalization, from a practical standpoint, it is safe to categorize spinal cord AVMs as either direct AVFs or nidus-associated AVMs.

Endovascular management

Endovascular and microsurgical treatment options are available for spinal cord AVMs for which treatment is indicated. The configuration and location of the spinal cord AVM or high-flow AVF could alter the level of risk. For lesions deemed equally accessible with similar expected cure rates and risk profiles by endovascular technique and microsurgery, it is now accepted practice to attempt endovascular embolization first or as part of a combined approach. Spinal cord AVFs are considered to be more favorable for surgical resection than for endovascular embolization, with the exception of lesions with large feeders and giant venous ectasia, which may pose considerable surgical risks. Good clinical outcome is generally the rule following successful treatment, endovascular or surgical, of SCAVFs.

Liquid adhesives, such as NBCA, are the preferred embolic agents. Flow-guided microcatheters may facilitate navigation in high-flow shunts. It would then be mandatory to reach beyond any vascular supply to the normal spinal cord, with the tip of the microcatheter in the specific sulcal artery to safely occlude the feeding pedicles and nidus. The ability to reach as close to the nidus as possible dictates the ease and success of embolization and avoidance of collateral injury. Migration of even minute amounts of embolic material into unintended vessels can cause devastating injury and neurological deficits. Exhaustive mapping of the shunt by selective and superselective injections, roadmapping technique, and meticulous comparison with control angiographic runs are the sine qua non of safe and successful endovascular embolization treatment. Whenever present, feeding pedicles from the radiculopial network should be preferentially chosen for embolization first, given the prominence of the anterior spinal axis in the arterial supply of the cord. Feeding pedicles, any arterial or intranidal aneurysms, venous pouches, or evidence of congestive venopathy should all be studied and addressed accordingly. When curative treatment is contraindicated by risk of substantial collateral injury, treatment must focus on ameliorating the risk from specific lesions such as aneurysms and varices. Emergency treatment is usually not indicated in intraspinal hemorrhage from spinal cord AVMs as the chance for spontaneous recovery is high; however, treatment options should be weighed to reduce the risk of recurrent hemorrhage. Liquid adhesives such as NBCA should be used whenever feasible. Embolization with particulate agents such as polyvinyl alcohol may serve as presurgical adjunct or in treatment of lesions that carry high risk with curative endovascular or surgical interventions. Given the difficulty of catheterizing specific radiculopial and radiculomedullary contributors, particle embolization may have to be resorted to, despite the possibility of recanalization and incomplete obliteration of the lesion. Particle embolization may be employed in conjunction with flow control and flow-reversal techniques to reduce the flow through the lesion, either for symptom palliation or in preparation prior to acrylic embolization of a more safely accessible collateral feeder or surgery.

Where surgical resection is feasible with minimal spinal cord damage, combined endovascular and surgical approaches may be employed. Such patients may benefit from partial obliteration of flow through the shunt with either particulate embolization or liquid acrylics in carefully selected feeding pedicles. Presurgical embolization facilitates subsequent surgical resection of the AVM, and may also improve spinal cord edema, reducing the morbidity of surgical procedures. In our center, presurgical endovascular embolization is seriously considered in all patients who are deemed to require surgery. Intraoperative electrophysiological monitoring is not routinely performed; the need is determined on an individual basis. Progressive venous thrombosis following partial or complete obliteration of the shunt may result in fatal ascending myelopathy. Therefore, it is advisable to consider short-term systemic anticoagulation (e.g., heparin) when compromised venous return is suspected, after excluding arterial aneurysms.

Results of endovascular treatment

Clinical outcome in the endovascular or surgical management of spinal intradural AVMs is related to the extent of spinal cord injury that the lesion has already inflicted. Therefore, an excellent angiographic result or postsurgical picture may still be associated with poor recovery or even subsequent deterioration from neural degeneration that has already set in. In a series of 114 patients, 69 (60%) underwent endovascular therapy exclusively and 21 (18%) surgery, with 24 (21%) deemed unsuitable for either modality [61]. Of the 69 patients treated by endovascular route, acrylic embolization was almost exclusively used (68 patients), and angiographic reduction of lesion size by more than 50% was seen in 59 (86%). Using the Karnofsky

Performance Scale score 15% of those patients experienced complete clinical recovery, 43% improved, and 25% remained unchanged in their clinical status during a mean follow up of 5.6 years [61]. In our experience of patients with intradural arteriovenous shunts treated by the endovascular method, either alone or in combination with surgery, four of six patients experienced good clinical recovery. However, two of these patients had subsequent gradual deterioration, presumably from recanalization of the shunt or from a degenerative cascade that may have commenced prior to intervention.

Spinal arteriovenous metameric syndrome

Metameric angiomatosis refers to vascular lesions involving structural derivatives of two or more related embryonic layers, classified by Lasjaunias and colleagues as genetic non-hereditary lesions with multiple shunts and metameric disposition [1,24]. Consequently, SAMS, analogous to cerebrofacial arteriovenous metameric syndromes, may involve any one or multiple segmental derivatives, including the spinal cord myelomere, the corresponding vertebrae and nerve roots, myotome, and dermatome. Metameric lesions correspond to group III malformations or juvenile AVMs described by Anson and Spetzler [21]. The expansive lesions in this type of AVM have been described as not being restricted by germinal boundaries. This can be etiologically explained by segmental or metameric design of the germ cell layers during embryonic neurovascular evolution. The involvement of two or more segmental derivatives is needed for a diagnosis of a metameric lesion. A more profound expression of this condition, where at least three of the segmental derivatives are involved (vertebra, spinal cord, and skin) is known as Cobb syndrome after its description by Cobb in 1915 [15]. A metameric pattern has not been demonstrated in Klippel–Trénaunay–Weber and Parkes–Weber syndromes, where lesions involve multiple germ cell layers in a non-segmental fashion (Fig. 21.3).

The incidence of metameric lesions among spinal vascular malformations can be as high as 14%; however, the full expression as in Cobb syndrome is quite rare. The presence of radicular AVM in association with spinal cord AVM should prompt careful evaluation for a metameric relationship between the lesions [1]. Although it is a clinical possibility, metameric angiomatosis in patients with hereditary hemorrhagic telangiectasia is quite rare in the reported literature. It should be noted that the cutaneous lesion may not correlate with the segmental dermatome associated with the triad of embryonic layers involved. The skin lesion may represent a separate dysplastic lesion [23,29]. The spinal components of the metameric lesions are approached in the same way as any other spinal vascular malformations in terms of diagnosis and treatment. Spinal cord involvement often poses the greatest morbidity and risk in these patients. The prognosis is generally poor and treatment should be conservative to ameliorate neurological deficits, with therapy targeted at the symptomatic lesion only.

Conclusions

The understanding of the anatomy of spinal arteriovenous shunts, their etiopathological basis, and arteriovenous configuration – and the therapeutic options for these – had improved remarkably by the turn of the last century. Selective catheter angiography remains the cornerstone in the diagnosis of this highly morbid condition, and it also plays a significant and rising role in management. A multidisciplinary approach, considering individualized endovascular and surgical options, will present the best and safest possible therapeutic plan for this complex disease.

References

1. Berenstein A, Lasjaunias P, terBrugge K. Spinal cord arteriovenous malformations. In Berenstein A, Lasjaunias P, terBrugge K, eds. *Surgical Neuroangiography*, Vol. 2. New York: Springer, 2003, pp. 737–872.
2. Hebold O. Aneurysmen der kleinstein ruckenmarksgefasse. *Arch Psychiat Nervkrankh* 1885;**16**:813–23.
3. Foix CH, Alajouanine T. La myélite nécrotique subaique: myélite central angéiphypertrophique a évolution progressive: paraplégie amyotrophique lentement ascendante, d'abord spasmodique, puis flasque, s'accompagnant de dissociation, albumino-cytologique. *Rev Neurol* 1926;**46**:1–42.
4. Skalski JH, Zembala M. Albert Wojciech Adamkiewicz: the discoverer of the variable vascularity of the spinal cord. *Ann Thorac Surg* 2005;**80**:1971–5.
5. Berenbruch J. Einfall von Multiplen Angio-Lipomen Kombiniert mit einem angiom des Ruckenmarks. Doctoral thesis, Universität Tübingen, 1890.
6. Black J. Spinal vascular malformations: an historical perspective. *Neurosurg Focus* 2006;**21**:E11.
7. Di Chiro G., Doppman J, Ommaya AK. Selective arteriography of arteriovenous aneurysms of spinal cord. *Radiology* 1967;**88**:1065–77.
8. Colas JF, Schoenwolf GC. Towards a cellular and molecular understanding of neurulation. *Dev Dyn* 2001;**221**:117–45.
9. Stemple DL. Structure and function of the notochord: an essential organ for chordate development. *Development* 2005;**132**:2503–12.
10. Gomez C, Ozbudak EM, Wunderlich J, *et al.* Control of segment number in vertebrate embryos. *Nature* 2008;**454**:335–9.
11. Tortori-Donati P, Fondelli MP, Rossi A, *et al.* Segmental spinal dysgenesis: neuroradiologic findings with clinical and embryologic correlation. *AJNR Am J Neuroradiol* 1999;**20**:445–56.
12. Carstens MH. Nerual tube programming and the pathogenesis of craniofacial clefts, Part I. The neuromeric organization of the head and neck. In Sarnat HB, Curatolo P, eds. *Handbook Of Clinical Neurology: Malformations of the Nervous System*. New York: Elsevier, 2008, pp.247–64.
13. Piscol K. [Blood supply of the spinal cord and its clinical importance.] *Schriftenr Neurol* 1972;81–91.

14. Thron AK, Rossberg C, Mironov A. *Vascular Anatomy of the Spinal Cord: Neuroradiological Investigations and Clinical Syndromes*. New York: Springer, 1988.

15. Cobb S. Haemangioma of the spinal cord: associated with skin naevi of the same metamere. *Ann Surg* 1915;**62**:641–9.

16. Santillan A, Nacarino V, Greenberg E, *et al*. Vascular anatomy of the spinal cord. *J Neurointerv Surg* 2012;**4**:67–74.

17. Tadie M, Hernet J, Aaron C. [Le dispositif proctecteur anti-reflux des veins de la moelle.] *Neruochirurgie* 1979;**25**:28–30.

18. van der Kuip M. Hoogland PV, Groen RJ. Human radicular veins: regulation of venous reflux in the absence of valves. *Anat Rec* 1999;**254**:173–80.

19. Virchow R. *Die Krankhaften Geschwulste*. Berlin: Virchow, 1865.

20. Wyburn-Mason R. *The Vascular Abnormalities and Tumours of the Spinal Cord and its Membranes*. St. Louis: Mosby, 1943.

21. Anson JA, Spetzler RF. Interventional neuroradiology for spinal pathology. *Clin Neurosurg* 1992;**39**:388–417.

22. Heros RC, Debrun GM, Ojemann RG, *et al*. Direct spinal arteriovenous fistula: a new type of spinal AVM. Case report. *J Neurosurg* 1986;**64**:134–9.

23. Berenstein A, Lasjaunias P. Spinal cord arteriovenous malformations. In Lasjaunias P, Berenstein A, terBrugge KG, eds. *Surgical neuroangiography, Vol. 5: Endovascular Treatment of Spine and Spinal Cord Lesions*. New York: Springer, 1992, pp. 24–109.

24. Rodesch G, Hurth M, Alvarez H, *et al*. Classification of spinal cord arteriovenous shunts: proposal for a reappraisal: the Bicêtre experience with 155 consecutive patients treated between 1981 and 1999. *Neurosurgery* 2002;**51**:374–9.

25. Govani FS, Shovlin CL. Hereditary haemorrhagic telangiectasia: a clinical and scientific review. *Eur J Hum Genet* 2009;**17**:860–71.

26. Strom RG, Derdeyn CP, Moran CJ, *et al*. Frequency of spinal arteriovenous malformations in patients with unexplained myelopathy. *Neurology* 2006;**66**:928–31.

27. Gilbertson JR, Miller GM, Goldman MS, *et al*. Spinal dural arteriovenous fistulas: MR and myelographic findings. *AJNR Am J Neuroradiol* 1995;**16**:2049–57.

28. Spain RI, Stuckert E, Sharan A, *et al*. Case report: spinal dural arteriovenous fistulas: MR and myelographic findings. *Hospital Physician* 2009;**45**:33–8.

29. Rosenblum B, Oldfield EH, Doppman JL, *et al*. Spinal arteriovenous malformations: a comparison of dural arteriovenous fistulas and intradural AVMs in 81 patients. *J Neurosurg* 1987;**67**:795–802.

30. Symon L, Kuyama H, Kendall B. Dural arteriovenous malformations of the spine. Clinical features and surgical results in 55 cases. *J Neurosurg* 1984;**60**:238–47.

31. Mourier KL, Gobin YP, George B, *et al*. Intradural perimedullary arteriovenous fistulae: results of surgical and endovascular treatment in a series of 35 cases. *Neurosurgery* 1993;**32**:885–91.

32. Lasjaunias P. *Vascular Diseases in Neonates, Infants and Children: Interventional Neuroradiology Management*. Berlin: Springer, 1997, pp. 531–64.

33. Kendall BE, Logue V. Spinal epidural angiomatous malformations draining into intrathecal veins. *Neuroradiology* 1977;**13**:181–9.

34. Tadie M, Hemet J, Freger P, *et al*. Morphological and functional anatomy of spinal cord veins. *J Neuroradiol* 1985;**12**:3–20.

35. Willinsky R, Lasjaunias P, terBrugge K, *et al*. Angiography in the investigation of spinal dural arteriovenous fistula. A protocol with application of the venous phase. *Neuroradiology* 1990;**32**:114–16.

36. Bowen BC, DePrima S, Pattany PM, *et al*. MR angiography of normal intradural vessels of the thoracolumbar spine. *AJNR Am J Neuroradiol* 1996;**17**:483–94.

37. Yaşargil MG, Symon L, Teddy PJ. Arteriovenous malformations of the spinal cord. *Adv Tech Stand Neurosurg* 1984;**11**:61–102.

38. McCutcheon IE, Doppman JL, Oldfield EH. Microvascular anatomy of dural arteriovenous abnormalities of the spine: a microangiographic study. *J Neurosurg* 1996;**84**:215–20.

39. Benhaiem N, Poirier J, Hurth M. Arteriovenous fistulae of the meninges draining into the spinal veins. A histological study of 28 cases. *Acta Neuropathol* 1983;**62**:103–11.

40. Manelfe C, Lazorthes G, Roulleau J. [Arteries of the human spinal dura mater.] *Acta Radiol Diagn (Stockh)* 1972;**13**:829–41.

41. Merland JJ, Riche MC, Chiras J. Intraspinal extramedullary arteriovenous fistulae draining into the medullary veins. *J Neuroradiol* 1980;**7**:271–320.

42. Criscuolo GR, Oldfield EH, Doppman JL. Reversible acute and subacute myelopathy in patients with dural arteriovenous fistulas. Foix–Alajouanine syndrome reconsidered. *J Neurosurg* 1989;**70**:354–9.

43. Toossi S, Josephson SA, Hetts SW, *et al*. Utility of MRI in spinal arteriovenous fistula. *Neurology* 2012;**79**:25–30.

44. Meder JF, Devaux B, Merland JJ, *et al*. Spontaneous disappearance of a spinal dural arteriovenous fistula. *AJNR Am J Neuroradiol* 1995;**16**:2058–62.

45. Muraszko KM, Oldfield EH. Vascular malformations of the spinal cord and dura. *Neurosurg Clin N Am* 1990;**1**:631–52.

46. Doppman JL, Di CG, Ommaya AK. Percutaneous embolization of spinal cord arteriovenous malformations. *J Neurosurg* 1971;**34**:48–55.

47. van Dijk JM, terBrugge KG, Willinsky RA, *et al*. Multidisciplinary management of spinal dural arteriovenous fistulas: clinical presentation and long-term follow-up in 49 patients. *Stroke* 2002;**33**:1578–83.

48. Sleiman M, Leclerc X, Lejeune JP, *et al*. [Clinical aspects and treatment of dural-spinal arteriovenous fistulas with perimedullary venous drainage. 10 cases.] *Neurochirurgie* 1999;**45**:276–85.

49. Szajner M, Weill A, Piotin M, *et al*. Endovascular treatment of a cervical paraspinal arteriovenous malformation via arterial and venous approaches. *AJNR Am J Neuroradiol* 1999;**20**:1097–9.

50. Kiyosue H, Tanoue S, Okahara M, *et al*. Spinal ventral epidural arteriovenous fistulas of the lumbar spine: angioarchitecture and endovascular treatment. *Neuroradiology* 2013;**55**:327–36.

51. Willinsky R, terBrugge K, Montanera W, *et al*. Spinal epidural arteriovenous fistulas: arterial and venous approaches

to embolization. *AJNR Am J Neuroradiol* 1993;**14**:812–17.

52. Hurth M, Houdard R, Djindjian R, *et al.* Arteriovenous malformations of the spinal cord. Clinical, anatomic, and therapeutic considerations. A series of 150 cases. *Prog Neurol Surg* 1978;**9**:238–66.

53. Rodesch G, Hurth M, Alvarez H, *et al.* Angio-architecture of spinal cord arteriovenous shunts at presentation. Clinical correlations in adults and children. The Bicêtre experience on 155 consecutive patients seen between 1981 and 1999. *Acta Neurochir (Wien)* 2004;**146**:217–26.

54. Kreppel D, Antoniadis G, Seeling W. Spinal hematoma: a literature survey with meta-analysis of 613 patients. *Neurosurg Rev* 2003;**26**:1–49.

55. Biondi A, Merland JJ, Hodes JE, *et al.* Aneurysms of spinal arteries associated with intramedullary arteriovenous malformations. II. Results of AVM endovascular treatment and hemodynamic considerations. *AJNR Am J Neuroradiol* 1992;**13**:923–31.

56. Aminoff MJ, Logue V. The prognosis of patients with spinal vascular malformations. *Brain* 1974;**97**:211–18.

57. Connolly ES, Jr., Zubay GP, McCormick PC, *et al.* The posterior approach to a series of glomus (type II) intramedullary spinal cord arteriovenous malformations. *Neurosurgery* 1998;**42**:774–85.

58. Djindjian M, Djindjian R, Rey A, *et al.* Intradural extramedullary spinal arterio-venous malformations fed by the anterior spinal artery. *Surg Neurol* 1977;**8**:85–93.

59. Rodesch G, Hurth M, Alvarez H, *et al.* Spinal cord intradural arteriovenous fistulae: anatomic, clinical, and therapeutic considerations in a series of 32 consecutive patients seen between 1981 and 2000 with emphasis on endovascular therapy. *Neurosurgery* 2005;**57**:973–83.

60. Lim SM, Choi IS, David CA. Spinal arteriovenous fistulas of the filum terminale. *AJNR Am J Neuroradiol* 2011;**32**:1846–50.

61. Rodesch G, Hurth M, Alvarez H, *et al.* Embolization of spinal cord arteriovenous shunts: morphological and clinical follow-up and results: review of 69 consecutive cases. *Neurosurgery* 2003;**53**:40–9.

Chapter

22 Radiosurgical basics for the treatment of arteriovenous malformations: indications and techniques

Jason P. Sheehan and Chun-Po Yen

Introduction

The concept of radiosurgery, proposed by Leksell [1] in 1951, was a milestone in contemporary neurosurgery and changed the management of many neurological pathologies including arteriovenous malformations (AVMs).

Leksell drew upon the experiences of his predecessors. The utilization of radiation to treat AVMs dated back to 1921 when Magnus operated for an AVM at the motor cortex [2]. Surgical removal was aborted because of the high possibility of neurological deficits. Following a decompressive craniectomy, the patient was treated with radium therapy and was free of seizures two years after radiotherapy. No imaging or histological study was available in this case.

Cushing and Bailey reported the first successful surgery for an AVM [3]. They explored a vascular tumor and felt that the lesion could not be attacked without fatal hemorrhage. The patient was treated with radiotherapy because of frequent epileptic seizures. When the lesion was re-explored three years later, the tangle of pulsating vessels previously encountered was largely thrombosed and transformed into a multitude of small bloodless shreds, which could be easily separated from the adjacent normal cortex.

This discovery led to intense interest in the use of radiation for AVMs, but the initial results were not encouraging [4–6]. Although some studies with small numbers of patients provided support for a possible value of ionizing radiation in treatment [7], most did not provide imaging or histology proof of the efficacy. Despite some occasional successes, radiotherapy was often used as a last resort and until 1970 it had been considered ineffective and abandoned [6].

With the introduction of the gamma knife, the potential value of radiation for AVMs was reassessed. Contributing factors included an increasing body of evidence that the cells constituting the vessel wall were responsive to ionizing radiation. Long-term angiographic follow-up of a small series of AVMs treated with fractionated radiation by Johnson in the 1950s revealed that the AVMs were obliterated in 45% of patients [8].

In 1970, Steiner *et al.* at the Karolinska Institute in Stockholm performed the first radiosurgical treatment for an AVM [9]. The patient refused surgery, and, given the patient's renal insufficiency, the risks of surgery were considered too high. Although the intention was to deliver focused radiation to the nidus, because only small collimators were available with the early gamma knife model, the feeding arteries were targeted and 25 Gy was given as the prescription dose to the 50% isodose line. On angiography 19 months after treatment, the feeding vessels were obliterated and the malformations no longer filled. Subsequently, large collimators were available to cover the AVM nidi and more patients were treated successfully. Today more than 50 000 patients with AVMs have been treated with gamma knife radiosurgery (GKS) and many more with linear accelerator-based radiosurgery. Stereotactic radiosurgery has been proven to be a safe and effective treatment alternative for AVMs.

Radiobiology of radiosurgery

While the controversy concerning the usefulness of radiation in the management of AVMs continued, a wealth of evidence on the effects of ionizing radiation beams on blood vessels became available.

Both X-rays and gamma rays induce ionization and a state of molecular excitation in any material they traverse and can trigger physical and chemical events at a cellular level. Ionizing radiation interacts with water molecules by stripping an electron from a hydrogen atom, resulting in a fast electron and an ionized water molecule. The resulting fast electrons interact with more water molecules through additional ionizing events. The positively charged water molecule exhibits a short half-life before dissociating into a hydrogen ion and a free hydroxyl radical. The hydroxyl radical is reactive and has sufficient energy to break chemical bonds in nearby molecules. The most sensitive target of ionizing radiation is the DNA. The manifestations of radiation damage at the cellular level are non-specific. The degree of responsiveness of cells to ionizing radiation defines the radiation sensitivity or resistance of the biological tissues.

Comprehensive Management of Arteriovenous Malformations of the Brain and Spine, ed. Robert F. Spetzler, Douglas S. Kondziolka, Randall T. Higashida, and M. Yashar S. Kalani. Published by Cambridge University Press.

Radiation effects on normal vessels

Early radiation-induced changes in small vessels include swelling, degeneration, and necrosis of endothelial cells. Hyperemia, thrombi, and fissuring of the vascular walls with punctate hemorrhages can be observed. The fibroblastic activity increases with subsequent fibrosis [10]. The initially scattered and subtle changes progress, with increasing areas of the small vessel undergoing degenerative and fibrotic changes. Degenerative intimal, medial, and adventitial changes also occur in medium-sized muscular arteries. However, the larger arteries are less severely damaged as are the arterioles and capillaries.

During the late period after radiation, progressive proliferation of the endothelial cells and subendothelial connective tissue result in narrowing or total occlusion of the lumen of small vessels. In large vessels, proliferation of smooth muscle within the media in addition to proliferation of endothelial linings may occur.

Histopathology of arteriovenous malformations after radiosurgery

Cushing and Bailey were the first to describe the histology of an AVM treated with fractionated radiation: "... the intima of the arteries greatly proliferated so that the lumen was occasionally completely occluded" [3].

The earliest pathological changes of vessels of AVMs following radiosurgery are endothelial or subendothelial. The endothelium either is denuded or the endothelial lining is disrupted from the underlying vessel wall. A few leukocytes, proteinaceous material, or debris are visible in the lacunes of the intima. There are proliferating or migrating spindle cells. The spaces in the intima are caused by leakage of fluid across the damaged endothelium into the intima.

Subsequent pathological changes are subendothelial and intimomedial proliferation of smooth muscle cells with elaboration of extracellular matrix components. Proliferation of intimal smooth muscle cells around the wall circumference produces concentric or eccentric narrowing of the vessel lumen.

In later stages, progressive cellular degeneration and increased matrix density in thickened vessel walls are visible. End-stage vessels display obliteration of the entire vascular structure by hyalinization. Occasionally, end-stage vessels contain one or multiple endothelium-lined small lumina containing erythrocytes. These histopathological changes are a function of time after radiosurgery and tend to occur in smaller vessels [11].

An important feature of the radiation-induced effects is that the pathological changes are concentric or eccentric involving all or nearly all of the vessel wall circumference. However, adjacent vessels of similar size sometimes show marked variation in radiation effects, suggesting that different vessels may have different radiation susceptibilities or develop changes at different rates. This may explain the occasionally non-uniform outcomes following radiosurgery in spite of using similar treatment parameters.

Decision making for radiosurgery

The decision to treat an AVM with GKS should take into consideration the following factors:

- the natural history of the disease and that patient's AVM
- whether the AVM ruptured or was incidentally diagnosed
- the parameters of the patient including age and medical and neurological status
- the variables of the AVM including its size and its relationship to surrounding brain structures as determined by MRI or CT, and the presence of intra- and perinidal aneurysms as well as draining veins (i.e., superficial, deep, or both)
- the anticipated benefit–risk ratio of the available therapeutic alternatives
- the expectation of the patient.

In general, radiosurgery is performed for small to medium-sized AVMs in deep brain locations. However, given its less invasive nature and favorable benefit–risk ratio, superficial AVMs amenable to surgery have been treated with radiosurgery. In an AVM that has no history of rupture, the risk of hemorrhage in the interval between treatment and subsequent cure is not high. Patients with a prior history of hemorrhage, however, are at a higher risk of repeated hemorrhage, particularly in the first year after the rupture. Also AVMs with certain angioarchitecture, such as peri- or intranidal aneurysms or draining vein stenosis, carry a higher risk of hemorrhage. Other options such as embolization or microsurgery should be explored. Radiosurgery may be recommended in AVMs that would require a difficult surgical approach, but microsurgery should never be easily discarded because it provides, if successful, immediate cure. Radiosurgery is also indicated in patients in whom other medical conditions preclude surgery or increase the risk of anesthesia. Finally, the patient's desire dictates the ultimate decision.

Modality of radiosurgery

The goal of radiosurgery for AVMs is to deliver a high radiation dose to the AVM nidus, typically in a single session, while largely sparing the surrounding brain of significant dose, thereby minimizing undesirable effects from the treatment. The modalities for delivering radiosurgery have increased over time. Reports in the literature exist for various radiosurgical modalities including the gamma knife, isocentrically mounted linear accelerators (e.g., Novalis, TrueBeam, Synergy) [12–15], charged particle accelerators (e.g., proton beam), and robotic linear accelerators (e.g., CyberKnife) [16]. Regardless of modality, radiosurgical devices achieve the desired characteristics of small fields, steep dose fall-off, and highly accurate targeting through the use of two fundamental principles: superposition of beams and stereotactic targeting.

Radiosurgery achieves highly conformal dose distributions by spreading the total energy delivered over a targeted volume, either through the superposition of many small beams on the target or through the use of non-coplanar arcs (where each arc can be thought of as a large number of small beams). The energy of any given single beam is too low to cause a significant biological effect. However, the superposition of all of the beams at the target delivers a substantial amount of radiation, sufficient to cause the desired biological changes and resulting in the occlusion of the AVM nidus.

The details of beam superposition vary by modality. In the case of the Gamma Knife 201 (or 192 depending on the model of the unit), individual beams are precisely aimed at a focal point to achieve this effect. The beams are collimated through individual beam channels cut into a tungsten collimator. In older units, this was achieved with a combination of internal primary and secondary collimation and external "helmet"-based final collimation. In the case of the newer gamma knife model, Leksell Gamma Knife Perfexion (Elekta Instruments, Atlanta, GA, USA), the collimator assembly is entirely within the main body of the unit [17].

For early linear accelerators adapted for radiosurgery, finely collimated beams were achieved through the use of circular collimator "cones" that could be attached to the accessory tray of the accelerator [18]. Many currently available accelerators are equipped with micro-multileaf collimators that can achieve irregularly shaped beams that can more precisely conform to the target morphology [19]. Both approaches are often used with a non-coplanar arc technique, which directs the fields at the target while spreading out the overall delivered energy [20].

The ability to create a focal, high-dose distribution does little good in itself if there is no way to precisely and accurately aim the radiation at the target. This problem is elegantly solved using the principles of stereotaxy. Traditionally in intracranial radiosurgery, a rigid frame is fixed to the skull. This frame defines a stereotactic space akin to a coordinate system by which any point within the brain can be localized. Fiducial markers, which are visible in stereotactic imaging as part of the procedure, are directly related to this coordinate system; the target can, therefore, be visualized and localized in "stereotactic space." Accuracy and precision of treatment are thus guaranteed by stereotactic frame placement and the assurance that this target will not move during a treatment because of the rigid head frame. More recent innovations in radiosurgery have included frameless stereotaxy [21]. In these systems image guidance plays an important role both before and during the procedure. Less invasive restraint systems such as thermoplastic masks are used in place of the rigid head frame, and periodic imaging is used to track and correct for patient motion. In non-rigid frames, movement along six degrees of freedom must be accounted for through expansion of the planned treatment volume and reregistration of the target related to the source of the ionizing radiation.

Technique of gamma knife radiosurgery

Preoperative management

At the University of Virginia, we perform AVM radiosurgery with the gamma knife. Patients are evaluated at least one day before the procedure. Antiepileptic medications are used for patients already on those medications and for patients with supratentorial AVMs. Dexamethasone, routinely given in the past during GKS, is generally used if there is pre-existing edema around the AVM nidus.

Frame placement

The placement of the head frame is performed in the operating room. The patients are placed in sitting position and given intravenous sedation, usually propofol and short-acting narcotics (e.g., fentanyl). The frame is held in position by a disposable strap fashioned with Velcro ends. This holds the frame in position while the pins are secured and eliminates the need for earplugs.

The space available within the gamma knife is limited as is the three-dimensional coordinate system within the head frame itself. For these reasons, care must be taken to shift the placement of the frame in the direction of the pathology if it is far off the center of the brain. The shifting of the frame is of less importance with the gamma knife model Perfexion, which has a much larger treatment volume than earlier gamma knife models.

Imaging and dose planning

The accuracy of radiosurgery is ultimately dependent on the neurosurgeon's ability to visualize the intended target. Consequently, the technique would be impossible without imaging studies that allow three-dimensional views of anatomical structures in the brain. In planning the treatment of an AVM, digital subtraction angiography remains the imaging modality of choice. As with MRI and CT, images are acquired using a fiducial system. However, digital subtraction angiography is based on projections (usually anteroposterior and lateral but occasionally oblique) rather than tomographic information. Images need to be geometrically corrected to account for the curvature of the image intensifier screen before importing the images into the treatment planning system. Gadolinium-enhanced MRI/MR angiography is also used to correlate the extent of the AVM nidus with angiography and additionally provides the contour of AVM nidus in axial plane. It helps to define the three-dimensional structure of the AVM and confirms angiographically obtained information (Fig. 22.1). However, it is sometimes difficult to differentiate the nidus from the feeding arteries and draining veins, and so MRI can overestimate the size of the AVM.

The gamma knife

The gamma knife models C and 4C have a body that contains the radiation sources and a treatment couch that moves the patient into the unit. Within the body are approximately 201 cobalt-60 source capsules, which are aligned with two internal collimators that direct the gamma radiation toward the center of the unit. A third external collimator helmet is attached to the treatment couch. Four external collimator helmets are provided and they have fixed diameter apertures that create an isocenter of diameters 4, 8, 14, or 18 mm. By changing external

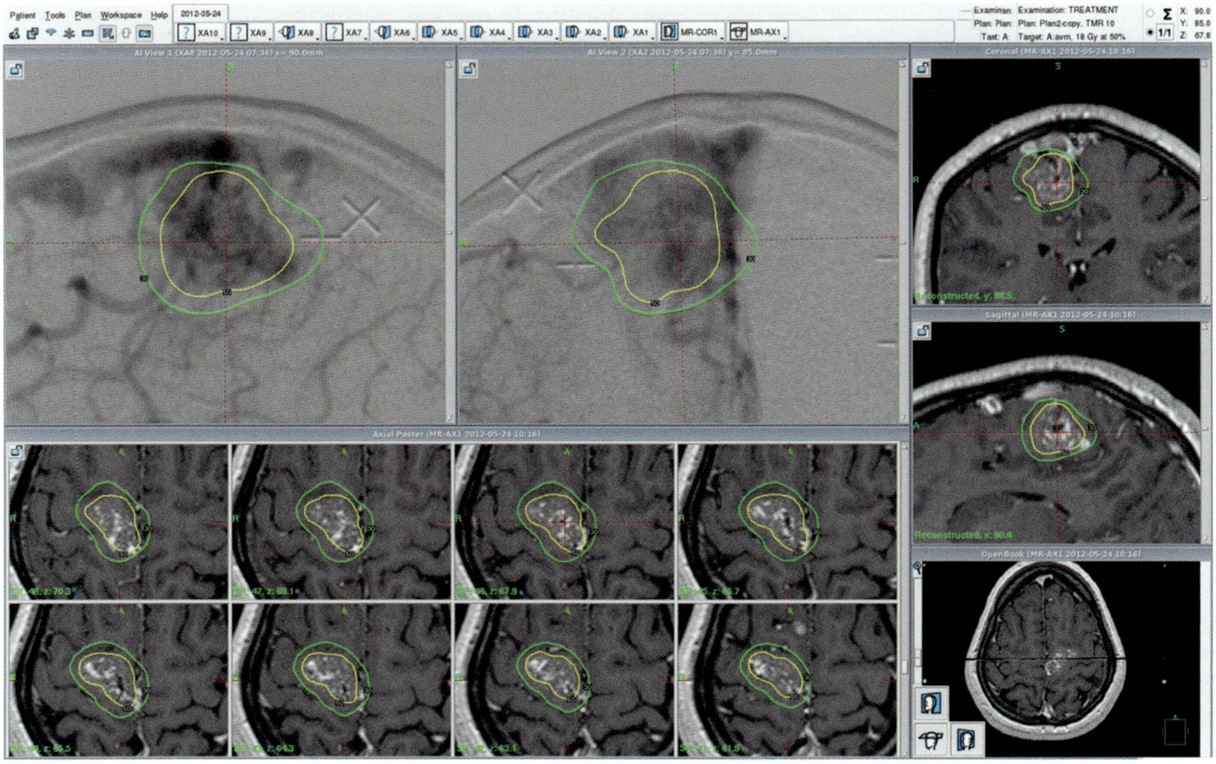

Fig. 22.1. A radiosurgical dose plan for use of the gamma knife to treat an arteriovenous malformation. The 50% isodose line is depicted by the yellow contour and the 30% isodose line by the green contour.

collimator helmets, the diameter of the roughly spherical isocenter can be varied. The 201 individual collimators within the helmet are machined to exact standards to direct the 201 beams of gamma radiation to a common point where they intersect, creating the isocenter (or shot). The frame attached to the patient's head is adjusted within the collimator helmet so that the area to be treated is at that point of intersection.

In Perfexion, the central body contains 192 cobalt-60 sources that are grouped into eight independent sectors and collimators are entirely internal to the radiation body. Each source sector is housed in an aluminum frame, which is attached to sector drive motors at the rear of the radiation body via linear graphite bushings. There are 576 collimators machined into 12 cm thick tungsten in five concentric rings to align with the source assembly configurations. Each source has three available collimators (4, 8, and 16 mm) as well as shielded positions ("blocked") to shield a critical structure. To achieve a particular collimation, the sector drive motors move the sources along their bushings to the correct position over the appropriate collimator opening. These changes allow a single isocenter composed of simultaneous differing beam diameters to optimize dose distribution shape for each individual shot.

Radiosurgical delivery

After the radiosurgical plan has been devised, the patient is moved onto the gamma knife couch and the y and z coordinates for the first exposure are set on the frame attached to the patient's head. The patient's head is then placed within the collimator helmet and secured on either side by trunions and the x coordinate is set. A gamma angle can also be set to adjust the patient's head relative to the collimator focal point. The patient's head is suspended by the frame within the helmet. The exposure time of the corresponding isocenter is entered at the control panel and the session then commences with the entire couch being mechanically pulled into the body of the gamma knife unit. The external collimator helmet locks into place with the internal collimators. After each exposure, the patient is withdrawn from the collimator helmet and the process is repeated. Necessary changes of the collimator helmet are made as needed according to the plan. The introduction of the automatic positioning system for the C and 4C models, a system that sets the coordinates by six independent motors just outside the radiation field, has led to shorter treatment times, enhanced selectivity, and better workflow.

In Perfexion, the treatment table itself acts as a positioning device (the patient position system). The stereotactic frame is attached to the treatment table via a removable frame adapter, which attaches to the frame and acts as an interface with the treatment table. Treatment execution with Perfexion is a fully automated process including set up of the stereotactic coordinates, alignment of different sector positions, and set up of exposure times. Obviously these changes will not affect the efficacy of the treatment but will make the process simpler for the operator.

Radiosurgery for AVMs is typically accomplished with 30 to 90 minutes of beam time in a gamma knife unit.

Postoperative care

At the end of the treatment the frame is removed from the patient's head. There is usually a sensation of tightening and discomfort reported by the patient during removal. At least two pairs of hands should be available to steady the frame and prevent injury by pins as they are removed. Venous bleeding when it occurs can be controlled with hand-held pressure for a few minutes. The occasional arterial bleeder might require a suture. After frame removal, steri-strips are used to oppose the skin edges for optimal cosmesis and a modest dressing is applied.

Follow-up

The need for adequate and thorough clinical and imaging follow-up cannot be overemphasized. Clinical and imaging responses as well as radiosurgery-related complications and hemorrhage during the latency period should be evaluated. We recommend that an MRI be performed at intervals of 6–12 months following radiosurgery until there are signs of AVM obliteration. When an MRI demonstrates AVM occlusion, follow-up cerebral angiography should be performed to confirm complete obliteration of the nidus. Thereafter, patients are advised to have further MRI every three to five years to rule out delayed adverse effects. To evaluate the outcome and causes of treatment failures, all the images are ideally analyzed by both the neurosurgeon and a neuroradiologist interested and experienced in the interpretation of MRI and angiography.

Degree of obliteration of arteriovenous malformations

Total obliteration of the AVM after radiosurgery was defined by Steiner and Lindquist as "complete absence of former nidus, normalization of afferent and efferent vessels, and a normal circulation time on high-quality rapid serial subtracted angiography" (Fig. 22.2) [22]. Any remaining nidus, regardless of its size, is considered partial obliteration. Subtotal obliteration of an AVM means the angiographic persistence of an early filling draining vein without a demonstrable nidus [23]. The early filling venous drainage suggests that some shunting still persists. Based on our experience and other published studies [23,24], no hemorrhage was observed in this subgroup of patients in spite of the fact that, by definition, the AVM nidus is still patent as indicated by the shunting.

Radiosurgery obliterates the AVM nidi in a delayed fashion. During the typical latency period of two to three years, patients remain at risk for hemorrhage. Whether radiosurgery changes the hemorrhage risk of a still-patent

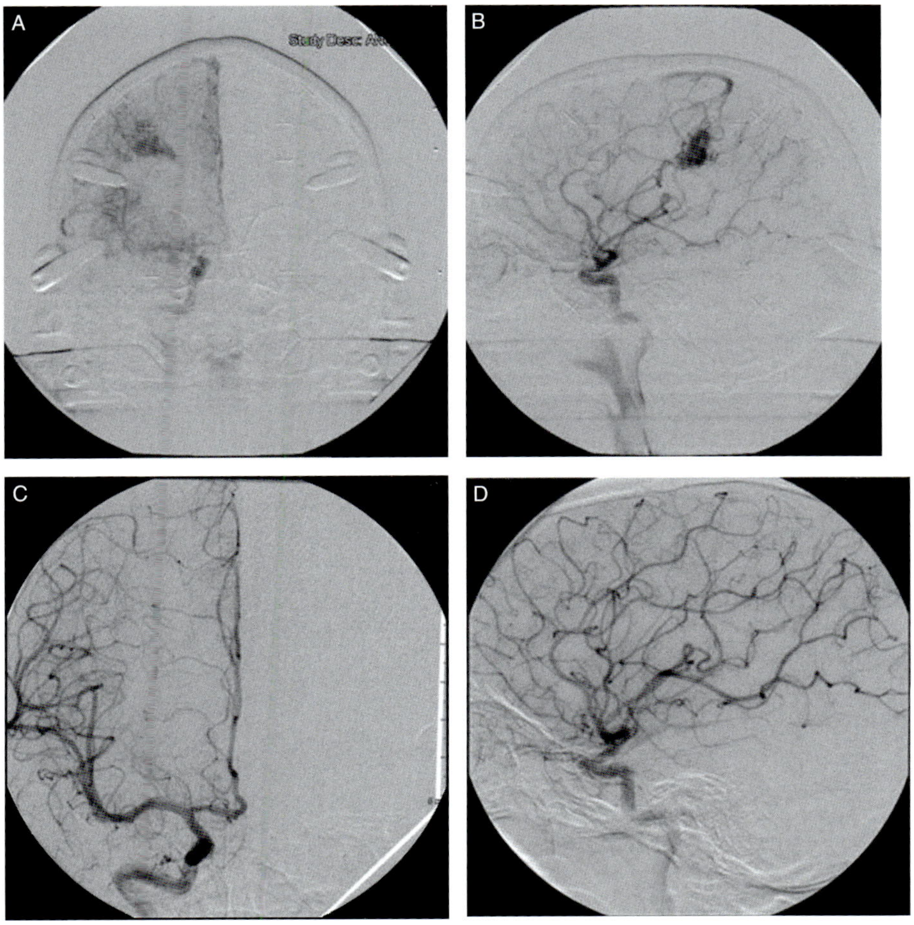

Fig. 22.2. Obliteration of an arteriovenous malformation by radiosurgery. (A,B) Angiography at the time of stereotactic radiosurgery. (C,D) Angiography 24 months after radiosurgery with the arteriovenous malformation obliterated. (A,C anterioposterior views; B,D, lateral views.)

AVM remains the subject of debate. Histopathological studies have shown that detectable radiation effects can occur as early as three months after radiosurgery and remain for years [11]. Thickness of the intima as well as proliferation and accumulation of subendothelial matrix decrease the tension of vessel wall [25]. Furthermore, thrombosis or occlusion of vascular channels in the nidi decreases the number of patent vessels and so there are fewer vessels prone to rupture. Recent studies demonstrated that the risk of AVM hemorrhage decreased even during the latency period [26,27]. Based on over 1200 patients with AVMs treated at the University of Virginia with long-term follow-up, the annual hemorrhage rate calculated between diagnosis and GKS of AVMs was 6.6% and the rate reduced to 2.5% following GKS. In the subgroup of patients with preradiosurgical hemorrhage, the postradiosurgical annual hemorrhage rate was 2.8%, significantly lower than the preradiosurgical hemorrhage rate of 10.4%. In the subgroup of patients who had never had a hemorrhage before GKS, the postradiosurgical annual hemorrhage rate was 2.2%, which is also lower than the 3.9% hemorrhage rate calculated during the period from the diagnosis of the AVM to the time of GKS.

In general, angiographic evidence of an absent nidus following radiosurgery indicates that the patient is no longer at risk of AVM-related hemorrhage. However, histological studies have demonstrated that obliterated vessels within the AVMs might contain small capillary-like spaces that are lined by a single layer of endothelial cells and contain red blood cells [11,28]. It is impossible to determine if this represents recanalization of end-stage occluded vessels or neovascularization. Because of their small caliber relative to the rest of vessels in the nidus, it is likely that their presence could not be detected by angiography. However, functionally the small vessels are probably of little significance, and they are at little risk for rebleeding because of their low flow. We interpret them as small vessels without opening and trapped in the hyalinization process of the nidus. Additionally, we have not noticed any patients having a hemorrhage after the AVM nidi are considered to be obliterated based on angiography.

There have been some rare but convincing case reports demonstrating that hemorrhage can occur after an AVM is no longer visible with angiography [29,30]. In two patients undergoing surgery because of hemorrhage and expanding cyst, histological studies demonstrated occlusion of AVMs by thickening of the intimal layer with dense hyalination [30]. Nevertheless, abnormal vessels maintained a small amount of blood flow through a tiny vasculature. The nature of the obliterated AVM nidus resembled that of an angiographically occult AVM in its hemodynamic status.

Recurrence of AVM after complete resection had been reported in surgical series and was also reported in radiosurgical series [29]. Redistribution of blood flow after progressive occlusion of the AVM may have affected immature vessels surrounding the malformations, giving rise to another AVM. These observations emphasize the necessity for continuing follow-up of patients with AVMs even where the nidus was proven to be obliterated. These angiographically occult lesions seem to continue to enhance on CT or MRI [29]. For the time being, MRI seems to be a reasonable screening tool for AVM recurrence.

Adverse effects of radiosurgery

Radiosurgery is a minimally invasive procedure with few adverse effects associated with the procedure during the acute stage. Patients might have headache or nausea with prolonged frame placement. However, mid- to long-term adverse effects do occur occasionally [31–33].

Increased signals on T_2-weighted MRI, usually interpreted as radiation-induced changes or brain edema, occur in one-third of patients, usually around a few months to one year following radiosurgery [31]. These changes can be just a few millimeters of increased signal without clinical significance or can be of moderate to severe extent, causing headache, seizure, or neurological deficits. Several mechanisms have been proposed to explain the radiation changes, including radiation injury of glial cells, endothelial cell damage followed by breakdown of the blood–brain barrier, excessive generation of free radicals, and autoimmune response. Given that radiation-induced changes occur more commonly in patients with AVMs than in those with tumors treated with radiosurgery, and quite often the extent of radiation changes develop beyond the high dose radiation field, vascular injury probably plays an important role [34]. We have reported patients with early draining vein thrombosis accompanying radiation-induced changes and brain edema [34]. Of note, the radiation-induced changes associated with draining vein thrombosis tend to be more extensive and this complication more likely happens in nidi with a single draining vein.

Cyst formation is another long-term adverse effect following radiosurgery. From our series of over 1200 patients with follow-up MRI, 1.6% have cyst formation. This is usually a self-limited condition, but on occasion the cyst can expand and pose neurological deficits. Breakdown of the blood–brain barrier with leakage of exudate is the possible cause of cyst formation, as we have observed that most patients had varying degrees of radiation changes before the development of a cyst [33]. Recently, microhemorrhage from angiomatous lesions developing within the degenerated nidus or adjacent brain have been reported to be the cause of some expanding cysts [35].

Secondary tumors following radiosurgery are a rare but concerning complication given that most patients with AVMs are treated at a relatively young age [32]. We have found meningiomas in two pediatric patients 12 years after GKS for AVMs. Another patient, who underwent proton beam radiotherapy and GKS for a posterior fossa AVM, developed a high-grade glioma 20 years after treatment. There are also several anecdotal cases reported in the literature [36,37]. Although these events are rare, given the large number of patients with AVMs treated with radiosurgery, one should be aware that a secondary tumor is a long-term event and most of the patients having radiosurgery do not have follow-up for longer than 10 to 20 years. Based on our material, the incidence of secondary tumors would be as high as 1.1% if we only consider patients who had MRI follow-up after 10 years.

Conclusions

In recent years, radiosurgery has become one of the most important treatment tools for AVMs. The neurosurgeons considering the best interests of a given patient will have to be familiar with the indications and technique of radiosurgery and decide when to use microsurgery, embolization, or radiosurgery, alone or in combination.

References

1. Leksell L. The stereotaxic method and radiosurgery of the brain. *Acta Chir Scand* 1951;**102**:316–19.
2. Yaşargil MG. *Microneurosurgery*. New York: Thieme, 1988.
3. Cushing H, Bailey P. *Tumors Arising from the Blood-Vessels of the Brain*. Springfield, IL: Charles C Thomas, 1928.
4. French LA, Chou SN, Story JL. Cerebrovascular malformations. *Clin Neurosurg* 1964;**11**:171–82.
5. McKissock W, Hankinson J. The surgical treatment of supratentorial angiomas. *Neurochir Bruxelles Acta Med* 1957;**15**:222–36.
6. Olivecrona H, Ladenheim J. *Congenital Arteriovenous Aneurysms of the Carotid and Vertebral Systems*. Berlin: Springer, 1957.
7. Kjellberg RN, Davis KR, Lyons S, *et al.* Bragg peak proton beam therapy for arteriovenous malformation of the brain. *Clin Neurosurg* 1983;**31**:248–90.
8. Johnson R. Radiotherapy of cerebral angiomas with a note on some problems in diagnosis. In Pia HW, Gleave JRW, Grote E, eds. *Cerebral Angiomas: Advances in Diagnosis and Therapy*. Berlin: Springer, 1975, pp. 256–66.
9. Steiner L, Leksell L, Greitz T, *et al.* Stereotaxic radiosurgery for cerebral arteriovenous malformations. Report of a case. *Acta Chir Scand* 1972;**138**:459–64.
10. Rubin P, Casarett G, Grise JW. The vascular pathophysiology of an irradiated graft. *Am J Roetgenol Radium Ther Nucl Med* 1960;**83**:1097–104.
11. Schneider BF, Eberhard DA, Steiner LE. Histopathology of arteriovenous malformations after gamma knife radiosurgery. *J Neurosurg* 1997;**87**:352–7.
12. Nataf F, Schlienger M, Lefkopoulos D, *et al.* Radiosurgery of cerebral arteriovenous malformations in children: a series of 57 cases. *Int J Radiat Oncol Biol Phys* 2003;**57**:184–95.
13. Schlienger M, Atlan D, Lefkopoulos D, *et al.* LINAC radiosurgery for cerebral arteriovenous malformations: results in 169 patients. *Int J Radiat Oncol Biol Phys* 2000;**46**:1135–42.
14. Voges J, Treuer H, Lehrke R, *et al.* Risk analysis of LINAC radiosurgery in patients with arteriovenous malformation (AVM). *Acta Neurochir Suppl* 1997;**68**:118–23.
15. Saunders WM, Winston KR, Siddon RL, *et al.* Radiosurgery for arteriovenous malformations of the brain using a standard linear accelerator: rationale and technique. *Int J Radiat Oncol Biol Phys* 1988;**15**:441–7.
16. Colombo F, Cavedon C, Casentini L, *et al.* Early results of CyberKnife radiosurgery for arteriovenous malformations. *J Neurosurg* 2009;**111**:807–19.
17. Lindquist C, Paddick I. The Leksell Gamma Knife Perfexion and comparisons with its predecessors. *Neurosurgery* 2007;**61**:130–40.
18. Friedman WA, Bova FJ. The University of Florida radiosurgery system. *Surg Neurol* 1989;**32**:334–42.
19. Benedict SH, Cardinale RM, Wu Q, *et al.* Intensity-modulated stereotactic radiosurgery using dynamic micro-multileaf collimation. *Int J Radiat Oncol Biol Phys* 2001;**50**:751–8.
20. Solberg TD, Boedeker KL, Fogg R, *et al.* Dynamic arc radiosurgery field shaping: a comparison with static field conformal and noncoplanar circular arcs. *Int J Radiat Oncol Biol Phys* 2001;**49**:1481–91.
21. Adler JR, Jr., Chang SD, Murphy MJ, *et al.* The CyberKnife: a frameless robotic system for radiosurgery. *Stereotact Funct Neurosurg* 1997;**69**:124–8.
22. Steiner L, Lindquist C, Steiner M. Radiosurgery. *Adv Tech Stand Neurosurg* 1992;**19**:19–102.
23. Yen CP, Varady P, Sheehan J, *et al.* Subtotal obliteration of cerebral arteriovenous malformations after gamma knife surgery. *J Neurosurg* 2007;**106**:361–9.
24. Abu-Salma Z, Nataf F, Ghossoub M, *et al.* The protective status of subtotal obliteration of arteriovenous malformations after radiosurgery: significance and risk of hemorrhage. *Neurosurgery* 2009;**65**:709–17.
25. Karlsson B, Lax I, Soderman M. Risk for hemorrhage during the 2-year latency period following gamma knife radiosurgery for arteriovenous malformations. *Int J Radiat Oncol Biol Phys* 2001;**49**:1045–51.
26. Yen CP, Sheehan JP, Schwyzer L, *et al.* Hemorrhage risk of cerebral arteriovenous malformations before and during the latency period after gamma knife radiosurgery. *Stroke* 2011;**42**:1691–6.
27. Maruyama K, Shin M, Tago M, *et al.* Radiosurgery to reduce the risk of first hemorrhage from brain arteriovenous malformations. *Neurosurgery* 2007;**60**:453–8.
28. Yamamoto M, Jimbo M, Kobayashi M, *et al.* Long-term results of radiosurgery for arteriovenous malformation: neurodiagnostic imaging and histological studies of angiographically confirmed nidus obliteration. *Surg Neurol* 1992;**37**:219–30.
29. Yun JH, Kwon DH, Lee EJ, *et al.* New nidus formation adjacent to the target site of an arteriovenous malformation treated by Gamma Knife surgery. *J Neurosurg* 2012;**117**(Suppl):120–5.
30. Shin M, Kawahara N, Maruyama K, *et al.* Risk of hemorrhage from an arteriovenous malformation confirmed to have been obliterated on angiography after stereotactic radiosurgery. *J Neurosurg* 2005;**102**:842–6.
31. Yen CP, Matsumoto JA, Wintermark M, *et al.* Radiation-induced imaging changes following Gamma Knife surgery for cerebral arteriovenous malformations. *J Neurosurg* 2013;**118**:63–73.

32. Sheehan J, Yen CP, Steiner L. Gamma knife surgery-induced meningioma. Report of two cases and review of the literature. *J Neurosurg* 2006;**105**:325–9.
33. Pan HC, Sheehan J, Stroila M, *et al.* Late cyst formation following gamma knife surgery of arteriovenous malformations. *J Neurosurg* 2005;**102**(Suppl):124–7.
34. Yen CP, Khaled MA, Schwyzer L, *et al.* Early draining vein occlusion after gamma knife surgery for arteriovenous malformations. *Neurosurgery* 2010;**67**:1293–302.
35. Shuto T, Ohtake M, Matsunaga S. Proposed mechanism for cyst formation and enlargement following gamma knife surgery for arteriovenous malformations. *J Neurosurg* 2012;**117**(Suppl):135–43.
36. Shamisa A, Bance M, Nag S, *et al.* Glioblastoma multiforme occurring in a patient treated with gamma knife surgery. Case report and review of the literature. *J Neurosurg* 2001;**94**:816–21.
37. Berman EL, Eade TN, Brown D, *et al.* Radiation-induced tumor after stereotactic radiosurgery for an arteriovenous malformation: case report. *Neurosurgery* 2007;**61**:E1099.

Chapter 23

Radiosurgery for brain arteriovenous malformations and fistulae

Hideyuki Kano, Douglas S. Kondziolka, L. Dade Lunsford, and John C. Flickinger

Introduction

Arteriovenous malformations (AVMs) of the brain can lead to intracranial hemorrhage, headache, and seizure. The management options include observation, surgical resection, embolization, and stereotactic radiosurgery (SRS). More than one option is often needed in each patient. Surgical resection is often the first procedure recommended for patients with smaller AVMs in non-critical areas of the brain. The Spetzler–Martin grading system has been accepted as an accurate method to predict patient outcomes when resection is performed at centers with extensive vascular expertise [1]. Microsurgical resection for AVMs has been reported to have a low risk of complications for Spetzler–Martin grade I and II AVMs [1]. Hemorrhagic AVMs with intracranial hematomas associated with elevated intracranial pressure may require early clot removal. Complete microsurgical resection has the advantage of eliminating repeat intracranial hemorrhage. Since endovascular embolization is rarely curative but may be effective in reducing AVM flow, it is best performed as a preoperative adjunctive therapy before resection [2].

Stereotactic radiosurgery has been widely used to manage patients with intracranial AVMs. The goal of radiosurgical management of intracranial AVMs is elimination of eventual intracranial hemorrhage risk without creating new neurological deficits. The overall risk of a hemorrhage from untreated intracranial AVM appears to range from 2 to 5% per year [3–6]. The primary disadvantage of SRS lies in the risk of hemorrhage during the latency interval between SRS and AVM total obliteration. Total obliteration appears to reduce the cumulative residual lifetime risk of hemorrhage to 1% or less [7].

Radiosurgery technique

Prior to radiosurgery, patients and their families speak to the treating neurosurgeon, a radiation oncologist, and radiosurgical nurse regarding the procedure. Many watch a teaching videotape available on our website (www.neurosurgery.pitt.edu). Patients older than 13 years of age undergo application of an imaging-compatible stereotactic head frame using local anesthesia supplemented by intravenous conscious sedation. Younger children usually undergo the procedure using general anesthesia. High-resolution axial plane contrast-enhanced stereotactic MRI (short repetition time images and volume-acquisition spoiled gradient-recalled sequences), and whole-head long repetition time imaging studies are then coupled with biplane stereotactic angiography in order to perform dose planning.

Radiosurgical dose planning is performed by the neurosurgeon in conjunction with a radiation oncologist and a medical physicist. For AVMs of irregular volume, multiple isocenter plans are created in order to conform the AVM nidus margin to the selected treatment isodose (usually 50%). The maximal dose is selected based on weighting of various factors such as the AVM volume, brain location, and pertinent clinical history. Through the use of the integrated logistic formula (which predicts a 3% risk of permanent radiation-related complications), a margin dose is selected. We attempt to choose an effective and tolerated dose by balancing the highest obliteration rates achievable with risk factors related to volume and location. Single or multiple isocenter radiation is then performed with a gamma knife (Fig. 23.1). Currently, we use either the Leksell Perfexion or 4C model (Elekta Instruments, Atlanta, GA, USA) to perform radiosurgery. As a last step, the stereotactic frame is removed and a local dressing is used to wrap the head. The patient is either transferred to the recovery room (if general anesthesia was required) or to the frame application room for frame removal. Since the development of the arterial quick-close techniques used during angiography, almost all patients are discharged home the same day. Therapeutic anticonvulsants such as levetiracetam are administered to patients with lobar AVMs. A single intravenous dose of methylprednisolone (20–40 mg) is administered immediately after radiosurgery.

Follow-up

We recommend MRI at 6, 12, 24, and 36 months after radiosurgery in order to assess both the vascular and the parenchymal response. Angiography is requested at three years after radiosurgery if the MRI studies indicate likely obliteration.

Comprehensive Management of Arteriovenous Malformations of the Brain and Spine, ed. Robert F. Spetzler, Douglas S. Kondziolka, Randall T. Higashida, and M. Yashar S. Kalani. Published by Cambridge University Press.

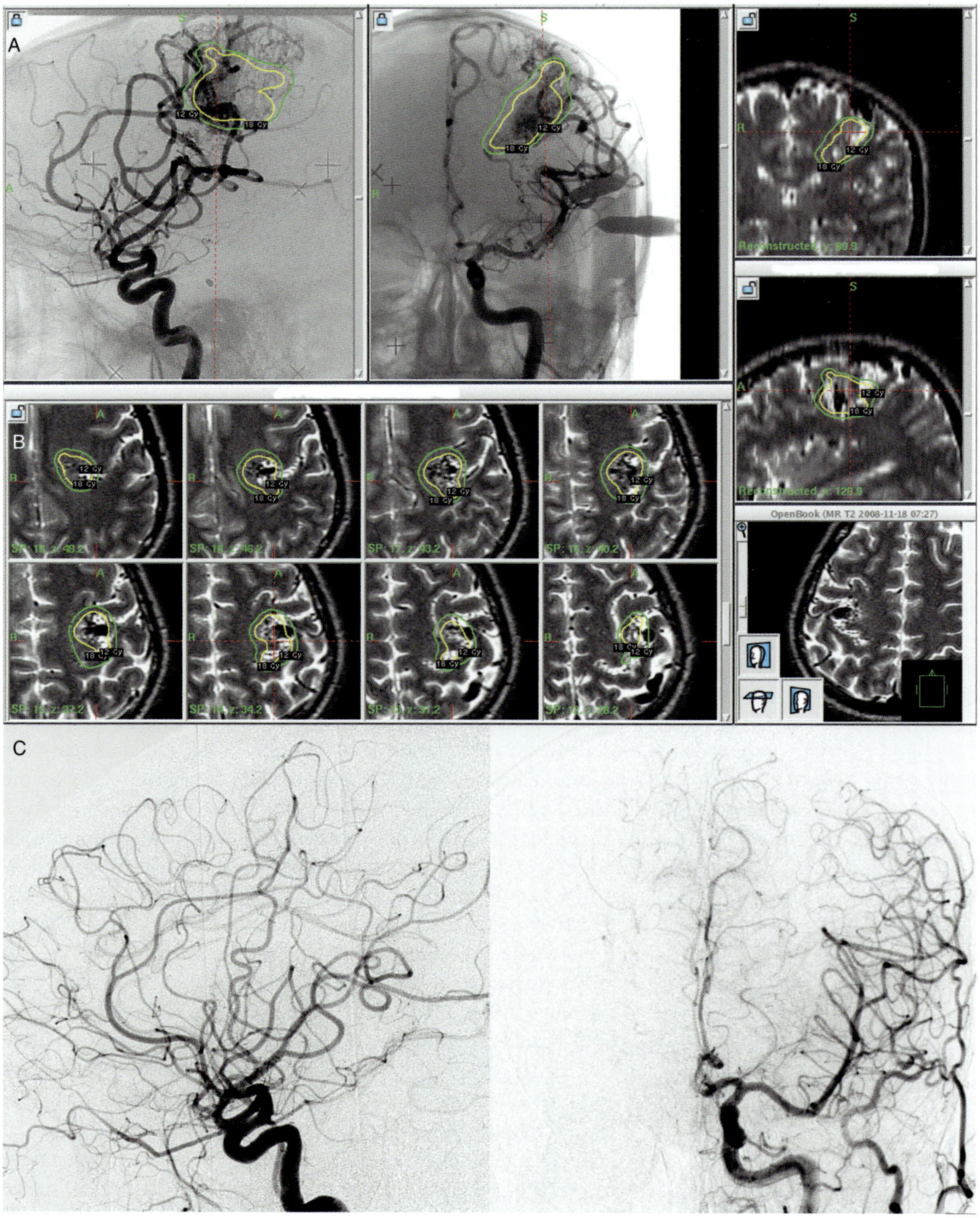

Fig. 23.1. A 26-year-old man with a left parietal arteriovenous malformation with a volume of 8.4 mL at the time of stereotactic radiosurgery. (A,B) Anterior and lateral carotid artery angiography (A) and radiosurgical dose plan (B). The 50% isodose line is depicted by the yellow contour and the 30% isodose line by the green contour. The margin dose was 18 Gy. (C) Anterior and lateral carotid artery angiography obtained 3 years after treatment showed the absence of nidus.

When complete obliteration, or only an early draining vein (a point-in-time finding that always resolves within 12 months), is identified on the follow-up angiography, no further treatment is necessary. For patients who have a small residual AVM nidus more than three to four years after radiosurgery, additional radiosurgery is usually required to complete obliteration.

Total arteriovenous malformations obliteration

The interval between SRS and total obliteration is usually three to four years. During our 25 years of experience with AVMs, we have come to understand that patients may not obtain the final angiography until three or more years have elapsed. The proportion of patients available for the final evaluation ranges from 36 to 82% in various reports [8–10]. Liscak *et al.* [9] reported that AVM obliteration was achieved in 222 of 330 patients (67%) after initial SRS. In their series of patients with a hemorrhage history before SRS, the obliteration rate was 63%. The four-year total obliteration rate after a single SRS was 81%. If a second procedure was required because of initial incomplete obliteration, 81% of those patients proceeded to obliteration. In most previous reports, total AVM obliteration was defined as disappearance of the nidus (AVM shunt) and absence of early venous drainage on angiography. Conventional cerebral angiography is the best technique to confirm that total AVM obliteration has been achieved by SRS. Unfortunately, not all patients are willing to undergo repeat angiography after MRI has shown that their AVM can no longer be visualized. The timing of confirmatory angiography is often delayed after the MRI shows obliteration, sometimes by many years. Pollock *et al.* [10] reported that serial MRI scans were predictive of total obliteration in 84% of patients. Over an additional observational interval, they documented a final predictive value of MRI-identified obliteration of 97%, since repeat angiography eventually showed the disappearance of features such as an early draining vein. In our previous reports [11–16], both MRI and angiographic data were included. The potential slight overestimation of obliteration rates by using MRI are balanced by the tendency to underestimate long-term obliteration rates when based only on early follow-up examinations. We believe it is both reasonable and necessary to use MRI evidence of obliteration to evaluate the outcomes of repeat SRS. The timing of documentation of obliteration is variable since patients may have delayed imaging performed months to years after the requested time of three years.

Our published reports can be summarized as follows. The four-year total obliteration on angiography or MRI after a single-session SRS procedure was 87% in patients with Spetzler–Martin grade I or II AVMs, 64% in children with AVMs, 70% in AVMs of the basal ganglia or thalamus, and 70% in AVMs of the brainstem. There was a higher chance of total obliteration for smaller-volume AVMs and for the application of a higher margin dose.

Subtotal obliteration

Subtotal obliteration of AVMs after SRS implies a complete angiographic disappearance of the AVM nidus but persistence of an early filling draining vein, indicating that residual shunting is still present. Initially there was concern that an early filling draining vein implied residual AVM shunting. Yen *et al.* reported that there was no AVM hemorrhage in 159 subtotally obliterated AVMs at mean follow-up of 3.9 years [17]. This observation that no patient with a subtotally obliterated AVM suffered a rupture (within the follow-up interval) is not compatible with the belief that a residual AVM has the same risk of hemorrhage until obliteration occurs. If additional studies confirm this observation, the data suggest that patients treated by radiosurgery have a reduced rate of hemorrhage even if the AVM is not completely eliminated.

Hemorrhage after stereotactic radiosurgery

Hemorrhages from AVM may range in seriousness from mild headache to a fatal event, with published annual hemorrhage rates in the range 2–5% for untreated AVMs [3–6]. A 24-year follow-up assessment for AVMs in the Finnish population reported an annual hemorrhage rate of 4%. In one natural history study, AVM bleeding was associated with an annual mortality rate of 1% and a combined risk of major morbidity including death of 2.7% each year [6]. After an initial hemorrhage, rebleeding rates varied between 6 and 18% per year [5,18–21]. Stapf *et al.* [22] reported that a hemorrhagic AVM presentation, increasing age, deep brain location, and exclusive deep venous drainage appeared to be independent predictors for AVM hemorrhage during additional years of observation. da Costa *et al.* [23] reported that a hemorrhagic presentation was a significant independent predictor of future bleeding, whereas associated aneurysms, deep venous drainage, and prior embolization were not significantly associated with future bleeding. Yamada *et al.* [24] reported that the annual rehemorrhage rate in patients with AVMs who presented with a bleeding event was 6.84%. In this report, bleeding hazard risks were increased in children (2.69), in women (2.93), and in patients with deep-seated AVMs (3.07).

A study of hemorrhage rates after SRS reported that the risk for hemorrhage decreased during the latency interval, with the annual hemorrhage rate in the first two years after SRS of 1.8% [25]. A retrospective analysis involving 500 patients with AVMs treated by radiosurgery reported a decrease in hemorrhage risk of 54% during the latency period and of 88% after total obliteration [26]. The calculated hemorrhage rate between the diagnosis of an AVM and its treatment by SRS was 10.4% [27]. The hemorrhage rate lessened to 2.8% after SRS until total obliteration of AVM in a subgroup of 605 patients with hemorrhage history. A meta-analysis considered 69 series of SRS for AVMs (gamma knife, 22; Linac SRS, 36; other radiosurgical modalities, 11) including 9436 patients [28]. Factors associated with lower hemorrhage rates included male sex, Spetzler–Martin grade I–III, smaller nidus size, and increased margin dose.

The optimal timing of SRS after AVM hemorrhage is unclear because SRS is usually performed at some point after the hematoma begins to resolve. A retrospective study of 211 patients with AVMs who presented with hemorrhage and underwent SRS as the initial treatment divided the patients into three groups according to the interval between the time of first hemorrhage and SRS: group 1, 0–3 months (70 patients); group 2, 3–6 months (62 patients); and group 3, >6 months (79 patients) [29]. After a median follow-up of 6.3 years, the rates of obliteration, hemorrhage after treatment, and complication were not significantly different between the three groups even though the patients with a longer interval before SRS (group 3) had more AVMs in eloquent areas and neurological deficits. However, the numbers of patients with preoperative hemorrhages in the interval before SRS was significantly higher in group 3 (1 patient in group 1, 3 in group 2, and 20 in group 3). The authors concluded that there was no benefit in waiting for hematoma volume reduction before SRS; because of higher hemorrhagic risk associated with waiting more than six months after hemorrhage, they recommended that SRS should be performed within six months after the bleeding event.

Other complications after stereotactic radiosurgery

Since immediate complications are rare after radiosurgery, many patients and physicians choose this modality because

Table 23.1. University of Pittsburgh experience using stereotactic radiosurgery for arteriovenous malformations

	No. patients	Median target volume (mL)	Median margin dose (Gy)	Total obliteration at 5 years (%)	Cumulative hemorrhage rate over 5 years (%)	Annual hemorrhage rate (%)	Adverse radiation effects (% permanent/ % temporary)	Rate of cyst formation (%)
Spetzler–Martin grade I or II	217	2.3	22	90	5.0	2.3	0/2.3	1
Pediatric	135	2.5	20	67	5.5	1.8	1.5/4.4	0.7
Repeat SRS	105	2.3	18	77	10.1	3.7	2.9/6.7	4.8
Basal ganglion or thalamus	133	2.7	20	72	11.2	4.7	4.5/5.3	0.8
Brainstem	67	1.4	20	70	3.0	1.9	10/6	3.0
Staged procedure	47	21.0	16	28	13.5	5.1	4.3/2.1	0
Embolization + SRS	120	6.6	18	55	7.7	2.7	2.5/5.8	0.8
Hemorrhagic presentation	407	2.3	20	80	6.6	1.3	N/A	N/A

N/A, not available; SRS, stereotactic radiosurgery.

a patient can rapidly return to regular activities and employment. The risk of major adverse radiation effects associated with long-term new neurological deficit is 2–3% in most reports [9,30]. Postradiosurgery seizures are rare when at-risk patients (patients with subcortical lobar AVMs) are treated with appropriate anticonvulsant medications. The meta-analysis study of van Beijnum *et al.* [28] found that the rate of acute complications after SRS was low. A higher risk of late complications was observed in earlier studies, in patients with older age and larger nidus size, in patient series with a higher number of ruptured AVMs, and in patients with high-grade AVMs or those located in critical brain regions.

A multicenter retrospective study reported that the risk of adverse radiation effects were higher in patients with brainstem AVMs than with AVMs in other locations [31]. The risk of symptomatic adverse radiation effects, including temporary and permanent neurological deficits, was reported to be 5% in patients with brainstem AVMs who underwent SRS [32]. The risk of a radiation injury resulting in a permanent neurological deficit varied between 4% and 11.9% in most reports of SRS for AVMs of the basal ganglia and thalamus [33–38].

Delayed cyst formation is a relatively rare long-term complication after radiosurgery for AVM. The incidence varies from as low as 0.4% to as high as 28% [39–41]. Prior embolization and radiation-related brain edema after the procedure increased the risk of delayed cyst formation [42]. The risk was elevated in patients who underwent repeat radiosurgery, with cyst development increasing in frequency from 1.3% in patients who had a single procedure to 10% of patients who underwent repeat procedures [40].

University of Pittsburgh experience

Between August 1987 and December 2006, 996 patients with AVMs underwent single-stage SRS using the Leksell Gamma Knife (Elekta Instruments) at our center (Table 23.1). Patients were evaluated, on average, five years after the procedure. For AVMs of smaller volume located in less critical brain areas (Spetzler–Martin grade I or II), the five-year total obliteration rate after a single SRS procedure was 90%. The five-year cumulative rate of AVM hemorrhage was 5.0% during the postprocedure latency interval. The risk of side-effects related to the procedure was 2% [16]. In 135 children, the five-year total obliteration rate after a single SRS procedure was 67%. Hemorrhages during the latency period developed in eight (6%). Permanent neurological deficits from treatment-related complications developed in two (1.5%). We found that SRS was a gradually effective and relatively safe management option for children who were considered to have excessive surgical risks [12]. Patients with deep-seated AVMs in critical brain areas (Spetzler–Martin grade III/IV) are often candidates for SRS as the primary management. In our experience of 56 patients with AVMs located in the basal ganglia and 77 with AVMs of the thalamus, the five-year total obliteration rate after one SRS was 72%; 15 patients (11%) had a hemorrhage during the latency interval and 6 (5%) died. Permanent neurological deficits from treatment-related side-effects developed in six patients (5%). The best results were noted in patients with AVMs of smaller volume located in the basal ganglia [14].

In 67 patients with grade VI (otherwise inoperable) AVMs located in the brainstem, the five-year total obliteration rate after a single procedure was 70%; four patients (6%) had a hemorrhage during the latency interval and two patients (3%) died. Permanent neurological deficits from treatment-related side-effects developed in seven patients (10%) after SRS; however, 25 patients (38%) who had neurological deficits at SRS from prior hemorrhage improved [15].

Repeat SRS was performed on 105 patients who had incompletely obliterated AVMs after an observation interval of three or more years. The five-year total obliteration rate after repeat SRS was 77%; 17 patients (16%) had hemorrhages after repeat SRS, 6 (6%) died, and treatment-related side-effects developed in 11 (10%). These results confirmed that repeat SRS for incompletely obliterated AVMs significantly increased the eventual obliteration rate. The best results were seen in patients with smaller AVMs, those who had more than 50% of volume reduction after the initial SRS, and those who had never sustained an AVM bleed [13].

Staged volume SRS at intervals of three to six months was used in 47 patients whose AVMs were >10 mL in volume. The five-year total obliteration rate after staged SRS was 36%. When dosage at each stage was >17 Gy, the obliteration rate increased to 62%. In 16 patients, additional SRS was performed after five years of observation and eight of these patients then obtained obliteration. After staged SRS, 10 patients (21%) bled, 5 (11%) died, and treatment-related side-effects were detected in 6 (13%). Our data suggest that prospective volume-staged SRS for large AVMs unsuitable for surgery has potential benefit if doses of ≥17 Gy are delivered to both anatomical components. In the future, prospective volume-staged SRS followed by embolization – to reduce flow, obliterate fistulae, and occlude associated aneurysms – may improve obliteration results and further reduce the risk of hemorrhage after SRS [11].

In the series of 120 patients with AVMs who underwent embolization followed by SRS, the five-year total obliteration rate after SRS was 55% and the annual hemorrhage rate after SRS was 2.7%. Using a case–control analysis, prior embolization reduced the rate of total obliteration after SRS but did not affect the hemorrhage risks during the latency interval [43]. In a series of SRS for hemorrhagic AVM in 407 patients, 25 patients had patent aneurysms (6 intranidal, 5 immediately prenidal, 14 circle of Willis) at the time of SRS. The five-year total obliteration rate after SRS was 80%. The presence of a patent aneurysm was significantly associated with an increased rehemorrhage risk after SRS (annual hemorrhage rate, 6.4%) compared with patients with a clipped or embolized aneurysm (annual hemorrhage rate, 0.8%). We recommend that when an aneurysm is identified in patients with AVMs selected for SRS, additional endovascular or surgical strategies should be considered after radiosurgery to reduce the risk of bleeding during the latency interval [44].

Dural arteriovenous fistulae

The decision to treat dural arteriovenous fistulae (DAVFs) depends on the severity of the symptoms, the angiographic characteristics, and the perceived risk for intracranial hemorrhage. The risk of hemorrhage from DAVFs is highly related to leptomeningeal cortical venous drainage and passive venous hypertension [45]. High-risk DAVFs (Borden grade II or III) warrant treatment because of their higher rate of intracranial hemorrhage [46]. Treatment modalities for DAVFs include surgical resection, embolization, SRS, and combined treatments using more than one approach.

Use of SRS is effective for selected DAVFs. We performed SRS in 40 patients with 44 DAVFs: 28 patients had upfront SRS before or after embolization and 12 patients underwent delayed SRS for recurrent or residual DAVFs after initial embolization [47]. The median SRS target volume was 2.0 mL (range, 0.2–8.2) and the median marginal dose was 21.0 Gy (range, 15–25). At a median follow-up of 45 months (range, 23–116), a total of 28 patients with 32 DAVFs had obliteration confirmed by imaging. There was an 83% obliteration rate in patients who had upfront SRS with embolization and a 67% obliteration rate in patients who only had SRS. One patient died of an intracerebral hemorrhage two months after SRS. Cavernous carotid fistulae were associated with higher rates of occlusion and symptom improvement than were fistulae of the transverse–sigmoid sinus. No patient had embolization or radiation-related morbidity. We suggest that embolization performed immediately before or after SRS (but still targeting the entire fistula volume) provides the best obliteration potential. Patients with DAVFs warrant management at centers where all treatment options exist. If direct surgery is not possible or is considered high risk, embolization provides early benefit and SRS provides late benefit during the management of these relatively rare vascular anomalies.

Conflict of interest notification

Drs. Lunsford and Kondziolka are consultants for AB Elekta and Dr. Lunsford is a stockholder.

References

1. Spetzler RF, Martin NA. A proposed grading system for arteriovenous malformations. *J Neurosurg* 1986;**65**:476–83.
2. Paulsen RD, Steinberg GK, Norbash AM, *et al.* Embolization of basal ganglia and thalamic arteriovenous malformations. *Neurosurgery* 1999;**44**:991–6.
3. Auger RG, Wiebers DO. Management of unruptured intracranial arteriovenous malformations: a decision analysis. *Neurosurgery* 1992;**30**:561–9.
4. Brown RD, Jr., Wiebers DO, Forbes G, *et al.* The natural history of unruptured intracranial arteriovenous malformations. *J Neurosurg* 1988;**68**:352–7.
5. Graf CJ, Perret GE, Torner JC. Bleeding from cerebral arteriovenous

malformations as part of their natural history. *J Neurosurg* 1983;**58**:331–7.

6. Ondra SL, Troupp H, George ED, *et al.* The natural history of symptomatic arteriovenous malformations of the brain: a 24-year follow-up assessment. *J Neurosurg* 1990;**73**:387–91.
7. Maruyama K, Shin M, Tago M, *et al.* Radiosurgery to reduce the risk of first hemorrhage from brain arteriovenous malformations. *Neurosurgery* 2007;**60**:453–8.
8. Inoue HK, Ohye C. Hemorrhage risks and obliteration rates of arteriovenous malformations after gamma knife radiosurgery. *J Neurosurg* 2002;**97**:474–6.
9. Liscak R, Vladyka V, Simonova G, *et al.* Arteriovenous malformations after Leksell gamma knife radiosurgery: rate of obliteration and complications. *Neurosurgery* 2007;**60**:1005–14.
10. Pollock BE, Flickinger JC, Lunsford LD, *et al.* Factors associated with successful arteriovenous malformation radiosurgery. *Neurosurgery* 1998;**42**:1239–44.
11. Kano H, Kondziolka D, Flickinger JC, *et al.* Stereotactic radiosurgery for arteriovenous malformations. Part 6: multistaged volumetric management of large arteriovenous malformations. *J Neurosurg* 2012;**116**:54–65.
12. Kano H, Kondziolka D, Flickinger JC, *et al.* Stereotactic radiosurgery for arteriovenous malformations. Part 2: management of pediatric patients. *J Neurosurg Pediatr* 2012;**9**:1–10.
13. Kano H, Kondziolka D, Flickinger JC, *et al.* Stereotactic radiosurgery for arteriovenous malformations. Part 3: outcome predictors and risks after repeat radiosurgery. *J Neurosurg* 2012;**116**:21–32.
14. Kano H, Kondziolka D, Flickinger JC, *et al.* Stereotactic radiosurgery for arteriovenous malformations. Part 4: management of basal ganglia and thalamus arteriovenous malformations. *J Neurosurg* 2012;**116**:33–43.
15. Kano H, Kondziolka D, Flickinger JC, *et al.* Stereotactic radiosurgery for arteriovenous malformations. Part 5: management of brainstem arteriovenous malformations. *J Neurosurg* 2012;**116**:44–53.
16. Kano H, Lunsford LD, Flickinger JC, *et al.* Stereotactic radiosurgery for arteriovenous malformations, Part 1: management of Spetzler–Martin grade I and II arteriovenous malformations. *J Neurosurg* 2012;**116**:11–20.
17. Yen CP, Varady P, Sheehan J, *et al.* Subtotal obliteration of cerebral arteriovenous malformations after gamma knife surgery. *J Neurosurg* 2007;**106**:361–9.
18. Forster DM, Steiner L, Hakanson S. Arteriovenous malformations of the brain. A long-term clinical study. *J Neurosurg* 1972;**37**:562–70.
19. Fults D, Kelly DL, Jr. Natural history of arteriovenous malformations of the brain: a clinical study. *Neurosurgery* 1984;**15**:658–62.
20. Itoyama Y, Uemura S, Ushio Y, *et al.* Natural course of unoperated intracranial arteriovenous malformations: study of 50 cases. *J Neurosurg* 1989;**71**:805–9.
21. Pollock BE, Flickinger JC, Lunsford LD, *et al.* Factors that predict the bleeding risk of cerebral arteriovenous malformations. *Stroke* 1996;**27**:1–6.
22. Stapf C, Mast H, Sciacca RR, *et al.* Predictors of hemorrhage in patients with untreated brain arteriovenous malformation. *Neurology* 2006;**66**:1350–5.
23. da Costa L, Wallace MC, terBrugge KG, *et al.* The natural history and predictive features of hemorrhage from brain arteriovenous malformations. *Stroke* 2009;**40**:100–5.
24. Yamada S, Takagi Y, Nozaki K, *et al.* Risk factors for subsequent hemorrhage in patients with cerebral arteriovenous malformations. *J Neurosurg* 2007;**107**:965–72.
25. Karlsson B, Lax I, Soderman M. Risk for hemorrhage during the 2-year latency period following gamma knife radiosurgery for arteriovenous malformations. *Int J Radiat Oncol Biol Phys* 2001;**49**:1045–51.
26. Maruyama K, Kawahara N, Shin M, *et al.* The risk of hemorrhage after radiosurgery for cerebral arteriovenous malformations. *N Engl J Med* 2005;**352**:146–53.
27. Yen CP, Sheehan JP, Schwyzer L, *et al.* Hemorrhage risk of cerebral arteriovenous malformations before and during the latency period after gamma knife radiosurgery. *Stroke* 2011;**42**:1691–6.
28. van Beijnum J, van der Worp HB, Buis DR, *et al.* Treatment of brain arteriovenous malformations: a systematic review and meta-analysis. *JAMA* 2011;**306**:2011–19.
29. Maruyama K, Koga T, Shin M, *et al.* Optimal timing for gamma knife surgery after hemorrhage from brain arteriovenous malformations. *J Neurosurg* 2008;**109**(Suppl):73–6.
30. Pollock BE, Meyer FB. Radiosurgery for arteriovenous malformations. *J Neurosurg* 2004;**101**:390–2.
31. Flickinger JC, Kondziolka D, Lunsford LD, *et al.* A multi-institutional analysis of complication outcomes after arteriovenous malformation radiosurgery. *Int J Radiat Oncol Biol Phys* 1999;**44**:67–74.
32. Massager N, Regis J, Kondziolka D, *et al.* Gamma knife radiosurgery for brainstem arteriovenous malformations: preliminary results. *J Neurosurg* 2000;**937**(Suppl 3):102–3.
33. Andrade-Souza YM, Zadeh G, Scora D, *et al.* Radiosurgery for basal ganglia, internal capsule, and thalamus arteriovenous malformation: clinical outcome. *Neurosurgery* 2005;**56**:56–63.
34. Kiran NA, Kale SS, Kasliwal MK, *et al.* Gamma knife radiosurgery for arteriovenous malformations of basal ganglia, thalamus and brainstem: a retrospective study comparing the results with that for AVMs at other intracranial locations. *Acta Neurochir (Wien)* 2009;**151**:1575–82.
35. Koga T, Shin M, Maruyama K, *et al.* Long-term outcomes of stereotactic radiosurgery for arteriovenous malformations in the thalamus. *Neurosurgery* 2010;**67**:398–403.
36. Nicolato A, Foroni R, Crocco A, *et al.* Gamma knife radiosurgery in the management of arteriovenous malformations of the basal ganglia region of the brain. *Minim Invasive Neurosurg* 2002;**45**:211–23.
37. Pollock BE, Gorman DA, Brown PD. Radiosurgery for arteriovenous malformations of the basal ganglia, thalamus, and brainstem. *J Neurosurg* 2004;**100**:210–14.
38. Sasaki T, Kurita H, Saito I, *et al.* Arteriovenous malformations in the basal ganglia and thalamus: management and results in 101 cases. *J Neurosurg* 1998;**88**:285–92.

39. Kihlstrom L, Guo WY, Karlsson B, *et al.* Magnetic resonance imaging of obliterated arteriovenous malformations up to 23 years after radiosurgery. *J Neurosurg* 1997;**86**:589–93.

40. Pollock BE, Brown RD, Jr. Management of cysts arising after radiosurgery to treat intracranial arteriovenous malformations. *Neurosurgery* 2001;**49**:259–64.

41. Yamamoto M, Jimbo M, Hara M, *et al.* Gamma knife radiosurgery for arteriovenous malformations: long-term follow-up results focusing on complications occurring more than 5 years after irradiation. *Neurosurgery* 1996;**38**:906–14.

42. Pan HC, Sheehan J, Stroila M, *et al.* Late cyst formation following gamma knife surgery of arteriovenous malformations. *J Neurosurg* 2005;**102**(Suppl):124–7.

43. Kano H, Kondziolka D, Flickinger JC, *et al.* Stereotactic radiosurgery for arteriovenous malformations after embolization: a case–control study. *J Neurosurg* 2012;**117**:265–75.

44. Kano H, Kondziolka D, Flickinger JC, *et al.* Aneurysms increase the risk of rebleeding after stereotactic radiosurgery for hemorrhagic arteriovenous malformations. *Stroke* 2012;**43**:2586–91.

45. Awad IA, Little JR, Akarawi WP, *et al.* Intracranial dural arteriovenous malformations: factors predisposing to an aggressive neurological course. *J Neurosurg* 1990;**72**:839–50.

46. Soderman M, Pavic L, Edner G, *et al.* Natural history of dural arteriovenous shunts. *Stroke* 2008;**39**:1735–9.

47. Yang HC, Kano H, Kondziolka D, *et al.* Stereotactic radiosurgery with or without embolization for intracranial dural arteriovenous fistulas. *Neurosurgery* 2010;**67**:1276–83.

Chapter 24

Radiosurgery for spinal arteriovenous malformations and fistulae

Syed Aftab Karim, Jacky T. Yeung, Scott G. Soltys, and Steven D. Chang

Introduction

Arteriovenous malformations (AVMs) of the spinal cord are rare vascular lesions first described by Gaupp *et al.* in 1888 [1]. Spinal AVMs are often mistaken for degenerative disease of the spine or other chronic neurological disorders. Mass effect from venous congestion along with ischemia or hemorrhage and spinal cord edema contribute to the presenting symptoms. Myelography, three-dimensional angiography, MRI, and CT allow prompt diagnosis of this disease entity. Embolization with or without surgical resection is the traditional treatment of choice for spinal AVMs [2,3]. Intramedullary spinal cords AVMs have an unfavorable natural history that characteristically involves myelopathy secondary to progressive ischemia and/or recurrent hemorrhage. Although intramedullary spinal AVMs can sometimes be managed successfully with embolization and/or surgery, nidus size, location, and angioarchitecture preclude treatment in many circumstances [4]. Advances in frameless devices for targeting spinal lesions have made stereotactic radiosurgery (SRS) an effective and attractive treatment modality for intramedullary spinal AVMs [5].

Clinical presentation and diagnosis

Spinal AVMs are broadly separated into intradural AVMs, extradural AVMs, and dural arteriovenous fistulae. Symptoms in patients with intramedullary AVMs typically present in the second decade of life whereas dural arteriovenous fistulae present in the fourth or fifth decade of life [6]. The incidence of spinal AVMs is independent of sex and age [7]. The natural history of spinal AVMs is poorly defined as they are rare disease entities. Exacerbation in symptoms can be seen with activity or a change in position, particularly in the thoracic or lumbar region [7]. Patients often present with painful radiculopathy and commonly experience progressive neurological symptoms over periods of months or years. The symptoms may be attributed to mass effect on the spinal cord from hemorrhage or vascular congestions, or from vascular steal resulting in hypoperfusion of neural tissue. Patients with spinal intradural AVMs can present acutely with subarachnoid hemorrhage, causing a sudden onset of a severe headache, meningismus, or photophobia [3]. Patients with signs and symptoms of subarachnoid hemorrhage and negative cerebral angiography should be evaluated for a spinal AVM [3].

A diagnosis of spinal AVM is suggested by MRI or myelography, which demonstrate flow voids or filling defects. Cord enhancement may be seen from venous congestion or venous infarction [8]. While CT angiography may be helpful, spinal angiography remains the gold standard for diagnosis and treatment planning [3,9]. The recent use of three-dimensional rotational spinal angiography helps to differentiate intramedullary lesions from perimedullary surface lesions [10]. Fusion of thin-cut postcontrast CT imaging with three-dimensional rotational spinal angiography is utilized to visualize the spinal AVM nidus for radiosurgical treatment planning [11].

Spinal cord vasculature

The pathophysiology and treatment of spinal AVMs is best understood by studying the normal blood supply to the spinal cord [3]. The aorta gives rise to segmental arteries, which subsequently supply the spinal medullary and radicular arteries. The medullary artery bifurcates into anterior and posterior divisions, which then merge and form the spinal arteries [12]. There are three main spinal arteries with one anterior and two posterior arteries running parallel to the spinal cord. The cervicothoracic region of the spinal cord is supplied by segmental vessels arising from the major aortic branches. The midthoracic region receives most of its segmental blood supply also from the aorta. The midthoracic region of the spinal cord is supplied mostly by collateral circulation, generating a watershed area that is susceptible to ischemia and infarction. The thoracolumbar region receives its blood supply from segmental vessels from the abdominal aorta and the iliac arteries. The artery of Adamkiewicz is the largest segmental artery, usually located between T9 and L2 spinal levels. Venous drainage of the spinal column is through the valveless Batson plexus, which permits anterograde and retrograde venous flow depending on venous pressures [12]. As with cerebral AVMs, spinal AVMs consist of abnormal vasculature and involve thick-walled arterial and

Comprehensive Management of Arteriovenous Malformations of the Brain and Spine, ed. Robert F. Spetzler, Douglas S. Kondziolka, Randall T. Higashida, and M. Yashar S. Kalani. Published by Cambridge University Press.

thin-walled venous vessels. Hemorrhage of a spinal AVM occurs when the arterial pressure exceeds the capacity of the venous walls.

Nomenclature for spinal arteriovenous malformations

Various classification systems for spinal AVMs exist, including the American/English/French Connection classification [8], Hôpital Bicêtre classification [13], and the Spetzler–Martin classification [2].

The original classification system for spinal AVMs included types I–IV, but in fact types I and IV are arteriovenous fistulae. A type I AVM is a slow-flow AVM found at the dural root sleeve, most commonly seen in the thoracolumbar spine, and is typically treated with surgical or endovascular obliteration of the fistula. Type II (spinal glomus) AVMs are intradural high-flow spinal AVMs, while type III (juvenile) spinal AVMs are both intra- and extradural high-flow AVMs. Type III AVMs are aggressive and can involve the vertebral bodies. The type IV intradural AVM is a direct fistula between the anterior or posterior spinal arteries and draining veins typically occurring in younger patients; it is sometimes referred to as a pial fistula.

A proposed nomenclature by Spetzler and colleagues classified spinal AVMs into extradural–intradural and intradural malformations [2]. The intradural category is further divided into intramedullary, intramedullary–extramedullary, and conus medullaris. Extradural–intradural AVMs are uncommon. This type of lesion is not bound by neighboring tissue structures and may involve the surrounding spinal cord, vertebral column, and extraspinal soft tissue. Intramedullary AVMs were previously classified as types II and III AVMs, as detailed above [14–21]. They can hemorrhage, compress neighboring structures, and cause vascular steal. Aneurysms can be seen with intramedullary AVMs [22]. The intramedullary nidus can also be divided into compact or diffuse.

A conus medullaris AVM is characterized by multiple feeding arteries, multiple nidi, and complex venous drainage, lending itself to possible recurrence. These lesions occur solely at the conus medullaris and cauda equina and they can involve both the intramedullary and the extramedullary space. They can present as progressive myelopathy, radiculopathy, or myeloradiculopathy from venous hypertension, ischemia, or local mass effect [2]. This type of lesion can cause insidious clinical deterioration [23].

Endovascular and surgical treatment

Symptomatic spinal AVMs generally require treatment and spontaneous occlusions have only rarely been reported [24–26]. There is currently no medical therapy available for the treatment of spinal AVMs. Endovascular surgery, open surgery, or a combination of both are offered to patients requiring intervention.

Type I spinal AVMs are often treated with open surgery [2]. However, endovascular treatment of type I spinal AVMs is possible if selective catheterization of the pedicle can be achieved without compromising the blood supply to the cord [3]. Type IV spinal AVMs can also be treated safely with embolization or surgery [3]. Extradural–intradural spinal AVMs can be treated with endovascular intervention, with surgery reserved for neural decompression and stabilization [2]. Intramedullary spinal AVMs and conus medullaris AVMs can be approached with a combined endovascular and open surgical approach [2,6].

Treatment of spinal AVMs with surgery or embolization resulted in a good outcome in approximately 90% of patients with dural spinal arteriovenous fistulae after nidus obliteration, while less than 50% of patients with intramedullary spinal AVMs improved after surgery or embolization [6]. Therefore, surgical treatments and endovascular intervention are often not optimal for intramedullary AVMs despite advances in microsurgery. This is largely because of the intraparenchymal spinal cord location of intramedullary AVMs with an anterior spinal artery blood supply [7,27].

The risk of complications from open surgical and endovascular therapies is not uncommon [7,16]. Poor surgical outcomes in patients with intramedullary spinal AVMs suggest a need for minimally invasive treatment modalities for this disease entity.

Radiosurgery

Stereotactic radiosurgery is a non-invasive treatment modality that delivers a high dose of ionizing radiation to a precise location and minimizes the dose to unaffected adjacent structures. Patients undergoing image-guided SRS typically receive MRI to assess the three-dimensional shape of the AVM and the anatomical relationship to the surrounding spinal cord. This imaging is limited in its ability to differentiate arterial and venous vessels. For this reason, conventional spinal angiography is applied to further define the AVM nidus and its associated blood supply [10]. Advancements in three-dimensional rotational spinal angiography have allowed improved spatial representation of the target compared with that achievable with biplanar stereotactic angiography. A fusion of axial slice reconstruction three-dimensional angiography with stereotactic contrast-enhanced CT scanning allows detailed characterization of an AVM nidus and its spatial relationship with adjacent skeletal landmarks [10]. Stanford University utilizes the CyberKnife stereotactic radiosurgical system (Accuray, Sunnyvale, CA, USA) as a major treatment modality for spinal AVMs.

Radiosurgical treatment planning is a joint effort between neurosurgeons, interventional radiologists, radiation physicists, and radiation oncologists. It involves the use of standard computerized drawing tools to contour the AVM nidus. The surrounding spinal cord is identified and isolated using the planning software to minimize the dose to normal tissue during treatment planning. Feeding arteries and draining veins are also excluded from the irradiation volume. The CyberKnife radiosurgical software utilizes an inverse treatment planning algorithm and calculates a plan through an iterative process to optimize coverage of the target nidus. The treatment process includes qualitative radiosurgical conformality and quantitative analysis of dose–volume histograms within the target volume and adjacent spinal cord.

Radiosurgical technique

An alpha cradle mold permits partial external immobilization of the patient. Thin-slice CT with contrast enhancement is fused with stereo MRI and three-dimensional angiography during patient simulation. The lesion is contoured and target and critical structure dose constraints are defined by the treating physicians. Once image-guided registration is performed, SRS is administered to an awake and usually unanesthetized patient [11]. Patients are given dexamethasone and antinausea medications as needed either before or after each treatment.

Radiosurgical dose prescription

Data from the use of radiosurgery for cerebral AVMs have provided the framework for radiation doses administered in spinal radiosurgery [28]. An understanding of dose constraints and toxicity was derived similarly based on experience with cerebral AVMs in critical regions [29]. In the initial phases of radiosurgery for spinal AVMs, a multisession approach was employed to minimize the risk of spinal cord injury, based on historical data from treatment with fractionated external beam radiotherapy for spinal AVMs [11]. Paradoxically, AVM obliteration is a late radiation effect and the goal of fractionation is to minimize late effects. The theoretical efficacy of single-session treatment, which may be greater than a multisession approach, is possibly offset by the higher potential risk of spinal cord injury.

A biological effective dose can be estimated from the following formula [29]:

$$nd[1 + d/(\alpha/\beta)]$$

where n is number of fractions (sessions), d is the dose per fraction (session), and α/β is a ratio estimating radiation sensitivity. A ratio of 3 is accepted to represent the value that estimates the sensitivity of late-responding tissue, whereas a value of 10 corresponds to early-responding tissue [11,28]. Hall and Brenner estimate the α/β ratio for AVMs to be somewhere between 0.2 and 5 [28].

Assuming an α/β ratio of 2, the multisession radiosurgical plans used early in our experience approached a biological effective dose comparable to a single session of 13 Gy, which is at the low end of dose used to treat intracranial AVMs in critical locations. This dose is estimated to result in an approximately 50% rate of in-field obliteration for intracranial AVMs [30]. However, as we gained experience in spinal AVM radiosurgery, we began to increase doses. Current radiosurgical doses for spinal AVMs are typically 20–22 Gy over two sessions or 16–18 Gy in a single session.

Spinal cord tolerance

Although less than one-third of patients achieve a complete obliteration of spinal AVM after radiosurgery, clinical improvement and some protective effect against hemorrhage are observed in most patients following spinal SRS for AVMs. Based on a clear dose–response curve for obliteration rates with intracranial AVMs, it is possible that higher spinal AVM obliteration rates may be achieved by dose escalation [30]. In our experience, gradual dose escalation could be performed without any increase in complication rate. Based on the safety of our experience with 20 Gy in two fractions, our current standard dose has been increased to 22 Gy in two fractions in an attempt to improve the obliteration rate. Selected small AVMs are treated with 16–18 Gy in a single fraction.

The true tolerance of the spinal cord to the partial volume dosimetry encountered in SRS remains unknown despite increasing utilization of spinal radiosurgery for the treatment of spinal metastases. We have been conservative in the dose escalation over the years for patients with spinal AVMs, as the spinal cord dosimetry of these treatment plans far exceeds any suggested guidelines regarding the tolerance of the cord. For example, the spinal cord dose constraints for the RTOG 0631 spinal radiosurgery trial for metastases (http://cancer.gov/clinicaltrials/RTOG-0631) are a volume of spinal cord greater than 10 Gy (V10) of <0.35 mL and <10%. Patients in our AVM series often had an AVM nidus that involved the entire cross-sectional area of the cord, with normal cord above and below the targeted nidus (Fig. 24.1). When treated with 20 Gy in two fractions, the entire cord received 10 Gy twice in two days (a V10 of 100% for both treatments), as opposed to the cited limits of a V10 of <10%. These spinal cord dosimetry data are in agreement with the tolerance data for spinal radiosurgery in a pig model [31]. Defining the true tolerance of the spinal cord to SRS should increase obliteration rates of spinal AVMs.

Contraindications

The major contraindications for radiosurgery in the treatment of spinal AVMs are large AVMs and diffuse involvement of the spinal cord and surrounding structures. Staged treatment of large spinal AVMs can be further studied once optimal dosing and cord tolerance becomes clearer [32]. Other considerations for radiosurgery include spinal instability and the presence of neurological deficits caused by bony or vascular compression of neural structures [32,33]. Previous irradiation to the affected area should be considered during the planning of radiosurgery given the radiation tolerance of critical structures. Patients with spinal arteriovenous fistulae are in general not candidates for SRS [2,6]

Outcomes with radiosurgery

Results from stereotactic radiosurgery for spinal AVMs have been promising. We follow patients after SRS for spinal AVMs with a contrast MRI at 6 months then yearly. Spinal angiography is considered at three years after SRS to determine the degree of obliteration, similar to the follow-up intervals for cranial AVMs [4,11]. Figure 24.1 shows an angiogram at 26 months after SRS confirming the complete obliteration of the nidus in a 17-year-old woman with an L1 AVM.

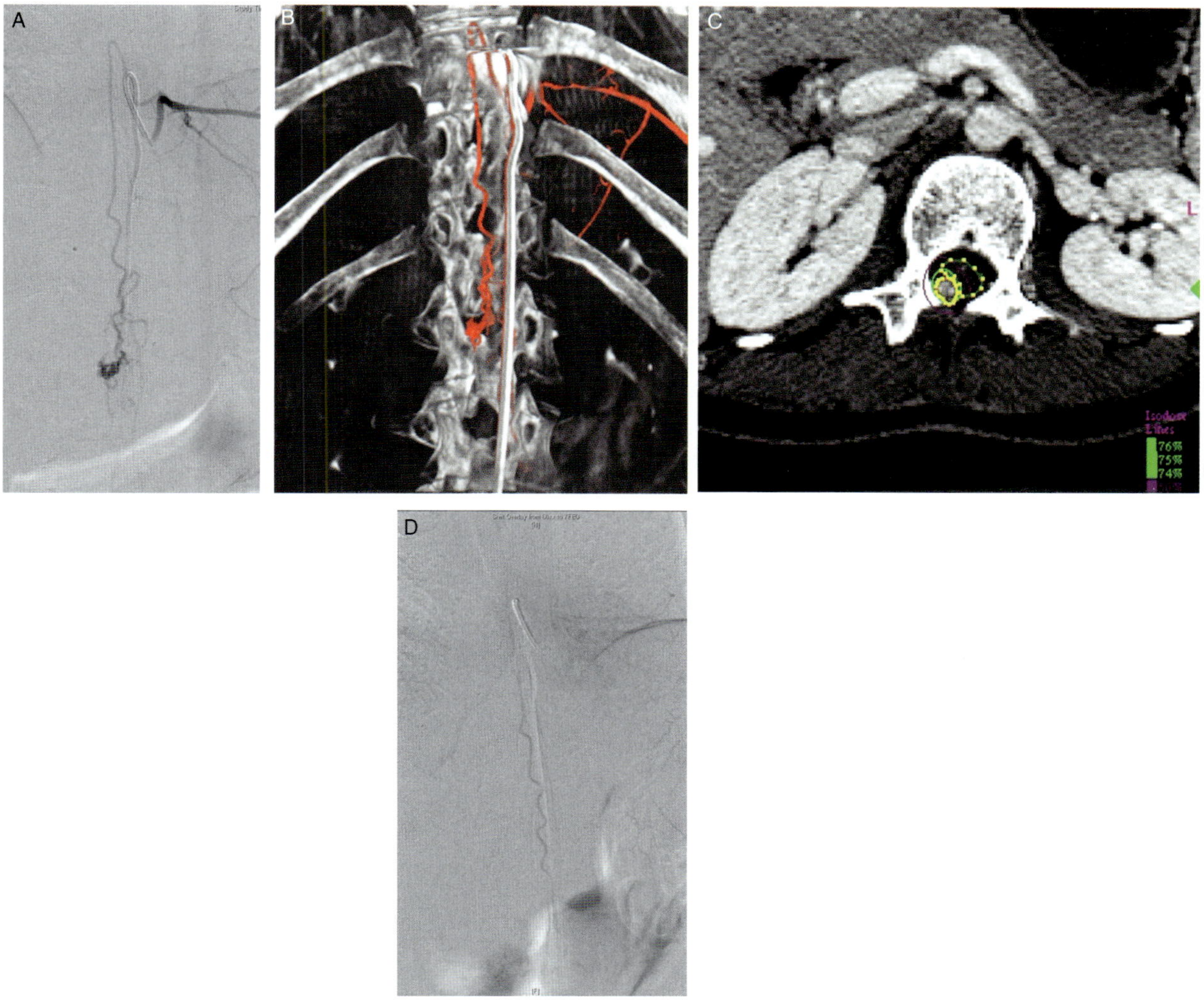

Fig. 24.1. A representative treatment plan in a 17-year-old woman with an L1 arteriovenous malformation (AVM), diagnosed following a hemorrhage associated with acute lower extremity paralysis. Her strength recovered fully and she underwent spinal radiosurgery for the AVM. Examples such as this patient highlight that the true radiation tolerance of the spinal cord is not known and is likely higher than the currently reported dose constraints. (A) Pretreatment angiography (right posterior) showing the L1 intramedullary AVM nidus. (B) Virtual reconstruction from CT, MRI, and three-dimensional digital rotational imaging. (C) The radiosurgical volume (solid yellow line) measured 0.3 mL and was treated with 18 Gy in a single fraction to the 75% isodose line (green line). Maximum dose was 24 Gy. Portions of the normal spinal cord (green contour with yellow dots) at the conus medullaris received the full prescription dose of radiation. D) Angiography 26 months following stereotactic radiosurgery confirmed complete obliteration. (Used with permission from Stanford University/Stanford Hospital and Clinics.)

Hida *et al.* have reported a 10-year experience treating 10 patients with spinal cord AVMs with hypofractionated linear accelerator-based SRS [34]. The AVMs were treated to a median of 36–40 Gy using daily doses of 1.8–2.0 Gy. Complete obliteration of spinal cord AVMs was not achieved; five patients had a partial volume reduction of the nidus on angiography, with a median follow-up of 49 months. There were no adverse reactions attributable to radiation and dose limits could not be identified.

At the Stanford University CyberKnife Radiosurgery Center, we have reported a series of 30 patients treated for intramedullary spinal cord AVMs with a median follow-up of 54 months (Table 24.1) [11]. Each patient received a total dose of 15–21 Gy administered in one to four sessions treated to the 70th to 90th percentile isodose line. The single fraction dose equivalent ranged from 10 to 18 Gy.

Table 24.1. Patient demographics for Stanford University CyberKnife Radiosurgery Center series

Demographic	
Sex	13M/17F
Mean time from diagnosis to radiosurgery (years [range])	8.3 (0.2–22)
Location (cervical/thoracic/conus)	18/9/3
Median age at radiosurgery (years [range])	33.0 (18–55)
Prior treatment modalities (No.)	
Surgical resection	6
Embolization	11
Repeat radiosurgery procedures	4

Source: with permission from Adler *et al.*, 2010 [4].

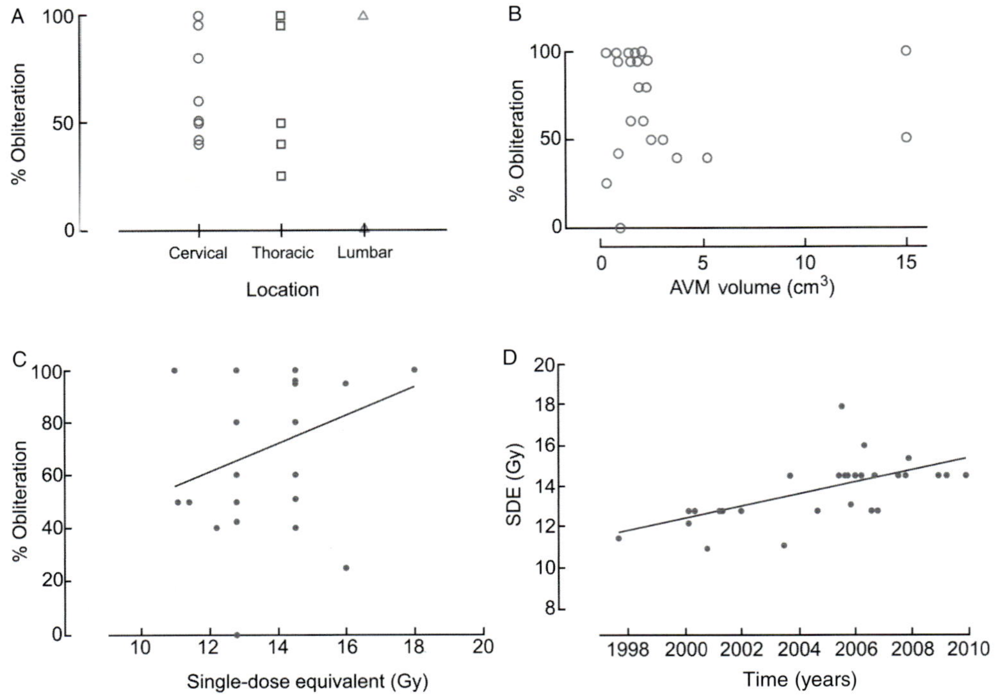

Fig. 24.2. Effect of radiosurgical dosage, spinal cord arteriovenous malformations (AVM) volume, and location. Calculation of the single dose equivalent (SDE) from the prescribed dose and number of fractions is described in the text. The percentage obliteration of the spinal AVM is plotted against location (A), lesion volume (B), and SDE (C). (D) Dose escalation with time. (Used with permission from Adler et al., 2010 [4].)

In the follow-up data from our original report, SRS resulted in a complete angiographic obliteration rate of 27%, a radiosurgical response rate of over 95%, and a complication rate of less than 10% [4,11]. There were no hemorrhages seen in any patients after SRS for intramedullary spinal cord AVMs in this series. There was one case of radiation-induced myelopathy within one year of radiosurgery. No correlations were found between spinal cord AVM single-dose equivalent, spinal cord AVM volume, and spinal cord AVM location (i.e., cervical, thoracic, or lumbar) in this study (Fig. 24.2). After SRS, improvement was observed in gait ataxia (70%), myelopathic weakness (50%), and pain (50%); in contrast, neuropathic pain is reportedly worse after open surgical treatment for spinal cord AVMs from the common surgical entry through the posterior column corridor [4]. Repeat radiosurgery was administered to 4 of the 30 patients because of incomplete response to the initial treatment, with two of these patients achieving complete obliteration of the spinal cord AVM after the second treatment.

Patients without prior hemorrhage were more likely to have improvement in pretreatment symptoms after radiosurgery than those with a bleeding history, suggesting that spinal cord damage from prior bleeding is less likely to recover [4]. The improvement of symptoms and lack of hemorrhage after radiosurgery for spinal cord AVMs suggest that radiosurgery has some clinical benefits despite a low rate (27%) of spinal cord AVM obliteration. Potential protective effect against post-treatment hemorrhage is also observed in reports for intracranial AVMs [35]. In our series, complete obliteration was not a prerequisite to clinical improvement in function. Larger series will be needed to determine the statistical significance of these data.

The difference between the results of Hida *et al.* [34] and Adler *et al.* [4] most likely reflects the dose escalation in the Stanford series reported by Adler *et al.*, particularly in the latter years of the Stanford experience. A better understanding of cord tolerance to SRS is needed to determine the dose–response curve for both optimization of obliteration of spinal cord AVMs and minimization of radiation-induced toxicity to the spinal cord.

Conclusions

The utilization of SRS as a treatment modality for spinal AVMs remains to be optimized despite our experience since the late 1990s. Overall obliteration rates of spinal AVMs after radiosurgery are significantly below reported rates in intracranial AVMs, which can approach 80–90% for lesions <3 cm in diameter [36,37]. This is likely to reflect the conservative doses used so far for spinal cord AVM radiosurgery. To date, the treatment plan for each patient remains highly individualized and there is still a lack of consensus on the optimal dose. Although efficacy appears to be limited for this treatment modality given the current data, the complication rates reported have also been low compared with those with open surgery and endovascular therapy [11,34]. In a large published microsurgical series of 27 patients with intramedullary AVMs, resection was achieved in 25 (92%), and 13 (53%) of those patients improved clinically following surgery [7]. Berenstein *et al.* reported on 47 patients with spinal AVMs treated with endovascular embolization, with excellent outcome, defined as normal neurological status after the procedure and complete obliteration, in 23 (49%). However, despite the overall positive clinical outcome in 36 patients (77%), a complication rate of 11% was reported [27]. In comparison, SRS has demonstrated both the relative safety and early evidence of efficacy for the treatment of spinal AVMs [4,11]. The safety of radiosurgery for this indication involves factors that are not currently well understood and may be related to spinal cord regional anatomy affected by the AVM, AVM volume, length of involved spinal cord, and the details of AVM blood supply [7]. Understanding the true spinal cord tolerance to radiosurgery will likely allow further dose escalation to achieve higher degrees of obliteration.

Longer follow-up and larger patient numbers are needed to optimize the treatment of spinal AVMs in order to improve obliteration rates and safety. The preliminary safety profile for radiosurgery for the treatment of intramedullary spinal AVMs suggests that this is a viable option and should be considered in a multimodality paradigm.

References

1. Gaupp J. Hamorrhoiden der Pia Mater Spinalis im Gebiet des Lendenmarks. *Beitr Pathol* 1888;**2**:516–18.
2. Kim LJ, Spetzler RF. Classification and surgical management of spinal arteriovenous lesions: arteriovenous fistulae and arteriovenous malformations. *Neurosurgery* 2006;**59**:S195–201.
3. Veznedaroglu E, Nelson PK, Jabbour PM, *et al.* Endovascular treatment of spinal cord arteriovenous malformations. *Neurosurgery* 2006;**59**: S202–9.
4. Adler J, Gupta G, Chang S. CyberKnife ablation for intramedullary spinal cord arteriovenous malformations (AVMs): a new promising new therapeutic approach. *Cureus* 2010;**2**:e14.
5. Ho AK, Fu D, Cotrutz C, *et al.* A study of the accuracy of CyberKnife spinal radiosurgery using skeletal structure tracking. *Neurosurgery* 2007;**60**: ons147–56.
6. Rosenblum B, Oldfield EH, Doppman JL, *et al.* Spinal arteriovenous malformations: a comparison of dural arteriovenous fistulas and intradural AVMs in 81 patients. *J Neurosurg* 1987;**67**:795–802.
7. Thompson B, Oldfield E. Spinal vascular malformation. In Carter L, Spetzler RF, Hamilton M, eds. *Neurovascular Surgery*. New York: McGraw-Hill, 1995, pp. 1167–95.
8. Greenburg M. Spinal vascular malformations. In Greenburg M, ed. *Handbook of Neuorsurgery*. New York: Thieme, 2010, pp. 507–9.
9. Doppman JL. Arteriography of the spinal cord. *Semin Roentgenol* 1972;**7**:231–9.
10. Prestigiacomo CJ, Niimi Y, Setton A, *et al.* Three-dimensional rotational spinal angiography in the evaluation and treatment of vascular malformations. *AJNR Am J Neuroradiol* 2003;**24**:1429–35.
11. Sinclair J, Chang SD, Gibbs IC, *et al.* Multisession CyberKnife radiosurgery for intramedullary spinal cord arteriovenous malformations. *Neurosurgery* 2006;**58**:1081–9.
12. Lasjaunias P, Berenstein A. *Surgical Neuroangiography:* Vol. 3: *Functional Vascular Anatomy of Brain, Spinal Cord, and Spine*. New York: Springer, 1990.
13. Rodesch G, Hurth M, Alvarez H, *et al.* Classification of spinal cord arteriovenous shunts: proposal for a reappraisal: the Bicêtre experience with 155 consecutive patients treated between 1981 and 1999. *Neurosurgery* 2002;**51**:374–9.
14. Anson JA, Spetzler RF. Surgical resection of intramedullary spinal cord cavernous malformations. *J Neurosurg* 1993;**78**:446–51.
15. Cogen P, Stein BM. Spinal cord arteriovenous malformations with significant intramedullary components. *J Neurosurg* 1983;**59**:471–8.
16. Connolly ES, Jr., Zubay GP, McCormick PC, *et al.* The posterior approach to a series of glomus (type II) intramedullary spinal cord arteriovenous malformations. *Neurosurgery* 1998;**42**:774–85.
17. Ommaya AK, Di CG, Doppman J. Ligation of arterial supply in the treatment of spinal cord arteriovenous malformations. *J Neurosurg* 1969;**30**:679–92.
18. Owen MP, Brown RH, Spetzler RF, *et al.* Excision of intramedullary arteriovenous malformation using intraoperative spinal cord monitoring. *Surg Neurol* 1979;**12**:271–6.
19. Raynor RB, Weiner R. Transthoracic approach to an intramedullary vascular malformation of the thoracic spinal cord. *Neurosurgery* 1982;**10**:631–4.
20. Wyburn-Mason R. *The Vascular Abnormalities and Tumours of the Spinal Cord and its Membranes*. London: Mosby, 1943.
21. Yaşargil MG, DeLong WB, Guarnaschelli JJ. Complete microsurgical excision of cervical extramedullary and intramedullary vascular malformations. *Surg Neurol* 1975;**4**:211–24.
22. Biondi A, Merland JJ, Hodes JE, *et al.* Aneurysms of spinal arteries associated with intramedullary arteriovenous malformations. I. Angiographic and clinical aspects. *AJNR Am J Neuroradiol* 1992;**13**:913–22.
23. Wilson DA, Abla AA, Uschold TD, *et al.* Multimodality treatment of conus medullaris arteriovenous malformations: 2 decades of experience with combined endovascular and microsurgical treatments. *Neurosurgery* 2012;**71**:100–8.
24. Gupta V, Rizvi T, Garg A, *et al.* Postangiographic thrombosis of a spinal arteriovenous malformation: case report. *J Neurosurg Spine* 2005;**2**:486–90.
25. Panciani PP, Fontanella M, Crobeddu E, *et al.* Spontaneous occlusion of a spinal arteriovenous malformation: is treatment always necessary? *J Neurosurg Spine* 2010;**12**:397–401.
26. Chun JY, Gulati M, Halbach V, *et al.* Thrombosis of a spinal arteriovenous malformation after hemorrhage: case report. *Surg Neurol* 2004;**61**:92–4.
27. Berenstein A, Lasjaunias P, terBrugge K. Spinal arteriovenous malformations. In Berenstein A, Lasjaunias P, terBrugge K, eds. *Surgical Neuroangiography*. Heidelberg: Springer, 2004, pp. 738–847.

28. Hall EJ, Brenner DJ. The radiobiology of radiosurgery: rationale for different treatment regimes for AVMs and malignancies. *Int J Radiat Oncol Biol Phys* 1993;**25**:381–5.

29. Steinberg GK, Fabrikant JI, Marks MP, *et al.* Stereotactic heavy-charged-particle Bragg-peak radiation for intracranial arteriovenous malformations. *N Engl J Med* 1990;**323**:96–101.

30. Flickinger JC, Kondziolka D, Maitz AH, *et al.* An analysis of the dose–response for arteriovenous malformation radiosurgery and other factors affecting obliteration. *Radiother Oncol* 2002;**63**:347–54.

31. Medin PM, Foster RD, van der Kogel AJ, *et al.* Spinal cord tolerance to reirradiation with single-fraction radiosurgery: a swine model. *Int J Radiat Oncol Biol Phys* 2012;**83**:1031–7.

32. Faul CM, Flickinger JC. The use of radiation in the management of spinal metastases. *J Neurooncol* 1995;**23**:149–61.

33. Gerszten PC, Welch WC. Current surgical management of metastatic spinal disease. *Oncology (Williston Park)* 2000;**14**:1013–24.

34. Hida K, Shirato H, Isu T, *et al.* Focal fractionated radiotherapy for intramedullary spinal arteriovenous malformations: 10-year experience. *J Neurosurg* 2003;**99**:34–8.

35. Maruyama K, Kawahara N, Shin M, *et al.* The risk of hemorrhage after radiosurgery for cerebral arteriovenous malformations. *N Engl J Med* 2005;**352**:146–53.

36. Pollock BE, Flickinger JC, Lunsford LD, *et al.* Factors associated with successful arteriovenous malformation radiosurgery. *Neurosurgery* 1998;**42**:1239–44.

37. Pollock BE, Gorman DA, Brown PD. Radiosurgery for arteriovenous malformations of the basal ganglia, thalamus, and brainstem. *J Neurosurg* 2004;**100**:210–14.

Chapter 25

Multidisciplinary treatment of arteriovenous malformations

Douglas J. Cook, Nitin Mukerji, and Gary K. Steinberg

Introduction

The modalities used to treat brain arteriovenous malformations (AVMs) in contemporary practice include surgical resection, stereotactic radiosurgery and intra-arterial embolization. Because single or combined treatments can be employed for any given patient, AVM management has evolved over the past three to four decades from a single surgeon, single modality approach to a multidisciplinary approach and management of AVMs in a multidisciplinary neurovascular clinic. Surgeons practice one or more subspecialties, including neurovascular surgery, stereotactic radiosurgery, and endovascular surgery. In this new model, surgeons with individual areas of expertise review patients as a group and discuss the advantages and limitations of each treatment modality to arrive at optimal treatment decisions. Bias from the therapeutic expertise of an individual practitioner is, therefore, balanced with colleagues' expertise and experience. This model has become the standard in neurovascular surgery.

Additional benefits of the multidisciplinary neurovascular clinic are the involvement of allied healthcare colleagues. Nursing staff, including nurse practitioners, may act as primary contacts for patients accessing the clinic. The nurse is a central and consistent interface between patients and the multiple physicians they may encounter in the course of their disease management. Psychosocial issues surrounding the treatment of AVMs include coping with neurological deficits, anxiety related to hemorrhage risk, and family dynamics. These can be addressed by allied health professionals, such as social workers, associated with the clinic and familiar with patients with AVMs. Many neurovascular clinics offer patient and family support groups to facilitate the development of coping skills related to psychosocial issues. Lastly, the clinic can coordinate referral through physiotherapy and rehabilitation medicine to trusted and experienced rehabilitation management personnel who are familiar with patients with AVMs and stroke rehabilitation.

Multidisciplinary AVM management allows practitioners to choose between a single or multimodality treatment based on AVM characteristics. Optimal AVM treatment maximizes the chance for complete lesion obliteration in the shortest possible timeframe and minimizes the chance of an adverse outcome, including treatment-related complications and lesion hemorrhage in the interval between treatment initiation and complete obliteration. A single modality approach generally best meets these criteria by avoiding the cumulative risk of multiple procedures. When feasible, surgery is preferred as immediate obliteration of the lesion can often be achieved. Radiosurgery is the most frequent single modality treatment for lesions that carry excessive surgical risk; however, the timeframe for lesion obliteration after radiosurgery is three years or longer. For the same reason, radiosurgery is more frequently used for unruptured AVMs and is generally reserved for inoperable ruptured AVMs. Embolization is less frequently used as a monotherapy to achieve complete obliteration, although in some surgeons' experience it is an effective approach for select lesions. Combined or multimodality treatment plans are employed in situations that cannot be addressed completely with a single modality or where one modality improves the risk profile of the subsequent definitive treatment. A minority of lesions require multimodality therapy. A population-based study from Sweden of the treatment modality selected for AVMs over 11 years found that 22 of 125 (17.6%) AVMs treated required multimodality therapy [1]. Multimodality therapy has allowed treatment of lesions previously deemed incurable and has led to an increase in the total number of lesions eligible for therapy. The larger Spetzler–Martin grade IV and V lesions as well as lesions in difficult anatomical locations are best treated by multimodality therapy [2]. At Stanford, which is referred a relatively high number of patients with large and complex AVMs, we have used multimodality therapy in 39% of over 1100 patients with AVMs treated over the last 23 years.

In summary, multidisciplinary management of AVMs provides multiple viewpoints in the discussion of AVM management with opinions and experience from experts in each treatment modality. The primary innovation that has arisen from multidisciplinary AVM management is multimodality AVM treatment. This approach fills three specific niches in contemporary practice: (1) to achieve complete obliteration of

Comprehensive Management of Arteriovenous Malformations of the Brain and Spine, ed. Robert F. Spetzler, Douglas S. Kondziolka, Randall T. Higashida, and M. Yashar S. Kalani. Published by Cambridge University Press.

AVMs that cannot be cured by a single modality based on an a priori plan set forth by the multidisciplinary team; (2) as an adjunctive therapy to improve the safety profile or efficacy of a primary, definitive treatment modality; and (3) to provide therapeutic options for incompletely treated AVMs following unsuccessful single modality treatment.

Multimodality therapy

Given the three therapeutic modalities for AVMs and the ability to apply a single modality multiple times in the treatment of AVMs, a number of permutations of treatment options can be applied to a given patient. The most common combination therapy includes preoperative and preradiosurgical embolization. Preoperative radiosurgery and surgery preceding radiosurgery or embolization are other – but far less commonly applied – applications. These methods are discussed for patients for whom the techniques have been applied.

Preoperative embolization

Preoperative embolization has become a common adjunct to surgery for AVMs. Embolization allows major AVM feeding vessels to be obliterated and the size of the AVM nidus to be reduced in size and flow (Fig. 25.1) [2–4]. The primary advantage of this technique is the reduction of nidus volume, particularly in large or diffuse AVMs, creating a compact nidus more practical for resection [5,6]. This involves the identification and selective injection of feeding arteries with the aim of achieving nidus penetration and occlusion of feeding arteries. Nidus penetration is generally most effectively achieved using liquid embolic materials. This process eliminates portions of the nidus in arterial distributions that are accessible and safe for embolization and leaves regions of nidus patent in remaining arterial distributions. This is particularly helpful for deep AVMs, including those in the basal ganglia and thalamus treatable with an acceptable risk profile using a multimodality approach [7]. During surgery, the embolic material is visualized in the nidus and feeding arteries. The embolized AVM and embolic material becomes hardened, sometimes making dissection and AVM mobilization more difficult; however, the benefit of decreased bleeding at surgery outweighs this disadvantage. Furthermore, embolic materials provide a means of nidus localization intraoperatively and may provide a starting point for the initiation of a resection. A major advantage of preoperative embolization is the occlusion of arterial feeding vessels not easily accessed via the surgical approach because of their anatomical location or positioning relative to the AVM nidus (Fig. 25.2) [8]. For example, large AVMs with dominant anterior circulation arterial supply and minor posterior circulation supply benefit from embolization of the posterior

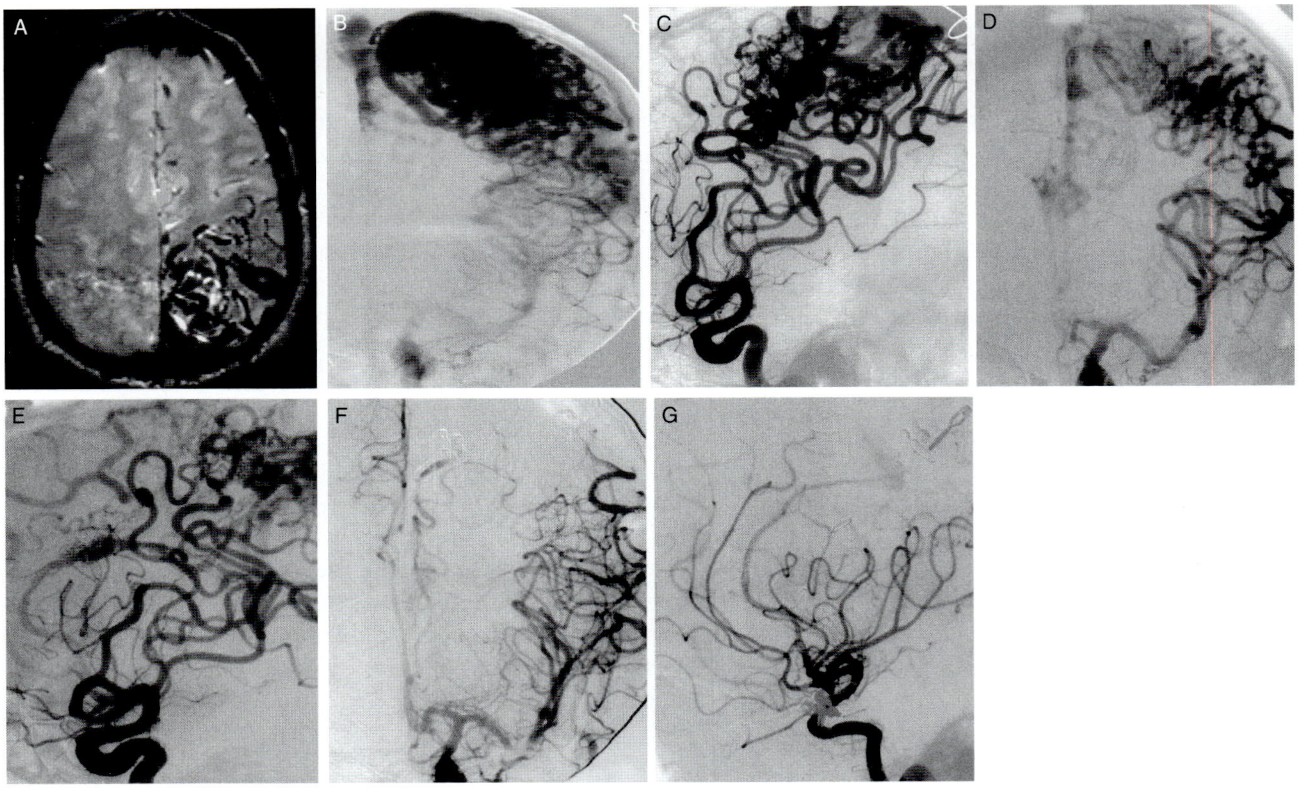

Fig. 25.1. A 25-year-old man presented with headaches, bruit, episodes of visual distortion, and memory difficulties. (A) Axial MRI showed a left parietal giant arteriovenous malformations (AVM). (B,C) Initial left carotid angiography showed the AVM filling (B, anteroposterior view; C, lateral view). His initial treatment was stereotactic radiosurgery at a dose of 18 Gy cobalt-60 equivalents. (D,E) Three years after radiosurgery, with no significant reduction in AVM volume, two courses of embolization were administered, resulting in a 40% reduction in AVM volume, as seen on left carotid angiography (D, anteroposterior view; E, lateral view). (F,G) In the operating room, intraoperative electrophysiological mapping showed that the AVM was posterior to the somatosensory cortex; left carotid angiography showed that a total resection was achieved (F, anteroposterior view; G, lateral view). The patient had initial mild right-sided lower extremity weakness and sensory deficit, which resolved completely during the next 6 months. (Reprinted from Chang *et al.*, 2003 [3], with permission from Wolters Kluwer Health.)

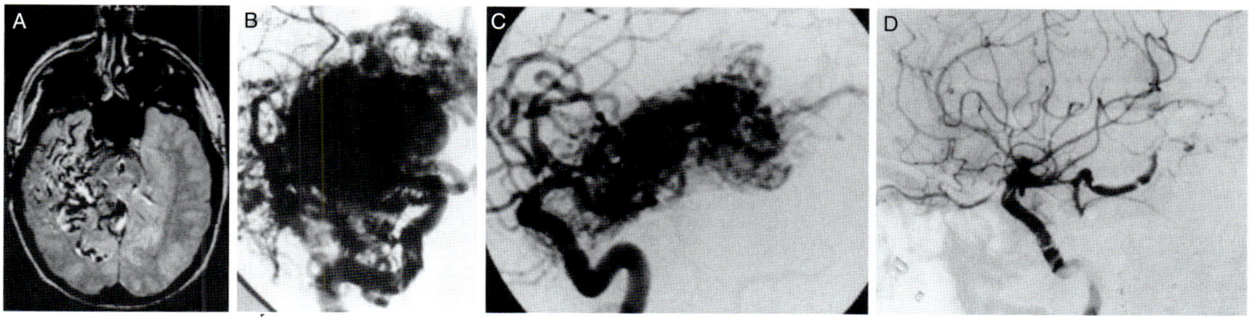

Fig. 25.2. A deep right temporo-occipital arteriovenous malformation (AVM) in a 34-year-old man. (A) Axial T_2-weighted MRI showed the extent of AVM. The patient was treated with 15 Gy to 47 500 mm^3. (B,C) Angiography 2 years after radiosurgery showed AVM filling from branches of the middle cerebral artery with no significant reduction in AVM size (B, anteroposterior view; C, lateral view). The patient subsequently underwent four staged embolizations (resulting in 70% obliteration) and then microsurgical resection. (D) Lateral view following surgical resection showed complete AVM obliteration. (From Steinberg *et al.*, 1996 [8], with permission from the American Association of Neurological Surgeons.)

circulation arterial feeders that are difficult to access or could only be accessed late in the procedure via an anterior supratentorial approach. Lastly, preoperative embolization has the advantage of reducing intraoperative blood loss [6,9].

The choice to use preoperative embolization must be balanced against the potential risk of this procedure. Known complications of AVM embolization include ischemic stroke; hemorrhage; venous hypertension and edema; visual loss, particularly via anastomotic ophthalmic arterial supply; pulmonary embolus; and the expected complications of an angiographic procedure [10]. Studies reporting the incidence of complications arising from embolization procedures have shown a wide range of long-term morbidity, ranging from 6 to 33% [6,11–13]. Reported mortality rates range from 0 to 3% in these studies.

There are few known determinants of successful preoperative embolization. Judging the success of a partial, preoperative or preradiosurgical therapy is difficult, particularly when few data exist that compare multidisciplinary and single modality treatments. In a study of 101 patients undergoing preoperative embolization, Vinuela *et al.* reported that at least 75% of AVM nidi had to be obliterated by embolization to produce a benefit for subsequent surgery [11]. This study suggested that limited embolization is of little value and should be avoided if only a small component of the AVM is expected to be treated with embolization. However, in specific cases where obliteration of a surgically inaccessible feeding artery or deep portion of nidus is possible, presurgical embolization may be considered. Data from 119 patients undergoing preoperative embolization were analyzed to determine predictive factors for AVM obliteration and complications at the completion of multimodality therapy [12]. Although there were insufficient patients to power a multivariate analysis, univariate analysis suggested that non-hemorrhagic presentation, large AVM size, deep venous drainage, and eloquent location were associated with elevated complication risks [12]. Unfortunately, determination of an independent relationship of any of these factors with embolization was not possible; however, these data confirmed findings by the group at the Barrow Neurological Institute with respect to risk factors for surgical excision of AVMs [13,14].

Preradiosurgery embolization

Embolization preceding radiosurgery is utilized to eliminate high-risk features, reduce nidus size, and to reduce flow to AVMs (Fig. 25.3) [2]. A common use of preoperative embolization and endovascular therapy is in the treatment of high-risk features, such as prenidal or intranidal aneurysms in both ruptured and unruptured AVMs, as these have been estimated to double the risk of rupture in unruptured AVMs and have a high rate of rerupture in ruptured AVMs [10,15]. In a large retrospective review of patients undergoing radiosurgery for AVMs, the Pittsburgh group demonstrated that the annual risk of rebleeding following radiosurgery in ruptured AVMs reduced from 6.4% to 0.8% by treating associated aneurysms using endovascular embolization or surgical clipping [16].

Radiosurgery is generally reserved for surgically inaccessible lesions as effects of radiosurgery progress to obliteration over a period of years and do not eliminate hemorrhage risk until complete obliteration occurs (Fig. 25.4) [3,17]. Nidus size is a limiting factor in selecting radiosurgery, as lesion diameter <3 cm has the best response from radiosurgery treatment. Therefore, preradiosurgical embolization is selected to reduce nidus volume to achieve this lesion diameter. However, given the relatively high recanalization rates of AVMs early after endovascular therapy, a potential criticism of preradiosurgical embolization is that recurrence could occur in non-radiated portions of the embolized AVM before the remainder of the radiated AVM is obliterated [18]. There have been reports that preradiosurgical embolization decreases obliteration rates compared with non-embolized lesions, supporting concerns about the durability of embolization during the interval of radiation response in AVMs subsequently treated with radiosurgery [19]. Additional proposed reasons for decreased radiosurgery efficacy in these patients include the notion that embolic materials may cause absorption or diffraction of radiation or image artifact on planning MRI and/or CT that could affect radiation dose delivery and skew targeting during radiosurgery [19–21]. Contrary to these concerns, it has been recently suggested that embolic procedures that reduce flow in fistulous AVMs and penetrate the nidus and venous drainage

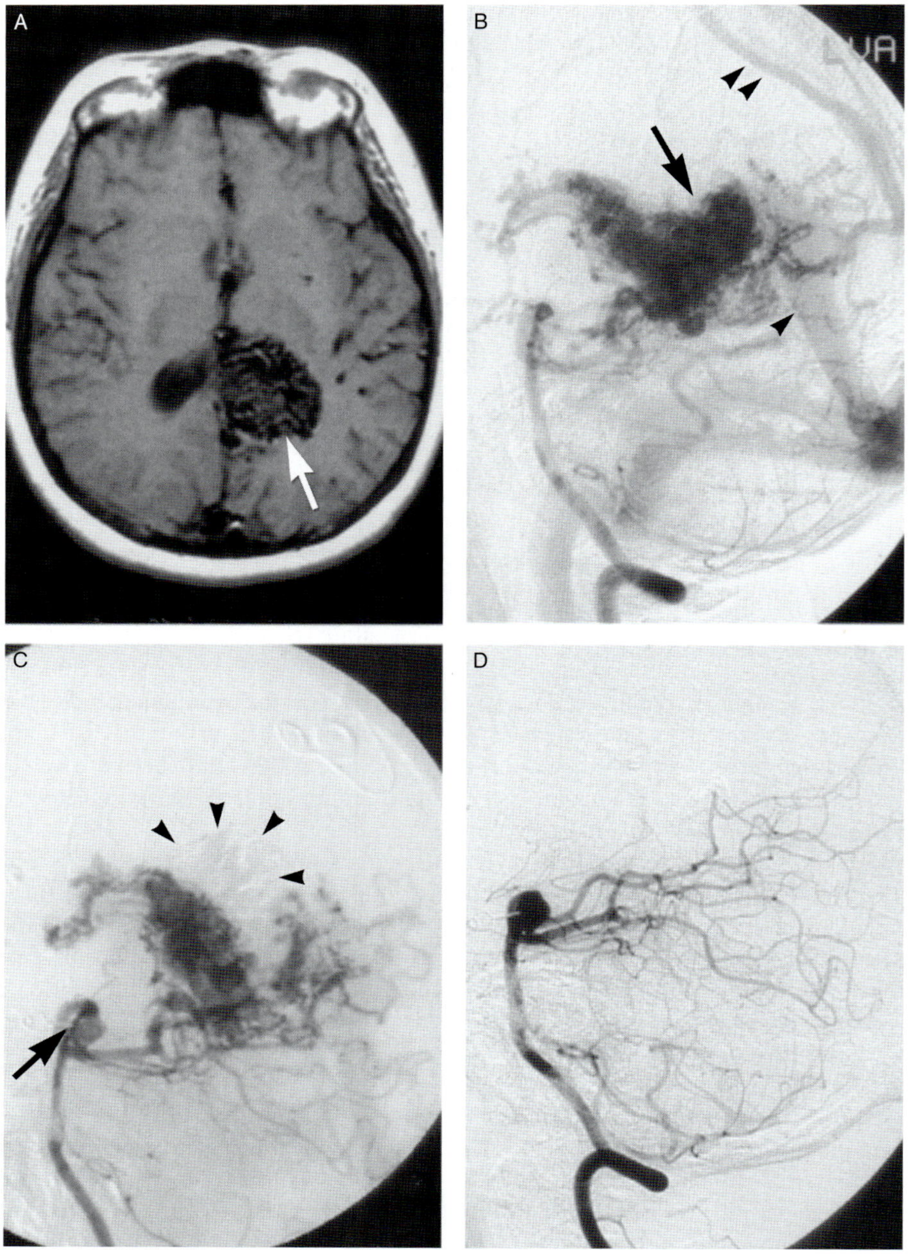

Fig. 25.3. A 36-year-old right-handed woman with a left medial parietal lobe arteriovenous malformation (AVM). (A) MRI showed the AVM (white arrow). (B) Angiography showed an AVM measuring 42 × 37 × 36 mm (black arrow), which is fed by the distal branches of the anteriorcerebral artery (not shown) and the posterior choroidal artery. Deep venous drainage was into the straight sinus (single arrowhead) and superficial venous drainage into the superior sagittal sinus via a cortical vein (double arrowhead). This was a Spetzler–Martin grade IV AVM. (C) Angiography after two embolization sessions shows a substantial reduction in the nidus size. The basilar artery aneurysm was clipped before management of the nidus (straight arrow). Arrowheads outline the embolized portion of the nidus. (D) Angiography taken 28 months after stereotactic proton beam radiosurgery with a dose of 25 Gy cobalt-60 equivalents. (From Fleetwood and Steinberg, 2002 [2], with permission from the Lancet Publishing Group.)

may be of benefit in high-flow AVMs [22]. Decreasing flow or encouraging stasis in the AVM theoretically decreases intranidal pressures and reduces shear stress on AVM vessel walls, which are responsible for lesion expansion, recanalization, and proliferation. The key to successful preradiosurgical embolization is achieving a durable result with the initial embolization procedure. This requires complete penetration of the portion of AVM nidus being treated, including penetration into the venous phase without obstructing drainage from the remaining nidus. In general, liquid embolics are required to achieve such a result [22].

Outcomes following preradiosurgery embolization have been reported by several groups. Gobin *et al.* published a series of 125 patients treated with embolization followed by radiosurgery [17]. In this series, 14 AVMs (11.2%) were totally occluded and did not go on to radiosurgery. Of the 111 AVMs that went on to radiosurgery, 72 (65%) were totally occluded after radiosurgery. For small AVMs (<2 cm), obliteration rates following embolization were better, with 79% of lesions obliterated [23]. There was a 12.8% permanent morbidity rate and a 1.6% mortality associated with this treatment plan; however, complications occurred only in patients with grade III or larger AVMs, with a positive correlation between morbidity severity and lesion size. There were no complications in patients with grade II AVMs. The authors attributed successful embolization to the use of liquid embolics and complete penetration of the portion of AVM nidus to be treated through to the venous phase. They attributed recanalization to incomplete nidus penetration and proximal occlusion permitting recanalization and proliferation of the AVM. In a small series of 20 patients treated with Onyx embolization followed by radiosurgery, Pierot *et al.* reported an overall occlusion rate of 58.8% with a follow-up

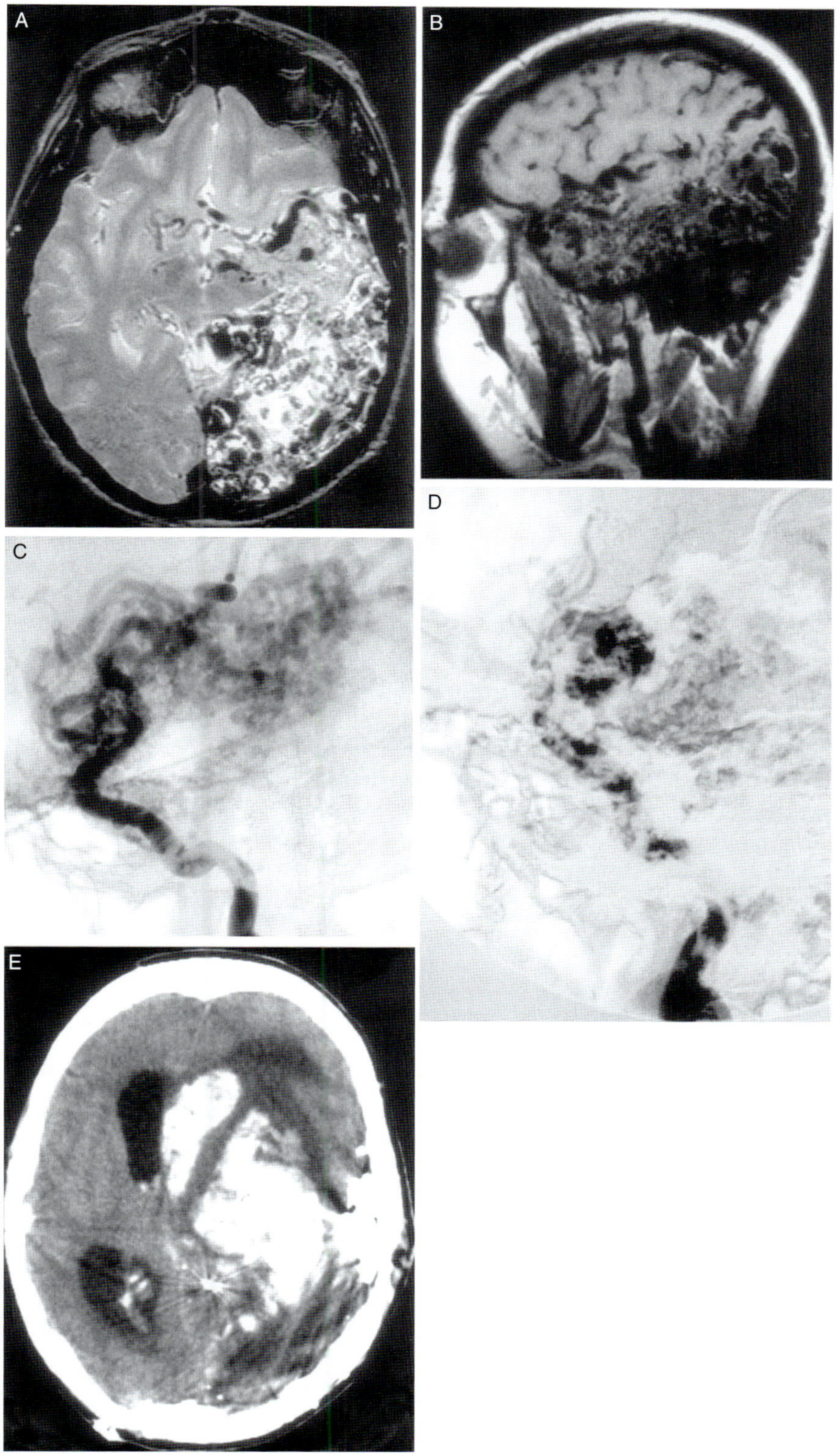

Fig. 25.4. A 26-year-old woman with a giant left temporo-occipital arteriovenous malformation (AVM) underwent proton beam radiosurgery. Her condition continued to deteriorate, however, with medically intractable seizures, progressive memory impairment, and a right homonymous hemianopsia. (A-C) Four years later, her AVM was unchanged angiographically from its preradiosurgical appearance, seen on axial (A) and sagittal (B) MRI and on lateral left internal carotid artery angiography (C). The patient underwent four embolization procedures. (D) Postembolization lateral left carotid angiography showed significant reduction in AVM volume. (E) The patient was scheduled for repeat heavy-particle radiosurgery but had a fatal hemorrhage, as shown on CT 1 week after the patient's last embolization procedure. (Reprinted from Chang *et al.*, 2003 [3], with permission from Wolters Kluwer Health.)

period ranging from two to five years following treatment [24]. In this series, larger AVMs (>3 cm) had a 50% occlusion rate and smaller lesions (<3 cm) had an 80% occlusion rate. The authors reported a 5% morbidity rate and attributed their low complication rate to the use of Onyx liquid embolic. While the authors made a case for increased safety with Onyx, this small study cannot be used to derive conclusions and larger studies will be required to confirm these findings. In a series of 24 patients with grade IV and V AVMs (all >3 cm in diameter) treated with embolization followed by radiosurgery, permanent neurological injury was sustained in three patients (14%) after embolization and in two (5%) after radiosurgery, but none had major neurological deficits [23]. Three year follow-up data was available for 16 patients in this series, with an an obliteration rate of 81%.

The Pittsburgh radiosurgery group published a retrospective series of 24 patients with large AVMs (>3 cm) embolized with particulate embolics and subsequently treated with radiosurgery where the three-year obliteration rate was 58% [18]. Based on these results, an overall obliteration rate using embolization followed by radiosurgery can be expected to be between 60 and 80%, with improved results in smaller lesions. There is an advantage to removing fistulous components of high-flow AVMs. Complete penetration of an AVM nidus is required to avoid recanalization during the three-year treatment interval of radiosurgery. Treatment of large AVMs, including those involving critical brain regions, is feasible using a staged endovascular and radiosurgical approach and has an acceptable risk profile and balanced risk–benefit ratio [25–27].

Preoperative radiosurgery

Preoperative radiosurgery is rarely intended a priori and is generally a result of failed radiosurgical treatment, partial radiosurgical treatment, lesion interval hemorrhage after radiosurgery, and radionecrosis. However, radiosurgery can be used to reduce the volume of the AVM nidus to facilitate surgical resection similar to the use of preoperative embolization (Fig. 25.5) [8]. At Stanford, we have resected AVMs in 77 patients following radiosurgical treatment. Radiosurgery results in vascular thickening and vessel thrombosis through hyalinization and mineralization of blood vessels [8]. There is brain atrophy related to brain necrosis and decreased tissue elasticity from gliosis. Vascular and tissue effects combine to produce a relatively solid, discrete mass with decreased vascularity and formation of tissue pseudoplanes at necrotic vessel–brain interfaces [8,28]. At the time of surgery, this produces a less vascular lesion that is more easily dissected from the surrounding brain. In many cases, this enables a more straightforward resection and significantly decreased blood loss [8]. Residual nidus can be contained within this gliotic mass or in the periphery and must be evaluated using catheter angiography in the preoperative stages to adequately plan for the resection.

There are limited outcome studies for this approach; however, those that are available suggest that radiosurgery preceding surgery is effective and safe. A case report describes a 57-year-old man with a grade V AVM who initially underwent eight embolization procedures and a failed craniotomy [29]. The residual large AVM was treated using three sessions of radiosurgery to fractionate portions of the nidus, followed by resection of the AVM three years later. The AVM was removed without major blood loss and the patient went on to make a good neurological recovery despite having four hemorrhages during the period of treatment [29]. The group from the University of California at San Francisco reported on 21 patients who underwent radiosurgery of large AVMs before surgical resection. They found that radiosurgery resulted in shorter wait times in the operating room, decreased blood loss, decreased morbidity, and decreased hospital stays when compared with a matched control cohort with surgically excised AVMs [30]. An additional benefit of resecting radiated AVMs is the opportunity to resect or debulk regions of tumefactive radionecrosis or proliferative endothelial hyperplasia that may become symptomatic following radiosurgery [31,32]. Timing of surgery of this nature was best undertaken soon after symptom onset to improve overall outcome.

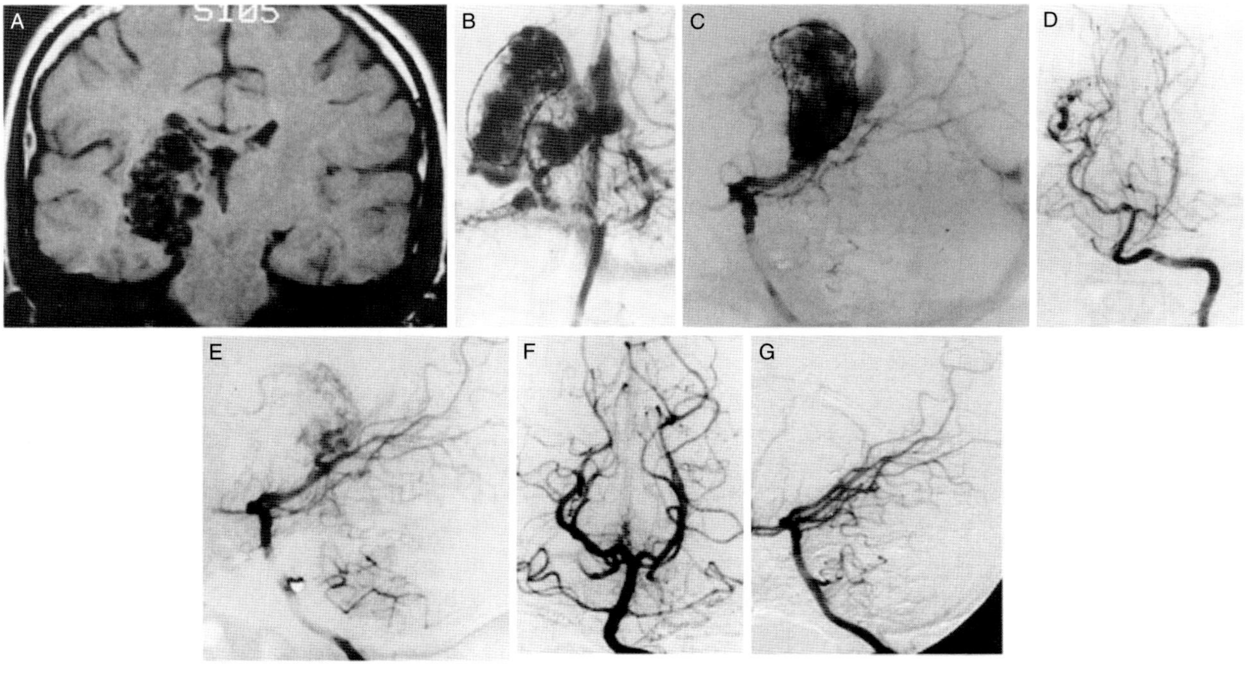

Fig. 25.5. A deep right thalamic arteriovenous malformation (AVM) in a 23-year-old woman presenting with hemorrhage. (A) Coronal MRI. (B,C) Angiography showed AVM blood supply from the posterior circulation. The areas of the AVM targeted for stereotactic radiosurgery are outlined (B, anteroposterior view; C, lateral view). (D,E) Angiography 2 years after radiosurgery (25 Gy cobalt-60 equivalents to 7000 mm^3) demonstrating approximately 80% obliteration of the AVM (D, anteroposterior view; E, lateral view). (F,G) Angiography after microsurgical resection showed complete resection of the AVM (F, anteroposterior view; G, lateral view). (From Steinberg *et al.*, 1996 [8], with permission from the American Association of Neurological Surgeons.)

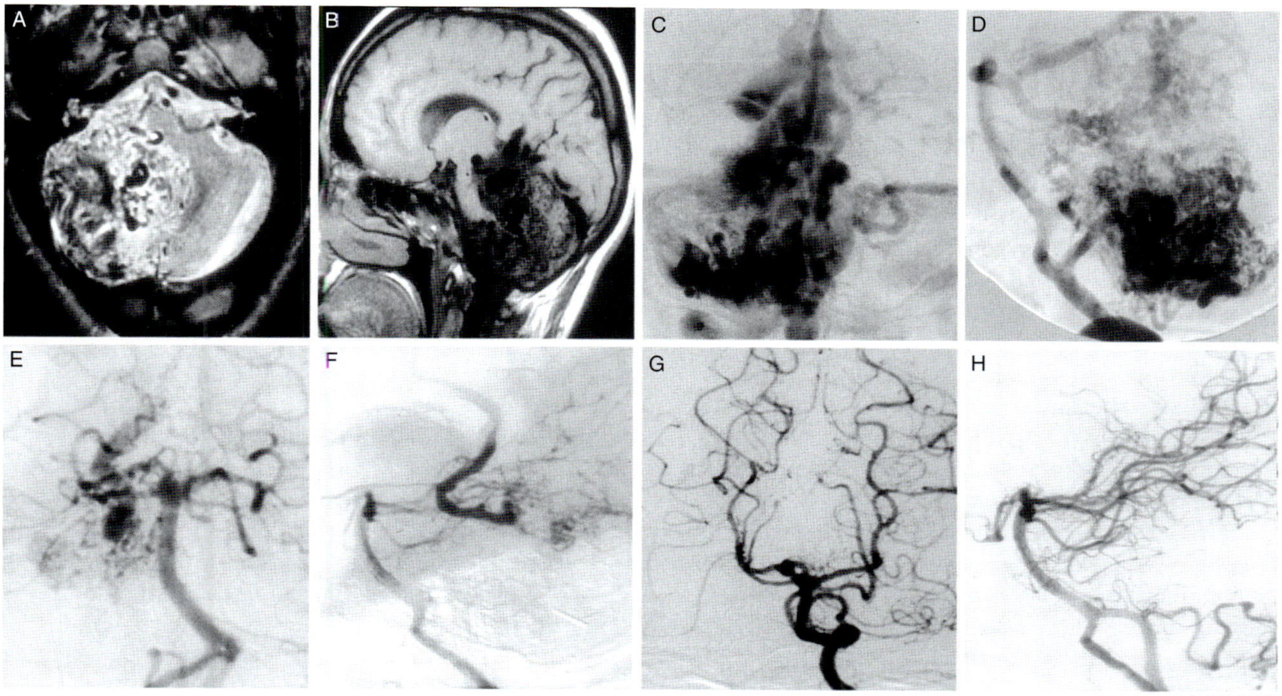

Fig. 25.6. A 33-year-old woman who presented with a 10-year history of diplopia, ataxia, and severe headache. (A,B) MRI showed a right posterior fossa giant arteriovenous malformation (AVM) (A, axial view; B, sagittal view). (C,D) Pretreatment vertebrobasilar angiography confirmed the presence of the AVM (C, anteroposterior view; D, lateral view). The patient underwent three sessions of embolization followed by subtotal resection of the AVM. She was then treated with 20 Gy cobalt-60 equivalents of stereotactic radiosurgery. (E,F) Follow-up vertebrobasilar angiography 3 years after radiosurgery showed a small residual AVM (E, anteroposterior view; F, lateral view). (G,H) Postoperative angiography after a second surgical resection showed complete obliteration of the AVM (G, anteroposterior view; H, lateral view). Clinically, the patient had resolution of her headaches but continued to experience baseline ataxia. (Reprinted from Chang *et al.*, 2003 [3], with permission from Wolters Kluwer Health.)

Partial resection preceding radiosurgery or embolization

The use of partial resection preceding the use of another treatment modality is rarely described. The main indication for this approach is in the compartmentalization of large or diffuse AVMs preceding a second or third treatment modality (Fig. 25.6) [3]. Some nidal components may be supplied by one or more arterial feeding vessels that are surgically accessible and secondary components may be supplied by separate arterial feeders that are anatomically impracticable to resect. This is generally seen in very large AVMs with complex angioarchitecture, which carry a high risk for periprocedural morbidity with any single therapy. In these cases, the concept of partial resection has been explored to reduce the overall size of the lesion. The portion of nidus supplied by a single feeding artery can be safely removed if the feeding artery is occluded and draining veins specific to this segment of nidus are removed, without affecting the drainage of adjacent portions of the AVM. Careful consideration of preoperative angiography in conjunction with interventional neuroradiology is required to do this. Selective injections of individual feeding arteries must also be considered to anatomically isolate the arterial distributions within a lesion. Once this anatomical segment is identified, it can be targeted and resected by occluding appropriate feeding arteries, removing the segment of nidus supplied by these feeders, and selectively taking only minor draining veins (veins that are independently draining the selected segment of AVM) and preserving major draining veins and veins draining adjacent portions of the malformations. Intraoperative angiography using indocyanine green or catheter angiography can be useful in confirming the localization of these types of resection. Reduction of the nidus volume can make the AVM amenable to subsequent radiosurgery or subsequent embolization/radiosurgery. In general, some embolization is undertaken before surgical resection in these patients.

Another scenario where partial surgical resection may be considered is in the case of a diffuse AVM where the nidus may have components that are within eloquent cortex or are widely distributed throughout the brain, making complete resection impossible. In diffuse AVMs, where lesion volume exceeds radiosurgical limitations, radiosurgery becomes impractical. In these situations, there may be components of the nidus that can be resected to reduce the overall volume of the malformations. Regions of compact nidus in or adjacent to diffuse nidi may also be managed in this fashion. For a ruptured AVM with diffuse components, regions with compact nidus or high-risk angioarchitectural features can be resected to theoretically reduce rebleeding risk during subsequent radiosurgery or a period of observation.

The goal of AVM surgery should be the complete removal of the malformations. Very rarely, residual AVM is left intentionally after microsurgical treatment. In the more common scenario of unintentional residual AVM, the lesion is usually discovered in the immediate postoperative period by angiography. In these cases, the patient is often taken back to the operating room in the acute phase to complete the resection. However, residual AVM has been demonstrated on later angiography despite initial negative angiography and may be related to persistent, slow flow or local compression of a nidus at the time of early postoperative angiography. Where a repeat operative procedure is feasible, this is generally pursued; however, where reoperation is not feasible because of the anatomical location, risk to eloquent brain, or concern about intraoperative localization in a deeply located, small residual, radiosurgery or embolization are potential options. Stereotactic radiosurgery is a convenient option for small residual AVMs in difficult locations as this technique utilizes preoperative MRI and angiography to locate the nidus in the planning stages of treatment. Endovascular embolization is an option in residual lesions with a single feeding artery. However, similar to primary treatment by embolization, AVM residuals with multiple arterial feeders or diffuse nidus have a high recurrence rate. For these reasons, embolization is reserved for residual AVMs that have one or two feeding vessels that can be selectively injected and occluded.

Outcomes following multimodality therapy

Few studies have reported the overall results of a multimodality treatment strategy for AVMs. Smith *et al.* from the Barrow Neurological Institute reported on a series of 54 patients with AVMs treated using a multimodality approach [33]. This series had 37 patients with adequate follow-up. Of these patients, there was a 35% overall obliteration rate with 27%, 58%, and 21% obliteration rates reported in grade V, IV, and III AVMs, respectively. There was one death and one patient with permanent morbidity, both related to hemorrhage.

Dehdashti *et al.* published a series of 135 patients with occipital AVMs treated in a multimodality clinic [34]. Within this cohort, 94 patients underwent treatment and 41 were observed. The observation group served as a control cohort for comparisons. In the treatment cohort, 60 patients had multiple treatment modalities, with surgery and embolization used in 33 patients, radiosurgery and embolization in 24 patients, and all three modalities in 3 patients. The overall obliteration rate in treated patients was 82%. There were two deaths related to embolization and no deaths related to surgical excision. The only interval hemorrhage in the treatment cohort was in a radiosurgery-treated patient (overall bleed rate in the treatment group was 0.1% per year). In the control cohort, there were two hemorrhages during the period of observation (4.6% per year hemorrhage rate). There were eight permanent neurological deficits associated with treatment overall; however, five patients with pre-existing visual field deficits had improvement of their visual fields after treatment. The authors concluded that there was a trend toward decreased hemorrhage rate and decreased mortality in the treatment group, although there was no statistically significant difference between the outcomes measured in the treatment and observation cohorts [34]. Sinclair *et al.* from Stanford University looked at a prospectively collected cohort of 55 patients treated for occipital AVMs [35]. In this cohort, 48 patients underwent multimodality therapy and 7 underwent radiosurgery alone. Complete obliteration was achieved in 42 of the 48 patients (88%) undergoing multimodality therapy. The most common treatment strategy utilized was embolization followed by microsurgery. Visual field outcomes were available for all 42 patients and revealed no change in 28 patients (67%), improvement in 6 (14%), and worsening in 8 (19%) when compared with preoperative examinations.

Hoh *et al.* reported the Massachusetts General Hospital experience in 141 patients with AVM-related seizures who underwent multimodality management [36]. In this study, 107 patients (76%) achieved Engel class I/II outcomes following treatment. No single treatment was associated with improved seizure outcome; however, complete obliteration of the lesion was associated with improved seizure outcome. This finding suggests that the primary goal for improved seizure outcomes is lesion obliteration by the modality or combination of modalities providing the lowest risk of complication. A series of 53 patients with giant AVMs (≥6.0 cm diameter) treated at Stanford University Medical Center using a multimodality approach achieved an overall 36% total obliteration rate [3]. In a cohort of 33 patients who had follow-up data three years following their latest radiosurgery, or had a complete obliteration after initial therapy, there was a 58% total obliteration rate. The permanent treatment-related morbidity in this series was 15%, with poor outcomes in 6%. There was 15% mortality in this series including five hemorrhages, one sagittal sinus thrombosis, one case of status epilepticus, and one case of sepsis.

Multimodality therapy for posterior fossa AVMs was evaluated utilizing prospectively collected data from the Stanford University AVM database [37]. A total of 76 patients with grade III–V AVMs were included in this study. In this cohort, there was an annual hemorrhage risk of 8.4% preceding treatment initiation, and 9.6% per year from the initiation of treatment to complete obliteration. Patients in this study were divided into a cohort that received radiosurgery in single or multiple sessions, and a cohort of patients that received multimodality therapy including radiosurgery, embolization, and surgery. In the radiosurgery cohort, there was a 21.4% cure rate with single treatment radiosurgery. This cure rate increased to 50% with multiple radiosurgery treatments. Despite improvements, these results are still inferior to the 61.8% cure rate with multimodality treatment. The overall complication rate for major neurological morbidity and death in this group was 18.8%, with no difference between treatment modality utilized. The study concluded that posterior fossa AVMs that are amenable should undergo multimodality therapy to maximize the likelihood of complete obliteration [37]. Radiosurgery remains a viable option for lesions involving the brainstem that are not surgically accessible; however, there is a lower obliteration rate using radiosurgery in single or multiple sessions.

Outcomes for multimodality therapy have also been studied in the pediatric population. Darsaut *et al.* treated 120 children (<18 years of age) with AVMs using a multimodality approach [38]. There were 76 patients with Spetzler–Martin grade I–III (low-grade) lesions, and 44 with grade IV–V (high-grade) lesions. The overall hemorrhage rate was 4% per year preceding treatment, and 3.2% per year following treatment initiation until complete obliteration. Single modality therapy led to complete obliteration in 76% of low-grade AVMs, and 9% of high-grade AVMs. Multimodality therapy improved obliteration rates to 87% and 26% in the low- and high-grade cohorts, respectively. The overall major neurological deficit and mortality rates were 5% in low-grade patients, and 28% in high-grade patients. A multivariate analysis looking at predictors of poor outcome revealed that high-grade AVMs, dominant hemisphere location, and poor initial clinical grade were predictors of poor outcome. The authors concluded that multimodality therapy increased the rate of complete obliteration and noted that balance must be struck in weighing the risk of intervention against the natural history of the disease, particularly in treating patients with large lesions and poor initial neurological function [38].

Overall obliteration rates of multimodality therapy are difficult to estimate based on the limited data in the literature. Studies reviewing the efficacy and complication profile of multimodality treatment should be undertaken to understand the advantages and disadvantages of this treatment option. Comparisons of treatment cohorts with observed cohorts or historical controls should be pursued to understand if an advantage is conferred by multimodality treatment.

Conclusions

There is no question that the multidisciplinary AVM clinic has advantages in the treatment of patients with complex AVMs, including the ability to consider each modality with focused expertise, a full understanding of treatment-related complications, and the option to utilize multiple modalities for a given patient. However, multimodality therapy comes with a cumulative risk associated with each modality used. This risk profile is not yet fully characterized in the literature for multimodality treatment and must be balanced against the natural history of hemorrhage or progressive neurological deficit for each patient. Furthermore, no protection against hemorrhage is conferred until there is complete obliteration of AVMs treated with radiosurgery [39,40] or partial embolization [17]. Therefore, it may not be worth embarking on multimodality therapy unless complete obliteration of the lesion is reasonably attainable, except where high-risk angioarchitecture is specifically addressed or for palliative embolization to treat venous hypertension, bruits, or intractable headache. Multidisciplinary AVM management has created options for addressing previously untreatable AVMs, particularly large and deeply situated lesions. Although multimodality AVM management does not currently confer obliteration rates achieved by single modality management of smaller, more accessible lesions, future applications of multimodality therapy and advances in each of the treatment modalities will likely lead to superior outcomes and improved risk profiles.

References

1. Hillman J. Population-based analysis of arteriovenous malformation treatment. *J Neurosurg* 2001;**95**:633–7.
2. Fleetwood IG, Steinberg GK. Arteriovenous malformations. *Lancet* 2002;**359**:863–73.
3. Chang SD, Marcellus ML, Marks MP, *et al.* Multimodality treatment of giant intracranial arteriovenous malformations. *Neurosurgery* 2003;**53**:1–11.
4. Nagashima H, Okudera H, Muraoka S, *et al.* Strategic embolisation for successful resection of a large cerebral arteriovenous malformation. *J Clin Neurosci* 2000;**7**(Suppl 1):86–7.
5. Spetzler RF, Martin NA, Carter LP, *et al.* Surgical management of large AVMs by staged embolization and operative excision. *J Neurosurg* 1987;**67**:17–28.
6. Taylor CL, Dutton K, Rappard G, *et al.* Complications of preoperative embolization of cerebral arteriovenous malformations. *J Neurosurg* 2004;**100**:810–12.
7. Fleetwood IG, Marcellus ML, Levy RP, *et al.* Deep arteriovenous malformations of the basal ganglia and thalamus: natural history. *J Neurosurg* 2003;**98**:747–50.
8. Steinberg GK, Chang SD, Levy RP, *et al.* Surgical resection of large incompletely treated intracranial arteriovenous malformations following stereotactic radiosurgery. *J Neurosurg* 1996;**84**:920–8.
9. Jafar JJ, Davis AJ, Berenstein A, *et al.* The effect of embolization with *N*-butyl cyanoacrylate prior to surgical resection of cerebral arteriovenous malformations. *J Neurosurg* 1993;**78**:60–9.
10. Krings T, Hans FJ, Geibprasert S, *et al.* Partial "targeted" embolisation of brain arteriovenous malformations. *Eur Radiol* 2010;**20**:2723–31.
11. Vinuela F, Dion JE, Duckwiler G, *et al.* Combined endovascular embolization and surgery in the management of cerebral arteriovenous malformations: experience with 101 cases. *J Neurosurg* 1991;**75**:856–64.
12. Hartmann A, Mast H, Mohr JP, *et al.* Determinants of staged endovascular and surgical treatment outcome of brain arteriovenous malformations. *Stroke* 2005;**36**:2431–5.
13. Hamilton MG, Spetzler RF. The prospective application of a grading system for arteriovenous malformations. *Neurosurgery* 1994;**34**:2–6.
14. Spetzler RF, Martin NA. A proposed grading system for arteriovenous malformations. *J Neurosurg* 1986;**65**:476–83.
15. da Costa L, Wallace MC, terBrugge KG, *et al.* The natural history and predictive features of hemorrhage from brain arteriovenous malformations. *Stroke* 2009;**40**:100–5.
16. Kano H, Kondziolka D, Flickinger JC, *et al.* Aneurysms increase the risk of rebleeding after stereotactic radiosurgery for hemorrhagic

arteriovenous malformations. *Stroke* 2012;**43**:2586–91.

17. Gobin YP, Laurent A, Merienne L, *et al.* Treatment of brain arteriovenous malformations by embolization and radiosurgery. *J Neurosurg* 1996;**85**:19–28.
18. Mathis JA, Barr JD, Horton JA, *et al.* The efficacy of particulate embolization combined with stereotactic radiosurgery for treatment of large arteriovenous malformations of the brain. *AJNR Am J Neuroradiol* 1995;**16**:299–306.
19. Andrade-Souza YM, Ramani M, Scora D, *et al.* Embolization before radiosurgery reduces the obliteration rate of arteriovenous malformations. *Neurosurgery* 2007;**60**:443–51.
20. Roberts DA, Balter JM, Chaudhary N, *et al.* Dosimetric measurements of Onyx embolization material for stereotactic radiosurgery. *Med Phys* 2012;**39**:6672–81.
21. Shtraus N, Schifter D, Corn BW, *et al.* Radiosurgical treatment planning of AVM following embolization with Onyx: possible dosage error in treatment planning can be averted. *J Neurooncol* 2010;**98**:271–6.
22. Taeshineetanakul P, Krings T, Geibprasert S, *et al.* Angioarchitecture determines obliteration rate after radiosurgery in brain arteriovenous malformations. *Neurosurgery* 2012;**71**:1071–8.
23. Blackburn SL, Ashley WW, Jr., Rich KM, *et al.* Combined endovascular embolization and stereotactic radiosurgery in the treatment of large arteriovenous malformations. *J Neurosurg* 2011;**114**:1758–67.
24. Pierot L, Kadziolka K, Litre F, *et al.* Combined treatment of brain AVMs with use of Onyx embolization followed by radiosurgery. *AJNR Am J Neuroradiol* 2013.
25. Jayaraman MV, Marcellus ML, Do HM, *et al.* Hemorrhage rate in patients with Spetzler–Martin grades IV and V arteriovenous malformations: is treatment justified? *Stroke* 2007;**38**:325–9.
26. Paulsen RD, Steinberg GK, Norbash AM, *et al.* Embolization of rolandic cortex arteriovenous malformations. *Neurosurgery* 1999;**44**:479–84.
27. Paulsen RD, Steinberg GK, Norbash AM, *et al.* Embolization of basal ganglia and thalamic arteriovenous malformations. *Neurosurgery* 1999;**44**:991–6.
28. Chang SD, Steinberg GK, Levy RP, *et al.* Microsurgical resection of incompletely obliterated intracranial arteriovenous malformations following stereotactic radiosurgery. *Neurol Med Chir (Tokyo)* 1998;**38**(Suppl):200–7.
29. Firlik AD, Levy EI, Kondziolka D, *et al.* Staged volume radiosurgery followed by microsurgical resection: a novel treatment for giant cerebral arteriovenous malformations: technical case report. *Neurosurgery* 1998;**43**:1223–8.
30. Sanchez-Mejia RO, McDermott MW, Tan J, *et al.* Radiosurgery facilitates resection of brain arteriovenous malformations and reduces surgical morbidity. *Neurosurgery* 2009;**64**:231–8.
31. Karamchandani J, Vogel H, Fischbein N, *et al.* Extravascular papillary endothelial hyperplasia mimicking neoplasm after radiosurgery: case report. *Neurosurgery* 2012;**70**:E1043–8.
32. Massengale JL, Levy RP, Marcellus M, *et al.* Outcomes of surgery for resection of regions of symptomatic radiation injury after stereotactic radiosurgery for arteriovenous malformations. *Neurosurgery* 2006;**59**:553–60.
33. Smith KA, Shetter A, Speiser B, *et al.* Angiographic follow-up in 37 patients after radiosurgery for cerebral arteriovenous malformations as part of a multimodality treatment approach. *Stereotact Funct Neurosurg* 1997;**69**:136–42.
34. Dehdashti AR, Thines L, Willinsky RA, *et al.* Multidisciplinary care of occipital arteriovenous malformations: effect on nonhemorrhagic headache, vision, and outcome in a series of 135 patients. *J Neurosurg* 2010;**113**:742–8.
35. Sinclair J, Marks MP, Levy RP, *et al.* Visual field preservation after curative multi-modality treatment of occipital lobe arteriovenous malformations. *Neurosurgery* 2005;**57**:655–67.
36. Hoh BL, Chapman PH, Loeffler JS, *et al.* Results of multimodality treatment for 141 patients with brain arteriovenous malformations and seizures: factors associated with seizure incidence and seizure outcomes. *Neurosurgery* 2002;**51**:303–9.
37. Kelly ME, Guzman R, Sinclair J, *et al.* Multimodality treatment of posterior fossa arteriovenous malformations. *J Neurosurg* 2008;**108**:1152–61.
38. Darsaut TE, Guzman R, Marcellus ML, *et al.* Management of pediatric intracranial arteriovenous malformations: experience with multimodality therapy. *Neurosurgery* 2011;**69**:540–56.
39. Betti OO, Munari C, Rosler R. Stereotactic radiosurgery with the linear accelerator: treatment of arteriovenous malformations. *Neurosurgery* 1989;**24**:311–21.
40. Friedman WA, Bova FJ, Mendenhall WM. Linear accelerator radiosurgery for arteriovenous malformations: the relationship of size to outcome. *J Neurosurg* 1995;**82**:180–9.

Chapter 26

Palliative treatment of inoperable arteriovenous malformations

Ayca Akgoz and Kai U. Frerichs

Introduction

Successful arteriovenous malformations (AVM) treatment is dependent upon achievement of the outcome of complete AVM nidus obliteration that leads to elimination of future hemorrhage risk. Eliminating this hemorrhage risk must be balanced with the risks and the morbidity and mortality associated with treating these lesions. Consequently, it is important to understand the natural history of these vascular malformations and be familiar with the risks and outcomes of each treatment modality: microsurgery, endovascular embolization, and stereotactic radiosurgery.

The widely used Spetzler–Martin grading system, which classifies AVMs based on their size, eloquence of adjacent brain, and patterns of venous drainage was specifically designed to estimate morbidity and mortality associated with AVM surgery [1]. Complete microsurgical excision of Spetzler–Martin grades I and II AVMs is associated with minimal morbidity and mortality rates. Indeed, most AVMs of grades I to III can be operated on with relative safety by experienced vascular neurosurgeons. However, the same cannot be said for grade IV and V AVMs. These large, critically located malformations require extensive dissection in close proximity to essential brain regions, and the resection could be complicated by difficulties with controlling fragile deep vessels. In addition, obliteration of a large AVM shunt exposes surrounding normal vessels to a sudden increase in perfusion, which may result in vasogenic edema or even hemorrhage (the phenomenon that has been termed as "normal perfusion pressure breakthrough"). Morbidity rates within the early postoperative period following complete surgical obliteration of grade IV and V AVMs, often using preoperative embolization, are 31% and 50%, respectively. Permanent major neurological morbidity rates of 21.9% and 16.7%, respectively, are noted on follow-up for these lesions [2]. With deep perforating arterial supply or deep meningeal recruitment, combined morbidity and mortality rates could be as high as 44% [3]. Given the unacceptably high rates of surgical morbidity and mortality, which exceed the risks determined by the natural history of AVM, it is a matter of debate whether these high-grade lesions should or should not be treated. According to Spetzler and Martin [1], inoperable AVMs are classified as grade VI lesions, which include extremely large diffuse AVMs that are dispersed through critical neurologically eloquent areas or malformations with a diffuse nidus encompassing critical structures such as the hypothalamus and the brainstem. Surgical resection of these lesions is almost always associated with a disabling deficit or death. However, in addition to grade VI lesions, some grade IV and V AVMs may also be considered unresectable, given associated high rates of surgical morbidity and mortality.

Combined therapeutic strategies utilizing preoperative embolization have potential in making large AVMs amenable to subsequent curative surgical or radiosurgical therapy [4]. Meanwhile, the limits of microsurgical therapy for AVMs also continue to expand. Potts *et al.* [5] reported their impressive surgical experience with 24 AVMs of the basal ganglia, with an overall 87.5% resection rate and only a 5% morbidity rate. Prospective staged volume radiosurgery could be also utilized as a therapeutic option for large AVMs. This approach has been used by Kano *et al.* for large AVMs unsuitable for resection, where treatment with prospective staged volume radiosurgery achieved a 36% obliteration rate and a 36% cumulative AVM hemorrhage rate at 10-year follow-up [6]. Kano *et al.* also published their results for brainstem, basal ganglia, and thalamic AVMs treated with stereotactic radiosurgery [7,8], achieving a 76% obliteration rate and 5.8% AVM hemorrhage rate for brainstem AVMs, and a 72% obliteration rate and 15.4% AVM hemorrhage rate for AVMs within the basal ganglia and thalamus. Patients remained at risk for hemorrhage during the latency interval until obliteration, which is probably the major problem with radiosurgical AVM treatment. Deep location of an AVM, which is a feature that makes an AVM unappealing from a surgical perspective, appears to be an independent risk factor for hemorrhage. Deep AVMs have reported annual rupture rates ranging from 3.1% to 4.4%, which is higher than the overall initial annual rupture rate of 2.2% for other lesions [9]. Some have postulated an association of deep AVM location with a greater tendency toward perforator involvement and a resultant higher rupture

Comprehensive Management of Arteriovenous Malformations of the Brain and Spine, ed. Robert F. Spetzler, Douglas S. Kondziolka, Randall T. Higashida, and M. Yashar S. Kalani. Published by Cambridge University Press.

rate because of the fragility of these vessels [10]. Management of these deep-seated AVMs is challenging and controversial. Higher rates of rupture and morbidity after hemorrhage, compared with AVMs situated within other locations if left untreated, may favor treatment over observation.

The decision to treat an AVM should be based on the natural history of the lesion, patient preference, and expertise of the treating team. Several studies have evaluated the natural history of AVMs with regard to risk of hemorrhage and found on average a 2–4% annual risk of rupture in all AVMs [11,12]. It is known that this risk may vary widely depending on certain characteristics of the AVM, such as previous hemorrhage, deep location, exclusively deep venous drainage, and associated aneurysms [9]. Because the purpose of Spetzler–Martin grade is to estimate the risk of AVM surgery, it has not been included in the hemorrhage risk calculations. Consequently, it is difficult to determine whether the natural history of grades IV and V AVMs is the same, worse, or better than that of grades I–III AVMs.

Three studies have specifically investigated the natural history of high-grade AVMs [13–15]. Han *et al.* [13] reported that the annual risk of hemorrhage in their series of 73 patients with high-grade AVMs was 1.5%, and therefore less than that usually reported for AVMs in general (2–4% per year). Moreover, among 59 patients who had received no previous treatment for their AVMs (true long-term natural history), the annual risk was even lower, at 1.0%. By comparison, the annual risk of hemorrhage was 10.4% among 14 patients who previously had received partial incomplete treatment. In contrast to these findings, Jayaraman *et al.* [14] observed a 10.4% annual rupture rate in their series of 61 patients with high-grade AVMs. Hemorrhagic presentation increased the risk of subsequent hemorrhage, with an annual rupture rate of 13.9% compared with 7.3% in patients with unruptured AVMs. Subsequently, Laakso *et al.* [15] published the Finnish data for these lesions, suggesting that, if ruptured, they may have a relatively malevolent course (with an overall 3.3% annual rupture risk increasing to 6.0% for ruptured grade IV or V AVMs). The discrepancy in hemorrhage rates reported by these three studies is hard to explain, but differences in patient selection, referral bias, or methods of calculation of annual hemorrhage rate could have contributed to the results.

In light of their results, Han *et al.* [13] recommended that no treatment should be performed for most grade IV and V AVMs. Complete treatment is only advised for patients who suffer recurrent hemorrhages with resultant progressive neurological deficits. An additional argument in favor of treatment of these ruptured high-grade AVMs is that in many patients the hemorrhage has already caused neurological deficits, sometimes permanent, which are not necessarily exacerbated by the treatment. Given that there is no evidence supporting that partial treatment of an AVM reduces the rate of hemorrhage, most teams do not recommend partial treatment of AVMs. In fact, partial treatment may worsen the natural history of an AVM.

Despite the lack of evidence in support of partial therapy, there are some instances when targeted treatment of high-risk features of an AVM may be indicated. Partial embolization, feeder ligation or associated aneurysm treatment only, and partial radiosurgery are sometimes performed in circumstances where the radical treatment of the AVM is not possible, or there is hesitancy to treat lesions in eloquent areas given high rates of morbidity and mortality associated with aggressive therapy [16]. Partial treatment is usually performed as a means of palliation with intention to decrease future hemorrhage risk, such as treatment of AVM-associated aneurysms, or to alleviate progressive non-hemorrhagic symptoms, such as progressive neurological deficits associated with vascular steal. Endovascular embolization is the most commonly utilized modality for partial or palliative treatment of AVMs. A representative case of partial embolization of an inoperable AVM is presented in Fig. 26.1. Miyamoto *et al.* [16] found an annual risk of hemorrhage of 14.6% in patients who underwent palliative treatment of brain AVMs. The rate of major neurological deficits was 23.3% and the mortality rate was 9.3%. Eleven patients who exhibited non-hemorrhagic onset experienced bleeding episodes for the first time after palliative treatments. Among 26 bleeding episodes in the 18 patients treated palliatively, 12 episodes were fatal or significantly morbid. The authors concluded that palliative treatments cannot prevent hemorrhage and may even worsen the natural history of an AVM. Kwon *et al.* [17] evaluated a group of 27 patients with inoperable AVMs to see if there was any potential benefit of palliative embolization, compared with medical treatment. The analysis of the long-term clinical follow-up (mean follow-up period was 99 ± 44 months) results showed no significant difference in either the risk of hemorrhage or the clinical status of the patients in the two treatment groups. Da Costa *et al.* [12] found similar results in the analysis of their cohort with no statistically significant change in hemorrhage risk in patients who underwent partial AVM embolization compared with patients without partial embolization. The risk of hemorrhage for brain AVMs that were partially embolized for any reason (preoperative, palliative, preradiosurgical, targeted, or in a failed cure attempt) was 3.95% per year, compared with 4.79% per year for AVMs not treated with embolization. Wikholm *et al.* [18] embolized AVMs with acrylic glue and often supplemented treatment with gamma radiation. No hemorrhages occurred in patients in whom there was ≥90% occlusion of the AVM. However, in patients with 90% rate of occlusion, the results were discouraging, with the rates of hemorrhage or mortality higher than what would be expected from the traditionally accepted annual rates of 4% hemorrhage and 1% for death based on the natural history of disease. These results underscore the fact that the ultimate goal of treatment should always be complete or near-complete eradication of the lesion, although this may require multiple sessions using various modalities. It is well known that if any residual portion remains, the risk of hemorrhage is unaltered. Therefore, if partial or palliative treatment is to be attempted, benefits should be well defined before proceeding. Each AVM should be considered individually. For each patient, consideration should be given to features such as the number of previous hemorrhages incurred, the clinical presentation, the patient's neurological status, the AVM Spetzler–Martin grade, the

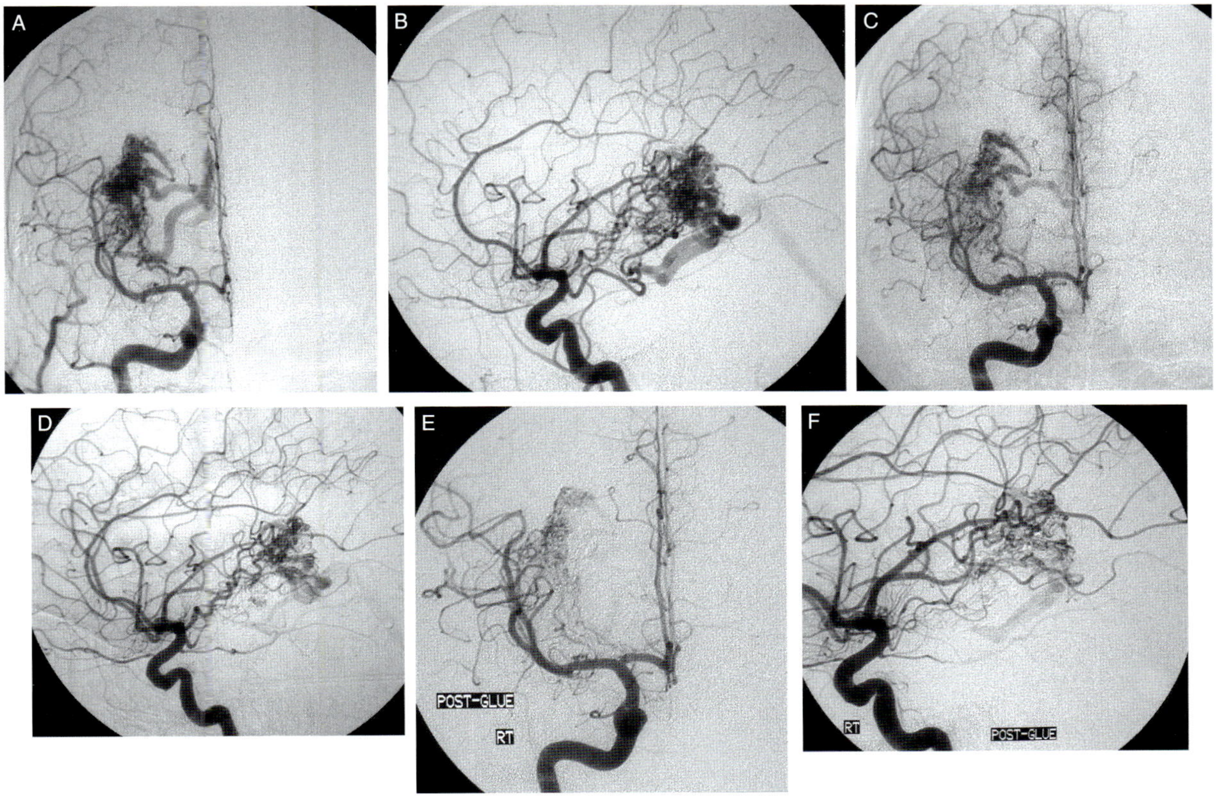

Fig. 26.1. A 24-year-old man who previously presented with intracranial hemorrhage from a right deep basal ganglia arteriovenous malformation (AVM) grade IV. (A,B) The AVM was supplied via a right anterior choroidal artery and right lenticulostriate perforator branches with venous drainage into the vein of Galen via two separate veins. This inoperable AVM was embolized with *N*-butyl cyanoacrylate in two stages. (C,D) During the first stage of embolization, the AVM was embolized via the right anterior choroidal artery feeder. This resulted in successful nidal penetration into the medial and inferior aspects of the AVM nidus, resulting in significantly decreased flow through the lesion. (E,F) The patient underwent a second stage of embolization 1 month later. This was carried out via the right M1 perforator feeders with further reduction of flow through the malformation. Embolization was followed by radiosurgery. The patient has been clinically asymptomatic since treatment.

amount of flow through the lesion, the degree of vascular steal from surrounding brain, the number and location of associated aneurysms, and previous treatments and their outcomes. Palliative treatment of high-grade AVMs could be considered in selected patients where there are angioarchitectural features associated with an increased risk of hemorrhage (e.g., aneurysms, high-flow shunts) or there are progressive non-hemorrhagic symptoms (e.g., progressive neurological deficits or intractable headaches).

Increased hemorrhage risk or progressive non-hemorrhagic symptoms

Radiographic and angioarchitectural features give an indication of AVMs with increased hemorrhage risk or progressive non-hemorrhagic symptoms.

Brain arteriovenous malformations with associated aneurysms

The incidence of aneurysms associated with AVMs reported in the literature has varied widely, with most series reporting an incidence between 10% and 20%, up to 58% [19]. Redekop *et al.* [19] classified these aneurysms as intranidal, flow related (proximal or distal), or unrelated to the AVM nidus. Aneurysms were described as intranidal if they were localized within the boundaries of the AVM nidus and filled early during angiography before substantial venous filling had occurred. Saccular aneurysms arising along the course of arteries supplying the AVM were defined as flow related. Intranidal aneurysms showed a high correlation with hemorrhagic clinical presentation and a 9.8% per-year risk of AVM hemorrhage, which is considerably higher than the 2–4% annual hemorrhage rate usually attributed to AVMs. Meisel *et al.* [20] reported similar findings in their patients with brain AVMs associated with intranidal aneurysms. They noted a higher rate of rebleeding before treatment (11%) compared with a group with no aneurysms (3%), confirming the potential risk represented by intranidal aneurysms and supporting the need to follow a prompt therapeutic strategy, particularly if complete surgical obliteration of the AVM is not possible.

By comparison, the need for treatment of flow-related aneurysms that are discovered incidentally in association with AVMs is a matter of some controversy. Some authors have suggested aggressive management strategies. Given the possibility that the hemodynamic changes associated with the abrupt elimination of an AVM may place associated aneurysms at immediate risk, Batjer *et al.* [21] recommended treatment of the aneurysm before proceeding with microsurgical resection of the associated AVM. Thompson *et al.* [22] also recommended a management protocol designed to treat the aneurysms by either surgical or endovascular means before administering definitive therapy for the AVM. However, specific intervention in all patients may not be necessary, as flow-related aneurysms may spontaneously regress following treatment of the AVM. Distal aneurysms have a high probability of regression with substantial or curative AVM treatment, with 80% completely regressing following AVM obliteration [19]. Proximal aneurysms regress infrequently, with only 17% decreasing in size and 4% disappearing after AVM cure. Patients with flow-related aneurysms in association with an AVM may present with hemorrhage from either lesion.

In the event of intracranial hemorrhage, the source of hemorrhage should be identified and eliminated. Feeding artery or intranidal aneurysms may warrant treatment irrespective of AVM size [13]. For unruptured proximal aneurysms, the decision could be based on size, as with general aneurysm treatment, and small proximal aneurysms could be followed while larger proximal aneurysms treated directly [23]. A clinical example of a patient with an AVM with an associated flow-related feeding pedicle aneurysm is presented in Fig. 26.2.

Intranidal high-flow shunts

An intranidal high-flow fistula implies a high-flow hole into the venous side. This may be suspected radiologically when large-caliber vessels with no intervening nidus are seen, and confirmed hydrodynamically when a microcatheter is placed in the artery and the contrast is seen to rapidly wash away [24]. Intranidal high-flow fistulae could be described as "weak spots" for hemorrhage [25] and could be chosen as targets for embolization in patients with unresectable brain AVMs. In addition, when a multimodality treatment is used to treat large AVMs, endovascular treatment of associated intranidal shunts may help to maximize the treatment effect. Recent reports have indicated that AVMs with a non-plexiform component, such as high-flow fistulae, appear to be more resistant to radiosurgery than other lesions. It is also known that AVMs with high-flow shunts are associated with an increased incidence of perioperative complications such as intra- or postoperative bleeding [26]. Meisel *et al.* [27] showed that partial targeted embolization with *N*-butyl cyanoacrylate reduced the long-term risk of hemorrhage by 31% at two years when weak

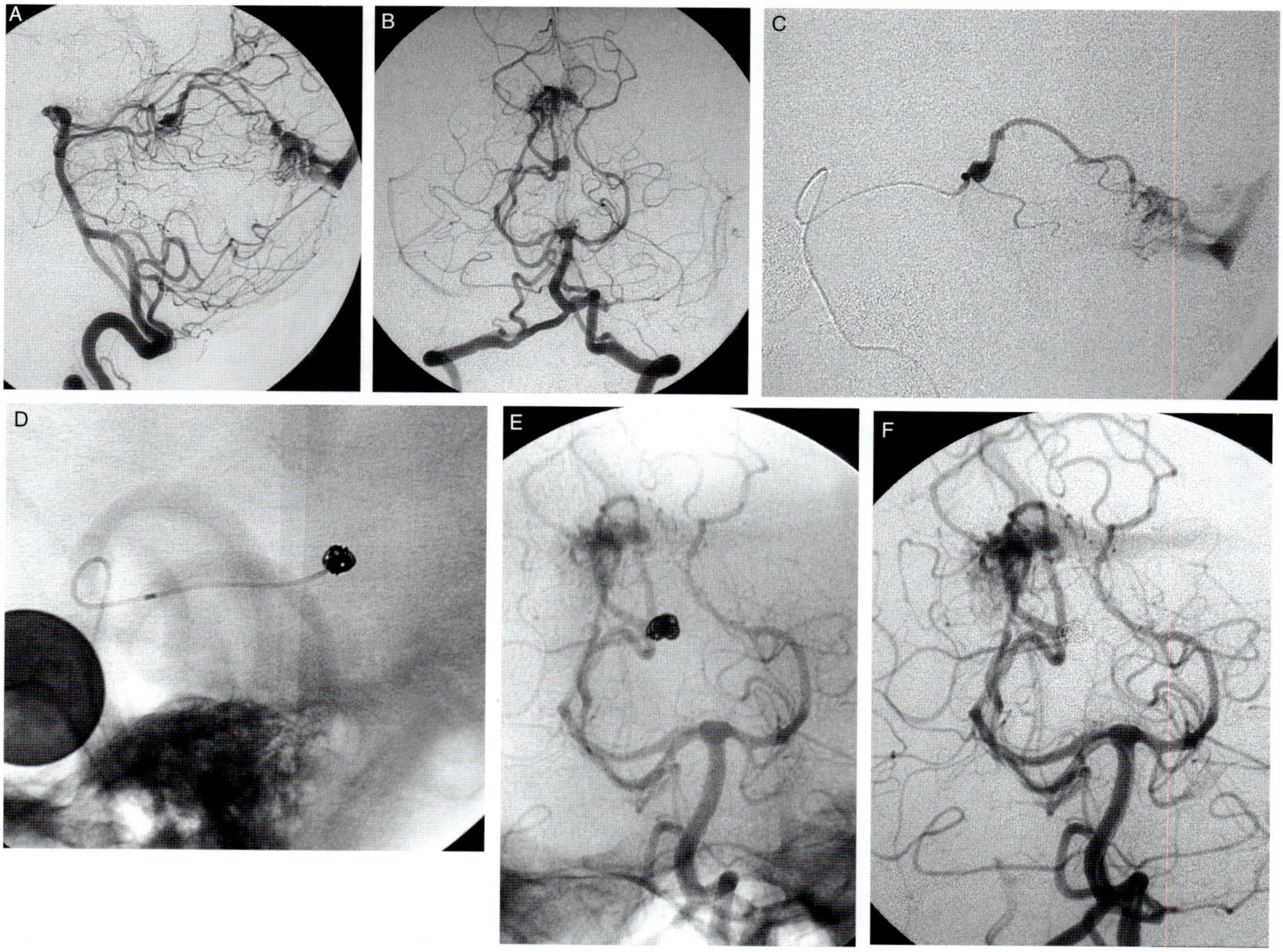

Fig. 26.2. A 58-year-old woman with a known right cerebellar arteriovenous malformation (AVM) presented with headache. (A,B) Angiography showed the AVM supplied via distal branches of the right superior cerebellar artery and the right posterior inferior cerebellar artery. The malformations drained into the torcula. A 3 × 2 mm saccular aneurysm was also seen arising from the midsegment of the right superior cerebellar artery. (C,D) The right superior cerebellar artery was superselectively catheterized and the proximal feeding artery aneurysm was embolized with multiple coils. (E,F) Postcoiling images demonstrated complete obliteration of the aneurysm.

spots within the AVM's angioarchitecture, such as intranidal aneurysms or fistulae, were targeted. Embolization of intranidal fistulae may not only reduce the rehemorrhage rate but also improve the seizure activity and headaches in patients when the target is decreasing venous flow.

Brain edema, venous drainage abnormalities, and venous stenosis

Brain edema in unruptured brain AVMs is rare [28–31]. Some reports mention venous outflow abnormalities and suggest that venous congestion is the cause of brain edema [28–30]. Kim *et al.* [31] found 13 patients (3.9%) with brain edema in 329 patients with unruptured AVMs. Neurological deficit was more frequently seen as a presenting feature in patients with edema, seen in 46.2% compared with 18.4% without edema. Venous thrombosis was present on imaging in 38.5% with edema versus 0.9% without edema. Venous ectasias (seen in 84.6%) and stenosis (seen in 38.5%) on angiography were also more frequent in patients with edema than in those without edema. Eight patients with brain edema received specific treatment (five embolization, two surgery, one radiosurgery). Clinical features correlated well with change in degree of edema in six of these patients. Three of five patients who were treated with embolization were stable or showed improvement after the procedure. On follow-up, however, intracranial hemorrhage developed in three, suggesting that palliative embolization may arrest the non-hemorrhagic symptoms in selected patients but it may not have an effect on hemorrhagic risk or may even worsen the natural history.

Although not formally confirmed in natural history studies, it is likely that stenosis of the drainage system is associated with an increased risk of hemorrhage [32,33]. Therefore, if possible, endovascular treatment options targeting treatment of venous stenosis or decreasing arterial inflow could be considered in selected patients with inoperable brain AVMs presenting with symptomatic congestive intracranial hypertension or progressive non-hemorrhagic symptoms. In case reports for four patients [34], two patients with inoperable brain AVMs presenting with symptomatic intracranial hypertension were treated with endovascular partial embolization, which effectively reduced intracranial pressure and achieved sustained patient recovery. One case report describes a patient with an inoperable pontine AVM, who presented with headache and neurological deficit and was treated with venous stenting, producing substantial clinical benefit [35].

Inoperable arteriovenous malformations with progressive non-hemorrhagic symptoms

Intractable headaches

Headache had been reported to be the first symptom in approximately 11–14% of patients with brain AVMs [36]; constant or migraine-like headaches may be described [37]. Galetti *et al.* [38] investigated the relationship between brain AVM location and nature of the headache, and found that the location of the malformations was strongly associated with migraine-like presentation. The occipital lobe was the predominant site associated with migraine-like headaches. Patients with occipital brain AVMs with significant or predominant posterior cerebral artery supply may also have visual disturbances and/or intermittent episodes of visual field deficits.

The headaches associated with various vascular distributions may relate specifically to the dural supply and/or external carotid participation in a vascular malformations [37]. These types of headache may have a precise distribution and are usually throbbing/migraine-like in nature. The frequency of dural arterial contribution is significantly higher in superficial AVMs, particularly in the temporal, parietal, and occipital regions. Larger lesions with higher shunting and steal phenomena on angiography are other factors favoring a meningeal arterial contribution [39]. Blood flow can be rerouted from the dural compartment to supply the malformations as part of the natural course of the disease, and this change may be present when the lesion is discovered or it may emerge later [40]. Transarterial embolization of a brain AVM via pial vessels supplying the lesion may promote the development of a transdural blood supply.

Endovascular embolization may relieve headaches of vascular origin. When the dural contribution to an AVM is properly embolized, associated headaches may resolve or diminish [37]. However, current literature lacks direct evidence to support a benefit of dural supply embolization in patients with brain AVM with intractable headaches. Also, it is usually difficult to correlate the origin of the patient's headache with the degree and extent of dural supply embolization, which would be a potential problem in assessing treatment response. Moreover, as transdural supply development is not always constant but could be a dynamic process, there is potential that dural supply embolization may alter the behavior and natural history of AVMs.

Progressive neurological deficits and seizures

Arteriovenous malformations may cause neurological deficits and seizures via vascular steal, occlusive changes, and direct or indirect mechanical compression [37]. The concept of vascular steal in angiography is based on non-visualization of vessels in a normal area of the brain that should have been visible at the time of the injection. However, careful angiographic evaluation will always demonstrate the non-visualized branches through leptomeningeal anastomosis from adjacent territories. Angiographic characteristics that have been found to correlate with cerebrovascular steal in AVMs are angiomatous change, large AVM size, and peripheral venous drainage [41]. Batjer *et al.* assessed the degree of vascular steal in patients with brain AVMs with single photon emission CT (SPECT) and correlated the degree of steal with clinical findings [42]. Patients presenting with a history of progressive deficits had increased severity of steal compared with those without progressive deficits. In selected patients with unresectable brain AVMs presenting with progressive neurological deficits, palliative partial AVM

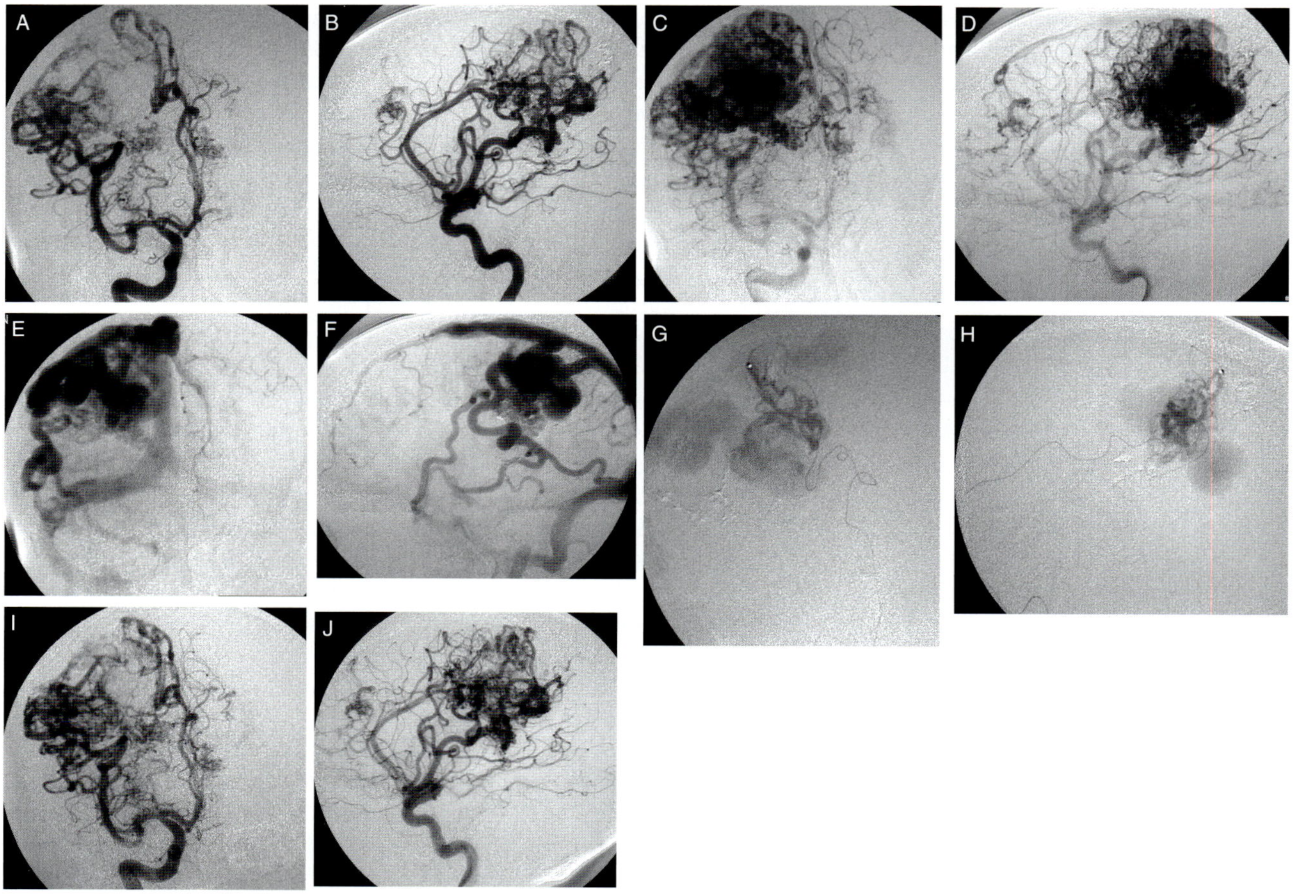

Fig. 26.3. A 55-year-old woman with a history of a grade V arteriovenous malformation (AVM) partially embolized at a different institution presented for consultation. The patient developed progressive difficulties with the use of her left hand, likely caused by a steal phenomenon. (A–D) The right internal carotid artery injection showed a large right parietal AVM supplied via branches of the right middle cerebral artery, particularly the right angular artery and distal branches of the right anterior cerebral artery, as well as left anterior cerebral artery contributors. (E,F) The venous drainage was into the superior sagittal sinus via multiple ectatic right parietal cortical veins, as well as into the right vein of Labbé and right sphenoparietal sinus. Initially, the right angular artery was catheterized; however, superselective injection via this branch showed en passage supply to the normal brain. (G,H) Superselective injection into the distal callosomarginal branch of the right anterior cerebral artery revealed significant nidal supply. The AVM was then embolized via this branch using *N*-butyl cyanoacrylate. (I,J) Postembolization arterial phase images demonstrate decrease in inflow to the malformation. Clinically, the patient has not had evidence of hemorrhage but remains significantly disabled.

embolization may stabilize or improve neurological deficits via enhancing perfusion of the normal brain [43,44]. Figure 26.3 shows a representative case of an attempt to manage a suspected steal phenomenon with partial embolization.

Trigeminal neuralgia and hemifacial spasm

Trigeminal neuralgia is rarely associated with an AVM within the posterior fossa [45,46]. The feeding arteries or draining veins of the AVM contacting the division(s) of the trigeminal nerve [45,47] or intrinsic AVMs within the nerve or brainstem itself [48] could be the cause of nerve irritation and trigeminal neuralgia. In patients with AVM-related trigeminal neuralgia, successful management includes invasive surgical AVM extirpation, or less commonly radiosurgery [49,50]. In unruptured high-grade AVMs, which are deemed inoperable because of an unacceptably high risk of morbidity and mortality of microsurgery, reducing the size of the feeding pedicles utilizing endovascular embolization may resolve trigeminal neuralgia [51,52]. A case report described a child with trigeminal neuralgia from a large posterior fossa AVM in whom repeated embolization of vascular feeders in contact with the V2 division provided only temporary relief [53]. Direct endovascular embolization of the artery of the foramen rotundum with Onyx (Covidien ev3 Neurovascular, Irvine, CA, USA), which provided minimal supply to the AVM, resulted in immediate and durable palliation of her trigeminal neuralgia symptoms with only a small area of hypesthesia of the left cheek.

Rarely, AVMs can also be associated with hemifacial spasm. A case report described a patient who was suffering severe chronic hemifacial spasm associated with a large temporo-occipital AVM; a dilated lateral mesencephalic vein lying in the vicinity of the facial nerve was identified on imaging [54]. This vein was transvenously embolized with coils, which resulted in complete long-standing remission of the patient's hemifacial spasm.

Conclusions

The management of inoperable AVMs continues to pose a significant clinical challenge. Palliative treatment of inoperable AVMs may be reasonable in selected patients for whom angioarchitectural features associated with an increased risk of hemorrhage are present. Partial embolization may also have a limited role in patients with progressive non-hemorrhagic symptoms, such as those with progressive neurological deficits related to vascular steal. Other than these special circumstances, partial treatment of an AVM is not indicated.

References

1. Spetzler RF, Martin NA. A proposed grading system for arteriovenous malformations. *J Neurosurg* 1986;**65**:476–83.
2. Hamilton MG, Spetzler RF. The prospective application of a grading system for arteriovenous malformations. *Neurosurgery* 1994;**34**:2–6.
3. Ferch RD, Morgan MK. High-grade arteriovenous malformations and their management. *J Clin Neurosci* 2002;**9**:37–40.
4. Blackburn SL, Ashley WW, Jr., Rich KM, *et al.* Combined endovascular embolization and stereotactic radiosurgery in the treatment of large arteriovenous malformations. *J Neurosurg* 2011;**114**:1758–67.
5. Potts MB, Chang EF, Young WL, *et al.* Transsylvian-transinsular approaches to the insula and basal ganglia: operative techniques and results with vascular lesions. *Neurosurgery* 2012;**70**:824–34.
6. Kano H, Kondziolka D, Flickinger JC, *et al.* Stereotactic radiosurgery for arteriovenous malformations. Part 6: multistaged volumetric management of large arteriovenous malformations. *J Neurosurg* 2012;**116**:54–65.
7. Kano H, Kondziolka D, Flickinger JC, *et al.* Stereotactic radiosurgery for arteriovenous malformations. Part 5: management of brainstem arteriovenous malformations. *J Neurosurg* 2012;**116**:44–53.
8. Kano H, Kondziolka D, Flickinger JC, *et al.* Stereotactic radiosurgery for arteriovenous malformations. Part 4: management of basal ganglia and thalamus arteriovenous malformations. *J Neurosurg* 2012;**116**:33–43.
9. Gross BA, Du R. Natural history of cerebral arteriovenous malformations: a meta-analysis. *J Neurosurg* 2013;**118**:437–43.
10. Hernesniemi JA, Dashti R, Juvela S, *et al.* Natural history of brain arteriovenous malformations: a long-term follow-up study of risk of hemorrhage in 238 patients. *Neurosurgery* 2008;**63**:823–9.
11. Brown RD, Jr., Wiebers DO, Forbes G, *et al.* The natural history of unruptured intracranial arteriovenous malformations. *J Neurosurg* 1988;**68**:352–7.
12. da Costa L, Wallace MC, terBrugge KG, *et al.* The natural history and predictive features of hemorrhage from brain arteriovenous malformations. *Stroke* 2009;**40**:100–5.
13. Han PP, Ponce FA, Spetzler RF. Intention-to-treat analysis of Spetzler–Martin grades IV and V arteriovenous malformations: natural history and treatment paradigm. *J Neurosurg* 2003;**98**:3–7.
14. Jayaraman MV, Marcellus ML, Do HM, *et al.* Hemorrhage rate in patients with Spetzler–Martin grades IV and V arteriovenous malformations: is treatment justified? *Stroke* 2007;**38**:325–9.
15. Laakso A, Dashti R, Juvela S, *et al.* Risk of hemorrhage in patients with untreated Spetzler–Martin grade IV and V arteriovenous malformations: a long-term follow-up study in 63 patients. *Neurosurgery* 2011;**68**:372–7.
16. Miyamoto S, Hashimoto N, Nagata I, *et al.* Posttreatment sequelae of palliatively treated cerebral arteriovenous malformations. *Neurosurgery* 2000;**46**:589–94.
17. Kwon OK, Han DH, Han MH, *et al.* Palliatively treated cerebral arteriovenous malformations: follow-up results. *J Clin Neurosci* 2000;7 (Suppl 1):69–72.
18. Wikholm G, Lundqvist C, Svendsen P. The Goteborg cohort of embolized cerebral arteriovenous malformations: a 6-year follow-up. *Neurosurgery* 2001;**49**:799–805.
19. Redekop G, terBrugge K, Montanera W, *et al.* Arterial aneurysms associated with cerebral arteriovenous malformations: classification, incidence, and risk of hemorrhage. *J Neurosurg* 1998;**89**:539–46.
20. Meisel HJ, Mansmann U, Alvarez H, *et al.* Cerebral arteriovenous malformations and associated aneurysms: analysis of 305 cases from a series of 662 patients. *Neurosurgery* 2000;**46**:793–800.
21. Batjer H, Suss RA, Samson D. Intracranial arteriovenous malformations associated with aneurysms. *Neurosurgery* 1986;**18**:29–35.
22. Thompson RC, Steinberg GK, Levy RP, *et al.* The management of patients with arteriovenous malformations and associated intracranial aneurysms. *Neurosurgery* 1998;**43**:202–11.
23. Almefty K, Spetzler RF. Arteriovenous malformations and associated aneurysms. *World Neurosurg* 2011;**76**:396–7.
24. Le Feuvre D, Taylor A. Target embolization of AVMs: identification of sites and results of treatment. *Interv Neuroradiol* 2007;**13**:389–94.
25. Soderman M, Andersson T, Karlsson B, *et al.* Management of patients with brain arteriovenous malformations. *Eur J Radiol* 2003;**46**:195–205.
26. Yuki I, Kim RH, Duckwiler G, *et al.* Treatment of brain arteriovenous malformations with high-flow arteriovenous fistulas: risk and complications associated with endovascular embolization in multimodality treatment. *J Neurosurg* 2010;**113**:715–22.
27. Meisel HJ, Mansmann U, Alvarez H, *et al.* Effect of partial targeted *N*-butyl-cyano-acrylate embolization in brain AVM. *Acta Neurochir (Wien)* 2002;**144**:879–87.
28. Miyasaka Y, Yada K, Kurata A, *et al.* An unruptured arteriovenous malformation with edema. *AJNR Am J Neuroradiol* 1994;**15**:385–8.
29. Shimizu S, Miyasaka Y, Tanaka R, *et al.* Pial arteriovenous malformation with massive perinidal edema. *Neurol Res* 1998;**20**:249–52.
30. Kurita H, Shin M, Ueki K, *et al.* Congestive brain oedema associated with a pial arteriovenous malformation with impaired venous drainage. *Acta Neurochir (Wien)* 2001;**143**:339–42.

31. Kim BS, Sarma D, Lee SK, *et al.* Brain edema associated with unruptured brain arteriovenous malformations. *Neuroradiology* 2009;**51**:327–35.
32. Vinuela F, Nombela L, Roach MR, *et al.* Stenotic and occlusive disease of the venous drainage system of deep brain AVMs. *J Neurosurg* 1985;**63**:180–4.
33. Miyasaka Y, Yada K, Ohwada T, *et al.* An analysis of the venous drainage system as a factor in hemorrhage from arteriovenous malformations. *J Neurosurg* 1992;**76**:239–43.
34. Rosenkranz M, Regelsberger J, Zeumer H, *et al.* Management of cerebral arteriovenous malformations associated with symptomatic congestive intracranial hypertension. *Eur Neurol* 2008;**59**:62–6.
35. Higgins JN, Kirkpatrick PJ. Stenting venous outflow gives symptomatic improvement in a patient with an inoperable brainstem arteriovenous malformation. *Br J Neurosurg* 2013;**12**:866–72.
36. Choi JH, Mohr JP. Brain arteriovenous malformations in adults. *Lancet Neurol* 2005;**4**:299–308.
37. Berenstein A, Lasjaunias P, terBrugge KG. *Surgical Neuroangiography.* Berlin: Springer, 2004.
38. Galletti F, Sarchielli P, Hamam M, *et al.* Occipital arteriovenous malformations and migraine. *Cephalalgia* 2011;**31**:1320–4.
39. Miyachi S, Negoro M, Handa T, *et al.* Contribution of meningeal arteries to cerebral arteriovenous malformations. *Neuroradiology* 1993;**35**:205–9.
40. Soderman M, Rodesch G, Lasjaunias P. Transdural blood supply to cerebral arteriovenous malformations adjacent to the dura mater. *AJNR Am J Neuroradiol* 2002;**23**:1295–300.
41. Marks MP, Lane B, Steinberg G, *et al.* Vascular characteristics of intracerebral arteriovenous malformations in patients with clinical steal. *AJNR Am J Neuroradiol* 1991;**12**:489–96.
42. Batjer HH, Devous MD, Sr., Seibert GB, *et al.* Intracranial arteriovenous malformation: relationships between clinical and radiographic factors and ipsilateral steal severity. *Neurosurgery* 1988;**23**:322–8.
43. Kusske JA, Kelly WA. Embolization and reduction of the "steal" syndrome in cerebral arteriovenous malformations. *J Neurosurg* 1974;**40**:313–21.
44. Al-Yamany M, terBrugge KG, Willinsky R, *et al.* Palliative embolisation of brain arteriovenous malformations presenting with progressive neurological deficit. *Interv Neuroradiol* 2000;**6**:177–83.
45. Garcia-Pastor C, Lopez-Gonzalez F, Revuelta R, *et al.* Trigeminal neuralgia secondary to arteriovenous malformations of the posterior fossa. *Surg Neurol* 2006;**66**: 207–11.
46. Figueiredo PC, Brock M, De Oliveira AMJ, *et al.* Arteriovenous malformation in the cerebellopontine angle presenting as trigeminal neuralgia. *Arq Neuropsiquiatr* 1989;**47**:61–71.
47. Sato K, Jokura H, Shirane R, *et al.* Trigeminal neuralgia associated with contralateral cerebellar arteriovenous malformation. Case illustration. *J Neurosurg* 2003;**98**:1318.
48. Edwards RJ, Clarke Y, Renowden SA, *et al.* Trigeminal neuralgia caused by microarteriovenous malformations of the trigeminal nerve root entry zone: symptomatic relief following complete excision of the lesion with nerve root preservation. *J Neurosurg* 2002;**97**:874–80.
49. Darsaut TE, Guzman R, Marcellus ML, *et al.* Management of pediatric intracranial arteriovenous malformations: experience with multimodality therapy. *Neurosurgery* 2011;**69**:540–56.
50. Anderson WS, Wang PP, Rigamonti D. Case of microarteriovenous malformation-induced trigeminal neuralgia treated with radiosurgery. *J Headache Pain* 2006;**7**:217–21.
51. Lesley WS. Resolution of trigeminal neuralgia following cerebellar AVM embolization with Onyx. *Cephalalgia* 2009;**29**:980–5.
52. Simon SD, Yao TL, Rosenbaum BP, *et al.* Resolution of trigeminal neuralgia after palliative embolization of a cerebellopontine angle arteriovenous malformation. *Cent Eur Neurosurg* 2009;**70**:161–3.
53. Levitt MR, Ramanathan D, Vaidya SS, *et al.* Endovascular palliation of AVM-associated intractable trigeminal neuralgia via embolization of the artery of the foramen rotundum. *Pain Med* 2011;**12**:1824–30.
54. Konan AV, Roy D, Raymond J. Endovascular treatment of hemifacial spasm associated with a cerebral arteriovenous malformation using transvenous embolization: case report. *Neurosurgery* 1999;**44**:663–6.

Chapter 27

Pediatric patients with arteriovenous malformations: special considerations

Edward R. Smith and R. Michael Scott

Introduction

Arteriovenous malformations (AVMs) are among the most important vascular anomalies in the nervous system of children; they are relatively common and usually require treatment. These children can present with hemorrhage, seizure, headache, progressive ischemia ("steal"), or the AVMs can be found incidentally. Treatment is predicated on obliteration of the lesion, which can be achieved by surgery, radiation, embolization, or a combination of therapies.

Closely related are vein of Galen malformations (VOGMs), involving pathological connections between the arteries of the limbic system and the vein of Galen. In addition to having typical AVM symptoms, infants with VOGMs can also sometimes present with high-output cardiac failure. These lesions are now nearly exclusively treated with embolization.

Basic vascular development and anatomy

Arteriovenous malformations

In an AVM, there are direct arterial-to-venous connections without intervening capillaries; they occur in the cerebral hemispheres, brainstem, and spinal cord. Functional neural tissue does not reside within the lesion [1]. Anomalies range from simple arteriovenous fistulae to complex tangled channels connecting enlarged feeding arteries to draining veins. The mechanism of expansion of AVM has been debated. One possibility is "mechanical" dilatation as the result of increased flow through poorly differentiated vessels and recruitment of collateral arterial feeders. Ischemia and surrounding microhemorrhages with resultant gliosis may promote enlargement of the AVM by destruction of the surrounding parenchyma.

Expansion of an AVM may also result from growth of new blood vessels (i.e., angiogenesis; a complex process regulated by a wide range of proteins, including metalloproteinases and related growth factors such as vascular endothelial growth factor [VEGF]) [2–8]. Immunochemical studies on resected cerebral AVMs have shown upregulation of VEGF, more prominently after preoperative embolization, supporting the concept that postnatal influences can affect the development and evolution of these lesions [6,8,9]. Both AVMs and cerebral cavernous malformations have been shown to produce VEGF and increased structural proteins in the endothelium and subendothelium and transforming growth factor-α in endothelial and perivascular layers [4]. A subsequent study confirmed upregulation of mRNA for these growth factors, receptors, and structural proteins [3]. These findings suggest that AVMs have the potential for postnatal growth. There are well-substantiated case reports describing the development of so-called "acquired" AVMs in the brain after cerebral infarction or trauma [10,11]. Likewise, AVMs in patients with hereditary hemorrhagic telangiectasia (HHT) and metameric AVMs are known to be progressive, likely because of hemodynamic effects superimposed upon genetically derived structural abnormalities.

Transgenic mice with one deletion of *ENG* (the gene that causes HHT and encodes an angiogenic protein endoglin) showed progressive destruction of the capillary bed related to endothelial cell nitric oxide synthetase deficiency [12]. Consequently, local or circulating angiogenic factors or a mutation in a component of the vascular bed can pose a lifelong risk for the development or recurrence of AVM, a finding particularly important in children.

Vein of Galen malformations

The most common lesions presenting with high output cardiac failure in the neonate and infant are the VOGMs. Further classification into mural and choroidal forms is helpful in terms of predicting prognosis and potential for successful treatment [13]. In general, VOGMs involve direct communication between arteries of the limbic system (predominantly choroidal branches of the posterior and anterior circulation) and a dilated central channel that is believed to be the embryonic precursor (the median vein of the prosencephalon) of the vein of Galen [14]. The median vein typically drains into an anomalous falcine sinus rather than the straight sinus. The presence of these embryonic structures infers that the defect arose in the third month of gestation. The severity of the associated cardiac volume overload is inversely proportional to the degree of obstruction of venous outflow. Likewise, the size of the varix

Comprehensive Management of Arteriovenous Malformations of the Brain and Spine, ed. Robert F. Spetzler, Douglas S. Kondziolka, Randall T. Higashida, and M. Yashar S. Kalani. Published by Cambridge University Press.

or "aneurysm" of the draining vein correlates with the flow and the severity of distal venous stenosis.

Choroidal VOGM is the most common form; the primitive vein of the prosencephalon or its choroidal tributary communicates with a large number of choroidal arteries, subependymal branches from the posterior circle of Willis, and dural arteries. The flow is usually unobstructed, resulting in dilatation of the draining falcine sinus and dural sinuses and with high-output cardiac failure. Over time, the dural sinuses may become obstructed, leading to intracranial hypertension. In the most severely affected neonates, ischemic changes in the developing CNS frequently occur, resulting in encephalomalacia or calcification and microcephaly, and consequent neurological and cognitive impairment.

The mural form of VOGM is characterized by a smaller number of fistulae between choroidal arteries and the wall of the dilated, often spherical, aneurysm of the vein of Galen or median vein of the prosencephalon. In most cases, there is some outflow obstruction of the draining vein, resulting in a varix. This tends to limit the severity of the cardiac volume overload but causes CNS problems in infancy, including development of hydrocephalus (from venous hypertension rather than compression of the aqueduct of sylvius), venous ischemia with cerebral atrophy, and herniation of the cerebellar tonsils (Chiari 1 malformations) [15]. This anomaly is less likely to be associated with developmental cerebral anomalies or ischemic changes at birth compared with the choroidal form; consequently, the prognosis for neurological development is better. Spontaneous thrombosis of the varix can occur [16].

Pediatric-specific treatment considerations

Pediatric-specific treatment considerations center on decisions to treat, methods of treatment, and the physiology of the child. With children, there is a strong impetus to provide definitive treatment, when possible, given the likelihood of a long life expectancy. Methods of treatment must be taken into consideration when formulating plans for children; specifically, the long-term effects of radiation exposure are important with the long potential lifespan of younger individuals. In addition, the risk of radiation exposure is greater in the developing brain than in the mature adult. The physiology of children is relevant in the plasticity of the brain, making it more resilient to injury than in an adult and adding the potential for tolerating insult at a greater level than older individuals. In addition, children may be more fragile surgical candidates, requiring greater attention to blood loss, blood pressure control, and medication dosing.

Pathophysiology

Arteriovenous malformations

Neurological signs and symptoms commonly relate to intracranial or subarachnoid hemorrhage from a vessel in the malformations or from a coexistent arterial aneurysm. Symptoms may also relate to cerebral ischemia caused by diversion of blood to the AVM from the normal cerebral circulation ("steal") or secondary to stagnation causing increased venous pressure secondary to the AVM. Enlarged anomalous vessels may compress or distort adjacent cerebral tissue or cause obstructive hydrocephalus by interfering with the normal circulation of cerebrospinal fluid. Communicating hydrocephalus can result from earlier hemorrhage or venous hypertension. There is an associated arterial aneurysm in 7–25% of patients with cerebral AVM [17–20]. An aneurysm can arise from hemodynamic stress caused by rapid flow in the AVMs. Therefore, there is often a close relationship between the site of the aneurysm and the vessels feeding the AVM. These flow-related aneurysms can spontaneously regress following the reduction in blood flow after treatment of the AVM [21,22].

Enlargement of an AVM seems to alter the adjacent brain. Functional MRI data have suggested that the presence of an AVM in an eloquent area of the brain may be associated with "migration" of the function to adjoining cortex or to the homologue on the contralateral hemisphere [23,24]. This migration or displacement of functional neuronal tissue has important implications for surgical planning.

Vein of Galen malformations

Pathophysiology of VOGMs is dependent on the type of lesion; high-flow VOGMs often present early in infancy with cardiac output failure and these patients may have "melting brain," in which gliosis of normal cortex occurs as a consequence of steal-related ischemia. Those with lesions with slower flow may present with hydrocephalus and signs of increased intracranial pressure. It is important to note that the hydrocephalus is a consequence of increased venous pressures, and so it should be treated by obliteration of the VOGM, not by shunting.

Incidence, epidemiology, and natural history

The most common symptomatic high-flow intracranial vascular abnormality in adults and children is the AVM [11]. In a large autopsy series, the overall frequency of detection for AVMs was 1.4% (46 among 3200 with brain tumors) [12]. In another report, the annual incidence of symptomatic AVMs was 1.1 per 100 000 [13]. The pediatric age group represents 12–18% of all AVMs presenting to major centers and the overall prevalence is about 0.02% of the pediatric population [14–17]. Most patients with AVMs present in adulthood, with a mean age of presentation approximately 30–40 years. Approximately 20% of all symptomatic patients with AVMs will present before 15 years of age [18]. There is no sex predilection for pediatric AVMs. A number of AVMs will be associated with underlying genetic conditions. The *RASA1* mutation, resulting in familial AVMs and/or cutaneous capillary malformations, has been associated with symptomatic cerebral AVMs in a small number of families [19]. HHT is a genetic condition that predisposes affected individuals to AVMs and 35% of children with AVMs have associated HHT. In HHT, 23% of patients have multiple AVMs, with mean age of presentation being 35 years [13].

Clinical presentation

Arteriovenous malformations

Patients with AVMs most commonly present with hemorrhage and seizure, but may also present with headache, focal neurological deficits, and cognitive decline. They may also be asymptomatic.

Hemorrhage in AVMs:

- is the presenting feature in 80–85% of all pediatric AVMs
- may present with seizures, headache, or focal neurological deficits
- is usually intraparenchymal because of the location of the AVM within the substance of the brain; a non-traumatic intraparenchymal hemorrhage should raise concerns for the presence of an AVM or tumor
- gives rise to major bleeding in 4.0% per year
- has a mortality rate of 1.0% per year; hemorrhagic AVMs have been associated with a 25% mortality rate
- is associated with rebleeding rates of approximately 6% for the first six months.

Deficits can arise from AVMs through a mass effect or through cerebral ischemia when blood is diverted to the AVM at the expense of normal cerebral circulation ("steal").

The presentation of symptoms with an AVM is generally acute if related to hemorrhage or seizure, often occurring within minutes to hours, or chronic over months if related to steal phenomenon or headache.

Vein of Galen malformations

Patients with VOGMs present with symptoms linked to flow rates. Those with:

- high-flow lesions usually present as infants with cardiac failure and "failure to thrive"
- slow-flow lesions may present with macrocephaly or hydrocephalus (or may be clinically silent).

Perioperative evaluation

If a child presents with symptoms suggesting an intracranial hemorrhage, CT should be performed. An AVM typically appears as a heterogeneous area of mixed density with serpiginous areas of enhancement after infusion of contrast material. Cerebral atrophy may sometimes be seen on the affected side. A large malformations or an intracerebral hematoma may distort the normal intracranial anatomy. Use of CT arteriography may be helpful for initial evaluation (Fig. 27.1A).

MRI is useful for three-dimensional anatomy and identification of chronic ischemia. Chronic ischemic changes, presumably a result of "steal" phenomenon or venous hypertension, may be identified on MRI as a bright signal of the surrounding brain on fluid-attenuated inversion recovery or T_2-weighted images (Fig. 27.1B,C). The typical MRI appearance is that of a latticework of signal-void spaces, highly contrasted against surrounding cerebral tissue on both T_1- and T_2-weighted sequences, intermixed with regions of various signal intensities corresponding to blood products in different stages of evolution, and occasionally calcium and hemosiderin [25,26]. The serpiginous shape of vessels may be distinctive, identified as flow voids, and relevant anatomy can be well visualized with MR angiography. Susceptibility imaging will sometimes disclose evidence of previous hemorrhage as a dark "bloom" around the nidus [27].

Digital subtraction angiography is the definitive investigation. It establishes the nature and extent of the lesion to its blood supply and its venous drainage [28]. Angiography entails bilateral injection of all potential arterial sources of supply to the AVM, both pial and dural (with 15% of cerebral AVMs receiving some blood supply from ipsilateral or contralateral meningeal arteries [29]). Typically at least the internal carotid arteries bilaterally as well as the ipsilateral external carotid and vertebral arteries, are injected. Three-dimensional angiography with computer-generated reconstruction is increasingly employed to depict lesional anatomy. The typical angiographic appearance of an AVM is that of distended, tortuous afferent and efferent vessels connecting with a tangled vascular mass, through which the circulation time is rapid because of arteriovenous shunting. Other vessels or structures are not displaced unless there is an intracerebral hematoma, which appears as an avascular mass (Fig. 27.1D,E).

A recent analysis of 241 consecutive pediatric patients assessed with catheter angiography revealed a 0% complication rate during the procedure and a 0.4% postprocedural complication rate [30]. Evaluation should look for:

- high-flow versus low-flow lesions
- outflow stenoses
- varices in subarachnoid or ventricular spaces
- number and location of feeding vessels
- aneurysms as approximately 7–25% of cerebral AVMs have an associated arterial aneurysm on a feeding pedicle; often these flow-related aneurysms will spontaneously regress following the reduction in blood flow after treatment of the AVM.

Standard preoperative laboratory studies (complete blood count), clotting times (prothrombin time/partial thromboplastin time), type and cross for blood bank, and a chemistry panel (Chem 7) should be considered as pretreatment studies for AVMs and VOGMs. Electroencephalography may be warranted if the concern for seizure exists.

Surgical approaches

Surgical treatment of VOGMs is now largely historical since the advent of embolization and will not be reviewed here.

Surgical technique

The operative goal is complete removal of the lesion. The decision to resect an AVM is based on several factors: (1) eloquence of cortical location (speech, motor function, and sensation), (2) pattern of venous drainage, (3) size, (4) associated

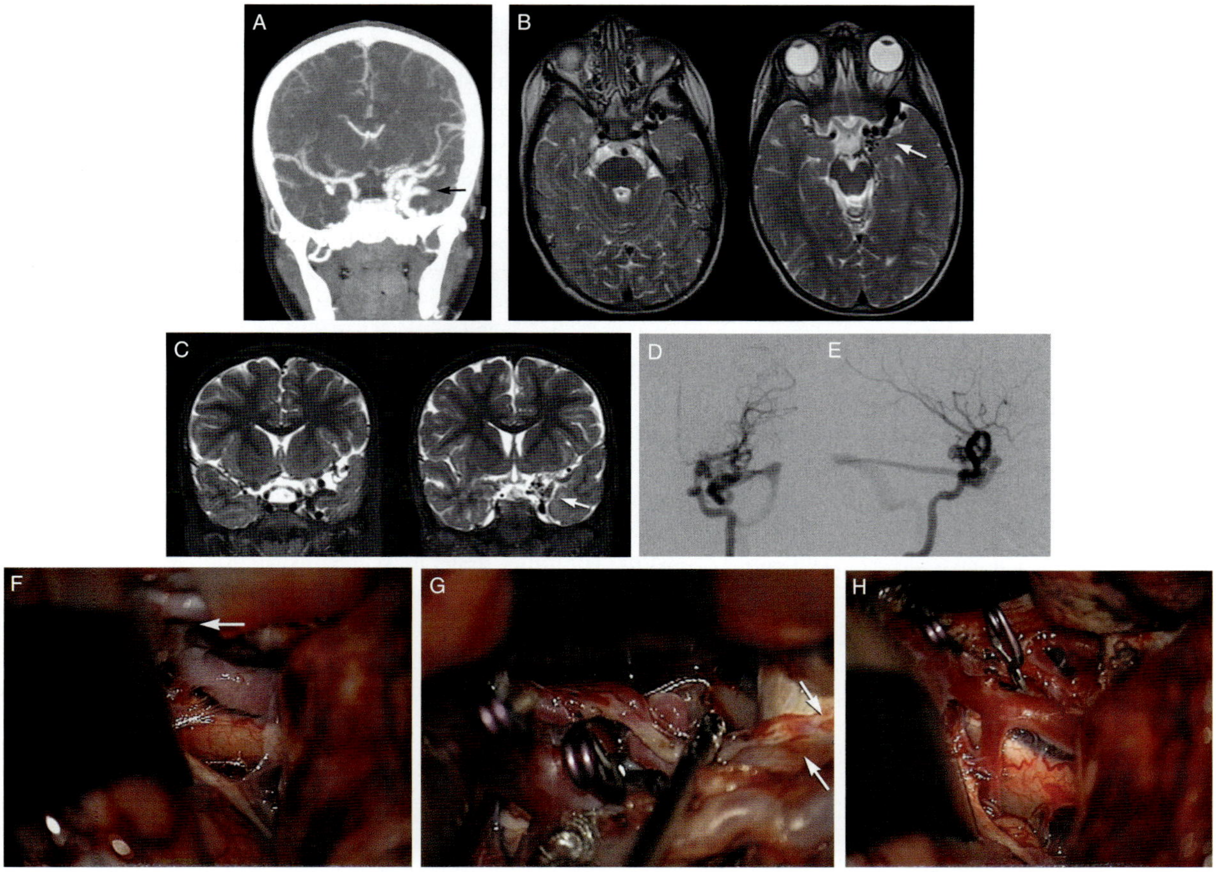

Fig. 27.1. A left mesial temporal arteriovenous malformation in a 4-year-old girl. (A) Coronal CT angiography. (B,C) Coronal T_2-weighted MRI (B, axial view; C, coronal view). (D) Catheter angiography with injection of internal carotid artery showing the high-flow lesion with feeders from the middle cerebral artery and rapid drainage to the venous circulation. (E) Postembolization images showed the marked reduction in flow and better resolution of anatomy. (F) Initial operative exposure of the AVM used a left pterional approach, revealing the internal carotid artery, the optic nerve, and AVM feeders (white arrow). (G) Diminished venous drainage was seen after skeletonization of the arterial feeders (arrows). (H) Postresection image showed the normal caliber of vessels and lack of swollen brain, indicative of lower risk of normal pressure perfusion breakthrough postoperatively.

aneurysms, (5) recent hemorrhage, (6) clinical deterioration, and (7) risk of complication from other modalities of therapy (e.g., radiation injury to the developing brain) [31,32]. Several of these factors are combined in the Spetzler–Martin grading system, which incorporates eloquence of location, pattern of venous drainage, and size and is considered predictive of outcome from surgical management [33]. In general, if a lesion is surgically accessible with minimal morbidity, it is reasonable to consider resection, given the expected lifespan of children and morbidity of hemorrhage, as outlined in the American Heart Association guidelines [34].

Positioning for surgery

Positioning is dependent on the location of the AVM and will vary widely. General principles include elevation of the head to maximize venous drainage, avoiding kinking of vessels in the neck, and maximizing access to the lesion by both the primary surgeon and the assistant. Rigid head fixation is preferable, although in the very young child (under 2 years of age), it may be necessary to employ a padded headrest.

Procedure

Given the wide variety of AVM sizes and locations, it is impossible to identify any single approach for AVM surgery. Specific approaches should be selected to maximize access to the lesion, avoid eloquent neurological cortex (if possible), and afford the surgeon visualization of feeding and draining vessels to permit proximal control of blood flow.

General principles

The operating room should be notified to prepare for surgery. Equipment should include the operating microscope, multiple suctions, bipolar electrocautery, an array of AVM/aneurysm clips, a craniotome (drill), and a retraction system. Anesthesia should be consulted and appropriate measures made to ensure that multiple large-bore intravenous access is present and adequate blood products are in the room. It is helpful to have the microscope draped and clips prepared prior to starting the procedure if possible, so that quick access can be obtained should unexpected bleeding occur during opening.

Craniotomy

Adequate exposure is critical to AVM surgery. It is important that the craniotomy is large enough to visualize the lesion safely. Use of frameless stereotaxy and other intraoperative navigation adjuncts (such as ultrasound) can help to minimize risk in these operations. At the time of bone flap removal, it is important to try to avoid tears in the dura in order to avoid injury to subjacent AVM vessels. When opening the dura, the surgeon should be cognizant of potential adhesions between the dura and vessels (Fig. 27.1F).

Once the dura is open, several general principles can be applied to nearly all AVM operations. A primary surgical principle for AVM resection is the obliteration of feeding arteries before occlusion of draining veins, as premature closure of outflow can lead to unexpected AVM rupture with uncontrolled bleeding. As AVMs are often wedge or cone shaped, resection can be performed in a circumferential pattern, staying close to – but not entering – the nidus. It is helpful to try to maintain an even depth of resection around the lesion (Fig. 27.1G) to avoid getting in a "hole" and caution must be taken to minimize retraction on draining vessels during dissection. Repeated inspection of the surrounding brain for swelling or bleeding can reduce complications by early identification of poorly placed retractors or clips. The vessels of an AVM may coagulate poorly and consideration should be given to clip application or gentle tamponade (if the bleeding is of small volume) if bipolar electrocautery is not working. Every attempt should be made to avoid operating within the nidus itself.

Closure

Inspection of the operative cavity for residual nidus is important, and perioperative angiography can be a useful adjunct to ensure complete resection (Fig. 27.1H). Evidence of brain swelling at closure may indicate occult bleeding, untreated hydrocephalus, or poorly compensated redistribution of blood flow, which can result in perfusion breakthrough hemorrhage. Causes for swelling should be thoroughly investigated and treated, if possible, prior to leaving the operating room. The temporalis is closed with interrupted vicryl sutures. Galea is also closed with vicryl sutures and skin is closed with a running rapide.

Complications

Bleeding is the most immediate complication of surgery and risks are magnified in smaller children, who have little reserve. The loss of one-quarter of blood volume can induce shock and there may be rapid decompensation in children, which mandates careful monitoring and replacement of blood products by the operative team. Normal perfusion pressure breakthrough is a phenomenon that is thought to occur after resection of high-flow AVMs in which the blood previously transmitted through the AVM is redirected to smaller, normal vasculature after the AVM has been removed, with subsequent inability of the vessels to handle the increased flow. This can result in brain swelling, increased intracranial pressure, seizure, neurological dysfunction, or hemorrhage. The problem may be minimized by staged preoperative embolization and rigorous blood pressure control postoperatively. Neurological deficit can occur following AVM resection, although specific rates are hard to derive given the wide variability in AVM size and location. Overall, there is low postoperative morbidity in low-grade Spetzler–Martin lesions (I–III; ranging from 0 to 12%), along with a high rate of complete obliteration (up to 100%), suggesting that surgical resection of these lesions is warranted, particularly when performed in experienced centers [32,35–37].

Alternative approaches

Radiation therapy

Conventional fractionated radiation is not helpful in the majority of AVMs; however, stereotactic radiosurgery offers cure rates of up to 90% in lesions <3 cm in size. This approach is beneficial for surgically inaccessible lesions or in patients who are high risk for surgery. Shortcomings of this approach include a delay of up to three years for lesion obliteration and exposure to radiation in children. Radiation has increased risk in younger populations, making its application less appealing in children under three years of age.

Complications

The long delay between treatment and lesion obliteration in radiosurgery for AVMs means that the child is at risk of the complication of bleeding during this interval. Patients with small (<3 cm diameter), deep-seated lesions (in the basal ganglia, internal capsule, and thalamus) are the best candidates for radiosurgery. A study of 42 children with lesions in these locations documented a 62% angiographic cure rate within two years [38]. However, after radiosurgery, these sites have shown a higher risk of rebleeding compared with AVMs treated in other areas of the brain [39].

Young children have risk of radiation-induced damage, including injury to the surrounding developing brain and potential for development of secondary malignancies. These risks limit radiation use to older children in most situations.

Embolization

Although not traditionally used as a stand-alone treatment for AVMs other than in rare lesions with a small nidus and a small number of feeding pedicles, there is a growing literature on the use of newer embolization agents (Onyx; Covidien ev3 Neurovascular, Irvine, CA, USA) for definitive treatment of brain AVM in adults. However, the situation in children is more complex and embolization is rarely used as a stand-alone modality, as the recurrence rate is higher and lesion immaturity may preclude complete visualization angiographically. Regardless, embolization is a significant aid in the treatment of AVMs, reducing their blood supply and facilitating operative approaches (usually <72 hours before surgery). Embolization also has a role in targeted treatment of non-operative lesions, by occluding areas at risk of hemorrhage such as aneurysms or high-risk varices (those that are intraventricular).

Outcomes

Outcome after surgery

In pediatric patients with grade I–III Spetzler–Martin AVMs treated by resection, good recovery was achieved in 90% and deaths occurred in 5%; the radiographic obliteration rate was 89% [37]. Although class I or II data are lacking, the combined class III data strongly support resection as a primary treatment for patients with Spetzler–Martin grade I or II AVMs. The relatively low postoperative morbidity in these lesions (ranging from 0 to 12%), along with a high rate of complete obliteration (up to 100%) suggests that chosing radiosurgery, with its inherent delay in control, might not be warranted [32,35–37].

Outcome after non-surgical treatments

For comparison, a similar group of patients treated with radiosurgery alone had a reported 80% efficacy of lesion obliteration at 36 months, with 4 out of 53 patients having recurrent hemorrhage post-treatment [40]. One large pediatric AVM study included 40 patients and confirmed radiographic obliteration of the AVM nidus in 35% [41]. The cumulative post-treatment hemorrhage rate was 3.2% per patient per year in the first year and 4.3% per patient per year over the first three years [41]. These rates of obliteration, which are notably lower than those reported in adult studies, were potentially complicated by a slightly larger than average size of treated AVM in the study group. In contrast, when a group of 53 pediatric patients was stratified by AVM size (<3, 3–10, and >10 mL), obliteration rates of 80% and 64.7%, respectively, were reported for the smallest and middle group [40]. Although class I and II data are lacking, the aggregate class III data strongly support the use of radiosurgery in the treatment of small (<3 cm diameter), deep-seated lesions in eloquent cortex. For Spetzler–Martin grade I and most grade II lesions, open resection is generally recommended over radiosurgery unless there are specific considerations that make the patient unsuitable for resection. Radiosurgery should only be used for larger lesions (grades II–V) if the objective is complete obliteration of the AVM [42].

Outcome after multimodal therapies

Multimodality therapy of AVMs has been advocated by several investigators [20,32,35,43]. Neurointerventionalists, radiation oncologists, and neurosurgeons work together to determine the best strategy for a particular patient. Using a multimodality approach, angiographic obliteration rates of 92.9% have been reported. The efficacy of multimodality treatment of large complex lesions is supported by results from a group of 53 children at three-year follow-up, in whom a 58% cure rate was noted for AVMs >6 cm in diameter [44].

In summary, the high likelihood of obliteration, coupled with low complication rates, make a convincing argument in favor of multimodality treatment of pediatric patients with AVMs. Although no class I or II data directly support this recommendation, the class III data are compelling and there is wisdom in pooling the skills of the concerned specialists.

Conclusions

Management of vascular malformations in the CNS begins with an accurate diagnosis, made by specialists with detailed knowledge of these lesions. Patients are best treated by a multidisciplinary team of physicians, including neurosurgeons, neurointerventional radiologists, and radiation oncologists. Recent advances in microsurgery, neurointerventional techniques, and delivery of therapeutic radiation have improved outcomes. Continued progress in this field requires basic research in the development and monitoring of these lesions and perhaps a discovery of pharmacological therapies to prevent recurrence.

References

1. Friedlander RM. Clinical practice. Arteriovenous malformations of the brain. *N Engl J Med* 2007;**356**:2704–12.
2. Sonstein WJ, Kader A, Michelsen WJ, *et al.* Expression of vascular endothelial growth factor in pediatric and adult cerebral arteriovenous malformations: an immunocytochemical study. *J Neurosurg* 1996;**85**:838–45.
3. Rothbart D, Awad IA, Lee J, *et al.* Expression of angiogenic factors and structural proteins in central nervous system vascular malformations. *Neurosurgery* 1996;**38**:915–24.
4. Kilic T, Pamir MN, Kullu S, *et al.* Expression of structural proteins and angiogenic factors in cerebrovascular anomalies. *Neurosurgery* 2000;**46**:1179–91.
5. Hashimoto T, Emala CW, Joshi S, *et al.* Abnormal pattern of TIE-2 and vascular endothelial growth factor receptor expression in human cerebral arteriovenous malformations. *Neurosurgery* 2000;**47**:910–18.
6. Sure U, Butz N, Schlegel J, *et al.* Endothelial proliferation, neoangiogenesis, and potential de novo generation of cerebrovascular malformations. *J Neurosurg* 2001;**94**:972–7.
7. Shenkar R, Elliott JP, Diener K, *et al.* Differential gene expression in human cerebrovascular malformations. *Neurosurgery* 2003;**52**:465–77.
8. Gault J, Sarin H, Awadallah NA, *et al.* Pathobiology of human cerebrovascular malformations: basic mechanisms and clinical relevance. *Neurosurgery* 2004;**55**:1–16.
9. Sure U, Butz N, Siegel AM, *et al.* Treatment-induced neoangiogenesis in cerebral arteriovenous malformations. *Clin Neurol Neurosurg* 2001;**103**:29–32.
10. Schmit BP, Burrows PE, Kuban K, *et al.* Acquired cerebral arteriovenous malformation in a child with moyamoya disease. Case report. *J Neurosurg* 1996;**84**:677–80.

11. Gonzalez LF, Bristol RE, Porter RW, *et al.* De novo presentation of an arteriovenous malformation. Case report and review of the literature. *J Neurosurg* 2005;**102**:726–9.
12. Jerkic M, Rivas-Elena JV, Prieto M, *et al.* Endoglin regulates nitric oxide-dependent vasodilatation. *FASEB J* 2004;**18**:609–11.
13. Lasjaunias P. *Vascular Diseases in Neonates, Infants and Children: Interventional Neuroradiology Management*. Berlin: Springer, 1997.
14. Raybaud CA, Strother CM, Hald JK. Aneurysms of the vein of Galen: embryonic considerations and anatomical features relating to the pathogenesis of the malformation. *Neuroradiology* 1989;**31**:109–28.
15. Zerah M, Garcia-Monaco R, Rodesch G, *et al.* Hydrodynamics in vein of Galen malformations. *Childs Nerv Syst* 1992;**8**:111–17.
16. Nikas DC, Proctor MR, Scott RM. Spontaneous thrombosis of vein of Galen aneurysmal malformation. *Pediatr Neurosurg* 1999;**31**:33–9.
17. Perret G, Nishioka H. Report on the cooperative study of intracranial aneurysms and subarachnoid hemorrhage. Section VI. Arteriovenous malformations. An analysis of 545 cases of cranio-cerebral arteriovenous malformations and fistulae reported to the cooperative study. *J Neurosurg* 1966;**25**:467–90.
18. Stapf C, Mohr JP, Pile-Spellman J, *et al.* Concurrent arterial aneurysms in brain arteriovenous malformations with haemorrhagic presentation. *J Neurol Neurosurg Psychiatry* 2002;**73**:294–8.
19. Kim EJ, Halim AX, Dowd CF, *et al.* The relationship of coexisting extranidal aneurysms to intracranial hemorrhage in patients harboring brain arteriovenous malformations. *Neurosurgery* 2004;**54**:1349–57.
20. Lee BB, Do YS, Yakes W, *et al.* Management of arteriovenous malformations: a multidisciplinary approach. *J Vasc Surg* 2004;**39**:590–600.
21. Hayashi S, Arimoto T, Itakura T, *et al.* The association of intracranial aneurysms and arteriovenous malformation of the brain. Case report. *J Neurosurg* 1981;**55**:971–5.
22. Watanabe H, Nakamura H, Matsuo Y, *et al.* [Spontaneous regression of cerebral arterio-venous malformation following major artery thrombosis proximal to dominant feeders: a case report.] *No Shinkei Geka* 1995;**23**:371–6.
23. Mine S, Hirai S, Yamakami I, *et al.* [Location of primary somatosensory area in cerebral arteriovenous malformation involving sensorimotor area.] *No To Shinkei* 1999;**51**:331–7.
24. Vates GE, Lawton MT, Wilson CB, *et al.* Magnetic source imaging demonstrates altered cortical distribution of function in patients with arteriovenous malformations. *Neurosurgery* 2002;**51**:614–23.
25. Leblanc R, Levesque M, Comair Y, *et al.* Magnetic resonance imaging of cerebral arteriovenous malformations. *Neurosurgery* 1987;**21**:15–20.
26. Smith HJ, Strother CM, Kikuchi Y, *et al.* MR imaging in the management of supratentorial intracranial AVMs. *AJR Am J Roentgenol* 1988;**150**:1143–53.
27. Chappell PM, Steinberg GK, Marks MP. Clinically documented hemorrhage in cerebral arteriovenous malformations: MR characteristics. *Radiology* 1992;**183**:719–24.
28. Pott M, Huber M, Assheuer J, *et al.* Comparison of MRI, CT and angiography in cerebral arteriovenous malformations. *Bildgebung* 1992;**59**:98–102.
29. Newton TH, Cronqvist S. Involvement of dural arteries in intracranial arteriovenous malformations. *Radiology* 1969;**93**:1071–8.
30. Burger IM, Murphy KJ, Jordan LC, Tamargo RJ, Gailloud P. Safety of cerebral digital subtraction angiography in children: complication rate analysis in 241 consecutive diagnostic angiograms. *Stroke* 2006;**37**:2535–9.
31. Fisher WS, III. Therapy of AVMs: a decision analysis. *Clin Neurosurg* 1995;**42**:294–312.
32. Hoh BL, Chapman PH, Loeffler JS, *et al.* Results of multimodality treatment for 141 patients with brain arteriovenous malformations and seizures: factors associated with seizure incidence and seizure outcomes. *Neurosurgery* 2002;**51**:303–9.
33. Spetzler RF, Martin NA. A proposed grading system for arteriovenous malformations. *J Neurosurg* 1986;**65**:476–83.
34. Roach ES, Golomb MR, Adams R, *et al.* Management of stroke in infants and children: a scientific statement from a Special Writing Group of the American Heart Association Stroke Council and the Council on Cardiovascular Disease in the Young. *Stroke* 2008;**39**:2644–91.
35. Humphreys RP, Hoffman HJ, Drake JM, *et al.* Choices in the 1990s for the management of pediatric cerebral arteriovenous malformations. *Pediatr Neurosurg* 1996;**25**:277–85.
36. Morgan MK, Rochford AM, Tsahtsarlis A, *et al.* Surgical risks associated with the management of grade I and II brain arteriovenous malformations. *Neurosurgery* 2004;**54**:832–7.
37. Kiris T, Sencer A, Sahinbas M, *et al.* Surgical results in pediatric Spetzler–Martin grades I–III intracranial arteriovenous malformations. *Childs Nerv Syst* 2005;**21**:69–74.
38. Andrade-Souza YM, Zadeh G, Scora D, *et al.* Radiosurgery for basal ganglia, internal capsule, and thalamus arteriovenous malformation: clinical outcome. *Neurosurgery* 2005;**56**:56–63.
39. Pollock BE, Gorman DA, Brown PD. Radiosurgery for arteriovenous malformations of the basal ganglia, thalamus, and brainstem. *J Neurosurg* 2004;**100**:210–14.
40. Levy EI, Niranjan A, Thompson TP, *et al.* Radiosurgery for childhood intracranial arteriovenous malformations. *Neurosurgery* 2000;**47**:834–41.
41. Smyth MD, Sneed PK, Ciricillo SF, *et al.* Stereotactic radiosurgery for pediatric intracranial arteriovenous malformations: the University of California at San Francisco experience. *J Neurosurg* 2002;**97**:48–55.
42. Ogilvy CS, Stieg PE, Awad I, *et al.* Recommendations for the management of intracranial arteriovenous malformations: a statement for healthcare professionals from a special writing group of the Stroke Council, American Stroke Association. *Circulation* 2001;**103**:2644–57.
43. terBrugge K, Lasjaunias P, Chiu M, *et al.* Pediatric surgical neuroangiography. A multicentre approach. *Acta Radiol Suppl* 1986;**369**:692–3.
44. Chang SD, Marcellus ML, Marks MP, *et al.* Multimodality treatment of giant intracranial arteriovenous malformations. *Neurosurgery* 2003;**53**:1–11.

Chapter 28

Management of residual or recurrent arteriovenous malformations

Mina G. Safain and Adel M. Malek

Introduction

Cerebral arteriovenous malformations (AVMs) are thought to arise from congenital failure of capillary development. An AVM is considered cured if complete obliteration of the nidus is demonstrated by cerebral angiography. Residual AVM may be found after treatment and, in rare cases, recurrence can be seen after angiographic cure. Appropriate management of residual and recurrent AVMs is a topic of relative controversy given the diversity of treatment options, the complexity of AVM treatment in general, and the paucity of literature on the specific topic of treatment of these AVM entities. Treatment of these lesions requires a center versed in multimodal management of AVM therapy, including surgical resection, endovascular embolization, and accurate stereotactic radiosurgery. This chapter presents the relevant literature on the management of residual and recurrent AVMs and discusses the treatment of these lesions.

Residual arteriovenous malformations

Management after surgical resection

Studies have found that unplanned residual AVM may be found on postoperative angiography in approximately 2–20% of patients [1–6]. In general, these residual lesions are small and may have been hidden under a thin layer of parenchyma not appreciated during surgical resection. In one case series, residual AVM was found in 6 out of 324 patients with operative treatments (1.8%) and all residual lesions were found to be <1 cm in diameter [3]. Many reasons have been cited for residual AVM being detected on postoperative angiography. One theory postulates that there may be angiographically occult areas of any given AVM that do not fill sufficiently to be seen on the preoperative angiogram, leading the surgeon to underestimate or even have a misrepresentation of the true size of the AVM [7]. This poor a priori detection can predispose the surgeon to misjudge the full extent of the AVM and, therefore, perform incomplete resection despite great care and technique. In addition, certain AVMs can have a rather large and diffuse nidus, which may lead the surgeon to underestimate the nidal transitional edge and leave residual AVM behind [2,3,5,7]. Although most residuals left behind tend to be small, these lesions seem to have an increased rate of hemorrhage, likely because of the impairment of venous outflow imparted by the surgical resection [2,3,8].

Surgeons have suggested certain intraoperative strategies to reduce the likelihood of leaving a residual after surgery, which include carrying out an intraoperative hypertensive challenge [2,3] using intraoperative microscopic indocyanine green fluorescence angiography [2,9,10] or performing catheter-based intraoperative angiography [2,3,9]. However, even when these strategies are employed, residual AVM remains a dreaded and potentially catastrophic complication of AVM therapy.

As has been previously reported [2,11], the detection of residual AVM poses a multifactorial clinical situation. Postoperative [2], postembolization, and even postradiosurgery [12–14] hemorrhage from residual AVM has been reported and can be significant, as well as life threatening. One Japanese series reported on 362 surgically resected AVMs, 35 of which were found to have a residual [15]. These patients were followed for an average of 9.2 years and the reported annual risk of hemorrhage was 2.9%, which did not differ from patients who had not undergone surgical resection. In the acute setting, one patient has been reported as having a large hemorrhage from residual AVM during transport from the operating room to the intensive care unit, and one patient had a major hemorrhage from residual AVM within 48 hours of surgery [2]. These case reports and the aforementioned case series confirm that complete AVM resection is essential in order to provide definite benefit to the patient; in fact, incomplete surgical resection may place patients at a higher risk of hemorrhage than no treatment at all.

The increased risk of hemorrhage from residual AVM has been postulated to arise from the presence of continued arteriovenous shunting through a nidus that, after operative management, has reduced venous outflow [8]. For this reason, most authors have suggested early angiography [2,3] with early or immediate return to the operating room for resection of any

Comprehensive Management of Arteriovenous Malformations of the Brain and Spine, ed. Robert F. Spetzler, Douglas S. Kondziolka, Randall T. Higashida, and M. Yashar S. Kalani. Published by Cambridge University Press.

residual nidus. This decision, however, is not simple if the residual is in eloquent cortex, and weighing the risk of hemorrhage versus causing additional neurological deficit can be complex and needs to be carried out for each individual patient.

At our center, we routinely perform postoperative angiography within 24 hours of surgical resection of cerebral AVMs. If residual AVM is detected, we recommend early return to the operating room to complete resection of the residual nidus. In nidus that resides within eloquent cortex after initial resection, a risk–benefit assessment must be conducted to balance the risk of causing permanent neurological deficit with additional immediate resection and the risk of hemorrhage in a lesion with decreased venous outflow. Patients who are found to have residual AVM should be maintained in a relative normotensive to hypotensive state compared with their baseline blood pressure to prevent postoperative hemorrhage from the altered venous drainage of the lesion [2,8]. We do not suggest management via embolization or radiosurgery in the immediate postoperative period given the high risk of hemorrhage linked to altered venous drainage [3,15,16].

Management after radiosurgery

Radiosurgery has been a useful treatment option for AVMs when surgical risks are thought to be excessive. Overall, the reported rate of angiographic AVM obliteration after radiosurgery has been demonstrated to vary from 60 to 85% at two to three years after treatment [13,14,17–23]. Additionally, in one series, approximately 20% of patients treated with radiosurgery had residual nidus at three years [17]. Radiosurgery-associated treatment failure has been correlated with many factors. The most frequent failure is targeting error [18,19,22,23]. Other factors include AVM volume >10 cm^3 [17,18,20–23], and suboptimal treatment doses (usually 15 Gy) [17,20,21,23]. Indeed several studies have demonstrated that smaller AVMs are more likely to be cured by radiosurgery alone [18,20,21,24].

At our center, we obtain post-treatment MRI with gadolinium and MR angiography every 6 months. Catheter-based angiography is performed at either two or three years to assess for nidus involution or regression once the MRI suggests no further shunting. Most treatment centers tend to defer treatment of any persistent AVM nidus until at least three years after radiosurgery to allow for sufficient time for the radiation dose to induce obliteration of an AVM nidus [17,18,20,21]. Furthermore, some authors have suggested that radiosurgery may have additional benefits at even 5 and 10 years after treatment [25,26].

Although uncommon, hemorrhage from residual nidus has been reported after radiosurgery and remains a major limiting factor [12–14,27,28]. Application of stereotactic radiosurgery thickens arteries and slows nidal flow, thereby decreasing the natural history risk of hemorrhage before complete AVM resolution occurs [12,27,28]. This risk, however, is not nullified. In addition, aggressive radiation to the venous drainage of AVMs has been associated with inducing a higher risk of hemorrhage than the natural history of untreated lesions [12,29]. In order to decrease the risk of residual AVM, most centers recommend employing as high a radiation dose as safely possible to the nidus while taking care to decrease the total radiation dose received by the lesion's venous drainage network. Additionally, the radiation dose must be calculated with consideration to limiting the amount of necrosis, cyst formation, and development of post-radiation edema. Furthermore, on post-treatment angiography, clinicians should be aware of the change of venous drainage patterns in addition to the decrease in size of the nidus. Major changes to venous drainage patterns with a visible nidus should alert the clinician to the need for retreatment or possible surgical or endovascular management.

The literature on the treatment of residual AVM after initial radiosurgery is limited to case reports [17,30–32]. Many authors have suggested that one of two methods be employed: resection of residual nidus after radiosurgery or repeat stereotactic radiosurgery. First, if at three years the residual nidus becomes an operative lesion based on Spetzler–Martin grade, some have suggested that an operative approach be employed [17]. The University of California at San Francisco group has reported that radiation induces intimal hyperplasia and medial hyalinization, causing nidal arteries to be thickened and sclerotic, which can make them less friable if subsequent surgical management is needed [33]. Additionally, blood flow within the nidus is usually significantly reduced and the adjacent brain tissue has a radiation-induced gliosis, making an easier plane for surgical dissection. The same group has demonstrated that patients with previous stereotactic radiosurgery had shorter operative times, reduced blood loss, decreased length of hospital stay, and a decreased need for staging in comparison with AVMs surgically managed without prior radiation. It has been suggested that AVMs that are not obliterated by stereotactic radiosurgery at the end of the latency period, and qualifying for surgical treatment based on Spetzler–Martin grade, should undergo surgical management instead of repeat radiosurgical treatment [33].

In addition to surgical management for residual AVM after initial stereotactic radiosurgery, repeat radiosurgical treatment has been advocated by the Karolinska group [34]. In their series of 101 patients, obliteration of a residual AVM by retreatment with stereotactic radiosurgery was only achieved in 63 patients (62%). This, however, is comparable to the rate found in primary radiosurgery treatment for an AVM. Others have replicated these studies: Yen *et al.* reported a 55% obliteration rate after a second radiosurgical treatment in 140 patients, with a low 3.6% radiation-induced deficit rate [35]. Stahl *et al.* reported a similar obliteration rate of 65% in 103 patients [31]. The literature, therefore, seems to support the assertion that it is not an unreasonable strategy to employ a repeat stereotactic treatment if at three years an AVM has not involuted and is still not considered to be an operative lesion (Fig. 28.1).

At our center, we follow AVMs managed with stereotactic radiosurgery for three years. If at this time point, an AVM is not obliterated, and if it is considered a surgical candidate based on Spetzler–Martin grade, we recommend microsurgical resection. If the lesion continues to be unfavorable for surgical resection, we proceed with repeat radiosurgical treatment.

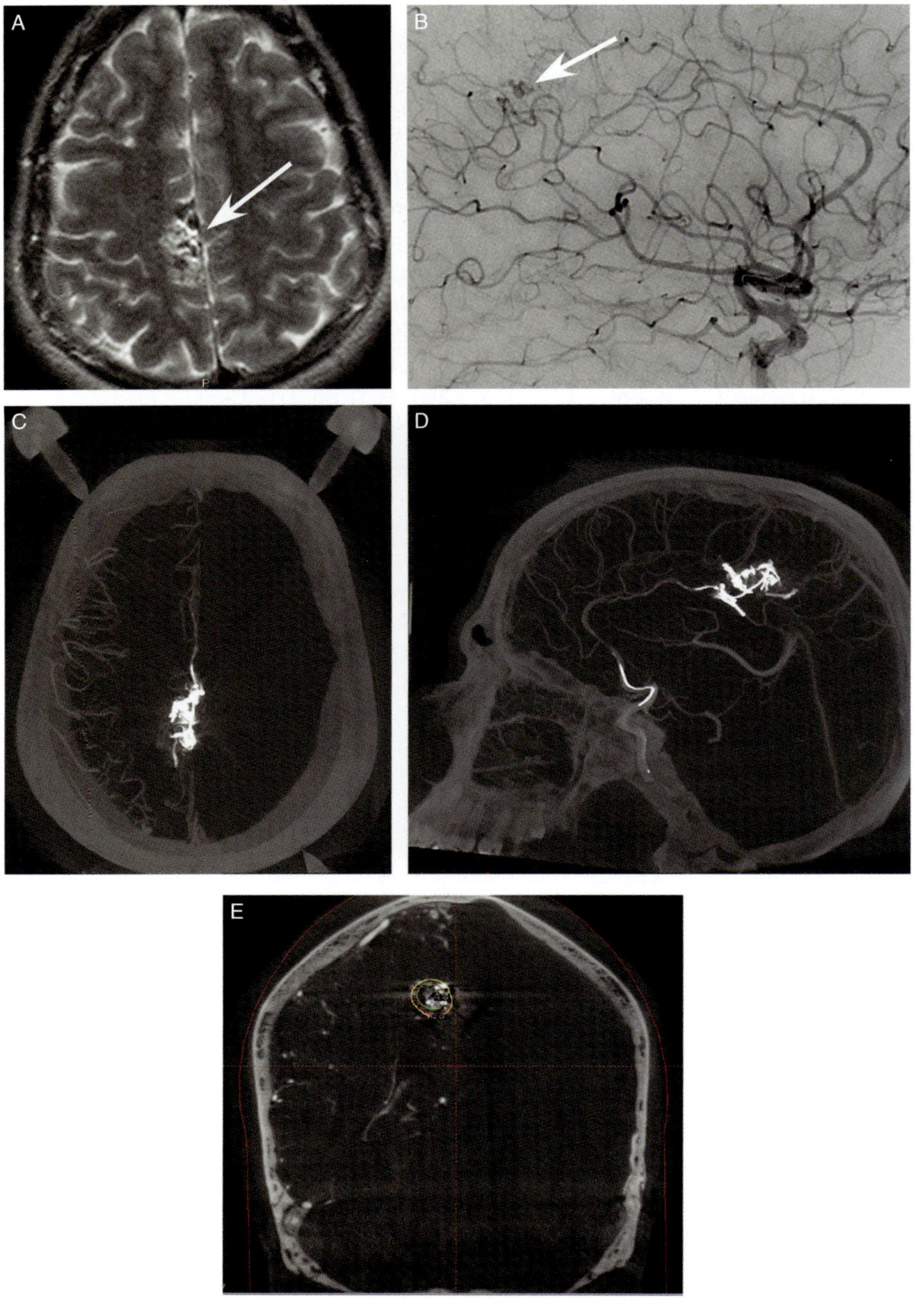

Fig. 28.1. A 13-year-old boy initially presented with severe headache and vomiting. He underwent three embolizations at outside institutions over a 6-year period. He continued to have residual arteriovenous malformation (AVM) and was referred to our center for gamma knife therapy. He had two different gamma knife therapies spaced 3 years apart. (A) At 6 years after initial presentation, axial T_2-weighted MRI demonstrated continued arteriovenous shunting in the medial frontal cortex adjacent to the motor strip (white arrow). Embolic material is apparent within parts of the nidus. (B) At 3 years after gamma knife therapy, lateral right internal carotid artery injection demonstrated a small residual nidus (white arrow). (C,D) Catheter-based cone-beam CT angiography demonstrated residual AVM and embolic material (C, axial view; D, sagittal view). (E) Coronal gamma knife treatment planning utilizing catheter-based cone-beam CT angiography. The residual AVM was reradiated with most embolic material and obliterated AVM excluded from the radiation field.

Surgical treatment is supplemented with presurgical adjunctive endovascular embolization if it is felt to have an appropriate risk–benefit profile.

Management after embolization

Angiographic embolization is a useful adjunct therapy both in the initial treatment of AVMs as well as in the treatment of residual AVMs (Figs. 28.1 and 28.2). It should be noted, however, that only a minority of AVMs can be cured by embolization alone [36–45]. These AVMs are characterized by a single feeder or simple feeder network in which the nidus, as well as the proximal venous outflow, can be completely cast [37]. Overall occlusion rates utilizing endovascular embolization as a curative treatment have been reported to range from 0 to 20%, with most studies suggesting rates in the 5–8% range [37,40, 46,47]. This suggests that the obvious advantage of managing an AVM with embolization is to allow decrease in the size of the nidus in order to make it suitable for either operative or stereotactic radiosurgical management. It is important not to sidestep the use of this modality as an adjunct to surgical and radiosurgical treatments. Angiographic embolization has been reported to improve cure rates by up to 25% by reducing the overall size and volume of a lesion, allowing a more precise plane for surgical resection or reducing the total radiation dose needed to obtain complete obliteration [46].

Although embolization has been shown to have benefit prior to microsurgical management, its use prior to stereotactic

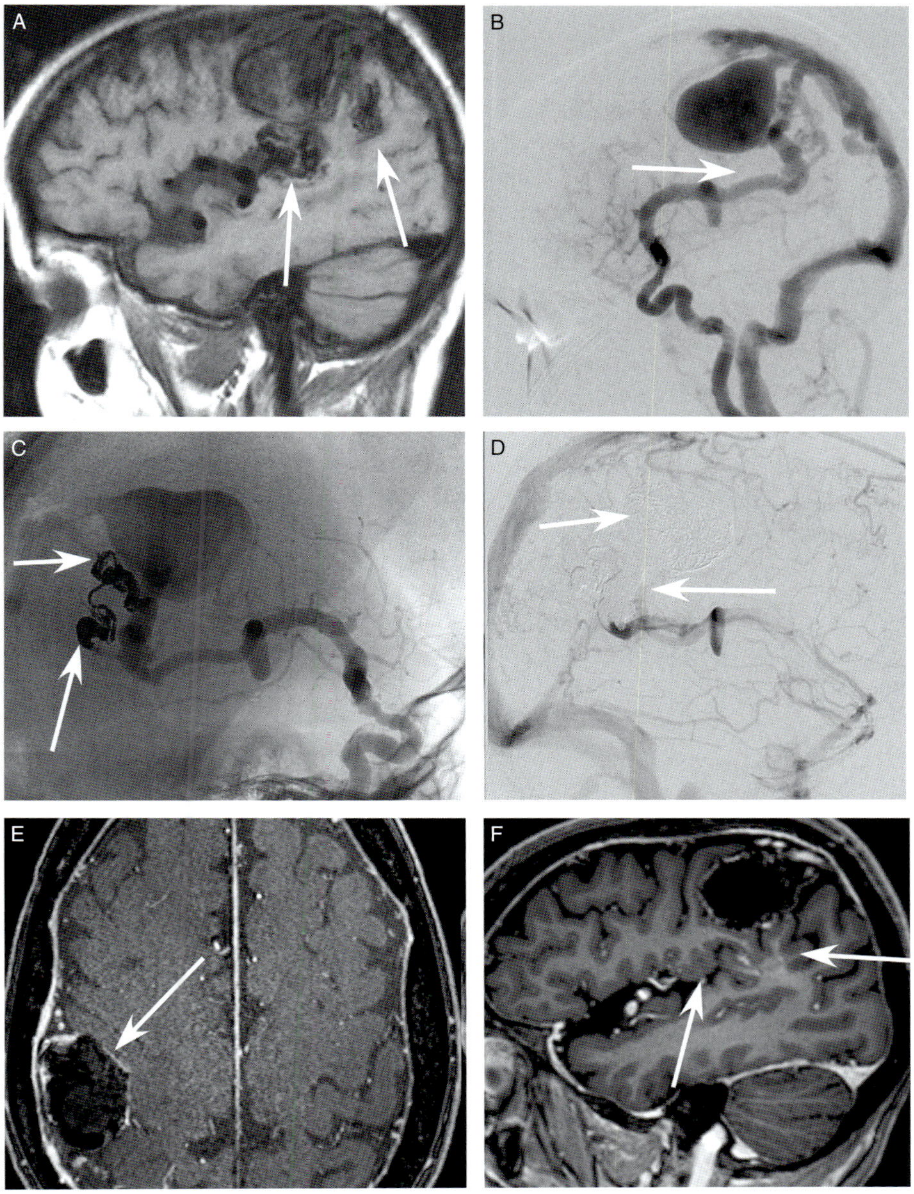

Fig. 28.2. A 31-year-old woman underwent imaging of the head for an endocrinological workup and was incidentally found to have a right sylvian fissure and parietal arteriovenous malformation (AVM) with a large venous varix. She underwent initial gamma knife therapy. (A) At 1 year after treatment, sagittal T_1-weighted MRI demonstrated two separate nidi of the AVM (white arrows). (B) At 3 years after treatment, angiography with right internal carotid artery (ICA) injection demonstrated obliteration of the sylvian fissure nidus (white arrow). The parietal nidus, as well as the venous varix, were still present. (C) Six months later, stage one of a staged coil embolization of the AVM occurred; non-subtracted right ICA injection angiography showed the AVM (white arrows). During this initial stage, the parietal arterial feeders were coil embolized. (D) At the second stage of embolization, lateral angiography demonstrated further coil embolization of the sylvian fissure arterial feeder, as well as the venous varix (white arrows). (E,F) At 4.5 years after gamma knife therapy, axial MR angiography demonstrated no flow within the venous varix (E, white arrow) and sagittal T_1-weighted MRI demonstrated no arterial feeders (F, white arrows) and an occluded venous varix.

radiosurgery has recently been debated and re-evaluated in the literature. Andrade-Souza *et al.* treated 61 patients with embolization prior to linear accelerator-based radiosurgery with an obliteration rate of 47% compared with 70% in case-matched controls undergoing stereotactic radiosurgery without prior embolization [25]. Kano *et al.* demonstrated that embolization decreased the overall total obliteration rate (55% at five years if embolized prior to radiosurgery, 76% in non-embolized patients) and did not alter the hemorrhage rate during the latency period when utilizing subsequent gamma knife radiosurgery [26]. Interestingly, in patients whose AVMs were embolized to volumes $<8\ cm^3$, embolization had a significant benefit in obliteration rates with subsequent radiosurgery. These data suggest that embolization should be mainly used as a volume-reducing adjunct.

Multiple reasons have been postulated for this decrease in obliteration rate when embolization is utilized. First, it has been suggested that embolization can alter the three-dimensional appearance of an AVM, resulting in an irregular volume for stereotactic targeting. Second, given that most areas embolized are not radiated, recanalization may occur in those areas, thus allowing for reconstitution of the nidus. It should be noted that these studies used older particle-based embolic agents. More recent studies have suggested that improved obliteration rates of approximately 20% and decreased complication rates are found when liquid embolic agents are used [48,49]. Further study is warranted with newer liquid embolic agents.

Overall, however, most literature supports the use of embolization as an adjunct in the treatment of cerebral AVMs. The major benefit of embolization may be in presurgical reduction of arterial feeders and the volume of blood flow to the nidus. Additionally, embolization can also be used to obliterate feeding artery aneurysms. We do not recommend the use of embolization as the primary modality in the management of residual

AVMs, except in select residuals containing a single arterial feeder. Its use as an adjunct therapy alongside surgical resection and stereotactic radiosurgery, however, should continue to be studied, particularly in light of the widespread use of newer liquid embolic agents [49,50].

Recurrent arteriovenous malformations

In the past, complete surgical resection had been thought to eliminate the recurrence of AVMs. However, there have been 25 reports in the English language of recurrence of surgically "cured" AVMs. Of these, 20 were children and 5 adults [51]. The true incidence of AVM recurrence, however, is unknown. Recurrence rates have been reported to range from 1 to 13%, occurring one to nine years after initial management [52–55].

In the largest series on this topic, comprising 808 patients with angiographically verified cured AVMs, five patients (all children) were found to have recurrent lesions [54]. Angiography indicated no residual nidus or early draining veins at seven days postoperatively in three patients, within 24 hours in one patient, and intraoperatively in the final patient. Most importantly, this study demonstrated that 5 out of 141 children and 0 out of 667 adults had a recurrence. A limitation of the study, however, is that no delayed angiography was obtained after the initial negative perioperative angiogram, mainly because of radiation concerns for the children. Although residual AVM not seen on early postoperative angiography (because of focal vessel spasm, thrombosis, or compressed residual through a mass effect) may be later misconstrued as a recurrent AVM, this study would still seem to suggest that there may be an association between the recurrence of an AVM and the inherent immaturity and plasticity of the pediatric vasculature. In addition, a recent literature review and case series [55] has reported that younger age, specifically younger than 20 years, and the presence of deep venous drainage are linked to higher recurrence rates after surgical resection, even in the setting of a normal delayed postoperative angiogram. For these reasons, this study concluded that patients of older age with normal postoperative angiography did not require long-term follow-up but that younger patients should be followed more closely.

Multiple theories have been proposed for the etiology of recurrent AVMs. "Recurrence" has been theorized to be a residual nidus that was not visualized on immediate postoperative angiography [52,56]. A variety of explanations have been put forward as causes for these lesions not being visualized immediately, including brain edema after surgical resection causing mass effect on the vasculature, temporary vessel spasm, or temporary thrombosis of the remaining vasculature. However, other data have shown that follow-up angiography in the period three to six months after treatment also failed to demonstrate residual AVM [52,57], thus ruling out these theories given the known resolution of these entities in the early postoperative period.

Several studies have suggested that there are unfilled areas of an AVM adjacent to the previously seen nidus [7,58]. These occult areas can subsequently grow and lead to hemorrhage or seizure. This "hidden compartment" theory hypothesizes that flow within the unseen portion of the AVM is augmented after treatment of the angiographically visible portion of the AVM [7], also proposed as a "reserve nidus" [58]. Finally, many others have suggested that there is an active vascular endothelial growth factor (VEGF)-mediated proliferation of vessels in areas adjacent to the AVM nidus that leads to the recurrence of AVM [59]. One immunohistochemical study analyzed VEGF in tissue samples from four children with recurrent AVMs (ages 8–11) compared with 15 with non-recurrent AVMs (seven in children aged 7 months to 18 years and eight in adults aged 19–58 years) [59]. All recurrent AVMs had a high level of VEGF in the AVM tissue compared with a high level in only one in the seven pediatric non-recurrent specimens and two in the eight adult specimens. The authors proposed that astrocytes associated with AVMs that express high levels of VEGF may still be supporting continued increases in vessel angiogenesis, and this may increase the risk of AVM recurrence even after complete surgical resection.

What seems to be clear, however, is that younger patients with AVMs need to undergo long-term follow-up in order to prevent hemorrhage from a recurrent AVM. Many authors have suggested that angiography be performed at one and five years after AVM resection. Follow-up may need to be extended further in children [52–54,56]. Given the limited numbers of recurrent AVMs reported in the literature, no detailed studies have been conducted on whether these lesions have a comparable risk of hemorrhage relative to the initial lesions. With this caveat, we advocate that recurrent AVMs should be treated aggressively given the altered arterial and venous state that these lesions are left in after initial treatment.

Conclusions

Residual and recurrent AVMs are complex entities that need an individualized assessment for optimal treatment. We have attempted to summarize the current literature on these lesions and to provide our center's management approach. Residual and recurrent AVMs are ideally managed at centers with the capability of multimodality therapy, including surgical resection, endovascular embolization, and stereotactic radiosurgery.

References

1. Reitz M, Schmidt NO, Vukovic Z, *et al.* How to deal with incompletely treated AVMs: experience of 67 cases and review of the literature. *Acta Neurochir Suppl* 2011;**112**:123–9.
2. Solomon RA, Connolly ES, Jr., Prestigiacomo CJ, *et al.* Management of residual dysplastic vessels after cerebral arteriovenous malformation resection: implications for postoperative angiography. *Neurosurgery* 2000;**46**:1052–60.
3. Hoh BL, Carter BS, Ogilvy CS. Incidence of residual intracranial AVMs after surgical resection and efficacy of

immediate surgical re-exploration. *Acta Neurochir (Wien)* 2004;**146**:1–7.

4. Deruty R, Pelissou-Guyotat I, Morel C, *et al.* Reflections on the management of cerebral arteriovenous malformations. *Surg Neurol* 1998;**50**:245–55.
5. Pikus HJ, Beach ML, Harbaugh RE. Microsurgical treatment of arteriovenous malformations: analysis and comparison with stereotactic radiosurgery. *J Neurosurg* 1998;**88**:641–6.
6. Majchrzak H, Kopera M, Majchrzak K, *et al.* [Treatment of deep brain arteriovenous malformations.] *Neurol Neurochir Pol* 2005;**39**:95–100.
7. Pellettieri L, Svendsen P, Wikholm G, *et al.* Hidden compartments in AVMs: a new concept. *Acta Radiol* 1997;**38**:2–7.
8. Bendok BR, Getch CC, Ali MJ, *et al.* Spontaneous thrombosis of a residual arteriovenous malformation in eloquent cortex after surgery. Case report. *Neurosurgery* 2002;**50**:1142–5.
9. Anegawa S, Hayashi T, Torigoe R, *et al.* Intraoperative angiography in the resection of arteriovenous malformations. *J Neurosurg* 1994;**80**:73–8.
10. Ng YP, King NK, Wan KR, *et al.* Uses and limitations of indocyanine green videoangiography for flow analysis in arteriovenous malformation surgery. *J Clin Neurosci* 2013;**20**: 224–32.
11. Barrow D, Cawley M. Surgical techniques for lobar arteriovenous malformations: frontal, temporal, parietal, occipital. In Batjer HH, ed. *Cerebrovascular Disease*. Philadelphia, PA: Lippincott-Raven, 1997.
12. Fujimoto M, Uno J, Ikai Y, *et al.* Risk of rebleeding in arteriovenous malformations due to impaired venous drainage after radiosurgery. *Neurol Med Chir (Tokyo)* 2011;**51**:585–7.
13. Friedman WA, Blatt DL, Bova FJ, *et al.* The risk of hemorrhage after radiosurgery for arteriovenous malformations. *J Neurosurg* 1996;**84**:912–19.
14. Pollock BE, Flickinger JC, Lunsford LD, *et al.* Hemorrhage risk after stereotactic radiosurgery of cerebral arteriovenous malformations. *Neurosurgery* 1996;**38**:652–9.
15. Shimamoto Y, Asada H, Onozuka S, *et al.* [Natural history for residual intracranial AVM: compared with that for conservatively treated AVM.] *No Shinkei Geka* 1992;**20**:931–6.
16. Guo WY, Karlsson B, Ericson K, *et al.* Even the smallest remnant of an AVM constitutes a risk of further bleeding. Case report. *Acta Neurochir (Wien)* 1993;**121**:212–15.
17. Foote KD, Friedman WA, Ellis TL, *et al.* Salvage retreatment after failure of radiosurgery in patients with arteriovenous malformations. *J Neurosurg* 2003;**98**:337–41.
18. Ellis TL, Friedman WA, Bova FJ, *et al.* Analysis of treatment failure after radiosurgery for arteriovenous malformations. *J Neurosurg* 1998;**89**:104–10.
19. Gallina P, Merienne L, Meder JF, *et al.* Failure in radiosurgery treatment of cerebral arteriovenous malformations. *Neurosurgery* 1998;**42**:996–1002.
20. Karlsson B, Lindquist C, Steiner L. Prediction of obliteration after gamma knife surgery for cerebral arteriovenous malformations. *Neurosurgery* 1997;**40**:425–30.
21. Pollock BE, Flickinger JC, Lunsford LD, *et al.* Factors associated with successful arteriovenous malformation radiosurgery. *Neurosurgery* 1998;**42**:1239–44.
22. Yamamoto M, Ide M, Jimbo M, *et al.* Neuroimaging studies of postobliteration nidus changes in cerebral arteriovenous malformations treated by gamma knife radiosurgery. *Surg Neurol* 1996;**45**:110–19.
23. Yamamoto M, Jimbo M, Hara M, *et al.* Gamma knife radiosurgery for arteriovenous malformations: long-term follow-up results focusing on complications occurring more than 5 years after irradiation. *Neurosurgery* 1996;**38**:906–14.
24. Touboul E, Al Halabi A, Buffat L, *et al.* Single-fraction stereotactic radiotherapy: a dose-response analysis of arteriovenous malformation obliteration. *Int J Radiat Oncol Biol Phys* 1998;**41**:855–61.
25. Andrade-Souza YM, Ramani M, Scora D, *et al.* Embolization before radiosurgery reduces the obliteration rate of arteriovenous malformations. *Neurosurgery* 2007;**60**:443–51.
26. Kano H, Kondziolka D, Flickinger JC, *et al.* Stereotactic radiosurgery for arteriovenous malformations after embolization: a case–control study. *J Neurosurg* 2012;**117**:265–75.
27. Maruyama K, Kawahara N, Shin M, *et al.* The risk of hemorrhage after radiosurgery for cerebral arteriovenous malformations. *N Engl J Med* 2005;**352**:146–53.
28. Maruyama K, Shin M, Tago M, *et al.* Management and outcome of hemorrhage after gamma knife surgery for arteriovenous malformations of the brain. *J Neurosurg* 2006;**105** (Suppl):52–7.
29. Gross BA, Ropper AE, Du R. Vascular complications of stereotactic radiosurgery for arteriovenous malformations. *Clin Neurol Neurosurg* 2013;**115**:713–17.
30. Kano H, Kondziolka D, Flickinger JC, *et al.* Stereotactic radiosurgery for arteriovenous malformations. Part 3: outcome predictors and risks after repeat radiosurgery. *J Neurosurg* 2012;**116**:21–32.
31. Stahl JM, Chi YY, Friedman WA. Repeat radiosurgery for intracranial arteriovenous malformations. *Neurosurgery* 2012;**70**:150–4.
32. Maesawa S, Flickinger JC, Kondziolka D, *et al.* Repeated radiosurgery for incompletely obliterated arteriovenous malformations. *J Neurosurg* 2000;**92**:961–70.
33. Sanchez-Mejia RO, McDermott MW, Tan J, *et al.* Radiosurgery facilitates resection of brain arteriovenous malformations and reduces surgical morbidity. *Neurosurgery* 2009;**64**:231–8.
34. Karlsson B, Kihlstrom L, Lindquist C, *et al.* Gamma knife surgery for previously irradiated arteriovenous malformations. *Neurosurgery* 1998;**42**:1–5.
35. Yen CP, Jain S, Haq IU, *et al.* Repeat gamma knife surgery for incompletely obliterated cerebral arteriovenous malformations. *Neurosurgery* 2010;**67**:55–64.
36. Blackburn SL, Ashley WW, Jr., Rich KM, *et al.* Combined endovascular embolization and stereotactic radiosurgery in the treatment of large arteriovenous malformations. *J Neurosurg* 2011;**114**:1758–67.
37. Frizzel RT, Fisher WS, III. Cure, morbidity, and mortality associated with embolization of brain arteriovenous malformations: a review of 1246 patients in 32 series over a

35-year period. *Neurosurgery* 1995;**37**:1031–9.

38. Fox AJ, Pelz DM, Lee DH. Arteriovenous malformations of the brain: recent results of endovascular therapy. *Radiology* 1990;**177**:51–7.
39. Jayaraman MV, Marcellus ML, Hamilton S, *et al.* Neurologic complications of arteriovenous malformation embolization using liquid embolic agents. *AJNR Am J Neuroradiol* 2008;**29**:242–6.
40. Lundqvist C, Wikholm G, Svendsen P. Embolization of cerebral arteriovenous malformations Part II. Aspects of complications and late outcome. *Neurosurgery* 1996;**39**:460–7.
41. Miyachi S, Negoro M, Okamoto T, *et al.* Embolisation of cerebral arteriovenous malformations to assure successful subsequent radiosurgery. *J Clin Neurosci* 2000; 7(Suppl 1):82–5.
42. Taylor CL, Dutton K, Rappard G, *et al.* Complications of preoperative embolization of cerebral arteriovenous malformations. *J Neurosurg* 2004;**100**:810–12.
43. Vinuela F, Dion JE, Duckwiler G, *et al.* Combined endovascular embolization and surgery in the management of cerebral arteriovenous malformations: experience with 101 cases. *J Neurosurg* 1991;**75**:856–64.
44. Weber W, Kis B, Siekmann R, *et al.* Preoperative embolization of intracranial arteriovenous malformations with Onyx. *Neurosurgery* 2007;**61**:244–52.
45. Wikholm G, Lundqvist C, Svendsen P. The Goteborg cohort of embolized cerebral arteriovenous malformations: a 6-year follow-up. *Neurosurgery* 2001;**49**:799–805.
46. Fisher WS, III. Therapy of AVMs: a decision analysis. *Clin Neurosurg* 1995;**42**:294–312.
47. Gobin YP, Laurent A, Merienne L, *et al.* Treatment of brain arteriovenous malformations by embolization and radiosurgery. *J Neurosurg* 1996;**85**:19–28.
48. Friedlander RM. Clinical practice. Arteriovenous malformations of the brain. *N Engl J Med* 2007;**356**:2704–12.
49. Weber W, Kis B, Siekmann R, *et al.* Endovascular treatment of intracranial arteriovenous malformations with onyx: technical aspects. *AJNR Am J Neuroradiol* 2007;**28**:371–7.
50. Schirmer CM, Zerris V, Malek AM. Electrocautery-induced ignition of spark showers and self-sustained combustion of Onyx ethylene–vinyl alcohol copolymer. *Neurosurgery* 2006;**59**:ons413–18.
51. Codd PJ, Mitha AP, Ogilvy CS. A recurrent cerebral arteriovenous malformation in an adult. *J Neurosurg* 2008;**109**:486–91.
52. Klimo P, Jr., Rao G, Brockmeyer D. Pediatric arteriovenous malformations: a 15-year experience with an emphasis on residual and recurrent lesions. *Childs Nerv Syst* 2007;**23**:31–7.
53. Andaluz N, Myseros JS, Sathi S, *et al.* Recurrence of cerebral arteriovenous malformations in children: report of two cases and review of the literature. *Surg Neurol* 2004;**62**:324–30.
54. Kader A, Goodrich JT, Sonstein WJ, *et al.* Recurrent cerebral arteriovenous malformations after negative postoperative angiograms. *J Neurosurg* 1996;**85**:14–18.
55. Morgan MK, Patel NJ, Simons M, *et al.* Influence of the combination of patient age and deep venous drainage on brain arteriovenous malformation recurrence after surgery. *J Neurosurg* 2012;**117**:934–41.
56. Freudenstein D, Duffner F, Ernemann U, *et al.* Recurrence of a cerebral arteriovenous malformation after surgical excision. *Cerebrovasc Dis* 2001;**11**:59–64.
57. Kondziolka D, Humphreys RP, Hoffman HJ, *et al.* Arteriovenous malformations of the brain in children: a forty year experience. *Can J Neurol Sci* 1992;**19**:40–5.
58. Sano K, Ueda Y, Saito I. Subarachnoid hemorrhage in children. *Childs Brain* 1978;**4**:38–46.
59. Sonstein WJ, Kader A, Michelsen WJ, *et al.* Expression of vascular endothelial growth factor in pediatric and adult cerebral arteriovenous malformations: an immunocytochemical study. *J Neurosurg* 1996;**85**:838–45.

Appendix: A note on the ARUBA trial

Jonathan J. Russin and Robert F. Spetzler

Hans Christian Andersen's tale of pluralistic ignorance warns of the dangers inherent in logical fallacies. The peer-review process can expose the naked truth about research methods, results, and their interpretation. However, once the literature reaches the readership it is assumed that the authors' conclusions have been blessed by the ranking authorities. Despite the details, the authors' conclusions can permeate general opinion and become embedded in practice.

Despite much effort, the question of how best to manage unruptured arteriovenous malformations (AVMs) remains unanswered. The long-term follow-up on ARUBA (A Randomised Trial of Unruptured Brain Arteriovenous Malformations) [1] provides little further clarity secondary to design flaws. Improving the care of patients harboring unruptured cerebral AVMs must be the goal. We are no closer to that goal than we were before ARUBA. With little clarity at hand, it is our responsibility to continue our investigations. Below we provide a critique of the recently published ARUBA trial.

ARUBA was designed as a prospective, multicenter, parallel design, randomized, controlled trial to assess the outcome of treatment (any modality) versus medical management for unruptured brain AVMs. In total, ARUBA investigators reviewed 1740 patients aged 18 years or older without a history of hemorrhage for inclusion in the study. Of those reviewed, 726 patients fitted the inclusion criteria but 226 were actually included in the study; 177 patients were treated outside the trial and 323 refused enrollment. The study had an attrition rate of 3%. The authors defined the primary outcome of the trial as death or symptomatic stroke, while clinical impairment, defined as a score of ≥2 on the modified Rankin Scale, was the secondary outcome. Although the authors planned to enroll 800 patients for an 87.5% power to detect a 40% reduction in risk of stroke or death, they ultimately decreased total enrollment numbers due to difficulties in enlisting patients. As noted, the final study enrolled only 226 patients, of whom 114 were randomized to treatment (any modality) and 109 were randomized to medical therapy. Despite the large number of patients screened, few were actually enrolled, and the authors fail to discuss the characteristics of those treated outside the trial.

One of the cardinal challenges with the ARUBA trial is the non-specificity of the intervention group. A recent meta-analysis of treated brain AVMs reports obliteration rates of 96% for surgical resection, 38% for stereotactic radiosurgery, and 13% for embolization [2]. The ARUBA study design included intervention as any modality – surgical, endovascular, or radiotherapy – deemed appropriate by the investigators. Interestingly, despite a preponderance of low-grade Spetzler–Martin AVMs in this study (76), for which the recommended therapy is surgery [3], only five patients were treated with neurosurgical procedures and most were treated with endovascular (30), radiation (31), or multimodality techniques (28). To our surprise, 30 patients were treated with embolization alone; embolization as a stand-alone treatment for brain AVMs is unorthodox and not standard practice. Furthermore, details on endovascular intervention and radiotherapy are not elaborated in the text. It is not clear what embolysates were used for the endovascular procedures, nor is it clear how many stages of embolization were used. As for radiation, information on the type of radiation, whether the radiation was fractionated, and dosing regimens are missing from the data and discussion. Given the heterogeneity of what the authors describe as the intervention arm, along with the lack of information on treatment plans and details on follow-up, it is difficult to know whether the conclusion of superiority of medical therapy versus intervention is sound and supported by the data presented in this study.

Another major challenge associated with the ARUBA trial is the relatively short period of follow-up; the mean follow-up in this study was 33 months. If one assumes that AVMs are congenital lesions and that the majority of these lesions do not become symptomatic until the second to fourth decades of life, than a mean follow-up of less than 33 months is an arbitrary, short, and meaningless representation of the natural history of these lesions.

As for an assessment of primary and secondary outcomes, the primary endpoint was achieved in 35 (30.7%) of the 114 patients randomized to intervention and in 11 (10.1%) of the 109 patients in the medical management arm. Based on this primary endpoint, the authors conclude that medical management is superior to intervention in preventing death or stroke in patients with unruptured brain AVMs, a conclusion that is hardly supported by the data.

The ARUBA trial highlights the challenges associated with the design and execution of randomized trials for rare pathologies such as brain AVMs. In summary, this trial represents an initial attempt to evaluate intervention versus medical management for unruptured brain AVMs. Unfortunately, due to errors in design and execution of the study, the authors' conclusions should be viewed with great caution. With a paucity of level I evidence, it is most important to base treatment recommendations on the best available literature. It is, therefore, most timely to summarize this literature on the treatment of brain and spine AVMs and gather treatment recommendations from the experts in the fields of interventional neuroradiology, radiation therapy, and neurological surgery. This book attempts to present one such multidisciplinary discourse on a topic of great controversy.

References

1. Mohr JP, Parides MK, Stapf C, for the International ARUBA Investigators. Medical management with or without interventional therapy for unruptured brain arteriovenous malformations (ARUBA): a multicentre, non-blinded, randomised trial. *Lancet* 2014;**383**:614–21.
2. van Beijnum J, van der Worp HB, Buis DR, *et al.* Treatment of brain arteriovenous malformations: a systematic review and meta-analysis. *JAMA* 2011;**306**:2011–19.
3. Spetzler RF, Ponce FA. A 3-tier classification of cerebral arteriovenous malformations. *J Neurosurg* 2011;**114**:842–9.

Index